Epigenomics

Anne C. Ferguson-Smith · John M. Greally ·
Robert A. Martienssen
Editors

Epigenomics

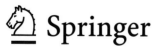

Editors
Dr. Anne C. Ferguson-Smith
Department of Physiology
  Development and Neuroscience
University of Cambridge
Downing Street
Cambridge CB2 3EG
UK

Prof. John M. Greally
Albert Einstein College of
  Medicine
1300 Marris Park Ave.
Bronx NY 10461
Ullman 921
USA

Dr. Robert A. Martienssen
Cold Spring Harbor Laboratory
I Bungtown Rd.
Cold Spring Harbor NY
1 1724-221 2
USA

ISBN: 978-1-4020-9186-5   e-ISBN: 978-1-4020-9187-2

DOI 10.1007/978-1-4020-9187-2

Library of Congress Control Number: 2008936212

© Springer Science+Business Media B.V. 2009
No part of this work may be reproduced, stored in a retrieval system, or transmitted
in any form or by any means, electronic, mechanical, photocopying, microfilming, recording
or otherwise, without written permission from the Publisher, with the exception
of any material supplied specifically for the purpose of being entered
and executed on a computer system, for exclusive use by the purchaser of the work.

Cover design: Boekhorst Design b.v.

Cover picture: From the article by Steven Henikoff, used with permission.

Printed on acid-free paper

9 8 7 6 5 4 3 2 1

springer.com

Preface

Now a popular and widely used term, "Epigenetics" has changed its meaning several times since "epigenesis" was debated by Greek philosophers as an alternative to existence of the homunculus (Aristotle, *On the Generation of Animals*). Waddington famously proposed that an "epigenetic landscape" underlies alternative cell fates, incorporating the idea, still novel at the time, that genes might contribute to this landscape. But it was the merging of embryology with non-Mendelian inheritance that ultimately led to the commonly accepted meaning of "Epigenetics" today. In this molecular age, we define epigenetics by what it is not – epigenetic changes are alterations in the hereditary material (usually chromosomes) that are not accompanied by changes in the DNA sequence. Certainly, epigenetics profoundly influences embryonic development, but equally it impacts chromosome organization, genome defense, heredity, gene expression and evolution.

Just as genetics allowed us the first glimpse of the genome in the form of linkage maps of genes and cytogenetic landmarks (Creighton and McClintock, 1931), so epigenetics allowed the first glimpse of the epigenome, with the discovery of widespread modifications of chromosomal material, including DNA and histones, associated with epigenetic regulation. Immunocytochemistry revealed striking correlations between, for example, histone H4 acetylation and dosage compensation, while molecular biology revealed correlations between, for example, DNA methylation and transposon inactivation. It was quickly realized that many of these modifications were conserved among most if not all eukaryotes, and were associated with a wide diversity of "epigenetic" phenomena. But it was only when the first whole genome sequences became available that the concept of the "epigenome" took hold. Just as DNA sequence can be aligned with the chromosome, so epigenetic modifications can be aligned with the DNA sequence. The epigenome has emerged at nucleosome and nucleotide resolution from genome profiling using high density programmable microarrays, chromatin immunoprecipitation and next generation DNA sequencing, as well as analytical procedures to detect and display significant associations. This volume commences with a section describing the current technologies employed in mapping epigenomes and the challenges associated with the analysis and visualization of these large datasets within their genomic context. The impact of the technology cannot be underestimated and as such, is recognised in many of the subsequent contributions.

In subsequent chapters, the current understanding of these epigenetic maps is reviewed within the context of epigenetic phenomena in eukaryotes. The role that model organisms have played in unveiling key conserved mechanisms is a general theme, as is the idea of an epigenetic "code", comprising histone and DNA modifications, guided by modifying enzymes, and in some cases RNA interference, and interpreted by histone and DNA binding proteins that recognize these modifications and signal their downstream effects. The relationship between epigenetic states, non-protein coding transcripts and sub-nuclear localization is also explored. The impact of these mechanisms on gene activity and repression, developmental memory, imprinting, X inactivation, genome defense and chromosome organization is reviewed in animals, plants and fungi. We also review the first glimpses of the human epigenome in differentiating cells and relate these mechanisms to human disease and development.

In the conclusion of his chapter describing the relevance of variant histones to epigenome function, Steven Henikoff reminds us that, since the completion of the draft human genome sequence, the 21st century is often referred to as the "post-genomics era". The combination of major advances in our understanding of model epigenetic processes and remarkable technological advances, as illustrated in this volume, have ushered in what he suggests might rather be considered an "epigenomics era". Whatever it is called, the integration of the epigenetic components required to consolidate DNA into its highly regulated chromatin context, is now recognized as profoundly important for understanding the functions of normal and compromised genomes. The development of effective new tools having the ability to modulate epigenetic states and influence genome function in clinical contexts, seems a realistic goal. We have witnessed the birth of a major new discipline in genetics that has taken us inside chromosomes to unfold multiple highly-regulated dynamic epigenetic landscapes within which a genome is parceled and to which it responds. We are grateful to all the authors of this volume for sharing their research, views and ideas, and for revealing these landscapes.

United Kingdom	Anne C. Ferguson-Smith
USA	John Greally
USA	Rob Martienssen

Contents

Part I Epigenomic Technologies and Analytical Approaches

Strategies for Epigenome Analysis 3
A.B. Brinkman and H.G. Stunnenberg

Sequencing the Epigenome 19
Alexander Meissner and Bradley E. Bernstein

Integrating Epigenomic Results 37
Suk-Young Yoo and R.W. Doerge

Visualising the Epigenome 55
Paul Flicek and Ewan Birney

Part II Roles of DNA, RNA and Chromatin in Epigenomics

The Expanding View of Cytosine Methylation 69
J.M. Greally

Structural and Biochemical Advances in Mammalian DNA Methylation .. 85
Xiaodong Cheng and Robert M. Blumenthal

Epigenetic Profiling of Histone Variants 101
Steven Henikoff

Epigenetic Phenomena and Epigenomics in Maize 119
Jay B. Hollick and Nathan Springer

**Epigenetic Silencing of Pericentromeric Heterochromatin by RNA
Interference in *Schizosaccharomyces pombe*** 149
Sarahjane Locke and Robert Martienssen

Describing Epigenomic Information in Arabidopsis 163
Ian R. Henderson

Role of Small RNAs in Establishing Chromosomal Architecture in Drosophila 177
James A. Birchler

MacroRNAs in the Epigenetic Control of X-Chromosome Inactivation ... 187
Shinwa Shibata and Jeannie T. Lee

Part III Epigenetic Control of Developmental Processes

Polycomb Complexes and the Role of Epigenetic Memory in Development 217
Yuri B. Schwartz and Vincenzo Pirrotta

Genomic Imprinting – A Model for Roles of Histone Modifications in Epigenetic Control 235
Kirsten R. McEwen and Anne C. Ferguson-Smith

The Epigenomic Landscape of Reprogramming in Mammals 259
Gabriella Ficz, Cassandra R. Farthing and Wolf Reik

Epigenetic Gene Regulation—Lessons from Globin 283
Ann Dean and Steven Fiering

Meiotic Silencing, Infertility and X Chromosome Evolution 301
James M.A. Turner

Part IV The Epigenome in Health and Disease

Genome Defense: The Neurospora Paradigm 321
Michael R. Rountree and Eric U. Selker

Integrating the Genome and Epigenome in Human Disease 343
Claes Wadelius

A Changing Epigenome in Health and Disease 369
Esteban Ballestar and Manel Esteller

Cancer Epigenomics 385
Christine Ladd-Acosta and Andrew P. Feinberg

Epigenetic Modulation by Environmental Factors 397
Mark R. Doyle and Richard M. Amasino

The Relevance of Epigenetics to Major Psychosis 411
Jonathan Mill and Arturas Petronis

Index 435

Contributors

R.M. Amasino Department of Biochemistry, University of Wisconsin-Madison, Madison, WI, USA

E. Ballestar Chromatin and Disease Group, Cancer Epigenetics and Biology Programme (PEBC), Catalan Institute of Oncology (ICO-IDIBELL), 08907 L'Hospitalet de Llobregat, Barcelona, Spain, eballestar@iconcologia.net

B.E. Bernstein Broad Institute of MIT and Harvard, 7 Cambridge Center, Cambridge MA 02142, USA; Molecular Pathology Unit and Center for Cancer Research, MGH, Charlestown, MA 02129, USA; Department of Pathology, Harvard Medical School, Boston, MA 02115, USA, Bernstein.Bradley@mgh.harvard.edu

J.A. Birchler Division of Biological Sciences, Tucker Hall, University of Missouri, Columbia, MO 65211, USA, BirchlerJ@Missouri.edu

E. Birney European Bioinformatics Institute, Wellcome Trust Genome Campus, Hinxton, Cambridge, CB10 1SD, UK, birney@ebi.ac.uk

R.M. Blumenthal Department of Medical Microbiology & Immunology, and Program in Bioinformatics & Proteomics/Genomics, University of Toledo Health Science Campus, Toledo, OH 43614-2598, USA

A.B. Brinkman Department of Molecular Biology, Nijmegen Centre for Molecular Life Sciences, Radboud University, The Netherlands, a.brinkman@ncmls.ru.nl

X. Cheng Department of Biochemistry, Emory University School of Medicine, Atlanta, GA 30322, USA, xcheng@emory.edu

A. Dean Laboratory of Cellular and Developmental Biology, NIDDK, NIH, Building 50, Room 3154, 50 South Drive, MSC 8028, Bethesda, MD 20892, USA, anndean@helix.nih.gov

R.W. Doerge Department of Statistics, Purdue University, 150 North University Street, West Lafayette, IN 47907 USA

M.R. Doyle Department of Biochemistry, University of Wisconsin-Madison, Madison, WI, USA

M. Esteller Cancer Epigenetics Group, Cancer Epigenetics and Biology Programme (PEBC), Catalan Institute of Oncology (ICO-IDIBELL), 08907 L'Hospitalet de Llobregat, Barcelona, Spain, mesteller@iconcologia.net

C.R. Farthing Laboratory of Developmental Genetics and Imprinting, The Babraham Institute, Cambridge CB22 3AT, UK

A.P. Feinberg Epigenetics Center, Institute for Basic Biomedical Sciences, and the Department of Medicine, Johns Hopkins University School of Medicine, Baltimore, MD 21205, USA, afeinberg@jhu.edu

A.C. Ferguson-Smith Professor of Developmental Genetics, Department of Physiology Development and Neuroscience, University of Cambridge, Physiology Building, Downing Street, Cambridge CB2 3EG, UK, afsmith@mole.bio.cam.ac.uk

G. Ficz Laboratory of Developmental Genetics and Imprinting, The Babraham Institute, Cambridge CB22 3AT, UK

S. Fiering Department of Microbiology/Immunology and Genetics, Dartmouth Medical School, Rubin 622, DHMC, Lebanon, NH 03756, USA, fiering@dartmouth.edu

P. Flicek European Bioinformatics Institute, Wellcome Trust Genome Campus, Hinxton, Cambridge, CB10 1SD, UK, flicek@ebi.ac.uk

J.M. Greally Einstein Center for Epigenomics, Department of Genetics, Albert Einstein College of Medicine, Bronx, NY USA

I.R. Henderson Department of Plant Sciences, University of Cambridge, Downing Street, Cambridge, CB2 3EA, UK, irh25@cam.ac.uk

J.B. Hollick University of California, Department of Plant and Microbial Biology, 111 Koshland Hall #3102, Berkeley CA, USA, hollick@nature.berkeley.edu

M. Jonathan Social, Genetic, and Developmental Psychiatry Research Centre, Institute of Psychiatry, King's College London, De Crespigny Park, London SE5 8AF, UK

C. Ladd-Acosta Epigenetics Center Institute for Basic Biomedical Sciences, and the Department of Medicine, Johns Hopkins University School of Medicine, Battimore, ND 21205, USA, claddac1@jhmi.edu

J.T. Lee Howard Hughes Medical Institute and Department of Molecular Biology, Massachusetts General Hospital, Simches 6.624, 185 Cambridge St., Boston, MA 02114, USA, lee@molbio.mgh.harvard.edu

S. Locke Cold Spring Harbor Laboratory, 1 Bungtown Road, Cold Spring Harbor NY 11724, USA, locke@cshl.edu

R. Martienssen Cold Spring Harbor Laboratory, 1 Bungtown Road, Cold Spring Harbor NY 11724, USA. martiens@cshl.edu

K.R. McEwen Department of Physiology Development and Neuroscience, University of Cambridge, Physiology Building, Downing Street, Cambridge CB2 3EG, UK, krm29@cam.ac.uk

A. Meissner Broad Institute of MIT and Harvard, 7 Cambridge Center, Cambridge MA 02142, USA; Department of Stem Cell and Regenerative Biology, Harvard University, Cambridge, MA 02138, USA, alex@broad.mit.edu

A. Petronis Krembil Family Epigenetics Laboratory, Centre for Addiction and Mental Health, 250 College street, Toronto ON M5T 1R8, Canada, arturas_petronis@camh.net

V. Pirrotta Department of Molecular Biology and Biochemistry, Rutgers University, 604 Allison Road, Piscataway, NJ 08854, USA, pirrotta@biology.rutgers.edu

W. Reik Laboratory of Developmental Genetics and Imprinting, The Babraham Institute, Cambridge CB22 3AT, UK; Centre for Trophoblast Research, University of Cambridge, Cambridge CB2 3EG, UK

M.R. Rountree Institute of Molecular Biology, University of Oregon, Eugene, OR 97403; USA, mrountree@molbio.uoregon.edu

Y.B. Schwartz Department of Molecular Biology and Biochemistry, Rutgers University, 604 Allison Road, Piscataway, NJ 08854, USA

E.U. Selker Institute of Molecular Biology, University of Oregon, Eugene, OR 97403; USA, selker@molbio.uoregon.edu

S. Shibata Department of Stem Cell Biology, Graduate School of Medical Sciences, Kanazawa University, 13-1 Takara-machi, Kanazawa, Ishikawa 920-8640, Japan, shinwa@med.kanazawa-u.ac.jp

N. Springer University of Minnesota, Department of Plant Biology, 250 Biosciences Center, 1445 Gortner Ave., Saint Paul MN 55105, springer@umn.edu

S. Henikoff Howard Hughes Medical Institute, Fred Hutchinson Cancer Research Center, 1100 Fairview Ave. N., Seattle, Washington 98109, USA, steveh@fhcrc.org

H.G. Stunnenberg Department of Molecular Biology, Nijmegen Centre for Molecular Life Sciences, Radboud University, The Netherlands, h.stunnenberg@ncmls.ru.nl

J.M.A. Turner Division of Stem Cell Research and Developmental Genetics, MRC National Institute for Medical Research, London NW7 1AA, UK

C. Wadelius Department of genetics and pathology, Rudbeck Laboratory, Uppsala University, SE-75185 Uppsala, Sweden, Claes.Wadelius@genpat.uu.se

S.-Y. Yoo Department of Statistics, Purdue University, 150 North University Street, West Lafayette, IN 47907 USA

Part I
Epigenomic Technologies and Analytical Approaches

Strategies for Epigenome Analysis

A.B. Brinkman and H.G. Stunnenberg

Abstract The eukaryotic genome is packaged into nucleosomes, which form the basal unit of chromatin, the physiological form of DNA within the nucleus. Apart from its function in compacting the immense nuclear DNA molecules, chromatin also serves as a platform onto which multiple signalling pathways converge to cooperate in determining the expression status of mRNAs and other (non-coding) RNA molecules. Epigenetic profile analysis aims to determine what changes on the nucleosomes cooperate to establish and maintain DNA sequence-independent heritable traits such as those determining cell identity.

Keywords Profiling · Histone modifications · DNA methylation · ChIP-on-chip · ChIP-seq

1 Introduction

Epigenetic changes can occur on all building blocks of the nucleosome to ultimately constitute the epigenome. They include (i) post-translational histone modifications; (ii) incorporation of histone variants; (iii) remodelling of the DNA-histone interaction; (iv) methylation of DNA; (v) association with transcription (co)factors; (vi) local changes in nucleosome density; (vii) changes in long-range chromatin interactions and compaction.

In this chapter we will focus on the different methods that are available to profile epigenetic changes. In particular, we will focus on methods that are suitable for high-throughput –or whole-genome– profiling, and we will discuss logical strategies to approach such profiling and consider aspects that we have found to be of importance.

The availability of highly specific antibodies for chromatin-modifying proteins and their resulting modifications, in combination with chromatin immunoprecipitation and immunofluorescence-based techniques has enabled mapping of epigenetic

---

A.B. Brinkman (✉)
Department of Molecular Biology, Nijmegen Centre for Molecular Life Sciences,
Radboud University, The Netherlands

changes. This has generated a wealth of information that drastically changed the concept of expression regulation from a transcription factor-based view into a system in which transcription factors and chromatin interact and cooperate. The advent of genomic tiling microarrays –and recently, massive parallel sequencing– have enabled global and whole-genome epigenetic profiling studies. Such large-scale analyses will allow the generation of new insights into how chromatin is utilized and shaped according to the cell's necessities, ultimately defining its epigenome.

The concepts outlined above are of particular importance for the development of novel treatment strategies for cancer. It has become clear that epigenetic alterations act as "surrogates" for genetic changes in cancer, and as epigenetic alterations are mitotically heritable, they play the same roles and undergo the same selective processes as genetic alterations in the development of cancer. However, epigenetic alterations are more feasible to be reversed than genetic aberrations, thus providing opportunities for therapeutic intervention.

2 ChIP

In 1988 a key publication from the Varshavsky laboratory (Solomon et al. 1988) demonstrated the use of chromatin immunoprecipitation (or ChIP) to study regulation of the Hsp70 genes in Drosophila. Modifications of the original protocol have been developed since, but the basic protocol includes the *in vivo* cross-linking of chromatin-bound proteins using formaldehyde, to 'freeze' the *in vivo* situation, and the generation of short random fragments of this chromatin using sonication. The obtained cross-linked chromatin fragments are subsequently used in an immunoprecipitation step using antibodies directed against the protein or histone modification of interest. After immunoprecipitation the isolated antibody-chromatin-complexes are decrosslinked and the DNA is purified. In parallel, the input material –or non-immunoprecipitated chromatin– is decrosslinked and DNA is purified likewise. Both fractions are subjected to quantitative PCR using primers specific for the genomic region of interest. In this way the magnitude of enrichment by ChIP is determined at a specific genomic position. Depending on the antibody, ChIP allows for profiling chromatin-associated factors, histone modifications, histone variants as well as local nucleosome density.

3 ChIP-on-Chip

Combining ChIP with genomic tiling array hybridization (CHIP-on-chip) or massive-parallel sequencing (ChIP-seq) instead of gene-specific PCR allows one to analyze larger genomic regions or even the whole genome. Several steps within such a procedure are of critical importance for a successful profiling experiment. In Fig. 1 we present a generalized strategy that can be followed to establish a ChIP-based profiling approach – the Roman numerals depict strategic points shown in Fig. 1. The strategy starts with a factor of interest, which is assumed to be a chromatin-associated protein (I).

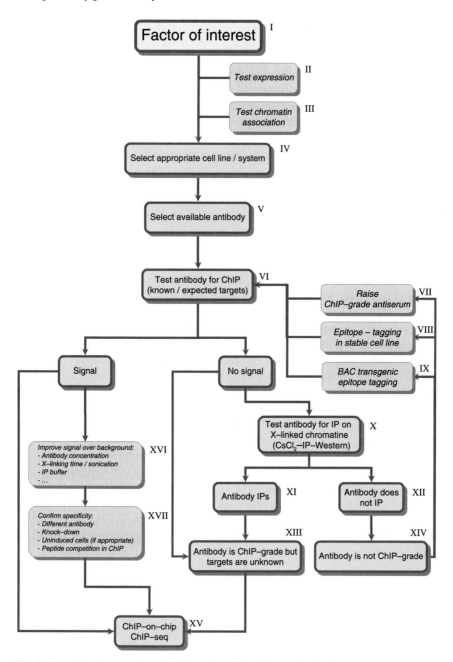

Fig. 1 Generalized strategy for a ChIP-based profiling. See text for further explanation

Since a ChIP experiment requires the availability of a relatively large amount of cells, the initial use of cultured cells is inevitable, but whenever conditions are optimized it should be possible to use primary cells or tissue-derived cells. The choice for a particular cell line (IV) most often depends on whether the protein is expressed or not (II). In addition, it may be relevant in this stage to confirm its chromatin-association (III). If an antibody is available, this can be done by cesium-chloride ($CsCl_2$)-density gradient centrifugation of formaldehyde-crosslinked material. Western blot analysis of the fraction containing crosslinked DNA-protein complexes (after decrosslinking) will reveal whether the protein of interest is chromatin-associated.

The most critical issue of ChIP is the availability of a high-quality ChIP-grade antibody (V). Commercial antibodies are available for many chromatin-associated proteins, and even though they may be specific in Western analysis or efficient in a normal immunoprecipitation, most of them are not ChIP-(profiling)-grade, even when marketed as such. A large-scale ChIP-profiling experiment requires substantial enrichment over background (a control region that is not enriched), even more than for a single ChIP-qPCR. Clearly, only a few ChIP-grade antibodies are also ChIP-profiling grade. In our experience, enrichment above 20-fold over background will give profiles of reasonable to good quality.

Whenever an antibody needs to be produced against the protein of interest (VII), generating a polyclonal antiserum against several different peptides (or a protein domain) will be preferred. A polyclonal antibody is directed against a range of different epitopes, which increases the chance for obtaining one that is ChIP-grade. In addition, the performance of a ChIP-grade polyclonal antibody will usually improve after affinity purification. An important constraint on immunogen selection is to avoid lysine residues within the amino acid sequence. Lysine residues are the primary targets for formaldehyde cross-linking, and epitopes containing lysines will be (at least partly) functionally destroyed by formaldehyde cross-linking. Most commonly used monoclonal antibodies against epitope-tags are not ChIP-grade for this reason (see Table 1). Although they have been successfully used by others, we have never reached substantial enrichment using MYC, and inconsistent results were obtained using FLAG. HA and HSV provide better alternatives because they lack lysines. We found that they are ChIP-grade, although

Table 1 Epitope tag sequences

Epitope tag	Amino acid sequence	ChIP-grade
MYC	EQKLISEEDL	-
FLAG	DYKDDDDK	+/−
VSV-G	YTDIEMNRLGK	Not tested
V5	GKPIPNPLLGLDST	Not tested
HA	YPYDVPDYA	+
HSV	QPELAPEDPED	+
TY-1	EVHTNQDPLD	+
2xTY-1	EVHTNQDPLDAEVHTNQDPLD	++
ERα	SLQKYYITGEAEGFPATV	++

the level of enrichment is not outstanding. We have recently exploited the use of two different universal epitope tags: TY-1 (and 2xTY-1) and ERα. For both epitopes monoclonal antibodies are available. Although a single lysine is present within the periphery of the ERα-tag, both tags show excellent performance in ChIP and also in ChIP-on-chip and ChIP-seq experiments. The use of the ERα-tag requires that ERα is not expressed endogenously or that its ligand is depleted from the culture medium, since we found only very low chromatin association of endogenous ERα in the latter case. Alternatively, a ChIP-reChIP approach using first TY-1 followed by ERα could be used, or vice versa.

Whenever epitope tagging is used one has to make sure that the tagged protein is expressed at (near-)endogenous levels. In our hands, ChIP profiles of overexpressed proteins contain many sites of enrichment that are otherwise absent in profiles of the endogenously expressed protein. For generating a stable cell line expressing a tagged protein (VIII), multiple independent clones should be screened for ones with near-endogenous expression levels.

An exploratory ChIP-qPCR experiment can be performed if one or more genomic target sites are known or can be predicted (VI). The absence of any signal over background (a genomic control region) could either mean that the antibody is not ChIP-grade (XIV) or that the wrong genomic targets were selected for qPCR (XIII). This can be analyzed by performing an immunoprecipitation on crosslinked chromatin that has been purified following cesium-chloride ($CsCl_2$)-density gradient centrifugation (X), which is used to remove non-crosslinked proteins. If the antibody precipitates the protein of interest from the crosslinked fraction –that is, a signal is obtained in Western blot– the antibody is most likely ChIP-grade, and one could proceed with a pilot ChIP-on-chip or ChIP-seq experiment to detect targets (XV). Whenever the exploratory ChIP experiment reveals sufficient enrichment over background, the ChIP protocol may need optimization (XVI). This may include antibody concentration, crosslinking and/or sonication time, and composition of the immunoprecipitation buffer, such as SDS concentration. Whenever the protein of interest is expected to be chromatin-associated through secondary interactions, additional protein-protein crosslinking may improve the level of enrichment (Zeng et al. 2006). In some cases it may be necessary to determine the specificity of the antibody in ChIP (XVII). This could involve the use of different antibodies against the same protein, RNAi-mediated knock-down of the protein, or performing a ChIP experiment using untreated/uninduced cells (e.g. in the case of many nuclear hormone receptors).

For ChIP-on-chip profiling, a number of additional (post-ChIP) aspects are of importance. First, ChIP DNA must be amplified to obtain sufficiently large amounts for labelling and array hybridization (typically several micrograms per microarray hybridization). Depending on the antibody the amount of ChIP DNA is within the nanogram range, and at least a 1000-fold amplification is necessary. Commonly used DNA amplification methods include linker-mediated PCR (LM-PCR), T7 polymerase-based linear amplification, and whole-genome amplification (WGA). In LM-PCR, linkers are ligated to both ends of the ChIP DNA fragments, which allows PCR amplification using universal primers (Ren 2000). In T7-based linear amplification, oligo-dT tails of defined length are added to the 3' termini of the DNA fragments, to which a T7-promoter sequence can be annealed. After conversion into dsDNA, the resulting DNA is used as a template for *in vitro* transcription using the T7 RNA polymerase. The transcribed RNA molecules are subsequently converted to dsDNA (Liu et al. 2003). WGA involves the proprietary GenomePlex® amplification technique (Sigma-Aldrich, St. Louis, MO, USA) in which DNA fragments are primed to generate a library of DNA fragments with defined 3' and 5' termini. This library is then replicated using linear amplification in the initial stages, followed by a limited round of geometric amplifications. We have used LM-PCR with some success for ChIPs against transcription factors or locally enriched histone marks like H3K4 tri-methylation and H3/H4 acetylation. However, the same procedure was not successful for histone marks that are distributed over larger regions, like H3K9 and H3K27 tri-methylation. In addition, we found that on complex samples (like human genomic DNA) LM-PCR amplification introduces a considerable bias. This is shown in Fig. 2. Upon hybridization of unamplified DNA, LM-PCR-amplified DNA and T7-amplified DNA, the obtained probe intensities were compared using scatter plots. Comparison of two unamplified genomic DNA samples shows that their probe intensities correlate well (Fig. 2A, R^2=0.85). When unamplified DNA is compared with the same DNA after LM-PCR amplification the correlation decreases dramatically (Fig. 2B, R^2= 0.52). In contrast, the correlation is maintained to a much greater extent when unamplified DNA is compared with T7 amplified DNA (Fig. 2C, R^2=0.75). This shows that T7 amplification is superior to LM-PCR, even upon multiple rounds of amplification (not shown). WGA has also been shown to eliminate bias problems (O'Geen et al. 2006), although we have not applied this technique in our laboratory.

Second, the choice of microarray platform is an important determinant for obtaining confident signal to noise ratios. Three different platforms have been mostly used for ChIP-on-chip analysis: Affymetrix, Nimblegen and Agilent. The main differences between these platforms are probe length, probe spacing and probe density. Whereas probe length ranges from 25 to 75 bp, probe densities currently vary from 2.4×10^5 to 6.5×10^6 probes per array. We have experienced that Nimblegen arrays with 50-bp probes provide good probe density and signal to noise ratios.

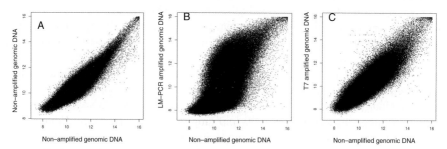

Fig. 2 Comparison of two random amplification methods used in ChIP-on-chip. Human non-amplified genomic DNA was hybridized against (**A**), human non-amplified DNA as a control; (**B**), human genomic DNA amplified using LM-PCR; (**C**), human genomic DNA amplified using T7-based linear amplification. Log^2 probe intensities are plotted

The 60-mer probe design of Agilent arrays shows better signal to noise ratios, but the number of probes per array is lower. Although it is possible to interrogate the whole human or mouse genome using tiling arrays, more directed analyses may be performed using promoter-tiling arrays or dedicated custom arrays containing selected genomic regions.

Third, data interpretation mostly starts with peak-calling: the assignment of enriched regions. Several independently developed peak recognition algorithms are available, e.g. MPeak (Zheng et al. 2007), TileMap (Ji and Wong 2005). In addition, array manufacturers provide similar software tools, e.g. Nimblegen's SignalMap. MPeak is a model-based method that assumes a triangular shape for enriched regions, while Tilemap uses test-statistics to define regions of enrichment and calculates statistically significant enriched regions between a sample and control dataset. Because of the different methodologies, the performance of these algorithms will vary depending on the factor to be profiled. For instance, MPeak may not be the method of choice in profiling H3K27 tri-methylation because of the presence of many non-triangular enrichment patterns. In contrast, for transcription factor profiling all methods mentioned have been used successfully in our laboratory. However, all algorithms will detect distinct but largely overlapping peak sets. Selecting peaks that are commonly found by all methods will significantly decrease the number of false-positives. The false-positive rate has to be determined empirically using ChIP-qPCR analysis of a number of randomly selected peaks (>50 for a genome-wide analysis). Such validation is of critical importance, because in our experience the number of detected peaks is subject to considerable variation just because of the selected method and its peak-detection settings.

4 ChIP-Seq

ChIP-seq represents a recent advance in epigenetic profiling. It involves direct massive parallel sequencing of individual DNA molecules obtained in a ChIP experiment. Counting of the number of sequence reads within a specific genomic region is proportional to the local level of enrichment. To date, a number of studies have described ChIP-seq approaches to profile histone-modifications (Mikkelsen et al. 2007, Barski et al. 2007) or transcription factors (Robertson et al. 2007, Johnson et al. 2007), using Solexa sequencing technology (Illumina Inc.). The technology starts with the generation of clusters of about 1000 identical DNA fragments, each originating from a single DNA molecule. Cluster generation is achieved by solid-phase DNA amplification onto a glass-surface. Up to 50 million clusters can be generated and sequenced in parallel, each producing a sequence read of 36 bases. Other platforms for massive-parallel sequencing are 454 Life Sciences and SOLiD. For ChIP, the advantages of massive-parallel sequencing over microarray hybridization are the increased throughput and dramatically increased signal to noise ratio. In Fig. 3, a comparison between a ChIP-on-chip profile and a ChIP-seq profile is shown. The screenshot shows the enrichment of a transcription factor at one of its target genes. While the enrichment of the ChIP-on-chip profile is displayed as the

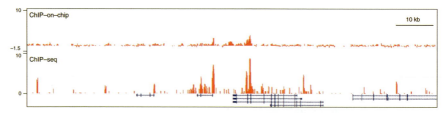

Fig. 3 Screenshot showing a comparison between a ChIP-on-chip profile (top panel, $\log^2$ of ChIP/input ratio) and a ChIP-seq profile (bottom panel, $\log^2$ of the number of sequence reads counted per 100 bp window) generated from the same cell line. The profile shows enrichment of a transcription factor at one of its target genes. Annotated genes are indicated at the bottom

ratio of ChIP DNA over non-immunoprecipitated (input) DNA, enrichment in the ChIP-seq profile is displayed as the number of sequence reads counted per 100-bp window within the ChIP DNA sample. The difference between enrichments represented in this way is over 40-fold: while ChIP-on-chip enrichment is maximally 2.9 (log2), ChIP-seq enrichment is 8.3 (log2). In addition, the average background enrichment within the regions flanking these peaks is clearly lower in the CHIP-seq profile. The increased signal to noise ratio obtained using ChIP-seq allows assignment of peaks with high confidence, and permits identification of binding sites that are not evident from the ChIP-on-chip profile. A single analysis-run (one out of eight lanes of a flowcell) using Solexa sequencing is able to provide genome-wide coverage for a ChIP experiment, although this is of course dependent on the factor to be profiled and the specificity of the used antibody. More sequence reads may be necessary to optimize the signal to noise ratio. Profiling of a widespread histone mark like H3K27 tri-methylation requires more sequence reads than profiling a transcription factor that has a limited number of binding sites throughout the genome, because of the difference in complexity of the ChIP DNA sample.

5 DNA Methylation

Within the last decades it has become clear that gene-silencing through DNA methylation involves multiple steps that cooperate to establish a gene-repressive state. Whereas the role of DNA methylation in gene-body and intergenic sequence is much less clear, promoter methylation has been strongly linked to gene-silencing. Roughly half of the human promoters are located within a CpG-island, a region in which the CpG dinucleotide motif is overrepresented relative to the average genome (Gardiner-Garden and Frommer 1987). While virtually all cytosine bases of a CpG are methylated, those within a CpG island are generally maintained methylation-free. However, within cancer cells a number of genes become inactivated through hypermethylation of their promoter CpG-islands. This phenomenon offers great potential towards the identification of cancer-specific epigenetic aberrations termed differentially methylated regions (DMRs). A model for DNA methylation-induced repression is shown in Fig. 4. DNA methyltransferases (DNMTs) are recruited

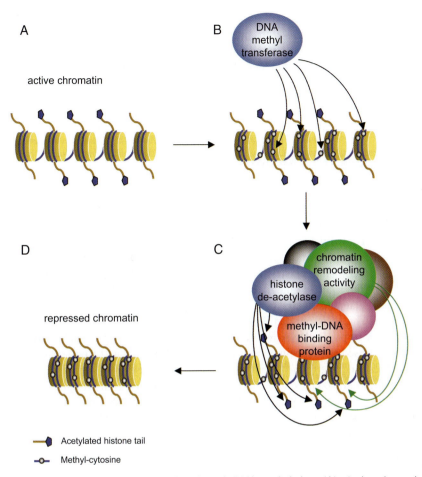

Fig. 4 General model for gene repression through DNA methylation. (**A**), Active chromatin, schematically displayed as open and acetylated. (**B**), DNA methyl transferases (DNMTs) are recruited to locally increase DNA methylation levels. (**C**), The methyl-DNA mark acts as a target for methyl-DNA binding proteins that specifically recognize and bind this mark. Methyl-DNA binding proteins are mostly part of multi-protein complexes that contain chromatin-modifying activity represented by histone-deacetylases (HDACs) and chromatin remodelers (e.g. MBD2-NuRD, (Le Guezennec et al. 2006, Feng and Zhang 2001, Ng et al. 1999)). (**D**), The recruited chromatin-modifying activities establish a repressive chromatin configuration, schematically shown as deacetylated and compacted chromatin

by currently poorly defined mechanism(s), and increase local DNA methylation. The DNA methylation marks act as targets for methyl-DNA binding proteins (MBPs) that specifically recognize and bind such sites. Some of these MBPs act as direct repressors through the presence of transcriptional repression domains, but their major repressive activity is exerted via associated proteins, including histone deacetylases (HDACs), chromatin remodelers, and histone methyltransferases (HMTs), which cooperate to establish a repressed chromatin state. HDACs remove acetyl groups from histone tails, which is closely associated with repressive chromatin. The various proteins with chromatin-modifying activities represent attractive targets for pharmacological inhibition of repression to reactivate repressed target genes. Indeed, a growing number of HDAC inhibitors are in development or are already in phase I-II clinical trials and effectively induce differentiation, growth arrest and/or apoptosis in tumorigenic cells, whereas normal cells appear to be less sensitive.

6 Profiling of DNA Methylation

In contrast to profiling of histone modifications, transcription factors and histone variants, for which ChIP is the most widely used method, profiling of DNA methylation is possible through a wide variety of techniques (at least 20 have been described). They differ in the resolution of methylation mapping, the ability to give qualitative rather than quantitative measurements, and in their potential to be used in global rather than gene-specific analysis. In this overview we will only discuss a selection of the available methods, focusing on the most widely used methods and those that are amendable for large-scale analysis (see also Chapter "Sequencing the Epigenome" by Meissner and Bernstein).

Methods to profile DNA methylation patterns can be roughly divided in three categories based on the principle of distinguishing methylated from unmethylated DNA. These include (i) bisulphite conversion, (ii) digestion with methylation sensitive restriction enzymes, and (iii) capture of methylated DNA fragments using a recombinant methyl-DNA binding protein domain (MBD) or a monoclonal anti-5-methyl-cytosine antibody.

6.1 Bisulphite Conversion Based Methods

Bisulphite sequencing (Frommer et al. 1992) provides quantitative information on methylation within the analyzed cell population at the basepair level. It involves chemical conversion of only the unmethylated cytosines to thymidines, followed by PCR amplification, cloning and sequencing of the obtained fragments. The latter steps however make it a relatively labour-intensive technique that can only be scaled up using a pipeline-infrastructure (Eckhardt et al. 2006). The design of primers that specifically amplify bisulphite-converted sequences puts constraints on the choice of genomic regions to be targeted, and only up to 250 bp-fragments can be analyzed at the time. This makes whole-genome coverage almost impossible. However, for validation purposes it is regarded as the 'golden standard'.

Bisulphite pyrosequencing (Colella et al. 2003) is a sequencing-by-synthesis technology in which nucleotide incorporation is measured using a luminescence signal. This is generated by pyrophosphate release through a cascade consisting of four enzymes. Bisulphite-converted DNA is subject to PCR amplification in which one of the two primers is biotinylated. The amplified DNA is immobilized on streptavidin beads, converted to ssDNA and sequenced. This method allows for quantitative analysis, but is limited to 25–30 bases in length, although modifications of the protocol have been shown to generate sequence reads of up to 75 bp (Dupont et al. 2004).

In Methylation-Specific PCR (MSP) (Herman et al. 1996) bisulphite conversion is combined with amplification by primer pairs that specifically amplify regions in which CpGs are methylated or unmethylated. MSP is a very fast and sensitive technique, although it should be regarded as a qualitative rather than a quantitative technique. It can only be scaled up to medium-throughput because it requires pre-selection of regions of interest for PCR amplification.

In COmbined Bisulphite Restriction Analysis (COBRA) (Xiong and Laird 1997) DNA is converted using bisulphite and amplified using gene-specific PCR. The amplified fragments are digested with *BstUI*, which recognition site is destroyed whenever overlapping CpGs are unmethylated. The digested DNA is subsequently analyzed using Southern blotting to determine the cut/uncut ratio. COBRA provides quantitative information on methylation and can be used for validation purposes, but like MSP it can only be scaled up to medium-throughput.

MethyLight (Eads et al. 2000) is a sensitive technology in which genomic DNA is converted using bisulphite. Subsequently, selected genomic regions are amplified using TaqMan amplification technology that requires two amplification primers flanking a fluorescent probe. MethyLight can be used in different ways: methylation-dependent sequence discrimination at the *probe* level (quantitative mode), discrimination at the *amplification primer* level (qualitative, similar to MSP), discrimination at both the *primer and probe* levels (semi-quantitative mode), or no methylation-dependent discrimination (control mode). Like MSP, MethyLight requires only low amounts of DNA of modest quality, which allows the analysis of material from various sources (e.g. fixed/fragmented patient material). MethyLight is a medium-throughput technology that requires target pre-selection, but it is more flexible than MSP.

The GoldenGate assay for methylation in combination with BeadArray technology (Ilumina Inc.) concomitantly interrogates over 1,500 individual CpGs in 96 samples (Laird, Illumina Application Note, www.illumina.com). The method is based on two specific probe pairs for a specific CpG site: one pair for the methylated state and one pair for the unmethylated state. The pairs are annealed to bisulphite-converted DNA, and the gap that remains between the oligo pair is extended and ligated, creating a PCR template that can be amplified using fluorescent primers. The resulting fragments are subsequently hybridized to beads that contain a known, probe-pair specific sequence tag that allows the fluorescent signal to be assigned to the specific CpG site in question. For every CpG site a two-channel fluorescent signal reports the methylated to unmethylated ratio. The GoldenGate assay is quantitative and amendable to high-throughput analysis.

6.2 *Restriction Enzyme Based Methods*

In Differential Methylation Hybridization (DMH) (Huang et al. 1999) adapters are ligated to MseI-fragmented genomic DNA, which are then cut with a methylation-sensitive restriction enzyme like *BstUI* or *McrBC*, although other enzyme combinations have been used as well (Nouzova et al. 2004). The uncut DNA is then PCR-amplified and hybridized onto microarrays. DMH compares samples with a reference sample so as to identify differentially methylated regions. The use of microarrays allows for high-throughput analysis. DMH is semi-quantitative.

HpaII tiny fragment Enrichment by Ligation-mediated PCR (HELP) (Khulan et al. 2006) involves digestion of genomic DNA by HpaII and in parallel its methylation-insensitive isoschizomer *MspI*. The two different populations of fragments are amplified and size-selected using LM-PCR and hybridized on genomic tiling microarrays. HELP allows both intragenomic profiling and intergenomic comparisons of DNA methylation and is quantitative.

6.3 Capture of Methylated DNA Fragments

Methylated-CpG Island Recovery Assay (MIRA) (Rauch et al. 2006, Rauch and Pfeifer 2005) is an affinity capture assay that is similar to those described in earlier studies in which the MBD domain of MeCP2 was used to capture methylated DNA fragments (Cross et al. 1994, Shiraishi et al. 1999). MIRA is a modification of this initial capturing method, and utilizes full-length GST-MBD2b complexed with His-MBD3L1. The latter stimulates the methyl-DNA binding affinity of MBD2. Genomic DNA is fragmented using *MseI*, linkers are ligated to the generated ends and methylated DNA is captured by the MBD2b/MBD3L1 protein complex. After washing, methylated DNA fragments are purified and analyzed using microarrays. Both CpG-islands and genomic tiling arrays have been used (Rauch et al. 2008). MIRA is a high-throughput method that could potentially be used to profile methylation along the complete genome. It is presumably unbiased, since no DNA sequence bias for MBD2's methyl-DNA binding activity has been reported, as opposed to that of MeCP2 (Klose et al. 2005). It is currently unknown whether the method is semi-quantitative or quantitative.

Methylated DNA ImmunoPrecipitation (MeDIP) is a capture assay that utilizes a monoclonal antibody that recognizes 5-methyl-cytosine. Despite the potential of various DNA methylation analysis methods for large-scale analysis, generation of whole-genome DNA methylation profiles had not been performed until the MeDIP technique became available. Studies using human cancer cells (Weber et al. 2005, 2007) and *Arabidopsis thaliana* (Zilberman et al. 2007, Zhang et al. 2006) demonstrated that MeDIP, when combined with whole-genome tiling arrays, provides a powerful solution for whole-genome methylation profiling. The application of MeDIP was first published by the Schübeler lab in 2005 (Weber et al. 2005). It includes the shearing of high-molecular-weight genomic DNA into 300–500 bp fragments using sonication, and subsequent immunoprecipitation using an anti-5-methyl-cytosine antibody. The captured DNA fragments are then analyzed using genomic tiling arrays. The basic principle of MeDIP is very similar to MIRA, but where MIRA uses recombinant proteins that recognize dsDNA, MeDIP uses an antibody that requires ssDNA. Both methods are ideally suited for whole-genome methylation profiling. We have extensively evaluated and optimized the MeDIP-on-chip approach, and we have no evidence for any sequence bias in MeDIP. A common problem with methyl-DNA (immuno)capturing approaches is that the efficiency with which DNA is captured is dependent on the number of methylated CpGs within the fragment. This "CpG-density factor" complicates quantification of methylation, assignment of an average "no-methylation" value, and cross-comparison between profiles of different samples. Our results indicate that MeDIP can be used in a quantitative manner by addition of exogenous control DNAs to the capturing step that serves normalization purposes. An additional advantage of capture over restriction-based methods is that it can be used to profile patient DNA samples even if these are fragmented. We have successfully used DNA isolated from paraffin-embedded fixed biopsies.

7 MeDIP-seq

When combined with massively parallel sequencing, MeDIP (or MIRA) would be a very powerful method to generate whole-genome DNA methylation profiles. The main problem with such approaches, however, is the presence of bulk quantities of highly methylated repetitive DNA among captured DNA fragments. Analyses in our laboratory have shown that in a typical MeDIP experiment several classes of repeats (e.g. ALUs, satellites) are recovered with high efficiency (up to 100%) due to the high methylation content of these elements. A genomic DNA sample that is to be randomly sequenced will normally yield mostly unique sequences that can be assigned to a single genomic locus. In contrast, a DNA sample that has been enriched using MeDIP will primarily yield sequence reads that correspond to (highly methylated) repetitive sequence, which cannot be assigned unequivocally to specific genomic regions. In order to detect sufficient numbers of unique sequences within such samples, the total number of sequence reads has to be increased dramatically. This represents a major challenge towards the analysis of MeDIP samples by massive parallel sequencing. In contrast to MeDIP-seq, MeDIP-on-chip does not have this problem since genomic tiling array probes are repeat-masked.

8 Concluding Remarks

The past decades have seen an enormous increase in the number of studies focused on epigenetic changes, both from a molecular and from a clinical point of view. It has become clear that epigenetic aberrations play an important role in disease, and rational 'epidrug' design will require an intimate knowledge of the epigenetic alterations that underlie disease pathways. Numerous examples of gene-by-gene studies have focused on epigenetic aberrations at 'usual suspect' genes, and have combined DNA methylation and ChIP analyses to provide mechanistic details on repression mechanisms. Nevertheless, it is currently poorly understood how (at a global scale) epigenetic marks such as DNA methylation are interpreted and translated into changes in gene expression. Several lines of evidence indicate that methyl-DNA binding proteins are functionally specialized (Hendrich et al. 2001), and their recruitment to genomic sites may not be determined only by recognition of methylated-DNA (Klose et al. 2005). Interestingly, a recent profiling analysis of MeCP2 –a prototype methyl-DNA binding protein with repressive activity– suggested that the majority of MeCP2-associated promoters are unmethylated and active (Yasui et al. 2007). In addition, the activities of various methyl-DNA binding proteins appears to be influenced by post-translational modifications of these proteins themselves (Chen et al. 2003, Le Guezennec et al. 2006, Tan and Nakielny 2006, Lyst et al. 2006). Together, this suggests the translation of the methyl-DNA mark into a repression signal is a highly regulated process involving many proteins and signalling pathways. Recently developed global profiling techniques for DNA methylation as well as ChIP provide opportunities for unbiased analyses to unravel molecular repression pathways at a global scale. Such approaches will allow comparative analyses of multiple different epigenomes. This kind of 'comparative epigenomics' will greatly increase our understanding of how epigenomes are shaped, and will provide opportunities to identify novel diagnostic/prognostic targets, and avenues for pharmacological interference with gene silencing.

References

Barski, A., et al., *High-resolution profiling of histone methylations in the human genome*. Cell, 2007. **129**(4): p. 823–37.
Chen, W.G., et al., *Derepression of BDNF transcription involves calcium-dependent phosphorylation of MeCP2*. Science, 2003. **302**(5646): 885–9.
Colella, S., et al., *Sensitive and quantitative universal Pyrosequencing methylation analysis of CpG sites*. Biotechniques, 2003. **35**(1): 146–50.
Cross, S.H., et al., *Purification of CpG islands using a methylated DNA binding column*. Nat Genet, 1994. **6**(3): 236–44.
Dupont, J.M., et al., *De novo quantitative bisulfite sequencing using the pyrosequencing technology*. Anal Biochem, 2004. **333**(1): 119–27.
Eads, C.A., et al., *MethyLight: a high-throughput assay to measure DNA methylation*. Nucleic Acids Res, 2000. **28**(8): E32.
Eckhardt, F., et al., *DNA methylation profiling of human chromosomes 6, 20 and 22*. Nat Genet, 2006. **38**(12): 1378–85.
Feng, Q. and Y. Zhang, *The MeCP1 complex represses transcription through preferential binding, remodeling, and deacetylating methylated nucleosomes*. Genes Dev, 2001. **15**(7): 827–32.
Frommer, M., et al., *A genomic sequencing protocol that yields a positive display of 5-methylcytosine residues in individual DNA strands*. Proc Natl Acad Sci U S A, 1992. **89**(5): 1827–31.
Gardiner-Garden, M. and M. Frommer, *CpG islands in vertebrate genomes*. J Mol Biol, 1987. **196**(2): 261–82.
Hendrich, B., et al., *Closely related proteins MBD2 and MBD3 play distinctive but interacting roles in mouse development*. Genes Dev, 2001. **15**(6): 710–23.
Herman, J.G., et al., *Methylation-specific PCR: a novel PCR assay for methylation status of CpG islands*. Proc Natl Acad Sci U S A, 1996. **93**(18): 9821–6.

Huang, T.H., M.R. Perry, and D.E. Laux, *Methylation profiling of CpG islands in human breast cancer cells.* Hum Mol Genet, 1999. **8**(3): 459–70.

Ji, H. and W.H. Wong, *TileMap: create chromosomal map of tiling array hybridizations.* Bioinformatics, 2005. **21**(18): 3629–36.

Johnson, D.S., et al., *Genome-wide mapping of in vivo protein-DNA interactions.* Science, 2007. **316**(5830): 1497–502.

Khulan, B., et al., *Comparative isoschizomer profiling of cytosine methylation: the HELP assay.* Genome Res, 2006. **16**(8): 1046–55.

Klose, R.J., et al., *DNA binding selectivity of MeCP2 due to a requirement for A/T sequences adjacent to methyl-CpG.* Mol Cell, 2005. **19**(5): 667–78.

Le Guezennec, X., et al., *MBD2/NuRD and MBD3/NuRD, two distinct complexes with different biochemical and functional properties.* Mol Cell Biol, 2006. **26**(3): 843–51.

Liu, C.L., S.L. Schreiber, and B.E. Bernstein, *Development and validation of a T7 based linear amplification for genomic DNA.* BMC Genomics, 2003. **4**(1): 19.

Lyst, M.J., X. Nan, and I. Stancheva, *Regulation of MBD1-mediated transcriptional repression by SUMO and PIAS proteins.* Embo J, 2006. **25**(22): 5317–28.

Mikkelsen, T.S., et al., *Genome-wide maps of chromatin state in pluripotent and lineage-committed cells.* Nature, 2007. **448**(7153): 553–60.

Ng, H.H., et al., *MBD2 is a transcriptional repressor belonging to the MeCP1 histone deacetylase complex.* Nat Genet, 1999. **23**(1): 58–61.

Nouzova, M., et al., *Epigenomic changes during leukemia cell differentiation: analysis of histone acetylation and cytosine methylation using CpG island microarrays.* J Pharmacol Exp Ther, 2004. **311**(3): 968–81.

O'Geen, H., et al., *Comparison of sample preparation methods for ChIP-chip assays.* Biotechniques, 2006. **41**(5): 577–80.

Rauch, T. and G.P. Pfeifer, *Methylated-CpG island recovery assay: a new technique for the rapid detection of methylated-CpG islands in cancer.* Lab Invest, 2005. **85**(9): 1172–80.

Rauch, T., et al., *MIRA-assisted microarray analysis, a new technology for the determination of DNA methylation patterns, identifies frequent methylation of homeodomain-containing genes in lung cancer cells.* Cancer Res, 2006. **66**(16): 7939–47.

Rauch, T.A., et al., *High-resolution mapping of DNA hypermethylation and hypomethylation in lung cancer.* Proc Natl Acad Sci U S A, 2008. **105**(1): 252–7.

Ren, B., et al., *Genome-wide location and function of DNA binding proteins.* Science, 2000. **290**(5500): 2306–9.

Robertson, G., et al., *Genome-wide profiles of STAT1 DNA association using chromatin immunoprecipitation and massively parallel sequencing.* Nat Methods, 2007. **4**(8): 651–7.

Shiraishi, M., Y.H. Chuu, and T. Sekiya, *Isolation of DNA fragments associated with methylated CpG islands in human adenocarcinomas of the lung using a methylated DNA binding column and denaturing gradient gel electrophoresis.* Proc Natl Acad Sci U S A, 1999. **96**(6): 2913–8.

Solomon, M.J., P.L. Larsen, and A. Varshavsky, *Mapping protein-DNA interactions in vivo with formaldehyde: evidence that histone H4 is retained on a highly transcribed gene.* Cell, 1988. **53**(6): 937–47.

Tan, C.P. and S. Nakielny, *Control of the DNA methylation system component MBD2 by protein arginine methylation.* Mol Cell Biol, 2006. **26**(19): 7224–35.

Weber, M., et al., *Chromosome-wide and promoter-specific analyses identify sites of differential DNA methylation in normal and transformed human cells.* Nat Genet, 2005. **37**(8): 853–62.

Weber, M., et al., *Distribution, silencing potential and evolutionary impact of promoter DNA methylation in the human genome.* Nat Genet, 2007. **39**(4): 457–66.

Xiong, Z. and P.W. Laird, *COBRA: a sensitive and quantitative DNA methylation assay.* Nucleic Acids Res, 1997. **25**(12): 2532–4.

Yasui, D.H., et al., *Integrated epigenomic analyses of neuronal MeCP2 reveal a role for long-range interaction with active genes.* Proc Natl Acad Sci U S A, 2007. **104**(49): 19416–21.

Zeng, P.Y., et al., *In vivo dual cross-linking for identification of indirect DNA-associated proteins by chromatin immunoprecipitation.* Biotechniques, 2006. **41**(6): 694, 696, 698.

Zhang, X., et al., *Genome-wide high-resolution mapping and functional analysis of DNA methylation in arabidopsis.* Cell, 2006. **126**(6): 1189–201.

Zheng, M., et al., *ChIP-chip: data, model, and analysis.* Biometrics, 2007. **63**(3): 787–96.

Zilberman, D., et al., *Genome-wide analysis of Arabidopsis thaliana DNA methylation uncovers an interdependence between methylation and transcription.* Nat Genet, 2007. **39**(1): 61–9.

Sequencing the Epigenome

Alexander Meissner and Bradley E. Bernstein

Abstract The term 'epigenome' refers to the complete description of chemical changes to DNA and histones as they map onto the genome in a given cell type. A comprehensive genomewide catalog of epigenetic control elements and how these vary across cell states could offer critical insight into the relationships between genotype, phenotype and environment, and serve as a catalyst for future studies of the epigenetic mechanisms that regulate normal physiology and human disease. Our ability to characterize mammalian epigenomes has been markedly enhanced by technological developments in recent years. In particular, the introduction of ultra high-throughput sequencing has improved the precision, comprehensiveness and throughput of techniques for mapping chromatin and DNA methylation. This chapter will largely focus on these new applications and their use for high resolution interrogation of mammalian epigenomes.

Keywords DNA methylation · Histone modifications · Epigenome · Bisulfite sequencing · ChIP-Seq

1 Introduction

1.1 Epigenetics

Epigenetic modifications provide essential regulatory information that does not alter the primary nucleotide sequence (Epi: on top or in addition to). DNA methylation is generally associated with repressive contexts and stably propagated through cell division by DNA methyltransferases. Despite being the most extensively studied epigenetic modification in mammals experimental data for its genome-wide distribution, it's dynamic role during differentiation and its relationship with histone modifications remain limited (Bernstein et al. 2007; Bird, 2002). Post-translational histone modifications are implicated in epigenetic regulatory pathways such as

---

A. Meissner(✉)
Broad Institute of MIT and Harvard, 7 Cambridge Center, Cambridge MA 02142, USA
e-mail: alex@broad.mit.edu

position effect variegation and Polycomb silencing, and play critical roles in transcriptional regulation and other genome functions (Kouzarides, 2007; Schuettengruber et al. 2007). Locus-specific and genome-scale studies in human cells and model organisms have identified specific patterns of histone modification that mark diverse functional genomic elements and reveal their activation states in a studied cell type. Cellular differentiation and lineage-commitment are associated with widespread changes in the chromatin landscape, consistent with genetic evidence documenting essential roles for genes encoding histone modifying enzymes and chromatin remodelers in embryonic development (Bernstein et al. 2007). Nevertheless, the precise mechanisms that underlie the regulatory and epigenetic properties of histone modifications remain obscure.

In addition to their critical roles in development and lineage-specification, epigenetic mechanisms contribute significantly to disease pathology. Characteristic changes in cancer include genomewide loss and aberrant local gain of DNA methylation, including at tumor suppressor gene promoters (Jones and Baylin, 2007). Epigenetic deregulation has also been implicated in congenital disorders, and may also provide a link between early environmental exposures and susceptibility to metabolic diseases such as diabetes later in life (Jirtle and Skinner, 2007). Global insight into the epigenetic mechanisms that regulate genome function could thus have wide-reaching implications for prevention, early detection and treatment of disease. Comprehensive characterization of epigenetic marks ('the epigenome') is thus a critical step towards a global understanding of the human genome in health and disease.

1.2 Next Generation Sequencing Technologies

Many previous larger-scale epigenome studies have applied microarrays to achieve increased genome coverage. While these continue to be powerful tools for certain applications (for instance screening large numbers of samples for a subset of loci), we will focus this chapter on more comprehensive genome-scale approaches using sequencing based technologies. Although the dominant methodology in sequencing over the past ten years has been ABI instruments running conventional Sanger chemistry, the last two years have seen a rapid migration to new 'single-molecule' sequencers. The new platforms offer dramatic increases in capacity and sizable cost-reductions. They include the Roche (454 Life Sciences) GS FLX, the Illumina GA (Solexa), the ABI Solid. Here we briefly describe the two most advanced systems that are already widely in use, but others are expected soon.

1.2.1 Roche GS FLX

The Roche GS FLX is based on a technology in which single DNA molecules are amplified and sequenced in miniaturized pyrosequencing reactions (Margulies et al. 2005). Individual molecules are amplified by emulsion PCR, attached to beads and deposited in a microtitre plate. The molecules are sequenced by a synthesis reaction in which different nucleotide bases are consecutively flowed across the plate, and incorporated into a complementary strand. The concomitant release of pyrophosphate is converted to a chemiluminescent signal which is captured by a CCD camera. The instrument throughput has consistently improved and currently generates ~400,000 reads of >250 bp for a total of >100 Mb per run. The GS FLX platform is well suited for reading cytosine methylation by shotgun sequencing of bisulphite-treated DNA (see Section 2.2.1) and has been already used for ultra-deep bisulfite sequencing of PCR amplicons (Korshunova et al. 2008; Taylor et al. 2007). An advantage of the platform (compared to classic bisulfite sequencing) is that it starts directly from libraries of fragmented DNA, and does not involve cloning in a bacterial host. Reads are of sufficient length for unique placement and detection of methylated (and unmethylated) cytosines.

1.2.2 Illumina GA Technology

The Illumina GA technology (formerly Solexa) is also based on single molecule amplification and synthesis on a surface. The ends of a single stranded library are annealed to complementary oligonucleotides on the flowcell. There are two different oligonucleotides, one complementary to each end of the construct. Bridge amplification (amplification in situ with oligos bound to the slide surface) is used to form double stranded clusters containing approximately 10 K molecules. Each of the 8 flowcell lanes contains ~5 million clusters. DNA in the clusters is then linearized by chemically cleaving one of the bound amplification primers from the glass surface. The remaining strands on the flowcell are blocked and the second strand of the linearized amplified library is denatured to leave clusters of single stranded library. The sequencing primer is then annealed to the single stranded clusters and first base incorporation is performed. This incorporation is used to QC primer annealing and to focus the instrument. Sequencing by synthesis is then performed with 36 consecutive cycles of polymerase-mediated reversible fluorescent nucleotide terminator incorporation (in contrast to 454 all four bases are added simultaneously; each base is labeled with a different dye), laser excitation of fluorescent nucleotide tag, image capture, cleavage of fluorescent tag and de-blocking of 3' hydroxyl group of nucleotide. Sequence reads are compiled, post-processed and aligned.

The Illumina GA has potential for notably increased capacity over the GS FLX, already routinely generating ~40 million reads of 35–51 (up to 100 bp possible), thereby yielding more than a billion bases of sequence per run at several hundred-fold lower cost than current Sanger technology. By generating paired-end reads, further improvements in the proportion of uniquely alignable reads may be possible.

2 Mapping DNA Methylation-Towards Comprehensive High Resolution Methylomes

2.1 Background

Of the chemical changes that define the epigenome, methylation of cytosines was the first to be recognized and studied in detail (reviewed in (Bird, 2002; Jaenisch, 1997; Jaenisch and Bird, 2003)). DNA methylation is established and maintained by at least three independent DNA methyltransferases: Dnmt1, Dnmt3a, and Dnmt3b. Dnmt1 acts to maintain methylation patterns after DNA replication, conferring heritability of this epigenetic mark, while Dnmt3a and 3b are considered de novo methyltransferases. The essential role of DNA methylation during development was demonstrated by the embryonic (Dnmt1 and Dnmt3b) and postnatal (Dnmt3a) lethality of the respective knockouts (reviewed in (Bestor, 2000; Bird, 2002)). Characteristic allele-specific patterns of methylation were found to be associated with genomic imprinting and X chromosome inactivation, with changes in methylation at some gene promoters correlating with gene expression changes during cell differentiation. DNA methylation patterns are dynamic in early development and during differentiation (Bird, 2002; Meissner et al. 2008; Reik, 2007; Reik et al. 2001). These physiologic patterns of cytosine methylation can be disrupted to cause disease, the best-studied example being cancer, in which abnormal methylation is common and implicated in pathologic events such as silencing of tumor-suppressor genes (Baylin and Bestor, 2002; Feinberg, 2004). Age and sex are also determinants of genomic methylation patterns, suggesting that other complex diseases may have epigenetic contributions that are as yet undiscovered. In vertebrates, the symmetric dinucleotide CpG is the primary target for DNA methylation. Global quantification of CG methylation by nearest neighbor analysis showed that the majority of CGs in the genome is methylated (70–80%) across cell types (Meissner et al. 2005; Ramsahoye et al. 2000). Loci at which CG dinucleotide density is increased are less likely to be methylated, leading to the definition of CpG islands using base compositional criteria. CpG islands cover roughly 0.5% and 0.7% of the mouse and human genomes, respectively. However, they contain 5% (mouse) and 7% (human) of the CG dinucleotides (Fazzari and Greally, 2004). Notably, the epigenetic role of the remaining CG dinucleotides not within CpG islands remains unclear. Individual methylcytosines can reportedly have biochemical and regulatory functions making high resolution maps an important goal (Attema et al. 2007; Chen et al. 2003; Takizawa et al. 2001).

Gene-specific and genome-wide studies have revealed dynamic patterns of cytosine methylation that define functional elements in the genome. CpG islands located at gene promoters have been reported to undergo some tissue-specific methylation in normal cells, while more extensive changes have been found in cancer. Changes in cancer include a global, genome-wide loss of methylation, but this is accompanied by local gains in methylation, notably at promoters of tumor suppressor genes, which typically results in their silencing. There is now compelling evidence that such aberrant changes play a central mechanistic role in tumor development (Baylin and Bestor, 2002; Feinberg, 2004, 2007; Gaudet et al. 2003; Jones and Baylin, 2002, 2007; Robertson, 2001). Differential methylation of non-promoter regions is another feature of functionally-important loci. Such loci may be differentially-methylated between alleles (imprinted (Bartolomei et al. 1993), X-inactivated (Pfeifer et al. 1990)), or between tissues (Shiota, 2004). Imprinted differentially-methylated loci can encode important *cis*-regulatory elements for sequences beyond the nearest gene, such as the CTCF-binding chromatin insulator upstream of H19 (Bell and Felsenfeld, 2000; Hark et al. 2000) and the *SNRPN* imprinting centre that regulates imprinting in the flanking (Horsthemke, 1997). The X inactivation center is also differentially-methylated (Boumil et al. 2006), with *cis*-regulatory effects that extend throughout the chromosome.

2.2 Mapping Cytosine Methylation

In the past years several new and improved methods of been reported that allow genome-scale methylation analysis. Most are based on combining traditional techniques with microarrays or new sequencing technologies (Table 1). While some are well-suited to high-throughput analysis, most current methods are inadequate for acquiring methylomes due to low resolution or limited scaling potential. Here we present a brief overview of selected techniques.

Table 1 Technologies for mapping DNA methylation

Approach	Comments
Restriction-enzyme based (MSRE)	Queries methylation status only at restriction sites, which limits resolution.
MeC-antibody-based (MeDIP)	Provides relative measure of methylation levels. Quality of antibody and IP variable. Genome-scale possible, max. resolution ~100 bp.
Chemical treatment (bisulfite-sequencing)	Gold standard. Genome-scale analysis possible with ultra high throughput sequencing. Single nucleotide resolution.

2.2.1 Bisulfite Sequencing

Bisulfite Sequencing is the most precise way to characterize DNA methylation as it provides nucleotide level, digital information. It relies on the relative resistance of methylcytosine to deamination by sodium bisulphite, whereas unmodified cytosines are converted to uracil (Frommer et al. 1992). Sequencing of the resulting product allows the methylation of each cytosine to be tested. This can be achieved with conventional technologies, or SNP quantification techniques such as pyrosequencing (Dupont et al. 2004) or MALDI-TOF mass spectrometry (Schatz et al. 2004). A sequencing approach can also detect SNPs and thereby allow allele-specific methylation patterns to be measured. The most comprehensive and detailed study using classic bisulfite sequencing to date was performed by the Sanger Centre and Epigenomics AG, generating 2,524 amplicons of sequences near known genes on human chromosomes 6, 20 and 22. DNA collected from 43 tissues was bisulfite-treated, followed by Sanger sequencing (Eckhardt et al. 2006). The study revealed striking insights with regard to quantitative intragenomic differences in cytosine methylation; for example, the study found 9.2% of CpG islands to have methylation values of >80%, a general decrease in methylation at transcription start sites compared with flanking sequences, and correlated degrees of methylation in cis within the genome, indicating that cytosine methylation/hypomethylation occurs over coordinately regulated clusters of CG dinucleotides. While the total number of CG dinucleotide reads was 1.88 million, this reflects the same loci tested in 43 different samples, indicating a total of 43,721 individual CG dinucleotides tested, which represent 1.6% of the 2,752,490 CGs on these chromosomes. Thus, even in an ambitious study such as this (with the explicit goal of generating a foundation for a Human Epigenome Project; see http://www.epigenome.org), the approach of locus-specific amplification, while revealing, can achieve only modest throughput.

2.2.2 Enrichment-Based Methods Coupled with Arrays

The selective digestion of genomic DNA by methylation-sensitive restriction enzymes (MSRE) can by exploited to enrich methylated or unmethylated DNA fractions. In combination with array hybridization this allows to generate genome-scale maps of relative DNA methylation levels (Zhang et al. 2006). The coverage of MSRE-based methods is dependent on the frequency and distribution of the recognition site of the particular enzyme used. This limits assay resolution and can lead to bias. An alternative and less biased enrichment strategy involves IP with methylcytosine antibodies followed by microarray hybridization (methyl-DNA IP or 'meDIP') (Keshet et al. 2006; Weber et al. 2005). While this technique is more comprehensive, antibody specificity and IP quality can be variable. Moreover, the effective coverage is restricted to sites with multiple methylated CpGs in close proximity, and resolution is limited by the size of IP fragments and array density. The *H*paII tiny fragment *E*nrichment by *L*igation-mediated *P*CR (HELP) approach for profiling DNA methylation also combines a restriction enzyme digest with microarrays (Khulan et al. 2006). HELP is a technically-simple assay that uses multiple internal controls and is amenable to sophisticated bioinformatic analysis that enable acquisition of high-confidence data. The major drawback is the inability of the assay to study more than the ~8% of CGs that are contained within *H*paII sites. As with other microarray-based methods, the HELP assay does not yield single CG dinucleotide resolution data. This illustrates the significant limitation of microarray-based techniques given an increasing body of evidence supporting the importance of low-density CGs in epigenetic regulation and the notion that much of the regulations occurs away from promoter regions.

2.3 Mapping DNA Methylation by Ultra High-Throughput Sequencing

Recent advances in next generation sequencing technologies have opened new avenues for analyzing DNA methylation patterns across genomes. Ultra-high throughput sequencing of enriched fractions (MSRE or meDIP) or bisulfite treated DNA can significantly increase genome-coverage, resolution and cost. High throughput bisulfite sequencing (HTBS) allows nucleotide level methylation analysis that involves "shotgun-sequencing" of bisulfite-treated DNA. This approach was recently used by Jacobsen and colleagues to map the entire Arabidopsis methylome at nucleotide resolution (Cokus et al. 2008). While technically feasible, the larger size of mammalian genomes makes it still too costly for comparative studies across many cell types. To overcome this limitation, we have recently combined reduced representation bisufite sequencing with high throughput sequencing (Meissner et al. 2008; see 2.3.3).

2.3.1 MeDIP-Seq

The combination of methylated DNA immunoprecipitation (MeDIP) and next-generation sequencing –termed MeDIP-Seq – presents an economical alternative to bisulfite sequencing-based approaches for DNA methylation profiling of whole genomes (methylomes), including mammalian-sized methylomes. Integrated with a novel computational algorithm (Batman), which uses a Bayesian deconvolution strategy to convert MeDIP enrichment data into absolute DNA methylation values, Down, Rakyan, Beck and colleagues have recently analyzed the methylome of human spermatozoa (Down et al. 2008). Extrapolating from this effort, the authors predict that up to two mammalian-sized methylomes of $\sim$100 bp resolution can be generated from a single run of an Illumina Genome Analyzer II. As in chromatin mapping (see Section 3.3; below), incorporation of sequencing offers improved resolution, specificity and genome coverage in DNA methylation studies. For chromatin marks the ideal resolution corresponds to a nucleosomal unit ($\sim$200 bases). In contrast for DNA methylation it may depend on the application. For some purposes nucleotide resolution may be essential, however, based on previous reports the lower resolution by meDIP may in many cases be sufficient. Thus meDIP-Seq presents a powerful tool for scanning whole methylomes (Beck and Rakyan, 2008).

2.3.2 Whole Genome Shotgun Bisulfite Sequencing

Sheared and adapter equipped genomic DNA can be subjected to bisulfite treatment followed by shotgun sequencing (Fig. 1b). The first whole genome shotgun bisulfite sequencing study to be reported is for a plant genome by the Jacobsen lab (Cokus et al. 2008). Cokus et al. used the Illumina GA (see Section 1.2.2) to sequence 3.8 Gb of bisulfite-converted DNA, and thereby generate the first nucleotide resolution methylome from the 120 Mb Arabidopsis thaliana genome. The data set includes 2.6 billion nucleotides that mapped to unique genomic locations covering 93% of all cytosines that could be theoretically covered. The methylome has been previously mapped using tiling arrays, however, the higher resolution provided additional important insights; (i) its higher sensitivity identified particular methylated CGs that had previously been missed, (ii) repetitive sequences including telomeric repeats could be analyzed, (iii) the approach allowed distinction of symmetric (CG and CHG) and asymmetric (CHH) DNA methylation, (iv) the single base resolution allowed identification of precise boundaries between methylated and unmethylated regions as shown for tandem repeats and flanking sequence. In principle the pipeline should be applicable for larger genomes. To this end Jacobsen and colleagues performed a small proof of principle experiment. 46 million bisulfite

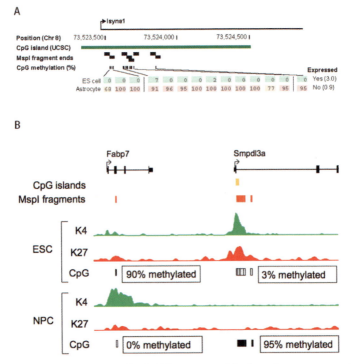

Fig. 1 HTBS and ChIP-Seq maps. (**A**) RRBS coverage of the *Isyna1* promoter associated CpG island. Shown are genomic location of *Isyna1* and the CpG island (green) surrounding its transcription start site (TSS). Think horizontal black bars indicate sequenced *Msp*I fragments and vertical bars the position of individual CpG dinucleotides. Inferred and color-coded (green=low methylation; red=high methylation) methylation values are shown for embryonic stem (ES) cells and ES-derived astrocytes. The expression status is shown on the right. (**B**) ChIP-Seq profiles (H3K4me3 and H3K27me3) and averaged methylation values (1.5 kb window around the TSS) for *Fabp7*, a low CpG promoter (LCP), and for *Smpdl3a*, a high CpG promoter (HCP) in ES cells and ES-derived neural progenitor cells (NPCs). *Fabp7* is not expressed in ES cells, but becomes highly induced upon neural differentiation. *Smpdl3a* is not expressed in ES cells and NPCs

converted bases from murine germ-cell tissue were aligned indicating that approximately 66% of the reads could be uniquely mapped back. This is highly consistent with our initial experiments (Meissner, Mikkelsen, Gnirke, Lander; unpublished) and with computational predictions for alignability of murine bisufite treated DNA (67%) compared to untreated (77%) with 36 bp reads. Notably, with 72 bp the difference becomes significantly smaller (84% for treated vs 87% for untreated). A similar increase in alignable reads is shown in Table 2 for the human genome. Solexa read length has already increased from 25 to 36 bp within the last year and now 51 bp reads can be routinely accomplished.

The Cokus et al. study is an exciting demonstration of the technology and provides novel insights, however significant differences exist between plant and mammalian methylation biology. Moreover, methylomes in all species are highly

Table 2 Whole-genome HTBS alignability. Synthetic reads were sampled randomly from the full human genome, bisulfite-converted, and then aligned back to the genome. To simulate sequencing errors (E), sampled reads were mutated with zero, one or two random subtitutions prior to alignment

Read length/ errors/read	$N = 36$	$N = 47$	$N = 72$
$E = 0$	72.5%	79.5%	87.4%
$E = 1$	69.4%	78.5%	86.9%
$E = 2$	64.1%	77.6%	86.1%

cell type-specific. Therefore, it will be important to generate similar DNA methylation maps of many distinct mammalian cell types.

2.3.3 Reduced Representation Bisulfite Sequencing

The reduced-representation method enables reproducible sampling of defined subsets of a mammalian genome (Altshuler et al. 2000; Meissner et al. 2005). The fraction can be controlled by the enzyme used and the size range of fragments selected. For instance, *Msp*I fragments of the size range 40–220 bp provide a significant enrichment of CpG islands (~90% are included) and promoter regions. Nonetheless, half of the fragments originate from lower CpG density regions including highly conserved non coding elements (HCNEs) and distal regulatory elements that have escaped previous array based studies (Meissner et al. 2008.). Because *Msp*I contains a CG within its recognition sequence (C'CGG) every read automatically contains at least one CG (Note: most of the genome is depleted of CG indicating that a large amount of shotgun reads will not include any CGs). End-sequencing of the terminal 36-bases of human *Msp*I fragments (size range 40–220 bp) provides data for ~3 million distinct CpG dinucleotides (~10% of all CpGs in the human genome) and includes sequence from over 90% of annotated CpG islands. Genome coverage can be increased by expanding the size range (expanding the *Msp*I library to 40–400 bp yields 3.8 million or ~15% of CpGs in the human genome) and coverage can be further increased by longer reads.

We have applied high-throughput bisulfite sequencing (HTBS) on the Illumina GA to acquire genome-scale DNA methylation maps for 17 murine cell types (Meissner et al. 2008.). Specifically, we combined HTBS with the reduced-representation approach to acquire 5.8 Gb of sequence and thereby determine absolute methylation levels of around one million CpGs in each cell type. The data provided several new insights; (i) DNA methylation is better correlated with histone methylation states than with sequence context, (ii) while it is known that CpG islands are susceptible to hypermethylation, the data show that the methylation occurs at a distinctive set of genes that are susceptible to this phenomenon, and that this susceptibility correlates with promoter CpG density and chromatin state. Moreover, this pattern bears a striking similarity to the pattern reported by other groups for genes frequently methylated in cancer, (iii) DNA methylation patterns are dynamic during cellular differentiation, and particularly so outside of CpG islands.

Alternative approaches in which target regions are captured using oligonucleotides in solution or on arrays (hybrid selection) provide another attractive route for shotgun bisulfite sequencing of defined regions. In summary, HTBS shows that (1) essentially complete genomewide bisulfite conversion (>99.9%) can be achieved; (2) restriction-based and hybrid selection-based methods can effectively reduce the sampled genomic space, thereby enabling deep coverage of CpG islands, promoters and other critical loci; and (3) 36 base reads of bisulfite-converted DNA can be readily aligned to about two thirds of the mouse or human genome, thereby enabling HTBS to scale genomewide with increasing sequencing capacity. We expect HTBS to rapidly emerge as the standard for genome-scale methylation analysis. With reduced-representations, 15% of CpG dinucleotides and a vast majority of CpG islands and promoters in the human genome can be interrogated by HTBS. Importantly, the cost of genome sequencing will continue to drop rapidly over the next years, which ultimately will lead to single nucleotide methylomes.

3 Mapping Histone Modifications by Ultra High-Throughput Sequencing

3.1 Background

The nucleosomal histones, H2A, H2B, H3 and H4, are subject to a large number of post-translational modifications, including acetylation, methylation, phosphorylation and ubiquitination. The modifications occur on specific lysines and other residues in the histone tails and cores. They are added and removed by families of histone acetylases, deacetylases, methylases, demethylases, kinases, phosphatases and ubiquitinases. The enzymes are recruited to promoters, enhancers and other genomic sites where they catalyze modification of proximal chromatin and can also spread along chromosomes. The recruitment mechanisms remain poorly understood but can involve interactions with RNAP II, transcription factors, repressors or other epigenetic marks (Kouzarides 2007; Margueron et al. 2005).

3.2 Chromatin Immunoprecipitation

Chromatin immunoprecipitation (ChIP) is the primary method used by researchers to query the modification state of histones at specific genomic sites (Table 3). The method involves treating cells with formaldehyde to cross-link DNA to nearby proteins, fragmenting the chromatin, and immunoprecipitating with antibody to a particular histone modification. Quantitative PCR can be used to determine whether a given DNA sequence is enriched in a ChIP assay, and thus associated in vivo with this modification. ChIP has been used to investigate many different histone modifications, and can also be used to test for association of other chromatin proteins or transcription factors. An advantage of the method is that the fixation step effectively preserves the modification states as they exist in the living cell. ChIP

Table 3 Technologies for mapping chromatin state

Approach	Comments
PCR (ChIP-PCR)	Gold-standard, but very low throughput.
Microarray (ChIP-chip)	Genome-scale. Ideal for targeted studies of promoters or specific genomic loci. Whole genome analysis requires multiple arrays and large quantities of DNA.
Sequencing (ChIP-Seq)	Genomewide, including most repeats. Sequencing requires just a few nanograms of DNA

can be combined with microarrays (ChIP-on-chip) for genome-scale or genome-wide analysis (Huebert et al. 2006). Here, DNA isolated by ChIP is amplified in a sequence-independent fashion, labeled and hybridized. Recent studies have used tiling oligonucleotide arrays that cover non-repetitive portions of entire chromosomes. These platforms are not restricted to currently annotated genes and may therefore detect epigenetic changes associated with uncharacterized transcriptional units or regulatory elements. Moreover, they generate continuous data along chromosomes and can thus identify genomic regions with modified histones as well as define their extents and boundaries. However, ChIP-chip is subject to a number of limitations as it (i) is insensitive to repetitive elements due to cross-hybridization, and thus can interrogate only $\sim 50\%$ of the genome; (ii) requires large quantities of DNA for hybridization and thus requires large numbers of cells and extensive bias-prone amplification; (iii) is expensive because genome-wide analysis requires parallel hybridizations to multiple arrays with high material, reagent and labor costs.

3.3 Sequencing-Based Methods for Mapping Chromatin

Many of the limitations of ChIP-on-chip can be addressed by a sequencing-based approach for mapping histone modifications. ChIP-Seq essentially involves sequencing DNA fragments in a ChIP sample and aligning the reads to the genome. The probability that a given genomic region is enriched in the ChIP sample (and hence associated with the relevant histone modification) can be determined from the number of sequencing reads that fall within the region. The sequencing approach (i) is inherently genome-wide; (ii) can detect repetitive elements and allele-specific changes; (iii) requires less DNA than array-based analysis; and (iv) capitalizes on remarkable recent advances in sequencing throughput. Recently, a few groups have developed tools for combining ChIP with high-throughput sequencing. In general, the key to effective genomewide mapping of mammalian chromatin is to acquire very large numbers of sequencing reads, just long enough to enable unique alignment, from a ChIP DNA library. Here we summarize some of the key findings.

3.3.1 ChIP-PET

Ruan and colleagues combined ChIP with a paired-end ditag strategy, and have used the approach to map p53 and other factors (Wei et al. 2006). The method uses cloning to generate sequencing libraries from ChIP DNA. An advantage is that it yields paired reads for each end of a given ChIP fragment. A potential disadvantage is that the method may be susceptible to cloning bias. The p53 sequencing study resulted in the identification of 65,572 unique ChIP DNA fragments, sufficient for the identification of roughly 500 binding sites. However, the study did not identify p53 sites with comprehensiveness due to an insufficient number of sequenced ditags (Ng et al. 2006).

3.3.2 ChIP SAGE

Roh and colleagues developed a 'SAGE-like' sequencing method to identify sites of histone modification (Roh et al. 2005). Initial studies focused on H3 acetylation in human T-cells and used conventional Sanger sequencing to sequence concatamerized tags from a ChIP DNA library. Roughly 670,000 tags were uniquely mapped to the human genome, revealing close to 50,000 acetylated sites (defined as sites with 2 or more clustered tags). Nearly all of these multiple tag sites were true positives (by qPCR). Though the study succeeded in identifying an unprecedented number of acetylated genomic sites, it still did not achieve comprehensiveness as many other acetylated sites, including those represented by single tags, could not be discriminated from background due to insufficient sequencing depth.

3.3.3 ChIP-Seq Using Ultra High-Throughput Sequencing

Although they can accurately identify significant numbers of true positive sites of binding or chromatin modification, ChIP-PET and ChIP-SAGE are non-ideal as they do not achieve comprehensiveness due to moderate sequencing depth. Chromatin mapping is a particularly demanding application because sites and extended regions of modification must be identified, and because certain modifications affect large proportions of the genome, thus distributing reads broadly. We estimate that mapping chromatin with precision and comprehensiveness requires millions of reads, depending on the degree of enrichment that can be achieved with a given antibody (Bernstein et al. 2007).

Conveniently, these kinds of read numbers can now be acquired with ultra high-throughput sequencing technologies. We and other have recently applied the Illumina Genome Analyzer to acquire millions of reads per ChIP sample and thereby map chromatin state (or transcription factor binding) comprehensively in mammalian cells (Mikkelsen et al. 2007; Mortazavi et al. 2006; Robertson et al. 2007).

Here we provide a brief overview of ChIP-Seq methodology as implemented by our research group. We use a standard cross-linking ChIP procedure and modification state-specific anti-histone antibodies to fractionate chromatin. Roughly one to ten nanograms of thus isolated ChIP DNA is then used to prepare a sequencing library. This is done by ligating sequencing adaptors to the ends of the ChIP fragments, gel purifying ligated fragments of appropriate length, and subjecting them to 18 cycles of PCR amplifications. Given the small quantities of ChIP DNA, the gel purification step is done 'blindly'. Completed libraries are subjected to ultra high-throughput sequencing on the Illumina Genome Analyzer according to standard protocols.

Sequence reads (typically 36 bases in length) are aligned using a general purpose computational pipeline that applies a seed-and-extend algorithm to align short reads with high sensitivity and specificity. We only retain "unique" alignments for which there is no alternative alignment of comparable accuracy. Genomewide maps that reflect relative ChIP enrichment are then computed by estimating the number of ChIP fragments that overlap any given position in the genome (Mikkelsen et al. 2007). We also generate binary maps of enriched intervals sites using a Hidden Markov Model (HMM), which takes into account nucleosome length and missing data due to low complexity sequences, and can effectively combine nearby enriched positions into continuous segments of modification (Mikkelsen et al. 2007; Richard Koche and B.E.B., unpublished data).

ChIP-Seq maps are highly consistent with data acquired by microarray-based methods, but offer greater genome coverage, a 'digital' readout of enrichment and higher resolution (Mikkelsen et al. 2007; Mortazavi et al. 2006). Comparisons with real-time PCR further indicate that the ChIP-Seq signal offers quantitative information about the relative enrichment of a region. Of course, signal and data quality are exquisitely dependent on the effectiveness of the upstream enrichment step which can vary substantially between different epitopes and antibodies. Further analysis and standardization is clearly needed to more precisely delineate the accuracy of the method, and how this depends on enrichment efficiency, read numbers and other factors. It should ultimately be possible to develop algorithms and metrics that accurately estimate sensitivity and specificity for a given ChIP-Seq experiment based on the number and distribution of sequence reads.

3.3.4 ChIP-Seq Studies of Mammalian Chromatin

Recent ChIP-Seq studies have offered notable insight into the chromatin landscape of mammalian cells. Barski et al mapped 20 chromatin epitopes genomewide in human T-cells. The investigators identified characteristic chromatin signatures associated with promoters, transcripts, insulators and enhancers (Barski et al. 2007). They also found that different methyl states of the same residue exhibited markedly different localizations; for example, whereas trimethylated histone H3 lysine 9 correlated with repression, monomethylated H3 lysine 9 associated with active loci. By providing a large number of datasets for distinct chromatin marks in a single cell type, the study offers a valuable resource for understanding the functions and inter-relationships among the many chromatin modifications.

Mikkelsen et al applied ChIP-Seq towards the study of chromatin state in pluripotent and lineage-committed murine stem cells (Mikkelsen et al. 2007). Five different lysine methylation marks were mapped genomewide in mouse embryonic stem cells, neural stem cells and embryonic fibroblasts. The chromatin maps revealed the locations and activation states of diverse functional genomic elements. In particular, histone H3 lysine 4 and lysine 27 trimethylation were found to be informative markers of promoter locations and activation states, while other patterns identified transcripts (H3 lysine 36 trimethylation), active transposons (H3 lysine 9 trimethylation) and imprinting control regions (combination of H3 lysine 9 and H3 lysine 4 trimethylation marking alternative alleles). Notably, the allele-specificity of the chromatin marks at imprinting control regions could be appreciated through direct analysis of the sequencing reads in the context of known single nucleotide polymorphisms. This potential for allele-specific chromatin analysis is another exciting attribute of the ChIP-Seq approach, though obtaining sufficient power for allele discrimination requires significant numbers of known polymorphisms and very large numbers of sequencing reads.

The Mikkelsen et al study also highlighted the capacity of chromatin state maps to inform on the developmental state and potential of a studied cell population. In particular, maps of lysine 4 and lysine 27 trimethylation offer insight into the activation states and the potentials of promoters genomewide. Monovalent lysine 4 trimethylated promoters show high activity. In contrast, monovalent lysine 27 trimethylated promoters are largely silent, consistent with the association of this methyl mark with the repressive Polycomb pathway. An additional set of 'bivalent' promoters carry both marks. The bivalent chromatin pattern is particularly prevalent in embryonic stem cells where it associates with many developmental genes that are silent but 'poised' to become induced upon differentiation. Remarkably, the fate of initially bivalent promoters in the committed cell types examined correlated with their known developmental potential. That is, the neural stem cells activated or kept bivalent a significant proportion of genes with neural-related functions, while the embryonic fibroblasts activated or kept bivalent many genes with functions in mesenchymal tissues.

The capacity of chromatin state maps to provide comprehensive insight into the epigenetic and developmental state of a given cell population should make ChIP-Seq a particularly powerful tool for the fields of development, cancer and stem cell biology, and regenerative medicine. To achieve maximal impact, further methodological innovations will be needed to make the ChIP-Seq procedure applicable to much smaller cell numbers as many biologically-critical cell populations can only be obtained in limited quantities.

4 Conclusion

With the completion of the human genome project, we now have the opportunity to contemplate and systematically decipher the next tier of information that controls how our genetic makeup becomes manifest. A full understanding of this epigenomic content (Qiu, 2006) will require significant effort, as every cell type has a distinct epigenetic state and environmental conditions may further increase this diversity. The technological developments and ultra high-throughput sequencing-based tools have provided substantial insights already and hold great promise for addressing this challenge with improvements in throughput, scale and resolution. These ambitious goals are also being enabled by collaborative research initiatives, including ENCODE (Birney et al. 2007), the Human Epigenome Project (Eckhardt et al. 2006;

Jones and Martienssen, 2005), and the NIH Roadmap. Unprecedented global views from these and other studies will greatly enhancer our understanding of the functions and inter-relationships among epigenetic marks, and provide deep insight into the relationships between genotype, phenotype and environment with implications for human health and disease.

References

Altshuler, D., Pollara, V.J., Cowles, C.R., Van Etten, W.J., Baldwin, J., Linton, L., and Lander, E.S. (2000). An SNP map of the human genome generated by reduced representation shotgun sequencing. Nature *407*, 513–516.

Attema, J.L., Papathanasiou, P., Forsberg, E.C., Xu, J., Smale, S.T., and Weissman, I.L. (2007). Epigenetic characterization of hematopoietic stem cell differentiation using miniChIP and bisulfite sequencing analysis. Proc Natl Acad Sci U S A *104*, 12371–12376.

Barski, A., Cuddapah, S., Cui, K., Roh, T.Y., Schones, D.E., Wang, Z., Wei, G., Chepelev, I., and Zhao, K. (2007). High-resolution profiling of histone methylations in the human genome. Cell *129*, 823–837.

Bartolomei, M.S., Webber, A.L., Brunkow, M.E., and Tilghman, S.M. (1993). Epigenetic mechanisms underlying the imprinting of the mouse H19 gene. Genes Dev *7*, 1663–1673.

Baylin, S., and Bestor, T.H. (2002). Altered methylation patterns in cancer cell genomes: cause or consequence? Cancer Cell *1*, 299–305.

Beck, S., and Rakyan, V.K. (2008). The methylome: approaches for global DNA methylation profiling. Trends Genet.

Bell, A.C., and Felsenfeld, G. (2000). Methylation of a CTCF-dependent boundary controls imprinted expression of the Igf2 gene. Nature *405*, 482–485.

Bernstein, B.E., Meissner, A., and Lander, E.S. (2007). The mammalian epigenome. Cell *128*, 669–681.

Bestor, T.H. (2000). The DNA methyltransferases of mammals. Hum Mol Genet *9*, 2395–2402.

Bird, A. (2002). DNA methylation patterns and epigenetic memory. Genes Dev *16*, 6–21.

Birney, E., Stamatoyannopoulos, J.A., Dutta, A., Guigo, R., Gingeras, T.R., Margulies, E.H., Weng, Z., Snyder, M., Dermitzakis, E.T., Thurman, R.E., *et al.* (2007). Identification and analysis of functional elements in 1% of the human genome by the ENCODE pilot project. Nature *447*, 799–816.

Boumil, R.M., Ogawa, Y., Sun, B.K., Huynh, K.D., and Lee, J.T. (2006). Differential methylation of Xite and CTCF sites in Tsix mirrors the pattern of X-inactivation choice in mice. Mol Cell Biol *26*, 2109–2117.

Chen, W.G., Chang, Q., Lin, Y., Meissner, A., West, A.E., Griffith, E.C., Jaenisch, R., and Greenberg, M.E. (2003). Derepression of BDNF transcription involves calcium-dependent phosphorylation of MeCP2. Science *302*, 885–889.

Cokus, S.J., Feng, S., Zhang, X., Chen, Z., Merriman, B., Haudenschild, C.D., Pradhan, S., Nelson, S.F., Pellegrini, M., and Jacobsen, S.E. (2008). Shotgun bisulphite sequencing of the Arabidopsis genome reveals DNA methylation patterning. Nature *452*, 215–219.

Down, T.A., Rakyan, V.K., Turner, D.J., Flicek, P., Li, H., Kulesha, E., Gräf, G., Johnson, N., Herrero, J., Tomazou, E.M., *et al.* (2008). A Bayesian deconvolution strategy for immunoprecipitation-based analysis of mammalian-sized DNA methylomes. Nature Biotechnology *26*, 779–785.

Dupont, J.M., Tost, J., Jammes, H., and Gut, I.G. (2004). De novo quantitative bisulfite sequencing using the pyrosequencing technology. Anal Biochem *333*, 119–127.

Eckhardt, F., Lewin, J., Cortese, R., Rakyan, V.K., Attwood, J., Burger, M., Burton, J., Cox, T.V., Davies, R., Down, T.A., *et al.* (2006). DNA methylation profiling of human chromosomes 6, 20 and 22. Nat Genet *38*, 1378–1385.

Fazzari, M.J., and Greally, J.M. (2004). Epigenomics: beyond CpG islands. Nat Rev Genet 5, 446–455.

Feinberg, A.P. (2004). The epigenetics of cancer etiology. Semin Cancer Biol 14, 427–432.

Feinberg, A.P. (2007). Phenotypic plasticity and the epigenetics of human disease. Nature 447, 433–440.

Frommer, M., McDonald, L.E., Millar, D.S., Collis, C.M., Watt, F., Grigg, G.W., Molloy, P.L., and Paul, C.L. (1992). A genomic sequencing protocol that yields a positive display of 5-methylcytosine residues in individual DNA strands. Proc Natl Acad Sci U S A 89, 1827–1831.

Gaudet, F., Hodgson, J.G., Eden, A., Jackson-Grusby, L., Dausman, J., Gray, J.W., Leonhardt, H., and Jaenisch, R. (2003). Induction of tumors in mice by genomic hypomethylation. Science 300, 489–492.

Hark, A.T., Schoenherr, C.J., Katz, D.J., Ingram, R.S., Levorse, J.M., and Tilghman, S.M. (2000). CTCF mediates methylation-sensitive enhancer-blocking activity at the H19/Igf2 locus. Nature 405, 486–489.

Horsthemke, B. (1997). Structure and function of the human chromosome 15 imprinting center. J Cell Physiol 173, 237–241.

Huebert, D.J., Kamal, M., O'Donovan, A., and Bernstein, B.E. (2006). Genome-wide analysis of histone modifications by ChIP-on-chip. Methods 40, 365–369.

Jaenisch, R. (1997). DNA methylation and imprinting: why bother? Trends Genet 13, 323–329.

Jaenisch, R., and Bird, A. (2003). Epigenetic regulation of gene expression: how the genome integrates intrinsic and environmental signals. Nat Genet 33 Suppl, 245–254.

Jirtle, R.L., and Skinner, M.K. (2007). Environmental epigenomics and disease susceptibility. Nat Rev Genet 8, 253–262.

Jones, P.A., and Baylin, S.B. (2002). The fundamental role of epigenetic events in cancer. Nat Rev Genet 3, 415–428.

Jones, P.A., and Baylin, S.B. (2007). The Epigenomics of Cancer. Cell 128, 683–692.

Jones, P.A., and Martienssen, R. (2005). A blueprint for a Human Epigenome Project: the AACR Human Epigenome Workshop. Cancer Res 65, 11241–11246.

Keshet, I., Schlesinger, Y., Farkash, S., Rand, E., Hecht, M., Segal, E., Pikarski, E., Young, R.A., Niveleau, A., Cedar, H., et al. (2006). Evidence for an instructive mechanism of de novo methylation in cancer cells. Nat Genet 38, 149–153.

Khulan, B., Thompson, R.F., Ye, K., Fazzari, M.J., Suzuki, M., Stasiek, E., Figueroa, M.E., Glass, J.L., Chen, Q., Montagna, C., et al. (2006). Comparative isoschizomer profiling of cytosine methylation: the HELP assay. Genome Res 16, 1046–1055.

Korshunova, Y., Maloney, R.K., Lakey, N., Citek, R.W., Bacher, B., Budiman, A., Ordway, J.M., McCombie, W.R., Leon, J., Jeddeloh, J.A., et al. (2008). Massively parallel bisulphite pyrosequencing reveals the molecular complexity of breast cancer-associated cytosine-methylation patterns obtained from tissue and serum DNA. Genome Res 18, 19–29.

Kouzarides, T. (2007). Chromatin modifications and their function. Cell 128, 693–705.

Margueron, R., Trojer, P., and Reinberg, D. (2005). The key to development: interpreting the histone code? Curr Opin Genet Dev 15, 163–176.

Margulies, M., Egholm, M., Altman, W.E., Attiya, S., Bader, J.S., Bemben, L.A., Berka, J., Braverman, M.S., Chen, Y.J., Chen, Z., et al. (2005). Genome sequencing in microfabricated high-density picolitre reactors. Nature. 437, 376–380.

Meissner, A., Gnirke, A., Bell, G.W., Ramsahoye, B., Lander, E.S., and Jaenisch, R. (2005). Reduced representation bisulfite sequencing for comparative high-resolution DNA methylation analysis. Nucleic Acids Res 33, 5868–5877.

Meissner, A., Mikkelsen, T.S., Gu, H., Wernig, M., Sivachenki, A., Zhang, X., Bernstein, B.E., Nusbaum, C., Jaffe, D.B., Jaenisch, R., et al. (2008). Genome-scale DNA methylation maps of pluripotent and differentiated cells. Nature, 7;454(7205), 766–770 (e-pub July 6) .

Mikkelsen, T.S., Ku, M., Jaffe, D.B., Issac, B., Lieberman, E., Giannoukos, G., Alvarez, P., Brockman, W., Kim, T.K., Koche, R.P., et al. (2007). Genome-wide maps of chromatin state in pluripotent and lineage-committed cells. Nature 448, 553–560.

Mortazavi, A., Leeper Thompson, E.C., Garcia, S.T., Myers, R.M., and Wold, B. (2006). Comparative genomics modeling of the NRSF/REST repressor network: from single conserved sites to genome-wide repertoire. Genome Res *16*, 1208–1221.

Ng, P., Tan, J.J., Ooi, H.S., Lee, Y.L., Chiu, K.P., Fullwood, M.J., Srinivasan, K.G., Perbost, C., Du, L., Sung, W.K., et al. (2006). Multiplex sequencing of paired-end ditags (MS-PET): a strategy for the ultra-high-throughput analysis of transcriptomes and genomes. Nucleic Acids Res *34*, e84.

Pfeifer, G.P., Tanguay, R.L., Steigerwald, S.D., and Riggs, A.D. (1990). In vivo footprint and methylation analysis by PCR-aided genomic sequencing: comparison of active and inactive X chromosomal DNA at the CpG island and promoter of human PGK-1. Genes Dev *4*, 1277–1287.

Qiu, J. (2006). Epigenetics: unfinished symphony. Nature *441*, 143–145.

Ramsahoye, B.H., Biniszkiewicz, D., Lyko, F., Clark, V., Bird, A.P., and Jaenisch, R. (2000). Non-CpG methylation is prevalent in embryonic stem cells and may be mediated by DNA methyltransferase 3a. Proc Natl Acad Sci U S A *97*, 5237–5242.

Reik, W. (2007). Stability and flexibility of epigenetic gene regulation in mammalian development. Nature *447*, 425–432.

Reik, W., Dean, W., and Walter, J. (2001). Epigenetic reprogramming in mammalian development. Science *293*, 1089–1093.

Robertson, G., Hirst, M., Bainbridge, M., Bilenky, M., Zhao, Y., Zeng, T., Euskirchen, G., Bernier, B., Varhol, R., Delaney, A., et al. (2007). Genome-wide profiles of STAT1 DNA association using chromatin immunoprecipitation and massively parallel sequencing. Nat Methods *4*, 651–657.

Robertson, K.D. (2001). DNA methylation, methyltransferases, and cancer. Oncogene *20*, 3139–3155.

Roh, T.Y., Cuddapah, S., and Zhao, K. (2005). Active chromatin domains are defined by acetylation islands revealed by genome-wide mapping. Genes Dev *19*, 542–552.

Schatz, P., Dietrich, D., and Schuster, M. (2004). Rapid analysis of CpG methylation patterns using RNase T1 cleavage and MALDI-TOF. Nucleic Acids Res *32*, e167.

Schuettengruber, B., Chourrout, D., Vervoort, M., Leblanc, B., and Cavalli, G. (2007). Genome regulation by polycomb and trithorax proteins. Cell *128*, 735–745.

Shiota, K. (2004). DNA methylation profiles of CpG islands for cellular differentiation and development in mammals. Cytogenet Genome Res *105*, 325–334.

Takizawa, T., Nakashima, K., Namihira, M., Ochiai, W., Uemura, A., Yanagisawa, M., Fujita, N., Nakao, M., and Taga, T. (2001). DNA methylation is a critical cell-intrinsic determinant of astrocyte differentiation in the fetal brain. Dev Cell *1*, 749–758.

Taylor, K.H., Kramer, R.S., Davis, J.W., Guo, J., Duff, D.J., Xu, D., Caldwell, C.W., and Shi, H. (2007). Ultradeep bisulfite sequencing analysis of DNA methylation patterns in multiple gene promoters by 454 sequencing. Cancer Res *67*, 8511–8518.

Weber, M., Davies, J.J., Wittig, D., Oakeley, E.J., Haase, M., Lam, W.L., and Schubeler, D. (2005). Chromosome-wide and promoter-specific analyses identify sites of differential DNA methylation in normal and transformed human cells. Nat Genet *37*, 853–862.

Wei, C.L., Wu, Q., Vega, V.B., Chiu, K.P., Ng, P., Zhang, T., Shahab, A., Yong, H.C., Fu, Y., Weng, Z., et al. (2006). A global map of p53 transcription-factor binding sites in the human genome. Cell *124*, 207–219.

Zhang, X., Yazaki, J., Sundaresan, A., Cokus, S., Chan, S.W., Chen, H., Henderson, I.R., Shinn, P., Pellegrini, M., Jacobsen, S.E., et al. (2006). Genome-wide High-Resolution Mapping and Functional Analysis of DNA Methylation in Arabidopsis. Cell *126*, 1189–1201.

Integrating Epigenomic Results

Suk-Young Yoo and R.W. Doerge

Abstract There has been growing interest in investigating epigenetic mechanisms as related to regulation of gene expression. DNA methylation and histone modifications are two types of epigenetic modifications that are highly correlated with regulation of gene expression, genome imprinting and gene silencing. Although epigenomic research has added to our understanding of biological phenomena, little work has been done to establish statistical methods that exploit the relationship between epigenetic modifications and gene expression. Here, we discuss the individual statistical hypotheses for differential expression, methylation and chromatin modification, and then suggest a simple statistical approach that integrates the results from each individual epigenomic experiment.

Keywords Epigenetics · Epigenomics · Methylation · Histone modification · Tiling array · Statistical bioinformatics · ANOVA model · Meta-analysis

1 Introduction

It has become increasingly evident that individuals who have the same DNA develop and react to stimuli, stresses, and diseases differently (Petronis 2006). Sometimes these differences are the result of environment, etc., but there are many situations where diseases (e.g., cancer) are the result of heritable changes in genome function that occur in the absence of changes to the DNA sequence itself. This area of science is referred to as epigenomics, and can be considered as the second-code of instruction that affects gene activity (i.e., regulation) in the absence of altered DNA sequence. With regard to functional genomics, epigenomics may turn out to be the missing link that supplies an explanation for the additional level of variation and regulation that has not been fully appreciated or understood up to this point (Richards 2006). How to design and statistically analyze epigenomic experiments

---

R.W. Doerge (✉)
Department of Statistics, Purdue University, 150 North University Street,
West Lafayette, IN 47907 USA
e-mail: doerge@purdue.edu

and data for the purpose of both understanding this variation and integrating the different levels of epigenomic information remains an open challenge.

Over the years microarray technologies and the experimental data that they produce have stimulated a great deal of interest from the statistics community with respect to normalization, statistical modeling, hypotheses testing, and multiple testing issues when determining statistically significant differential expression. The majority of this interest has been centered specifically on the analysis of gene expression data, with less attention being paid to the statistical issues surrounding the study of epigenomics. Although there are similarities in the statistical models that are used to test for differential gene expression, testing for epigenomic phenomena is quite different since it uses a different type of microarray than traditional cDNA or oligonucleotide microarrays and asks biologically different questions. The application of microarray technology to epigenomics is a good example of when testing the incorrect hypothesis will lead to less informative, if not wrong biological conclusions. Toward this end, the identification of statistically significant epigenomic states will be discussed for the purpose of acknowledging and defining the differences in hypotheses that test for differential expression, methylation and chromatin modification, respectively. The statistical and biological conclusions that follow once the hypotheses are established and tested supply a basis of judgment for the significance of the particular epigenomic result.

Epigenetic status such as DNA methylation and histone modification (i.e., acetylation, phosphorylation, and methylation) play an important role in regulation of gene expression, genome imprinting and gene silencing. For example, histone lysine methylation is associated with transcriptional stimulation or repression. In fact, methylation of lysine 9 and 27 of histone H3 is generally correlated with transcriptional repression and gene silencing, whereas methylation of lysine 4 and 36 of histone H3 is associated with active transcription (Zhang and Reinberg 2001; Kim et al. 2003; Stewart et al. 2005). In humans, epigenetic alternations have been associated with cancer, syndromes relating chromosomal instabilities and mental retardation. For some of these situations DNA methylation suppresses gene activity and abnormal methylation of CpG islands in gene promoter regions is strongly associated with silencing of transcription and inactivation of tumor suppressor genes (Jones and Laird 1999; Jones and Baylin 2002; Herman and Baylin 2003; Baylin 2005). In plants there are similar phenomena where changes in epigenomic states affect gene expression. For instance, cytosine methylation is associated with expression of genes in developing seeds, control of flowering time and floral morphogenesis. Specifically, the Flowering Locus C (FLC), a repressor for flowering, is down regulated under low levels of methylation (Finnegan et al. 2005). DNA methylation has also been associated with silencing of transposable elements in *Arabidopsis* (Lippman et al. 2004). Finally in plants, histone phosphorylation has been associated with the activation of transcription, DNA repair, recombination, and replication (Nelissen et al. 2007) and as such has stimulated an increasing interest in understanding global epigenetic mechanisms associated with regulating gene expression.

To date, assessing changes in gene expression, methylation, and/or chromatin modifications consists of conducting independent experiments using a range of technologies, often microarray technology. Once the data are gained, each experiment (i.e., transcription, methylation or chromatin modification) is typically analyzed separately. Biological connections may be inferred based on the results gained from the individual analyses, but a statistical assessment or analysis that combines the different levels of epigenomic data and/or results is uncommon, if not unheard of. Usually the results, in the form of fold-changes or p-values, from the epigenomic experiments are aligned graphically, and visually correlated by recognizing patterns of say, increased expression with methylation loss, or histone modification(s) (Fig. 1) for specific tiles or regions of the chromosome.

In situations where different microarray technologies (e.g., microarrays and tiling arrays) are employed, the benefits of visual correlation allow these different technologies to lend their results easily to the more general epigenomic conclusions. In situations where the same array, specifically tiling arrays, are employed the same tiles are being assessed for biologically different reasons, yet the generalization of their combined results may be of interest. Relying on an area of statistical specialization known as meta-analysis (Hedges and Olkin 1985) we propose a simple statistical approach that takes advantage of results that are gained from testing the correct epigenomic hypothesis in independent epigenomic experiments. By combining the results from differential expression, methylation, and chromatin immunoprecipitation (ChIP) experiments as gained from the same array technology, statistically significant assessments of epigenomic relationship can be made. The challenge presented by combining results from epigenomic experiments using unique technologies remains an open question and requires an alignment of features between technologies prior to the integration of results.

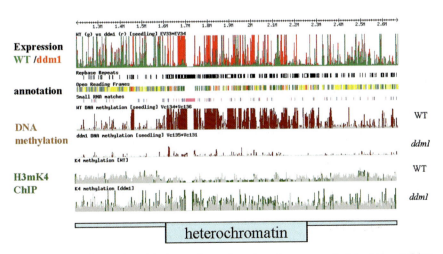

Fig. 1 A genomic illustration of the heterochromatic region, chromosome 4 of *Arabidopsis* (Lippman et al. 2004). The results for two genotypes, wild type (WT) and a mutant known to have decreased DNA methylation (*ddm1*), are reported. Differential expression is illustrated in green (WT) and red (*ddm1*). The genome annotation is followed by statistically significant tiles that are the result of individual analyses of DNA methylation, and H3mK4 ChIP-chip

2 Tiling Arrays and Hypothesis Testing

2.1 Tiling Microarrays

DNA microarray technologies can be used to monitor the simultaneous expression levels for thousands of genes. Using a similar technology, tiling microarrays have become popular for studying whole genomes with high-density probes. A tiling array is composed of sequences of DNA that cover a genomic region, a chromosome, or an entire genome. Tiles, sometimes called probes, include both annotated and unannotated regions of the genome and are systematically placed (tiled) from one end of a genomic region to the another in an unbiased manner (Mockler and Ecker 2005; Royce et al. 2005). Depending on the type of tiling array, tiles may be placed end-to-end or have some overlap or gaps between tiles. Furthermore, some tiles may be repetitive as their sequence represents more than one genomic location. It is important to realize that when used to measure expression, differential analysis is performed on a per-tile basis which is in sharp contrast to the probe-sets that in the past have uniquely identified a gene and are typically used for traditional differential expression studies. Genomic tiling microarrays have been used for exploring a multitude of situations: the human genome (Emanuelsson et al. 2007); differential expression in plants (Yamada et al. 2003; Jiao et al. 2005); the identification DNA methylation (Shi et al. 2003); and chromatin immunoprecipitation of transcription factor-bound genomic DNA (ChIP-Chip) to examine targets of DNA-binding proteins (Buck and Lieb 2004).

2.2 Hypothesis Testing

Analysis of variance models (ANOVA) or linear models (Lippman et al. 2004) have been successfully used to analyze tiling microarray data for a variety of epigenomic situations. The ANOVA model under a common variance assumption (i.e., all tiles have the same level of variation) is:

$$\log(y_{ijkgr}) = \mu + A_i + D_j + T_k + G_g + AG_{ij} + DG_{jg} + TG_{kg} + \epsilon_{ijkgr} \qquad (1)$$

where $i = 1, \ldots, n_a$; $k = 1, 2$; $g = 1, \ldots, n_{ug}$, $r = 1, \ldots n_g$, n_a is number of arrays, n_{ug} is number of unique tiles, and n_g is number of replicates of each tile. Specifically, μ is the grand mean, and A, D, T and G the array, dye, treatment and tile effects, respectively. Moreover, AG, DG and TG are the interactions between array and tile, dye and tile, and treatment and tile, respectively. Without loss of generality, if no dye-labeling of samples occurs, then the dye (D) terms and all corresponding interactions are removed from the model. Finally, the error is denoted ϵ_{ijkgr} and is an independent random variable from a normal distribution with mean 0 and variance σ^2.

2.2.1 Differential Expression

Using a linear model Eq. (1) differential expression for each tile is easily tested. The hypotheses for identifying differentially expressed (i.e., transcription) tiles are:

$$H_0 : T_1 + TG_{1g} = T_2 + TG_{2g} \text{ versus } H_1 : T_1 + TG_{1g} \neq T_2 + TG_{2g} \quad (2)$$

where T and G are the treatment/condition effect and the tile effect, respectively (Black 2002). For situations where the average treatment effects (T_1 and T_2) are not the same, the inclusion of the treatment effect (T) in the hypotheses assures that testing for differential expression using the interaction between the treatment and tile is beyond the average treatment effects. A two-sided t-test is used to test for differential expression, and the multiple testing issue is typically accommodated using a false discovery rate of 0.05 (Benjamini and Hochberg 1995).

2.2.2 Methylation

To identify methylated tiles, consider data from an experiment that allows such comparisons. For example, samples digested with the enzyme McrBC (methylation-dependent restriction enzyme) can be compared with untreated or control samples. In order to test for methylation of each tile the hypotheses, which are different from differential expression (2), need to be formulated. Control tiles are chosen *a priori* based on their native state of no methylation. Any unexpected affect of the treatment/condition beyond the intended methylation status is accommodated by determining the methylation status of tiles relative to the control tiles. Therefore, the hypotheses for identifying methylated tiles are:

$$H_0 : (T_1+TG_{1g})-(T_2+TG_{2g}) = \mu_0 \text{ versus } H_1 : (T_1+TG_{1g})-(T_2+TG_{2g}) > \mu_0 \quad (3)$$

where $\mu_0 = \text{median } \{(T_1 + TG_{1g}) - (T_2 + TG_{2g}), \text{ g control tiles}\}$.

A one-tailed t-test can be employed to test for methylation Eq. (3). In contrast to testing for differential expression using a two-sided test that acknowledges that tiles can remain unchanged, or either up- or down-regulated, methylation is either present or absent (relative to the control tiles). Once all tiles are tested the multiple testing problem is typically accommodated for by using a false discovery rate of 0.05.

2.2.3 Chromatin Immunoprecipitation (ChIP-chip)

ChIP-chip experiments involve samples that are treated and untreated with any one of a variety of antibodies. Similar to testing methylation, the hypotheses for testing chromatin modifications are relative to control tiles. Furthermore, the statistical test for enrichment or depletion of a protein is accomplished with a two-sided t-test, and the false discovery rate controlled at 0.05. Specifically,

$$H_0 : (T_1+TG_{1g})-(T_2+TG_{2g}) = \mu_0 \text{ versus } H_1 : (T_1+TG_{1g})-(T_2+TG_{2g}) \neq \mu_0 \quad (4)$$

where $\mu_0 = $ median $\{(T_1 + TG_{1g}) - (T_2 + TG_{2g}),$ g control tiles$\}$.

When the same tiling array is employed to statistically test and identify statistically significant tiles that are differentially expressed, methylated, or modified the independent results of each hypothesis test Eqs. (2)–(4) are typically represented as p-values or fold-changes. Visual inspection of the results (e.g., expression, methylation, chromatin immunoprecipitation) may indicate correlations, however these correlations or trends of significant results are not supported by any type of formal statistical procedure that integrates the results into a single evaluation of significance. With this in mind, we are motivated to rely on an area of Statistics known as meta-analysis.

3 Meta-Analysis

Like many areas of Statistics, meta-analysis was motivated by applications in agriculture where the goal is to combine evidence from different studies. There are two general and different approaches that one takes when combining evidence across studies. The first approach, and the one that fits an epigenomic application, integrates results from independently tested hypotheses. The second approach focuses on estimating treatment effects across experiments. Because our interests are in integrating results from independently tested hypotheses of expression, methylation and chromatin modification, the latter approach fails to suit the epigenomic application since the estimated treatment effect within each experiment is different and completely incomparable, let alone combinable.

Combining results from independent epigenomic studies is straightforward when each study employs the same array technology. However, this is not to say that using a variety of technologies for each of the expression, methylation and chromatin modification experiments is impossible. One would first need to gain results using a statistical model, hypothesis, and testing, and then align the genes and/or tiles across technologies. Once the alignment is accomplished, then a proper meta-analysis can be implemented since the tests that are involved do not depend on the technology, data themselves, or the statistical distribution of the data. In fact, the only requirement of a meta-analysis that combines results is that the p-values from each individual experimental data analysis are uniformly distributed between zero and one under the respective null hypothesis regardless of the statistical test and/or distribution used to gain the p-values. The relaxed restrictions on testing combined p-values across experiments make them highly flexible and applicable to individual tests that investigate different biological hypotheses.

3.1 Vote Counting

Vote counting is a specific meta-analysis method that allows the results of independent studies to be combined by counting the number of statistically significant positive results or the number of positive results. The vote counting approach requires either knowledge about the sign of mean difference or correlation, or knowledge about whether a hypothesis test yields a statistically significant result. If a large proportion of studies obtain statistically significant results (per tile, in this application) then it can be inferred that the effect is not zero. On the contrary, if few studies achieve statistically significant results then it is difficult to declare that the integrated result has nonzero effect (Gibbons et al. 1977; Hedges and Olkin 1985).

To carry out a vote counting analysis in an epigenomic arena, we assume the technology is the same across experiments and refer to the proportion of significant (per-tile) results as the counting estimator which can be gained from each epigenomic experiment. The experimental design may differ between epigenomic experiments. Specifically, each tile on the array may not be represented equally (e.g., one tile may be represented two times while another tile may be represented four times), and/or the number of arrays may be different across experiments, such that the sample size for each tile may different across results. To accommodate these issues, as well as missing data, the square mean root (SMR) for unequal sample sizes (Gibbons et al. 1977) is recommended

$$n_{SMR} = \left(\frac{\sqrt{n_1} + \cdots + \sqrt{n_k}}{k} \right)^2,$$

where k is number of studies being integrated and n_i the sample size of study i.

In general the null hypothesis in a vote counting analysis is that there is no relationship between the independent variable and the dependent variable for each analysis in a collection of independent analyses. In this context the null hypotheses Eq. (2)–(4) for differential expression, methylation and histone modification are not correlated. The effect size, θ, is the standardized mean difference between two treatments or conditions as specified by the null hypothesis in Eqs. (2)–(4). Let $T_1, \ldots, T_k$ be the estimators or test statistics of parameters $\theta_1, \ldots, \theta_k$ of k experiments as defined by the hypotheses Eqs. (2)–(4). The important feature of the vote counting approach is that test statistics $T_1, \ldots, T_k$ are not observed. However, the number of test statistics for which null hypothesis of each experiment is rejected is observed. Letting U be the number of experiments for which the null hypothesis is rejected, the sample proportion, U/k, is the maximum likelihood estimate of the probability that the null hypothesis of vote counting analysis is rejected, $p(\theta)$. Since $p(\theta)$ is a monotone function of θ, confidence intervals for $p(\theta)$ can be translated to confidence intervals for θ. Using this as the foundation it is possible to test the null hypothesis of a vote counting per tile analysis using a 95% confidence interval based on the proportion of significant results, $\hat{p} = U/k$, using either a normal approximation or a χ^2 distribution. For normal approximation method, if the variance $p(1-p)/k$ is estimated by $\hat{p}(1-\hat{p})/k$ then $100(1-\alpha)$ % confidence interval (p_L, p_U) is given by

$$P_L = \hat{p} - C_{\alpha/2}\sqrt{\hat{p}(1-\hat{p}/k}, \quad P_U = \hat{p} + C_{\alpha/2}\sqrt{\hat{p}(1-\hat{p}/k} \quad (5)$$

where C_α is the two-tailed critical value of the standard normal distribution. Similarly, the chi-square distribution can be used to obtain a confidence interval for $\hat{p}$ by setting $k(\hat{p} - p)/p(1 - p) = C_\alpha$ where C_α is the upper critical value of the chi-square distribution with one degree of freedom. Then $100(1 - \alpha)\%$ confidence interval (p_L, p_U) can be obtained by

$$p_L = \frac{2\hat{p} + b - \sqrt{b^2 + 4b\hat{p}(1-\hat{p})}}{2(1+b)}, \quad p_U = \frac{2\hat{p} + b - \sqrt{b^2 + 4b\hat{p}(1-\hat{p})}}{2(1+b)} \quad (6)$$

where $b = C_\alpha/k = \chi^2_\alpha(1)/k$. Using a table of $p(\theta)$ as a function of θ produced by Hedges and Olkin (1985) a confidence interval for the proportion of significant results from each tile, (p_L, p_U) can be converted to the confidence interval for the effect size of each tile, (θ_L, θ_U), by solving $p(\theta_L) = p_L$, $p(\theta_U) = p_U$. If the confidence interval for an effect size of a specific tile contains zero, then the null hypothesis is not rejected and it is concluded that the tile for which the results were being combined is not statistically significant. In this case, both the normal approximation (5) and the chi-square distribution (6) confidence intervals yield the same results.

4 Application

To demonstrate the utility of a meta-analysis for epigenomic applications, epigenomic data from three different experiments (Lippman et al. 2004) are employed. A tiling array of the short arm of chromosome 4 was used to assess wild type (WT) and homozygous *ddm1* (decrease in DNA methylation 1) *Arabidopsis* plants (Columbia ecotype) for differential expression. Methylation and chromatin modification experiments were also conducted for both WT and *ddm1*. A 1.5Mb region of chromosome 4 was tiled using 1724 unique tiles that were represented two to six times on a tiling array (Lippman et al. 2004). Although the experimental design differed between the expression, methylation, and histone modification experiments, the same tiling array was employed in each study. Due to the varying number of replicate tiles on the array, a total 5748 or 3822 tiles are interrogated for each epigenomic study.

4.1 Differential Expression Experimental Design

The differential expression experiment consisted of two biological samples of both wild type (WT) and *ddm1*. A portion of the experiment was based on a duplicated dye swap experimental design (i.e., 4 arrays) where the first biological sample of WT was labeled with a Cy5 dye and compared to *ddm1* Cy3 labeled sample using a single array. The labels were then switched and a second array was hybridized. Technical samples (i.e., subsamples) of the first biological replicates of WT and *ddm1* were labeled in a similar manner, and provided a second dye swap (i.e., arrays 3 and 4). A single dye swap experiment was used for the second biological sample of both WT and *ddm1*. For two biological samples of WT and *ddm1*, a total of six arrays provided the data for the differential expression study.

4.2 DNA Methylation Experimental Design

Similar to the expression study, a dye swap experimental design was employed for the DNA methylation experiments. In order to detect methylation of CpG dinucleotides, the DNA sample was divided into two equal subsamples. One subsample acted as the control while the other was digested with the methylation-dependent restriction enzyme McrBC. Since the goal is to identify methylated tiles, the McrBC treated sample was compared with total DNA (the untreated sample) for both WT and *ddm1*, respectively. Specifically, McrBC treated and untreated samples of WT (or *ddm1*) were labeled with Cy3 and Cy5 and hybridized on an array. The dyes were switched, and the dye swap completed. The *ddm1* samples were handled the same way. For both WT and *ddm1* two dye swap experiments were completed (i.e., 4 arrays each; Table 1).

Table 1 For each Lippman et al. (2004) study (i.e., expression, DNA methylation, ChIP-chip) the number of arrays, total number of tiles, and number of unique tiles are detailed. For the differential expression tiling array study, wild type (WT) and *ddm1* were hybridized together on the same array. For the DNA methylation and ChIP-chip tiling array experiments, wild type and *ddm1* were treated with McrBC and an antibody (H3mK4), respectively. The treated and untreated samples were hybridized to the tiling array for both wild type and *ddm1*

		Number of arrays	Number of unique tiles	Total number of tiles
Expression	WT/*ddm1*	6	1724	5748
DNA methylation	WT	4	1722	3822
	ddm1	4	1722	3822
H3mK4	WT	4	1724	5748
	ddm1	4	1724	5748

4.3 Chromatin Immunoprecipitation (ChIP) Experimental Design

Chromatin immunoprecipitation (ChIP) is an approach that allows one to investigate interactions between proteins and DNA. When ChIP is combined with DNA microarray (chip) technology, ChIP-chip experiments can be designed to study DNA binding sites for any given protein (Buck and Lieb 2004). The design and analysis of ChIP-chip experiments are similar to those of DNA methylation microarray experiment. For the Lippman et al. (2004) experiment H3 lysine-4 di-methylation (H3mK4) was considered. WT and *ddm1* samples were individually split into subsamples with one subsample of each treated with antibodies to H3mK4. The untreated and treated samples of WT were labeled and hybridized to an array. The dye labels were then switched and a second hybridization conducted. Similarly, untreated and treated samples of *ddm1* were labeled and hybridized to an array using a dye swap design. For H3mK4 four arrays (two biological samples, each dye swapped) for both WT and *ddm1* were employed (Table 1).

4.4 Control Tiles

The unique difference between testing for differential expression and DNA methylation or histone modifications lies in what is being hybridized to the array, and thus what is being compared. In differential expression experiments expression is compared relative to two samples (i.e., WT and *ddm1*) (2). However, in DNA methylation (3) or histone modification (4) experiments the sample (i.e., WT or *ddm1*) is treated as to alter the DNA of the sample. Therefore, in order to compare treated to untreated sample the difference must be relative to something that is either known to be unchanged, or relative to the average of all tiles on the array. In the case of chromosome 4 of *Arabidopsis*, the heterochromatic region of the chromosome is known to be highly methylated, thus the euchromatic region can be employed to represent the average of all tiles across the chromosome. Euchromatin has been defined as lightly staining chromosomal material and generally more easily transcribed, while heterochromatin is deeply staining (Martienssen et al. 2005; Grewal and Jia 2007). Additionally, in many eukaryotes it is known that heterochromatin consists primarily of repetitive DNA sequence such as satellite repeats and transposons, and that these regions are heavily methylated (Lippman et al. 2005). To investigate epigenetic modifications between heterochromatin and euchromatin Lippman et al. (2004) chose 800 control tiles from the euchromatic region which were largely lacking both DNA methylation and histone modifications.

4.5 Data Quality

For the Lippman et al. (2004) data, a background correction was performed by subtracting the background median intensity from the foreground median intensity for both red and green (i.e., Cy5 and Cy3) channels in all three (expression, methylation, and histone modification) analyses. Negative results were set to 1 and the natural log transformation of all background-corrected intensities taken. MA plots (Dudoit et al. 2002) illustrated any dye effect. Specifically, there were no significant patterns found in either the expression MA plots or the methylation tiling array data for *ddm1*. However, for both the WT methylation tiling array data and the ChIP-chip data a significant dye effect was detected. To reduce the dye effect, the data were normalized using a robust local regression (Cleveland and Devlin 1988). After normalization, MA plots were re-checked and the dye effect was reduced substantially.

4.6 Integrating Epigenomic Results

Normalized data from each of the expression, DNA methylation, and histone modification experiments were analyzed using the general linear model Eq. (1) and the respective hypotheses Eqs. (2)–(4) as discussed previously. The results of the individual analyses are reported in Table 2. Recall that differential expression is tested using hypotheses Eq. (2) that compare wild type to *ddm1*, while methylation or histone modification is tested using hypotheses Eqs. (3) or (4) that compare treated (i.e., McrBC or antibodies) with untreated for both wild type and *ddm1* samples.

Using the previously described vote counting meta-analysis, combinations of results from the individual expression, DNA methylation, and histone modification analyses were statistically combined for the purpose of providing an integrated epigenomic assessment of statistically significant tiles. Because there are differences in the experimental design for each experiment (i.e., the number of biological and/or technical replicates) the number of observations for each tile takes one of three values, $n = 50, 24$, or 21 depending on the number of replicates on the array and the number of arrays used in each study. It is important to remember that the results from the differential expression analysis between wild type and *ddm1* contribute to the meta-analyses for both wild type and *ddm1* equally. When employing the vote counting approach to combine three results (expression, methylation and H3mK4), it is necessary to calculate the 95% confidence intervals Eq. (5)–(6). If the proportion of significant results per tile is greater than 0.67 when integrating results from three experiments, then the 95% confidence intervals for effect size (standardized mean difference between two conditions or treatments being compared Eqs. (2)–(4)) do not contain zero and there is a significant relationship between the results that were combined for that tile. The 95% confidence intervals for all experimental settings (i.e., number of tiles on the array, number of experimental results combined, and the confidence interval method) are summarized in Table 3.

Table 2 The number of statistically significant tiles from independent analyses of wild type (WT) and/or *ddm1* genotypes

		Expression	Methylation	H3mK4
Number of significant tiles	WT	785	743	380
	ddm1		152	25

Table 3 Confidence intervals of effect size, θ, for vote counting method meta-analysis using both the normal approximation Eq. (5) and chi-square distribution Eq. (6). The number of observations for each tile is denoted as n in each study, p is the proportion of significant results for a tile, and k is the number of studies integrated

			95% Confidence Intervals for Effect Size	
	p	k	Normal approximation	Chi-square distribution
$n=50$	0.67	3	(0.0740, >1.0)	(0.1644, 0.6720)
$n=24$	0.67	3	(0.1470, >1.4)	(0.2424, 0.9447)
$n=21$	0.67	3	(0.1585, >1.4)	(0.2602, 1.0067)

Table 4 The number of unique statistically significant tiles that resulted from a vote counting analysis of wild type (WT) and *ddm1* expression, DNA methylation, H3mK4 ChIP-chip experiments. The number in parentheses is the number of unique statistically significant tiles from the heterochromatic region of chromosome 4 in *Arabidopsis*

	Integrated results from expression, methylation and H3mK4	
Chromosome 4 Meta-Analysis Data	Number of unique significant tiles	
expression, methylation and H3mK4	WT	*ddm1*
expression, methylation, H3mK4	198 (161)	5 (3)
expression and methylation	217 (128)	77 (49)
Expression and H3mK4	28 (3)	3 (0)
Methylation and H3mK4	125 (94)	10 (8)
Total	568 (386)	95 (60)

Using the number of experiments whose results are combined, along with the confidence intervals of Table 3, the statistically significant tiles that result from the vote counting meta-analysis are reported in Table 4 for both wild type and *ddm1*. In total 568 unique tiles were found to have nonzero effect size (i.e., statistically significant) when significant p-values from WT expression, methylation, and ChIP-chip of H3mK4 experiments were integrated; 386 of these significant tiles are in the heterochromatic region of chromosome 4. On the other hand, for *ddm1* 95 (60 in the heterochromatin) unique tiles were identified as significant in the vote counting meta analysis. More specifically, 198 unique tiles (161 in the heterochromatin) in WT were significantly expressed, methylated and modified with H3mK4. In contrast only 5 unique tiles (3 in the heterochromatin) were significant in all three individual analyses in the *ddm1* genotype which is not surprising since *ddm1* (decreased DNA methylation) has dramatically reduced cytosine methylation

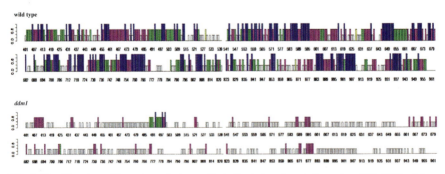

Fig. 2 Significant per-tile meta-analysis results in the heterochromatic region (401–961) of *Arabidopsis* chromosome 4 illustrates that *ddm1* silences via DNA and histone methylation. Integrated results from individual analyses of expression, methylation, H3mK4. *Top*: wild type (WT). *Bottom*: *ddm1*. Blue represents tiles with significant result in all three analyses. Yellow represents tiles with significant results in expression and H3mK4. Pink represents tiles with significant results in expression and methylation. Green represents tiles with significant results in methylation and H3mK4

in DNA. These results also reveal that the majority of tiles that are statistically significantly differentially expressed between WT and *ddm1* are also methylated in both genotypes (i.e., 217 for WT and 77 for *ddm1*). The meta-analysis results from the voting counting analysis of wild type revealed that methylation and H3mK4 were significantly related in many tiles when H3mK4 was combined with significant differential expression and methylation results. Table 4 and Fig. 2 illustrate the results from the described vote counting approach. These results demonstrate the usefulness of meta-analysis in revealing statistically significant per tile results that in turn integrate complex epigenomic activity. Specifically, Fig. 2 illustrates the per tile relationship between differential expression between WT and *ddm1*, and methylation and H3mK4 in heterochromatin region of either wild type or *ddm1*.

5 Discussion

Since it is known that epigenetic modifications such as methylation and histone modifications are related with transcriptional regulation, it is valuable to explore relationships between differential expression and epigenetic modifications. Genome-wide analyses using tiling microarray technology have been used to investigate relationships between methylation and differential expression of *Arabidopsis*. It was shown that enriched methylation was detected in heterochromatin regions and the distribution of methylation was correlated with transcription of genes. By comparing met1 (DNA methyltransferase) mutant plants with wild type plants, the loss of methylation in met1 plants influenced the increased regulation of gene expression in the heterochromatic region which is known to contain massive pseudogenes and transposons (Zhang et al. 2006; Vaughn et al. 2007; Yazaki et al. 2007; Zilberman et al. 2007). As an illustrative example of epigenomic meta-analysis for both wild type and *ddm1* mutants of *Arabidopsis* provided a comparison of the heterochromatic region contained in the short arm of chromosome 4. The status of methylation and H3mK4 was estimated using the tiles in euchromatin as controls. Results from a meta-analysis using the vote counting approach demonstrate consistent results from previous studies. Namely, that hypermethylation in heterochromatin is associated with repression of gene expression (Figs. 1 and 2). These results indicate a strong connection between depletion of H3mK4 and presence of methylation in heterochromatin of wild type. When compared, the statistically significant vote counting results for the *ddm1* were sufficiently less than that of wild type.

By integrating statistically significant results from individual epigenomic studies, it is possible to statistically investigate how the results are correlated with each other. Meta-analysis has great potential to integrate quantitative estimates from a great number of experiments while accounting for the variation between analyses. Vote counting in particular accumulates significant and null results/effects by counting and thus is not capable of providing a direct pooled estimate of effect size. Although the effect sizes can be approximated, there are restrictions and practice limitations to their use. This aside the disadvantages to vote counting that apply in a general sense are not necessarily negatives in this context since no other approach seems capable of providing similar capabilities.

A vote counting method only requires information pertaining to whether the hypothesis at hand was rejected. It does not incorporate sample size or test statistics into any of its calculations, and it does not provide an effect size estimate. In integrating epigenomic results the standardized mean difference can be used as the effect size, and the test of statistical significance accomplished using the confidence intervals of the effect size. However, it is worth noting that in the most general applications of meta-analysis, the results that are combined are from several similar experiments and can be combined to conclude an overall decision. For example, different laboratories may conduct gene expression profiling experiments to test for differential expression of genes in a specific tissue type. Through the application of meta-analysis there is more power for detecting significantly differentially expressed genes by integrating the results across laboratories since the sources of variation, which include laboratory, can be included in the analysis.

While meta-analysis is an approach that integrates statistically significant results from different studies, integrating epigenomic information itself into tests of differential expression is an approach that may have promise. Recently, statistical methods that exploit the linear order of tiles across the genome have made good strides in improving the power of detecting significant tiles for individual analyses of expression, methylation and histone modifications. Li et al. (2006) applied a hidden Markov model (HMM) for analyzing ChIP-chip tiling arrays, and Ji and Wong (2005) combined a hierarchical empirical bayes model with a moving average method, or hidden Markov model (HMM), to merge information from neighboring tiles. Moreover, Johnson et al. (2006) proposed a model-based analysis of tiling array (MAT) data which considers characteristics of ChIP-chip data and Park et al. (2007) suggested error pooling based statistical methods to shrink error estimates and to provide better statistical power for testing hypotheses.

In tiling arrays the tiles typically are overlapped, or in linear order, such that information from adjacent tiles can be used in the hypotheses when results from expression, methylation, and chromatin modification are combined. Yoo (2008) has developed an approach that employs information from neighboring tiles to estimate more accurate relationships between differential expression and epigenetic modifications. Specifically, a two-stage analysis that employs HMMs and linear models combines data and results from both methylation tiling and expression tiling arrays. In the first stage, the methylation status of each tile is estimated using a hidden Markov model and in the second stage a linear model analysis is conducted to test for per-tile expression differences for the purpose of identifying significantly differentially expressed tiles given the state of methylation in the samples that are tested for differential expression. There are benefits to using a hidden Markov model since both biological and technical variation from the estimated methylation status can be adjusted, and information from neighboring tiles utilized. Once the HHM step is complete, differential expression is evaluated between two samples by fitting a linear model that incorporates results from the first stage while testing for differential expression. Simulation studies provided by Yoo (2008) demonstrate that integrating results from the first stage (i.e., methylation) into the second stage analysis of differential expression give rise to more precise estimates of per-tile differential expression.

Epigenomic research is providing exciting information about the complex landscape of genomes. The majority of epigenomic investigations are not in isolation and entail the integration of multiple levels (e.g., expression, methylation, chromatin modifications) of genome information using cutting edge technologies that provide vast multidimensional datasets. Because both the data and the hypotheses that are tested are completely different in their biological focus, yet correlated in their endpoint, it is not possible to combine the actual epigenomic data into a single statistical or mathematical analysis for the purpose of providing clues as to how gene expression is affected by methylation and/or histone modifications. Therefore, integrating the results from individual statistical analyses of the different layers of epigenomic phenomena provides a useful statistically sound means for accumulating all epigenomic knowledge at a particular tile, gene, or region of the genome. Although this particular introduction integrated only three studies, one can imagine taking a large number of results from many laboratories and integrating the results across the genome to surmise statistically significant regions of the epigenomic landscape.

Acknowledgments We thank Professor Rob Martienssen and his laboratory at Cold Spring Harbor Laboratory for providing the *Arabidopsis* data, and many appreciated discussions. This work was funded in part by a National Science Foundation Grant (0501712) to RWD, and Purdue University Bilsland Fellowship to S-Y Yoo.

References

Baylin, S. B., 2005. DNA methylation and gene silencing in cancer. Nature Clinical Practice Oncology 2:s4–s11.
Benjamini, Y. and Hochberg Y., 1995. Controlling the false discovery rate: a practical and powerful approach to multiple testing. Journal of the Royal Statistical Society, Series B 57:289–300.
Black, M. A., 2002. Statistical issues in the design and analysis of spotted microarray experiments. Ph.D. Thesis, Department of Statistics, Purdue University, West Lafayette, IN, USA.
Buck, M. J. and Lieb, J. D., 2004. ChIP-chip: consideration for the design, analysis, and application of genome-wide chromatin immunoprecipitation experiments. Genomics 83:349–360.
Cleveland, W. S. and Devlin, S. J., 1988. Locally-Weighted Fitting: An Approach to Fitting Analysis by Local Fitting . Journal of the American Statistical Association, 83:596–610.
Dudoit, S., Yang, Y. H., Speed, T. P. and Callow, M. J., 2002. Statistical methods for identifying differentially expressed genes in replicated cDNA microarray experiments. Statistica Sinica 12(1): 111–139.
Emanuelsson, O., Nagalakshmi, U., Zheng D., Rozowsky, J. S., Urban, A. E., Du, J., Lian, Z., Stolc, V., Weissman, S., Snyder, M. and Gerstein, M. B., 2007. Assessing the performance of different high-density tiling microarray strategies for mapping transcribed regions of the human genome. Genome Research 17:886–897.
Finnegan, J.E., Kovac, K.A., Jaligot, E., Sheldon, C.C., Peacock, W.J. and Dennis, E.S., 2005. The downregulation of FLOWERING LOCUS C (FLC) expression in plants with low levels of DNA methylation and by vernalization occurs by distinct mechanisms Plant Journal 44(3): 420–432, doi: 10.1111/j.1365-313X.2005.02541.x
Gendrel, A.-V., Lippman, Z., Martienssen, R. and Colot, V., 2005. Profiling histone modification patterns in plants using genomic tiling microarrays. Nature methods 2:213–218.

Gibbons, J. D., Olkin, I. and Sobel, M., 1977. Selecting and ordering populations: a new statistical methodology. New York, Wiley.

Grewal, S. I. S, and Jia, S., 2007 Heterochromatin revisited. Nature Reviews Genetics 8:35–46.

Hedges, L. V. and Olkin, I., 1985. Statistical methods for meta-analysis. New York, Academic Press.

Herman, J. G. and Baylin S. B., 2003. Gene silencing in cancer in association with promoter hypermethylation. The New England Journal of Medicine 349:2042–2054.

Ji, H. and Wong W. H., 2005. TileMap: create chromosomal map of tiling array hybridizations. Bioinformatics 21(18):3629–3636

Jiao, Y., Jia, P., Wang, X., Su, N., Yu, S., Zhang, D., Ma, L., Feng, Q., Jin, Z., Li, L., Xue, Y., Cheng, Z., Zhao, H., Han, B. and Deng, X. W., 2005. A tiling microarray expression analysis of rice chromosome 4 suggests a chromosome-level regulation of transcription. The Plant Cell 17:1641-15-657.

Johnson, W. E., Li, W., Meyer, C. A., Gottardo, R., Carroll, J. S., Brown, M. and Liu, X. S., 2006. Model-based analysis of tiling-arrays for ChIP-chip. PNAS 103(33):12457–12462.

Jones, P. A. and Baylin, S. B., 2002. The fundamental role of epigenetic events in cancer. Nature Review Genetics 3:415–428.

Jones, P. A. and Laird P. W., 1999. Cancer epigenetics comes of age. Nature Genetics 21:163–167.

Kim, J., Jia, L., Tilley, W. D. and Coetzee, G. A., 2003. Dynamic methylation of histone H3 at lysine 4 in transcriptional regulation by the androgen receptor. Nucleic Acids Research 31(23):6741–6747.

Li, W., Meyer, C. A. and Liu, X. S., 2006. A hidden Markov model for analyzing ChIP-chip experiments on genome tiling arrays and its application to p53 binding sequences. Bioinformatics 21(Suppl.1):i274–i282.

Lippman, Z., Gendrel, A-V., Black, M., Vaughn, M. W., Dedhia, N., McCombie, W. R., Lavine, K., Mittal, V., May, B., Kasschau, K. D., Carrington, J. C., Doerge, R. W., Colot, V. and Martienssen, R., 2004. Role of transposable elements in heterochromatin and epigenetic control. Nature 430:471–476.

Lippman, Z., Gendrel, A.-V., Colot, V. and Martienssen, R., 2005. Profiling DNA methylation patterns using genomic tiling microarrays. Nature Methods 2:219–224.

Martienssen, R. A., Doerge, R. W. and Colot, V., 2005. Epigenomic mapping in *Arabidopsis* using tiling microarrays. Chromosome Research 13:299–308.

Mockler, T. C. and Ecker, J. R., 2005. Applications of DNA tiling arrays for whole-genome analysis. Genomics 85(1):1–15.

Nelissen, H., Boccardi, T., Himanen, K., Van Lijsebettens, M., 2007. Impact of core histone modifications on transcriptional regulation and plant growth. Crit Rev Plant Sci 26: 243–263.

Park, T., Kim, Y., Bekiranov, S., and Lee, J. K., 2007. Error-pooling-based statistical methods for identifying novel temporal replications profiles of human chromosomes observed by DNA tiling arrays. Nucleic Acids Research 35(9) e69.

Petronis, A., 2006. Epigenetics and twins: three variations on the theme. Trends in Genetics 22(7):347–350.

Richards, E.J., 2006. Inherited epigenetic variation -revisiting soft inheritance. Nature Genetics Reviews 7:395–401.

Royce, T. E., Rozowsky, J. S., Bertone, P., Samanta, M., Stolc, V., Weissman, S., Snyder, M. and Gerstein, M., 2005. Issues in the analysis of oligonucleotide tiling microarrays for transcript mapping. Trend in Genetics 21(8):466–475.

Shi, H., Maier, S., Nimmrich, I., Yan, P. S., Caldwell, C. W., Olek, A. and Huang, T. H-M, 2003. Oligonucleotide-based microarray for DNA methylation analysis: principles and applications. Journal of Cellular Biochemistry 88:138–143.

Stewart, M. D., Li, J. and Wong, J., 2005. Relationship between histone H3 lysine 9 methylation, transcription repression and heterochromatin protein 1 recruitment. Molecular and Cellular Biology 25(7):2525–2538.

Vaughn, M., Tanurdzic, M., Lippman, Z., Jiang, H., Carrasquillo, R., Colot, V., Doerge, R.W., and Martienssen, R.A. 2007. Epigenetic natural variation in *Arabidopsis* thaliana. Public Library of Science (PLoS) Biology. 5(7): e174.

Yamada, K. et al. Empirical analysis of transcriptional activity in the *Arabidopsis* genome. Science 302:842 (2003).

Yazaki, J., Gregory, B. D., and Ecker, J. R., 2007 Mapping the genome landscape using tiling array technology. Current Opinion in Plant Biology 10:534–542.

Yoo, S-Y. 2008. A two-stage statistical approach for integrating epigenomic results with gene expression data using tiling array technology. Ph.D. Dissertation. Purdue University. West Lafayette, IN, USA.

Zhang, Y. and Reinberg D., 2001. Transcription regulation by histone methylation: interplay between different covalent modifications of the core histone tails. Genes & Development. 15:2343–2360.

Zhang, X., Yazaki, J., Sundaresan, A., Cokus, S., Chan, S. W.-L., Chen, H., Henderson, I. R., Shinn, P., Pellegrini, M., Jacobsen, S. E., and Ecker, J. R., 2006 Genome-wide high-resolution mapping and functional analysis of DNA methylation in *Arabidopsis*. Cell 126:1189–1201.

Zilberman, D., Gehring, M., Robert, T. K., Ballinger, T. and Henikoff, S., 2007 Genome-wide analysis of *Arabidopsis* thaliana DNA methylation uncover an interdependence between methylation and transcription. Nature Genetics 39(1):61–69.

Visualising the Epigenome

Paul Flicek and Ewan Birney

Abstract The epigenome describes the collection of chromatin modifications that are stable through cell division and are apparently indicative of cell type. Epigenetic features include DNA methylation, histone modifications, and other aspects of chromatin organisation. Genome browsers were developed as part of the human genome project to visualise and organise genomic data and analysis using the common index of the genome sequence. These browsers and other tools are now being expanded to support the growing collection of epigenomic data. Ideally viewing data in genome browsers allows researchers to better understand their own data, draw new scientific conclusions, and present their data to others in a visually appealing and intuitive way.

Keywords Genome browser · Data visualisation

1 Introduction

The sequencing of the human genome, in parallel with dramatic increases in computer power and the expansion of the World Wide Web, led to an explosion of interactive bioinformatics applications. Among the most widely used of these applications are general-purpose genome browsers such as Ensembl (Flicek et al. 2008), the UCSC Genome Browser (Kuhn et al. 2007) and Map Viewer at NCBI (Wheeler et al. 2007). Each of these applications represents an integrated mechanism for researchers to interact with the very large genomic data sets created first by the human (International Human Genome Sequencing Consortium 2001, Venter et al. 2001) and mouse (Mouse Genome Sequencing Consortium 2002) genome projects. Today genome browsers include many different data types in an effort to provide a comprehensive and integrated resource for biomedical researchers. Data types include mammalian genome sequences from platypus to macaque,

P. Flicek (✉)
European Bioinformatics Institute, Wellcome Trust Genome Campus, Hinxton, Cambridge, CB10 1SD
e-mail: flicek@ebi.ac.uk

gene expression atlases (Lein et al. 2007), extensive resequencing (Cunningham et al. 2006) and phenotype data (Giardine et al. 2007), haplotype maps (International HapMap Consortium 2005), and functional and epigenetic data from projects such as ENCODE (ENCODE Project Consortium 2007). In each case, genome browsers provide both data organised in such a way as to facilitate the use of the data in other analysis and a visualisation of the data in a way that, ideally, helps researchers better understand their data and present their results.

All of the major on-line integrated genome browsers, as well as deployable genome browser applications such as gBrowse (Stein et al. 2002), take advantage of the linear nature of the DNA sequence to create an interface based on either a vertical or horizontal axis with the DNA sequence serving as an index on which other annotated genomic features such as genes, repeats, or regulatory regions are placed (See Fig. 1). Such an interface is both flexible and scalable as most genome features, such as genes, can themselves be represented by linear annotations with defined positions in the genome. This characteristic makes their display on a linear genome browser both sensible and conceptually easy to understand. Moreover the linear nature of the display makes it possible to assess data and draw conclusions, such as the genomic positions of certain histone modifications (Koch et al. 2007, Mikkelsen et al. 2007), even before rigorous statistical analysis of the data.

Epigenetic data, while often linear, is conceptually different than genes, SNPs, or most other data types displayed by genome browsers. Epigenetic data has several extra dimensions that make display of the data a challenge. These extra dimensions include tissue specific epigenetic marks (Imamura et al. 2001), effects of the environment on the epigenome (Whitelaw and Whitelaw 2006) and the analogue nature of epigenetic marks.

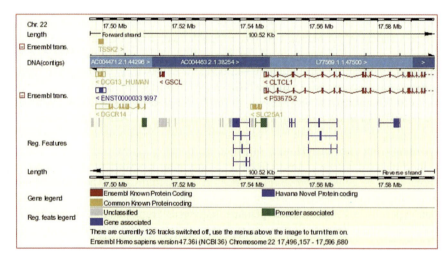

Fig. 1 A view of the genome from the Ensembl genome browser showing genes and regulatory regions from a section of chromosome 22. Genes are displayed on both the forward and reverse strand and are identified by specific transcript names

As an example of how the nature of the epigenome differs from traditional genome annotation and visualisation, consider the difference between identifying the exon-intron structure of a given protein coding gene and identifying a differentially methylated region upstream of that gene. The gene structure, encoded in the DNA sequence, is consistent across all tissue types and in all environmental conditions and can often be correctly annotated with expressed sequence data (such as a cDNA) from only one tissue. (We will ignore the complication of alternatively spliced isoforms and tissue specific gene expression levels). A differentially methylated region is a relative measurement that requires comparing the assay results from many different tissue types and requires the determination of the average DNA methylation rate at the possible sites of methylation across the assayed sample.

In the rest of this chapter, we will discuss how the specific characteristics of high-throughput epigenome mapping techniques help to determine the visualisation decisions for the data, describe several methods for viewing epigenetic data at scales from individual base pairs to the entire genome, present ways to visually link epigenetic and genetic data, and finally identify future ways to create and organise comprehensive views of the active epigenome.

2 Experimentally Mapping the Epigenome

The epigenome is the biological mechanism that establishes and maintains heritable chromosomal conformations, gene expression patterns, and other tissue specific genome functions without a change to the DNA sequence. We will concentrate on two major recognised epigenetic phenomena: DNA methylation and histone modifications. DNA methylation, always of cytosine and normally at CpG dinucleotides, has the largest known effect at CpG island promoter regions that are apparently unmethylated in the germ line and where methylation results in the inactivation of the promoter. Histone modifications include the methylation, acetylation, and other observed and possible post-translational modifications to the histone protein tails. These modifications have been shown to be associated with gene expression, regions of heterochromatin, and other features of the genome such as transcription start sites and repeats. For a more in-depth review see Bernstein et al. (2007) and references therein.

Recent technological advances have made unbiased mapping of the epigenome experimentally feasible. These include the development of whole genome tiling microarrays for use with chromatin immunoprecipitation (ChIP-chip) experiments for producing genome-wide maps of histone modifications and DNA protein interactions (Horak and Snyder 2002, Buck and Lieb 2004, Kim et al. 2007) and ChIP-seq, a related technique that uses high-throughput sequencing technologies rather than tiling microarrays to identify the genomic location of a given histone modification isolated by ChIP (Mikkelsen et al. 2007, Barski et al. 2007). Similar developments have occurred in the area of DNA methylation mapping with techniques such as meDIP (Weber et al. 2005) isolation of methylated DNA, which can then be assessed using microarrays (Rakyan et al. 2008) or sequencing (Down et al. 2008) (See also Chapter "Strategies for Epigenome Analysis").

From a data analysis point of view, these techniques reduce the computational problem of epigenome mapping to one of determining enrichments on arrays (Johnson et al. 2006) or of counting DNA sequences (Johnson et al. 2007). For the near future it seems nearly certain that mapping with high-throughput sequencing technologies will be the dominant experimental technique. Visualisation techniques are needed to display both existing and new experimental data in their appropriate genomics context.

Even with all of the advances in technologies, from a visualisation point of the view the epigenome is an analogue signal rather than a digital one. That is, instead of the digital value of the DNA sequence at the same location in the genome (either A, C, G or T), the epigenome at the same location will be the result of a counting experiment and may need to be compared in a relative way to other regions of the genome. The use of thresholds will allow the creation, for example, of genome-wide maps of DNA methylation or histone modifications, but the information in the relative modification levels between areas of the genome will be important for truly understanding the relationship between the genome and the epigenome. Moreover, even if or when technology allows for the measurement of the epigenome of a single cell, the information will have to be considered in the context of the tissue average. Put more simply, if the epigenome of each of the approximately 75 trillion cells in a human individual could be measured, it would be impossible to display this data except in an aggregate, averaged form.

There is potentially a difference between visualising the epigenome and visualising the experimental assessment of the epigenome. In our current state, with limited genome-wide epigenetic data, the best visualisation tool for discovery is probably a display relatively close to the experimental data itself. However, displays using many graphical elements including colour, lines, shapes, and plots to summarise the various and disparate data types must be the way forward for the multitude of data in the future.

3 Visualising the Epigenome

The focused nature of DNA methylation means that most of the experimental assays of methylated DNA have been focused at CpG islands (Eckhardt et al. 2006) and thus specialised visualisation systems were designed to both identify the assayed regions and, in those regions, provide base pair resolution. One of these methods is the MVP ("methylation variable position") viewer (Rakyan et al. 2004) shown in Fig. 2. The MVP viewer displays DNA methylation data collected using traditional Sanger-style sequencing of specific amplicons after bisulphite conversion (Olek et al. 1996) with coverage over a limited portion of the genome. Figure 2A of the MVP viewer shows the location of the sequenced amplicons in the context of SYNGAP1 gene. Exact base pair level data are also available for each of the assayed CpGs though the MVP viewer (Fig. 2B).

Visualising the Epigenome 59

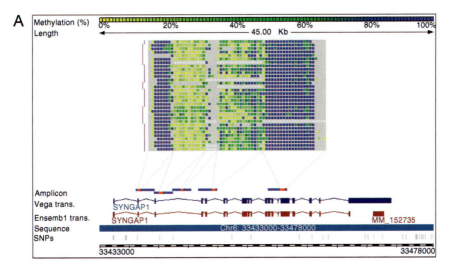

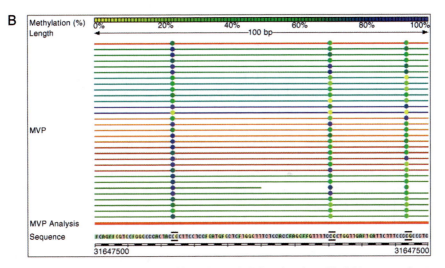

Fig. 2 (**A**) Region and base pair specific DNA methylation data from bisulphite sequencing as visualised by the MVP viewer, which identifies assayed regions of the genome in the context of important genomic features including genes and SNPs. (**B**) A zoomed in view from the MVP viewer showing DNA methylation at base pair level resolution. (from Vakyan et al. 2004. DOI: 10.1371/journal.pbio.0020405.g003)

As described above, experimental technology for DNA methylation detection has evolved to use genome wide microarrays in conjunction with techniques that are able to isolate DNA regions that are methylated such as meDIP (Weber et al. 2005). The DNA, once isolated, can be mapped to the genome using whole-genome tiling microarrays or high throughput DNA sequencing methods. Genome-wide methylation patterns developed from meDIP or similar techniques mean reduced requirements for visually identifying which chromosomes have data or which specific regions within those chromosomes have data; we can expect the data to appear all across the genome, especially in regions with genes and in regions immediately upstream of genes (i.e. where CpG islands are most likely to occur).

Using meDIP data from 16 human cell and tissue types, we have recently developed an integrated resource for analysis and visualisation of DNA methylation profiles (Rakyan et al. 2008). The visualisation component of this resource is built into the Ensembl genome browser (see Fig. 3). Following the colour scheme of the MVP viewer, Ensembl displays array-based DNA methylation values determined with the BATMAN algorithm (Down et al. 2008), the analysis component of the integrated resource. Briefly, BATMAN performs a Bayesian deconvolution of the enrichment signal on the meDIP arrays and the neighbourhood CpG density in a window around a specific probe on the microarray, which is able to estimate the absolute methylation level of the CpG dinucleotides for each probe. The visualisation infrastructure is designed to work flexibly with data either incorporated into the Ensembl databases or with data available external to the Ensembl genome browser using the DAS protocol (Dowell et al. 2001). Data available via DAS allows individual researchers to display and share their data in the context of all of the other annotations that are available on the Ensembl genome browser.

The colour-gradient visualisation of both the MVP browser and the Ensembl genome browser provides a way to graphically demonstrate which fraction of the experimental sample is methylated. The colour-gradient display also allows for the rapid visual identification of tissue-specific differentially methylated regions, for example, or regions of the genome where the methylation signal changes across the sequence (see Fig. 3).

Extending the Ensembl-based visualisation to genome-wide meDIP-sequencing data is a straightforward process requiring the generalisation of the probe-windowing concept described above to an arbitrary window size on the genome. These generalisations are built into the infrastructure of the BATMAN algorithm and the Ensembl displays.

Like DNA methylation, histone modifications are generally represented by visual displays based on the experimental data itself. These types of displays feature real-valued data, plotted vertically, indexed on the genome sequence, and commonly know as a "wiggle track" following the name introduced by the UCSC Genome Browser (Karolchik et al. 2003). Wiggle track visualisation is now available on all of the major genome browsers (see top-most track on Fig. 3) and in a number of popular stand-alone applications such as SignalMap (NimbleGen, Inc. Madison, USA). The ability to a continuous epigenetic signal across potentially large regions of the genome in the context of all of the other data types available on the major genome browsers (such as genes, evolutionary conservation, etc.) makes the wiggle track data visualisation particularly effective for quickly assessing and understanding the data.

However, almost every display of any size on the genome will have more data points than pixels on the screen. This mismatch between data density and pixel density can reach extreme situations when viewing an entire chromosome at once.

Visualising the Epigenome

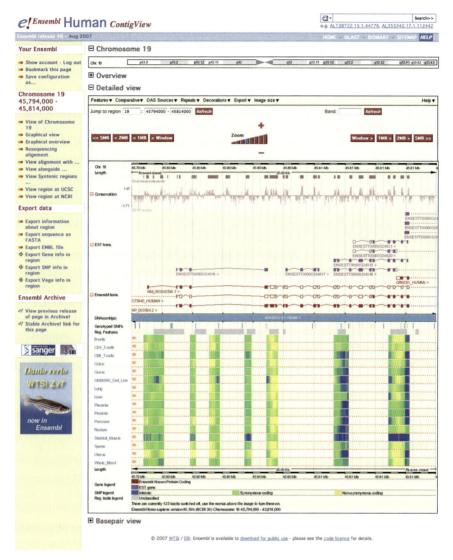

Fig. 3 A screen shot from the Ensembl genome browser showing a region of chromosome 19 including the integrated colour gradient display for DNA methylation assayed by meDIP and analysed by BATMAN. In this image, a tissue-specific differentially methylated region (tDMR) can be observed on the right hand side of the display in the skeletal muscle sample

Addressing the mismatch between data density and pixel density to produce visually useful displays for research discovery and data visualisation is one of the key challenges for genome browsers attempting to visualise the epigenome. To address this, most wiggle track implementations use variations on a procedure that selects the most significant value rather than taking the average of multiple values when displaying overlapping data points. This is an effective method to deal with the mismatch in data density and pixel size because this type of overlap function preserves the contrast between the highest and lowest values in the data making signal peaks (i.e. locations of histone modifications) visible even at high zoom levels such as visualisations covering tens of megabases.

One complication for the visualisation of continuous epigenetic data across regions of the genome is the observation that distinct functional domains occur across the genome at scales larger than the size of genes (ENCODE Project Consortium). These have been classified as regions of active and repressed chromatin using a variety of epigenetic data types (Thurman et al. 2007). Other studies have observed that many epigenetic features have distinctive genomic spans, for example Mikkelsen et al. reported that both focused and widespread histone modification are associated with active genes; specifically H3K4me3 focused at the transcription starts site and H3K36me3 present over the entire transcribed region (Mikkelsen et al. 2007).

As a part of functional domain classification described above, Thurman et al. introduced a wavelet transformation as robust analysis method to process the experimental results prior to using them as input into a hidden Markov model of genome organisation. (Thurman et al. 2007). Wavelets provide for a consistent mathematical description of data types that are correlated on many different scales and the wavelet images display these correlations in the data at many length scales simultaneously. Thus, wavelet images may become valuable tools for visually understanding large scale epigenetic organisation and potentially provide new insights into structure of the epigenome.

4 Future Directions

As more epigenetic data is produced through projects such as the NIH Roadmap Epigenomic Program, the tools to visualise the epigenome will also have to evolve. Improvements in epigenome visualisation will no doubt proceed in tandem with both discoveries made in epigenetics and new methods for epigenetic data analysis. These discoveries will point to effective ways to create visual summaries from extensive supporting data. To use an example from comparative genomics, multispecies alignments incorporating dozens of component genome sequences are now commonly distilled into summary statistics at nearly base pair resolution with analysis programs such as GERP (Cooper et al. 2005) or PhastCons (Miller et al. 2007), which allow for both compact and intuitive display of a large amount of data. For the epigenome, available experimental data and discoveries will help design specialised displays both in dedicated visualisation tools and in specially designed views in major genome browsers. For example, analogous displays to Ensembl's GeneView pages may be produced for imprinted regions or other centers of epigenetic regulatory control. These may include visualisation tools for a variety of epigenetic data types and resolutions.

A second probable future development in epigenome visualisation is analysis tools capable of identifying and displaying data with dynamic resolution, so that the pictures created always provide the most informative way to display the data no matter what window size or resolution is selected. For example, image displays may be precalculated at several resolutions or (like wavelets) exist natively at all resolutions. Such an algorithm could determine the optimal resolution by, for example, information content and then choose the display automatically so that each region of the genome has the most useful epigenome visualisation. In a sense this is the next generation of wiggle track displays.

The ability to understand the epigenome requires effective tools to transform assays of the epigenetic state into visualisations that allow researchers to present their data in a way that illustrates their conclusions and drives future hypotheses. As the genome is the foundation for the epigenome, our current genome-focused displays provide a strong base for expanding and incorporating a view on the epigenome.

References

Barski A, Cuddapah S, Cui K, Roh TY, Schones DE, Wang Z, Wei G, Chepelev I, Zhao K: High-resolution profiling of histone methylations in the human genome. *Cell* 2007, **129**:823–837.

Bernstein BE, Meissner A, Lander ES: The mammalian epigenome. *Cell* 2007, **128**:669–681.

Buck MJ, Lieb JD: ChIP-chip: considerations for the design, analysis, and application of genome-wide chromatin immunoprecipitation experiments. *Genomics* 2004, **83**:349–360.

Cooper GM, Stone EA, Asimenos G, NISC Comparative Sequencing Program, Green ED, Batzoglou S, Sidow A: Distribution and intensity of constraint in mammalian genomic sequence. *Genome Res* 2005, **15**:901–913.

Cunningham F, Rios D, Griffiths M, Smith J, Ning Z, Cox T, Flicek P, Marin-Garcin P, Herrero J, Rogers J, van der Weyden L, Bradley A, Birney E, Adams DJ: TranscriptSNPView: a genome-wide catalog of mouse coding variation. *Nat Genet* 2006, **38**:853.

Dowell RD, Jokerst RM, Day A, Eddy SR, Stein L: The distributed annotation system. *BMC Bioinformatics* 2001, **2**:7.

Down TA, Rakyan VK, Turner DJ, Flicek P, Li H, Kulesha E, Gräf S, Johnson N, Herrero J, Tomazou EM, Thorne NP, Bäckdahl L, Herberth M, Howe KL, Jackson DK, Miretti MM, Marioni JC, Birney E, Hubbard TJP, Durbin R, Tavaré S, Beck S. 2008. A Bayesian deconvolution strategy for immunoprecipitation-based DNA methylome analysis. *Nat Biotechnol.* 2008 Jul, **26**(7): 779–85.

Eckhardt F, Lewin J, Cortese R, Rakyan VK, Attwood J, Burger M, Burton J, Cox TV, Davies R, Down TA, Haefliger C, Horton R, Howe K, Jackson DK, Kunde J, Koenig C, Liddle J, Niblett D, Otto T, Pettett R, Seemann S, Thompson C, West T, Rogers J, Olek A, Berlin K, Beck S: DNA methylation profiling of human chromosomes 6, 20 and 22. *Nat Genet* 2006, **38**:1378–1385.

ENCODE Project Consortium: Identification and analysis of functional elements in 1% of the human genome by the ENCODE pilot project. *Nature* 2007, **447**:799–816.

Flicek P, Aken BL, Beal K, Ballester B, Caccamo M, Chen Y, Clarke L, Coates G, Cunningham F, Cutts T, Down T, Dyer SC, Eyre T, Fitzgerald S, Fernandez-Banet J, Gräf S, Haider S, Hammond M, Holland R, Howe KL, Howe K, Johnson N, Jenkinson A, Kähäri A, Keefe D, Kokocinski F, Kulesha E, Lawson D, Longden I, Megy K, Meidl P, Overduin B, Parker A, Pritchard B, Prlic A, Rice S, Rios D, Schuster M, Sealy I, Slater G, Smedley D, Spudich G, Trevanion S, Vilella AJ, Vogel J, White S, Wood M, Birney E, Cox T, Curwen V, Durbin R,

Fernandez-Suarez XM, Herrero J, Hubbard TJ, Kasprzyk A, Proctor G, Smith J, Ureta-Vidal A, Searle S. 2008. Ensembl 2008. *Nucleic Acids Res.* 2008, **36**(Database issue): D707-14.

Giardine B, Riemer C, Hefferon T, Thomas D, Hsu F, Zielenski J, Sang Y, Elnitski L, Cutting G, Trumbower H, Kern A, Kuhn R, Patrinos GP, Hughes J, Higgs D, Chui D, Scriver C, Phommarinh M, Patnaik SK, Blumenfeld O, Gottlieb B, Vihinen M, Väliaho J, Kent J, Miller W, Hardison RC: PhenCode: connecting ENCODE data with mutations and phenotype. *Hum Mutat* 2007, **28**:554–562.

Horak CE, Snyder M: ChIP-chip: a genomic approach for identifying transcription factor binding sites. *Methods Enzymol* 2002, **350**:469–483.

Imamura T, Ohgane J, Ito S, Ogawa T, Hattori N, Tanaka S, Shiota K: CpG island of rat sphingosine kinase-1 gene: tissue-dependent DNA methylation status and multiple alternative first exons. *Genomics* 2001, **76**:117–125.

International HapMap Consortium: A haplotype map of the human genome. *Nature* 2005, **437**:1299–1320.

International Human Genome Sequencing Consortium: Initial sequencing and analysis of the human genome. *Nature* 2001, **409**:860–921.

Johnson DS, Mortazavi A, Myers RM, Wold B: Genome-wide mapping of in vivo protein-DNA interactions. *Science* 2007, **316**:1497–1502.

Johnson WE, Li W, Meyer CA, Gottardo R, Carroll JS, Brown M, Liu XS: Model-based analysis of tiling-arrays for ChIP-chip. *Proc Natl Acad Sci U S A* 2006, **103**:12457–12462.

Karolchik D, Baertsch R, Diekhans M, Furey TS, Hinrichs A, Lu YT, Roskin KM, Schwartz M, Sugnet CW, Thomas DJ, Weber RJ, Haussler D, Kent WJ, University of California Santa Cruz: The UCSC Genome Browser Database. *Nucleic Acids Res* 2003, **31**:51–54.

Kim TH, Abdullaev ZK, Smith AD, Ching KA, Loukinov DI, Green RD, Zhang MQ, Lobanenkov VV, Ren B: Analysis of the vertebrate insulator protein CTCF-binding sites in the human genome. *Cell* 2007, **128**:1231–1245.

Koch CM, Andrews RM, Flicek P, Dillon SC, Karaöz U, Clelland GK, Wilcox S, Beare DM, Fowler JC, Couttet P, James KD, Lefebvre GC, Bruce AW, Dovey OM, Ellis PD, Dhami P, Langford CF, Weng Z, Birney E, Carter NP, Vetrie D, Dunham I: The landscape of histone modifications across 1% of the human genome in five human cell lines. *Genome Res* 2007, **17**:691–707.

Kuhn RM, Karolchik D, Zweig AS, Trumbower H, Thomas DJ, Thakkapallayil A, Sugnet CW, Stanke M, Smith KE, Siepel A, Rosenbloom KR, Rhead B, Raney BJ, Pohl A, Pedersen JS, Hsu F, Hinrichs AS, Harte RA, Diekhans M, Clawson H, Bejerano G, Barber GP, Baertsch R, Haussler D, Kent WJ: The UCSC genome browser database: update 2007. *Nucleic Acids Res* 2007, **35**:D668-D673.

Lein ES, Hawrylycz MJ, Ao N, Ayres M, Bensinger A, Bernard A, Boe AF, Boguski MS, Brockway KS, Byrnes EJ, Chen L, Chen L, Chen TM, Chin MC, Chong J, Crook BE, Czaplinska A, Dang CN, Datta S, Dee NR, Desaki AL, Desta T, Diep E, Dolbeare TA, Donelan MJ, Dong HW, Dougherty JG, Duncan BJ, Ebbert AJ, Eichele G, Estin LK, Faber C, Facer BA, Fields R, Fischer SR, Fliss TP, Frensley C, Gates SN, Glattfelder KJ, Halverson KR, Hart MR, Hohmann JG, Howell MP, Jeung DP, Johnson RA, Karr PT, Kawal R, Kidney JM, Knapik RH, Kuan CL, Lake JH, Laramee AR, Larsen KD, Lau C, Lemon TA, Liang AJ, Liu Y, Luong LT, Michaels J, Morgan JJ, Morgan RJ, Mortrud MT, Mosqueda NF, Ng LL, Ng R, Orta GJ, Overly CC, Pak TH, Parry SE, Pathak SD, Pearson OC, Puchalski RB, Riley ZL, Rockett HR, Rowland SA, Royall JJ, Ruiz MJ, Sarno NR, Schaffnit K, Shapovalova NV, Sivisay T, Slaughterbeck CR, Smith SC, Smith KA, Smith BI, Sodt AJ, Stewart NN, Stumpf KR, Sunkin SM, Sutram M, Tam A, Teemer CD, Thaller C, Thompson CL, Varnam LR, Visel A, Whitlock RM, Wohnoutka PE, Wolkey CK, Wong VY, Wood M, Yaylaoglu MB, Young RC, Youngstrom BL, Yuan XF, Zhang B, Zwingman TA, Jones AR: Genome-wide atlas of gene expression in the adult mouse brain. *Nature* 2007, **445**:168–176.

Mikkelsen TS, Ku M, Jaffe DB, Issac B, Lieberman E, Giannoukos G, Alvarez P, Brockman W, Kim TK, Koche RP, Lee W, Mendenhall E, O"Donovan A, Presser A, Russ C, Xie X, Meissner A, Wernig M, Jaenisch R, Nusbaum C, Lander ES, Bernstein BE: Genome-wide maps of chromatin state in pluripotent and lineage-committed cells. *Nature* 2007, **448**:553–560.

Miller W, Rosenbloom K, Hardison RC, Hou M, Taylor J, Raney B, Burhans R, King DC, Baertsch R, Blankenberg D, Kosakovsky Pond SL, Nekrutenko A, Giardine B, Harris RS, Tyekucheva S, Diekhans M, Pringle TH, Murphy WJ, Lesk A, Weinstock GM, Lindblad-Toh K, Gibbs RA, Lander ES, Siepel A, Haussler D, Kent WJ. 2007. 28-way vertebrate alignment and conservation track in the UCSC Genome Browser. *Genome Res.* 2007 Dec, **17**(12): 1797-808. Epub 2007 Nov 5.

Mouse Genome Sequencing Consortium: Initial sequencing and comparative analysis of the mouse genome. *Nature* 2002, **420**:520–562.

Olek A, Oswald J, Walter J: A modified and improved method for bisulphite based cytosine methylation analysis. *Nucleic Acids Res* 1996, **24**:5064–5066.

Rakyan VK, Down TA, Thorne NP, Flicek P, Kulesha E, Gräf S, Tomazou EM, Bäckdahl L, Johnson N, Herberth M, Howe KL, Jackson DK, Miretti MM, Fiegler H, Marioni JC, Birney E, Hubbard TJ, Carter NP, Tavaré S, Beck S. 2008. An integrated resource for genome-wide identification and analysis of human tissue-specific differentially methylated regions (tDMRs). *Genome Res.* 2008 Sep, **18**(9):1518-29. Epub 2008 Jun 24.

Rakyan VK, Hildmann T, Novik KL, Lewin J, Tost J, Cox AV, Andrews TD, Howe KL, Otto T, Olek A, Fischer J, Gut IG, Berlin K, Beck S: DNA methylation profiling of the human major histocompatibility complex: a pilot study for the human epigenome project. *PLoS Biol* 2004, **2**:e405.

Stein LD, Mungall C, Shu S, Caudy M, Mangone M, Day A, Nickerson E, Stajich JE, Harris TW, Arva A, Lewis S: The generic genome browser: a building block for a model organism system database. *Genome Res* 2002, **12**:1599–1610.

Thurman RE, Day N, Noble WS, Stamatoyannopoulos JA: Identification of higher-order functional domains in the human ENCODE regions. *Genome Res* 2007, **17**:917–927.

Venter JC, Adams MD, Myers EW, Li PW, Mural RJ, Sutton GG, Smith HO, Yandell M, Evans CA, Holt RA, Gocayne JD, Amanatides P, Ballew RM, Huson DH, Wortman JR, Zhang Q, Kodira CD, Zheng XH, Chen L, Skupski M, Subramanian G, Thomas PD, Zhang J, Gabor Miklos GL, Nelson C, Broder S, Clark AG, Nadeau J, McKusick VA, Zinder N, Levine AJ, Roberts RJ, Simon M, Slayman C, Hunkapiller M, Bolanos R, Delcher A, Dew I, Fasulo D, Flanigan M, Florea L, Halpern A, Hannenhalli S, Kravitz S, Levy S, Mobarry C, Reinert K, Remington K, Abu-Threideh J, Beasley E, Biddick K, Bonazzi V, Brandon R, Cargill M, Chandramouliswaran I, Charlab R, Chaturvedi K, Deng Z, Di Francesco V, Dunn P, Eilbeck K, Evangelista C, Gabrielian AE, Gan W, Ge W, Gong F, Gu Z, Guan P, Heiman TJ, Higgins ME, Ji RR, Ke Z, Ketchum KA, Lai Z, Lei Y, Li Z, Li J, Liang Y, Lin X, Lu F, Merkulov GV, Milshina N, Moore HM, Naik AK, Narayan VA, Neelam B, Nusskern D, Rusch DB, Salzberg S, Shao W, Shue B, Sun J, Wang Z, Wang A, Wang X, Wang J, Wei M, Wides R, Xiao C, Yan C, Yao A, Ye J, Zhan M, Zhang W, Zhang H, Zhao Q, Zheng L, Zhong F, Zhong W, Zhu S, Zhao S, Gilbert D, Baumhueter S, Spier G, Carter C, Cravchik A, Woodage T, Ali F, An H, Awe A, Baldwin D, Baden H, Barnstead M, Barrow I, Beeson K, Busam D, Carver A, Center A, Cheng ML, Curry L, Danaher S, Davenport L, Desilets R, Dietz S, Dodson K, Doup L, Ferriera S, Garg N, Gluecksmann A, Hart B, Haynes J, Haynes C, Heiner C, Hladun S, Hostin D, Houck J, Howland T, Ibegwam C, Johnson J, Kalush F, Kline L, Koduru S, Love A, Mann F, May D, McCawley S, McIntosh T, McMullen I, Moy M, Moy L, Murphy B, Nelson K, Pfannkoch C, Pratts E, Puri V, Qureshi H, Reardon M, Rodriguez R, Rogers YH, Romblad D, Ruhfel B, Scott R, Sitter C, Smallwood M, Stewart E, Strong R, Suh E, Thomas R, Tint NN, Tse S, Vech C, Wang G, Wetter J, Williams S, Williams M, Windsor S, Winn-Deen E, Wolfe K, Zaveri J, Zaveri K, Abril JF, Guigó R, Campbell MJ, Sjolander KV, Karlak B, Kejariwal A, Mi H, Lazareva B, Hatton T, Narechania A, Diemer K, Muruganujan A, Guo N, Sato S, Bafna V, Istrail S, Lippert R, Schwartz R, Walenz B, Yooseph S, Allen D, Basu A, Baxendale J, Blick L, Caminha M, Carnes-Stine J, Caulk P, Chiang YH, Coyne M, Dahlke C, Mays A, Dombroski M, Donnelly M, Ely D, Esparham S, Fosler C, Gire H, Glanowski S, Glasser K, Glodek A, Gorokhov M, Graham K, Gropman B, Harris M, Heil J, Henderson S, Hoover J, Jennings D, Jordan C, Jordan J, Kasha J, Kagan L, Kraft C, Levitsky A, Lewis M, Liu X, Lopez J, Ma D, Majoros W, McDaniel J, Murphy S, Newman M, Nguyen T, Nguyen N, Nodell M, Pan S, Peck J, Peterson M, Rowe W, Sanders R, Scott J, Simpson M, Smith T, Sprague A, Stockwell T,

Turner R, Venter E, Wang M, Wen M, Wu D, Wu M, Xia A, Zandieh A, Zhu X: The sequence of the human genome. *Science* 2001, **291**:1304–1351.

Weber M, Davies JJ, Wittig D, Oakeley EJ, Haase M, Lam WL, Schübeler D: Chromosome-wide and promoter-specific analyses identify sites of differential DNA methylation in normal and transformed human cells. *Nat Genet* 2005, **37**:853–862.

Wheeler DL, Barrett T, Benson DA, Bryant SH, Canese K, Chetvernin V, Church DM, DiCuccio M, Edgar R, Federhen S, Geer LY, Kapustin Y, Khovayko O, Landsman D, Lipman DJ, Madden TL, Maglott DR, Ostell J, Miller V, Pruitt KD, Schuler GD, Sequeira E, Sherry ST, Sirotkin K, Souvorov A, Starchenko G, Tatusov RL, Tatusova TA, Wagner L, Yaschenko E: Database resources of the National Center for Biotechnology Information. *Nucleic Acids Res* 2007, **35**:D5–12.

Whitelaw NC, Whitelaw E: How lifetimes shape epigenotype within and across generations. *Hum Mol Genet* 2006, **15 Spec No 2**:R131-R137.

Part II
Roles of DNA, RNA and Chromatin in Epigenomics

Part I

The Expanding View of Cytosine Methylation

J.M. Greally MB PhD

Abstract We are currently in an era of increased interest in the role of the epigenome in normal cellular physiology and its role in human disease. Part of this increased interest is driven by new technologies that have allowed us to gain insights never previously possible. Our view of cytosine methylation is expanding not only in terms of how much of the genome we can study at a time, but also in terms of what we think cytosine methylation might be doing functionally. While DNA methylation in mammalian cells has been studied for more than 45 years at this point (Srinivasan 1962), new insights are revealing the sobering reality that we understand much less about its functional consequences than we may have believed. In this review, the insights gained from new technologies to study cytosine methylation are examined so that we can redefine the paths for further exploration of this intriguing molecular regulator.

Keywords Cytosine methylation · Epigenetic · CpG island · CG di

1 Introduction

The methylation of cytosine is the major recognizable covalent modification of DNA in animals. The cytosines targeted are almost exclusively followed by a guanine in mammalian cells with a small number of cytosines not located at CG dinucleotides also modified (Clark et al. 1995), although not to the extent manifested in plants, where non-CG methylation is found most frequently at CHG or CHH trinucleotides (H = A/C/T) (Cokus et al. 2008). Biochemically, the methyl group is located in the context of double-stranded DNA protruding into the major groove, where DNA-binding proteins normally find their cognate sequence motifs. The methyl group can interfere with the binding of these sequence-specific proteins, but can also act as a ligand for methyl-binding proteins that interact with single (Hendrich and Tweedie 2003) or multiple adjacent (Filion et al. 2006) methylated cytosines.

J.M. Greally (✉)
Einstein Center for Epigenomics, Department of Genetics, Albert Einstein College of Medicine, Bronx, NY USA

Cytosine methylation is one of the ensemble of regulators of gene expression collectively and loosely referred to as epigenomic. Research into the epigenome has tended to divide into that studying the physiology of the epigenome and that focused on epigenomic dysregulation in disease. In addition, when studying epigenomic regulators, there is a tendency of investigators to divide into those specializing in the study of cytosine methylation and those studying chromatin using immunoprecipitation techniques. The assortment within the matrix created tends to be non-random, with disease studies mostly performed with the focus on cytosine methylation, whereas epigenomic physiology has tended to be studied using chromatin immunoprecipitation (ChIP) techniques.

This bias reflects a couple of practical problems. Samples of tissue from subjects with disease tend to be limited in quantity and poorly suited to ChIP, whereas DNA is more readily obtained and stable. Furthermore, the technologies to study the genome-wide distributions of chromatin components enriched using ChIP have advanced more quickly than those for cytosine methylation, allowing genome-wide maps to be created using microarray or massively-parallel sequencing technologies. Cytosine methylation assays, on the other hand, have proven more difficult to scale genome-wide, as will be discussed below.

One outcome of this divergence of emphases has been the relative dearth of information about the physiology of cytosine methylation. While cytosine methylation has been studied for much longer a period of time than histone modifications, we now know more about the latter field in terms of genomic distribution characteristics and changes during differentiation. For example, while we now have chromatin maps in multiple cell types for many histone modifications, DNA-binding proteins and for RNA polymerase II (Bernstein et al. 2006, Heintzman et al. 2007, Mikkelsen et al. 2007, Kim et al. 2007), very few studies have looked genome-wide at cytosine methylation. The analysis of cytosine methylation was a noticeable omission from the otherwise very comprehensive ENCODE project (The ENCODE Project Consortium 2007) designed to determine the function of all nucleotides in 1% of the human genome. As a result, while cytosine methylation as a transcriptional regulator has been studied for a long time (Bird 1986) and the histone code hypothesis is a relatively new idea (Strahl and Allis 2000), the role of histone modifications in processes such as stem cell differentiation is now reasonably well-described (Bernstein et al. 2006) when compared with cytosine methylation studies of similar processes, which remain quite limited. Compounding the relative deficiency is the absence of cytosine methylation in simpler eukaryotes such as yeast, in which very powerful experiments can been performed to define the role of chromatin constituents in the regulation of transcription and other processes.

The functional role of cytosine methylation can be predicted with reasonable certainty in specific situations, for example when a promoter is methylated, which appears to be a good predictor of the silencing of the gene regulated by that promoter (Pfeifer et al. 1990). Unfortunately, the absence of methylation of a promoter does not have the same regulatory predictive capacity, as transcriptionally-inactive genes can have constitutively hypomethylated promoters (Bird et al. 1987, Walsh and Bestor 1999, Weber et al. 2007). Promoter methylation has been sought and found in human disease states, demonstrating inappropriate methylation and silencing of genes as part of neoplastic processes (Feinberg and Tycko 2004) and potentially other diseases (Hatchwell and Greally 2007). In addition, as described previously (Fazzari, and Greally 2004) and below, the vast majority of CG dinucleotides in the genome are not located at promoters, so we have very little idea how to interpret changes in methylation at those sites. As technologies have improved, we are now faced with the recognition that many changes in cytosine methylation take place during differentiation and in disease at these non-promoter sites, challenging us to understand how these changes are related to new properties of the cell. In this review, the role of cytosine methylation in mammalian species is the focus, although it should be appreciated that additional facets of this interesting phenomenon arise when studying its role in plants (Matzke et al. 2006) and fungi (Selker 2004).

2 Advances in Technologies to Study Cytosine Methylation

The new technologies that have created insights into chromatin composition and dynamics have been used to study cytosine methylation also. In the last several years these technologies were based on the use of microarrays, but recently the advent of massively-parallel sequencing technologies has allowed alternative and probably more powerful analytical systems. Genome-wide DNA methylation profiling has been the subject of excellent reviews (Laird 2003, Zilberman et al. 2007) which summarise the current state of the art and describe the many approaches taken to profile the 'methylome' (see also Chapter "Sequencing the Epigenome").

Before considering the specific technologies available at present, it is worth taking into account what we require of the ideal cytosine methylation assay. The assay should test methylation at every individual CG dinucleotide in the genome, quantitatively with reasonable accuracy and sufficiently cost-effectively that multiple samples can be tested. No technology performs all of those functions today. In Table 1 the assays available are presented in three major categories, a genome-wide low resolution approach (Discovery), a local nucleotide-resolution quantitative approach (Comprehensive) and a high sample throughput approach (Population), with examples of each.

The assays can be used in a manner that is complementary – if cytosine methylation is studied using the Discovery approach, loci can be identified that can be targeted for the Comprehensive analyses, allowing validation of the genome-wide approach and identification of specific CG dinucleotides that can be used in Population assays of large numbers of samples.

At present, the Discovery approach is allowing us to gain new insights into the normal physiology of cytosine methylation and its dysregulation in disease. All of these approaches have been published with microarrays reporting the methylation patterns, so the insights gained depend on the design of the microarray used. If the microarray targets CpG islands (Gardiner-Garden and Frommer 1987) in the genome, then information will be restricted to those genomic sequences. Some

Table 1 The three categories of cytosine methylation assays and examples of each. The quantitative ability of the Comprehensive assays represents the gold standard for these studies. Each platform has relative advantages in terms of genomic coverage and sample throughput. The sample throughput figures are approximated by estimating the typical cost for <10 Discovery assays and then calculating how many assays could be performed for the same cost for each of the other categories

	Proportion of genome tested	Number of CG dinucleotides tested	Quantitative ability	Sample throughput per typical experiment	Examples of assays
Discovery	All (unique)	Majority	Poor	<10	HELP (Khulan et al. 2006), mcrBC (Lippman et al. 2005), meDIP (Weber et al. 2005)
Comprehensive	30–600 bp	1–50	Excellent	<100	Pyrosequencing (Dupont et al. 2004), MassArray (Ehrich et al. 2005)
Population	Single nucleotides	1	Good	>>100	MSP (Herman et al. 1996), MethylLight (Trinh 2001), Infinium (Illumina)

studies have looked at promoters (Weber et al. 2007, Hatada et al. 2006, Hoque et al. 2008, Kuang et al. 2008, Schilling and Rehli 2007) or CpG islands (Flanagan et al. 2006, Gebhard et al. 2006) in the genome, with a few studies tiling contiguous sequences within the genome (Khulan et al. 2006, Hayashi et al. 2007, Kerkel et al. 2008), with the result that studies of CG-depleted regions are still uncommon.

Each of the Discovery approaches has inherent limitations. Anything based on restriction enzymes is directly testing only a subset of CGs in the genome, while affinity approaches generate signal based on regional populations of CGs, causing CG density to influence the outcome (Weber et al. 2007, Down et al. 2008) and increasing the analytical burden for subsequent quantitative validation assays. Alleviating these technical concerns is an innate characteristic of cytosine methylation, its tendency to exist in co-ordinate states *in cis* within the genome. Another way of putting this is that the methylation state of one CG tends to predict the methylation of adjacent CGs. When this was tested formally using extensive bisulphite sequencing data, this distance was calculated to be up to 1,000 basepairs in length (Eckhardt et al. 2006). Not only does this allow restriction enzyme approaches to test indirectly a much greater proportion of the genome than at their recognition sites, it also allows a subset of CGs to be tested when validating results of affinity techniques, without having to test all of the CGs in the region. Thus the Discovery assays are all reasonably good in their individual ways at identifying loci for subsequent testing using Comprehensive assays.

Recently, massively-parallel ("next-generation") sequencing has been used to study cytosine methylation. The chapter by Meissner and Bernstein (Chapter "Sequencing the Epigenome") describes this in detail. A relatively simple approach is to use these technologies to perform the assays previously accomplished by cloning and Sanger sequencing, as used in a study of leukaemias and lymphomas (Taylor et al. 2007). In a study testing the biomarker potential of cytosine methylation, a comparison of DNA from breast cancer and free DNA in serum showed complex patterns of cytosine methylation when studied using these sequencing techniques (Korshunova et al. 2008). In each case, PCR was used to generate a limited subset of the genome, allowing much deeper coverage than would be possible with a whole-genome study. Similar enrichment strategies have proven successful using restriction enzymes and Sanger sequencing (Meissner et al. 2005) and more recently with massively-parallel sequencing (Meissner et al. 2008). Such enrichment is not needed when studying smaller genomes, allowing the first comprehensive, nucleotide-resolution studies of cytosine methylation in *Arabidopsis thaliana* (Cokus et al. 2008, Reinders et al. 2008). While massively-parallel sequencing technologies used to study cytosine methylation are accelerating at a rapid rate, at present the cost of these assays is such that enrichment strategies remain practically necessary in larger genomes such as those of mammals.

3 Insights from New Technologies

While technology development continues to gain momentum, we are already beginning to get insights into the epigenome that were not previously possible or were based on extremely limited information. An example is the variability of methylation in different cellular states such as differentiation (see Chapter "The Epigenomic Landscape of Reprogramming in Mammals"). Previously we gained insights into such variability through the restriction landmark genomic scanning (RLGS) technique which assays a limited number of sites that are mostly within CpG islands (Fazzari and Greally 2004). Even these approaches showed tissue-specific methylation (Kremenskoy et al. 2003, Shiota 2004, Song et al. 2005) or changes in cancer (Smith et al. 2007), but the limited sampling involved made it difficult to assess the significance of these changes. Our use of the HELP assay testing HpaII sites showed very extensive changes in methylation in a tissue-specific manner (Khulan et al. 2006), reinforcing the RLGS insights with more extensive sampling of the genome.

In the same study (Khulan et al. 2006), we tested methylation at Hox gene clusters in the mouse genome. In Fig. 1 we show the Hox D domain on chromosome 2. The major finding for this region (and other Hox domains, not shown) is a substantial block of hypomethylated DNA of >100 kb in size extending throughout the Hox gene cluster. This is sufficiently unusual that we refer to it as a 'broad'

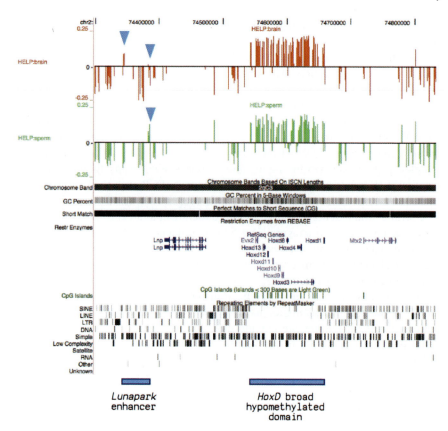

Fig. 1 The data shown were generated as part of a previously published study (Khulan et al. 2006). Hypomethylation is represented by positive (upward) values, methylation by negative (downward) values. Brain (red) and spermatogenic cell (green) cytosine methylation data are represented for the ~536 kb at the *HoxD* gene cluster. Two major findings are evident. Firstly, the *HoxD* gene cluster is diffusely hypomethylated, which we refer to as a 'broad hypomethylated domain'. This lab has also found the same patterns at other *Hox* clusters, isolated homeobox-encoding genes and genes critical for early development (data not shown). The second finding is of the pair of loci manifesting hypomethylation downstream from the *Lunapark* (*Lnp*) gene (blue arrowheads). These loci map within the known enhancer for *HoxD* expression (Spitz et al 2003), suggesting that these non-promoter, non-CpG island, distinctively hypomethylated loci should be considered candidate *cis*-regulators

domain of hypomethylation, in contrast with the more focal patterns we usually see in the genome. Distinctive broad domains of histone modifications (H3K4me) have also been seen for Hox gene clusters (Bernstein et al. 2005), suggesting that these transposon-sparse, highly-conserved and developmentally-critical gene clusters are unusual in terms of their epigenomic organization.

The other finding from data shown in Fig. 1 is non-promoter hypomethylation located 3′ and centromerically to the *Lnp* gene. The two hypomethylated loci are <40 kb apart and map exactly to a *cis*-regulatory enhancer sequence responsible for the *Ulnaless* mutation in mouse (Spitz 2003). It should also be noted that neither of these sites is located at a CpG island, nor do any genomic annotations show any evidence for genes at these sites. This example suggests that non-promoter, non-CpG island hypomethylation can be a means of identifying *cis*-regulatory sites in the genome.

The idea that methylation changes outside promoters or CpG islands can be informative in understanding the dysregulation of the epigenome in disease is substantiated by other genome-wide approaches. The methyl DNA immunoprecipitation (meDIP) technique applied to the study of cancer cells showed CG-depleted regions to be strikingly hypomethylated, manifesting a degree of change greater than those at the CpG islands tested in the same experiment (Weber et al. 2007). RLGS studies of methylation changes in cancer showed marked changes in 3′ UTRs of genes (Smith et al. 2007), while the mcrBC-based MethylScreen assay applied to breast cancer showed one of the most discriminatory loci to be >0.2 Mb from the nearest annotated gene (Ordway et al. 2007).

It remains to be determined whether these intergenic changes in cytosine methylation have functional consequences in terms of gene expression or other outcomes. In order to assess this, we need to understand more about the patterns of cytosine methylation in normal cells and their capacity to change when cells differentiate. The reduced representation bisulphite sequencing approach described by Meissner *et al.* was designed to focus on CG-dense promoter regions of the genome, but they also included CG-depleted, distal elements, where they observed relatively greater frequencies of change in methylation during differentiation (Meissner et al. 2008). The bivalent chromatin domains characteristic of embryonic stem cells (Bernstein et al. 2006) were notable in the same study for being consistently hypomethylated. When the cells studied were tested for cell culture-induced changes, even the CG-dense promoters started to acquire methylation over time, suggesting a model associated with the changes observed in neoplastic transformation (Meissner et al. 2008). The authors propose that CG density is a critical determinant of the mechanism by which methylation acts at that sequence. The emerging picture appears to be one of CG-depleted regions encoding sites at which tissue-specific variability in cytosine methylation occurs, with CG-dense regions being relatively more stably hypomethylated. It will be interesting to integrate the data from chromatin immunoprecipitation (ChIP) experiments to see whether the distinctive patterns of chromatin composition and post-translational modifications at putative *cis*-regulatory sites compared with promoters (Heintzman et al. 2007) define similar CG-depleted, constitutively hypomethylated regions.

While the results of the reduced representation bisulphite sequencing study would suggest CG-dense promoters to be very stable and invariant in terms of their cytosine methylation, Methylated CpG island Amplification in combination with Microarrays (MCAM) data show a subset (4%) of the promoter CpG islands to be methylated in normal cells, associated with the silencing of transcription of those genes (Shen et al. 2007). This is a valuable observation for the cancer epigenomics field, as it emphasizes the need to test whether methylation at a promoter CpG island detected in a tumour specimen is, in fact, an abnormal finding.

These observations represent a sampling of studies that demonstrate the value of high-throughput, genome-wide studies in the Discovery category. We find that some of our preconceptions about cytosine methylation are confirmed, such as the generally stable hypomethylation at CG-dense promoter regions, but we are challenged to understand the significance of robust findings of methylation changes at other locations. This raises the fundamental question of how cytosine methylation is targeted to specific sequences in the genome when the known mediators of cytosine methylation have no innate sequence specificity of their own.

4 Sequence-Specificity of Cytosine Methylation

DNA methyltransferases (DNMTs) catalyse the addition of the methyl group to cytosine using a donor molecule from S-adenosyl methionine (SAM). These enzymes have been extensively studied for some time and are the subject of a number of excellent reviews (Bestor 2000, Cheng and Blumenthal 2008). What is not addressed by these insights into the DNMTs is how they target certain sequences for methylation, sparing other sequences, and change this repertoire of targeting in situations such as those described above, such as differentiation and cancer. DNMTs do not have innate sequence-specificity in terms of their genomic localization, although it was recently described that the Dnmt3a-Dnmt3L complex favours the methylation of CG dinucleotides spaced 8–10 bp apart (Jia et al. 2007).

There are multiple means by which variable targeting may be mediated. One involves the interaction with the modifiers of chromatin, the second with sequence-specific molecules themselves. The modifiers of chromatin implicated in this potential interaction include the PRC2 (polycomb repressive complex 2) which includes the Ezh2 histone methyltransferase that methylates lysine 27 of histone H3 (H3K27me). As DNMTs were found to be associated with the same PRC2 complex (Vire et al. 2006), this provided an attractive model for co-operativity of this repressive histone modification with DNA methylation. Likewise, the H3K9me established by the G9a histone methyltransferase allows heterochromatin protein 1 (HP1) to bind and recruit DNMT1, linking another repressive histone modification with DNA methylation (Smallwood et al. 2007). On the other hand, H3K4me is negatively associated with DNA methylation (Okitsu and Hsieh 2007), which is reasonable given their opposing roles in transcriptional regulation, H3K4me being associated with active transcription (Heintzman et al. 2007). A histone methyltransferase that adds methyl groups to H3K4 is MLL, which contains a CXXC protein domain that binds selectively to unmethylated CG dinucleotides (Allen et al. 2006). It is logical that MLL should be preferentially targeted to CG-dense, unmethylated sequences through this domain, explaining this association. It also follows that the action of Ezh2 or G9a should influence cytosine methylation locally. Whereas the MLL paradigm is one in which cytosine methylation directs the histone modification, the Ezh2 and G9a examples represent mechanisms by which the histone modification directs cytosine methylation. As Ezh2 and G9a exist in multiprotein complexes that include DNA-binding proteins (Vire et al. 2006, Cao and Zhang 2004, Esteve et al. 2006), the sequence-specificity of the combination of epigenetic regulatory events could thus be mediated by the binding specificities of these proteins, allowing a mechanism for targeted cytosine methylation events.

This is a relatively simple means of framing the problem of sequence-specific patterns of cytosine methylation based on biochemical observations. The potential for these approaches to illuminate the targeting problem is immense. However, even at present it is apparent that the entire picture will be extraordinarily complex, with influences of non-catalytic DNMT family members on histone associations exerting additional influences (Ooi et al. 2007) and new observations of loci exhibiting hemimethylation and cyclical cytosine methylation requiring explanation (Kangaspeska et al. 2008, Metivier et al. 2008). In plants a further mechanism of targeting of cytosine methylation has been observed to be mediated through RNA processed by the Dicer-Argonaut pathway (Pikaard 2006). This may explain the targeting of transcribed sequences by cytosine methylation in non-vertebrate species (Suzuki et al. 2007, Zilberman et al. 2007). Some evidence for similar RNA-directed DNA methylation exists in mammalian cells (Morris et al. 2004) although as reviewed recently (Suzuki and Bird 2008) it will be difficult to identify targeting of transcribed sequences in vertebrates by cytosine methylation given the global methylation of the entire genome.

Finally, an obvious omission from the discussion above is the targeting of demethylation of cytosines as a means of sequence specificity. Global hypomethylation has been observed in early embryogenesis at a rate suggestive of an active process (Barton et al. 2001), and recent studies suggest that the cyclical demethylation of a mammalian promoter is mediated by DNMT3A and DNMT3B causing deamination of the methylcytosines, leading to their recognition by the DNA repair machinery and replacement by unmethylated nucleotides (Metivier et al. 2008). However, as described in a recent comprehensive review (Ooi and Bestor 2008), this model has some theoretical problems in terms of the biochemical efficiency of conversion needed and the absence of obvious dysregulation of cytosine methylation in genetic backgrounds that might be considered likely to influence this process. The issue of whether active demethylation occurs and how it might be targeted is intriguing but remains at an early stage of understanding.

5 Disease Associations

With the advanced technologies available and insights into the normal epigenome, the next scientific question is to ask how patterns of cytosine methylation are dysregulated in human pathological states. The dysregulation of the cancer epigenome has provided the paradigm for such avenues of enquiry. It appears that every cancer studied has shown aberrant cytosine methylation to be a feature of the disease. Interestingly, these studies often did not require an antecedent Comprehensive assay to screen for informative loci throughout the genome, but rather focused on promoter sequences at candidate genes to identify these patterns. While acquisition of methylation at normally unmethylated promoter CpG islands at tumour suppressor genes is the typical outcome, there have also been abnormally hypomethylated loci identified that represent putative oncogenic loci (Esteller 2007). A subset of colorectal carcinomas displays an unexpected pattern of global hypomethylation with de novo methylation of CpG islands, the CpG Island Methylator Phenotype (CIMP) (Issa 2004), suggesting a redistribution rather than merely a global acquisition or loss of methylation. This brings us back to the need to understand how methylation is targeted to specific sequences as discussed above, as the failure of normal targeting mechanisms may be the major pathological event in at least this subset of cancers.

When thinking about the role of methylation in human disease, it is useful to consider why this normal physiological process could be going wrong. The epigenome is fundamentally a means of buffering our fixed genetic properties in variable environments. With excessive or prolonged stress on this buffering capacity, a decompensatory response is possible. The response of the gastric mucosa to *Helicobacter pylori* infection is an intriguing example of such a potential decompensation. In this study, abnormal methylation was found at promoters of tumour-suppressor genes known to become methylated in gastric cancer, the malignancy associated with *H. pylori* infection. It is plausible that the inflammatory response and associated increased epithelial turnover favoured the selection of cells silencing growth-suppressing genes, as a model. With antibiotic treatment, the methylation disappeared in some but not all individuals (Maekita et al. 2006). The implications of this study were that the role of *H. pylori* to cause gastric neoplasia may be mediated through epigenomic changes, and that the altered methylation had to be encoded in a stem cell in order to allow its survival in the long term.

Other potential stressors are now being studied, including diet (Waterland 2006, Waterland and Jirtle 2003), age (Fraga et al. 2005), sex (Sarter et al. 2005) and drugs (Gottlicher et al. 2001). It is also being recognized that at least some instances of epigenetic abnormalities are constitutive throughout the body and can be inherited through the germ line (Suter 2004). With the increasing availability of technologies to study the epigenome, different stressors and categories of disease can now be tested to test whether they manifest epigenomic changes (reviewed in (Hatchwell and Greally 2007)).

An attractive aspect to the study of epigenomic dysregulation in human disease is that epigenetic changes should be reversible, whereas genetic mutations are difficult to complement with gene therapy approaches. At present, the drugs available are globally active and include DNA methyltransferase and histone deacetylase inhibitors (Hellebrekers 2007), whereas the changes in the disease might be limited to a subset of the genome. As we understand more about the normal targeting of epigenomic changes in the genome, we will be establishing a foundation for more precise targeting of therapeutic reagents to reverse the specific changes observed. However, it should be stressed that even the non-selective genome-wide therapeutic agents available to us are proving to be effective in a number of cancers (Hellebrekers 2007), creating a sense of optimism that our insights into human disease have a realistic chance of leading to successful therapeutic strategies.

6 Reference Epigenomes and the Future

At this point, we are in a period of imminent transition regarding the study of cytosine methylation. The information from high-throughput assays is revealing the normal epigenome to have patterns of methylation that are not readily predicted from DNA sequence annotations – no longer can we assume that CG-dense regions, however defined (Gardiner-Garden and Frommer 1987, Glass et al. 2007), invariably predict hypomethylated sequences, nor does it appear that other constitutively hypomethylated loci are identifiable *a priori* from DNA sequence features. Only 7% of CG dinucleotides are located within CpG islands, with 41% located in non-repetitive, non-CpG island sequences (Fazzari and Greally 2004). Within this vast amount of CG-depleted genome exist loci that manifest hypomethylation constitutively or tissue-specifically and are candidates for having *cis*-regulatory effects, but are not obviously distinctive in terms of their genomic annotations. While bioinformatic approaches have been developed that should allow us to predict these sequences (Bhasin et al. 2005, Bock et al. 2006, Feltus et al. 2003), they require that a certain amount of data to be collected at the outset for modeling purposes. This is an example of the need to define reference epigenomes, a need recognized by the NIH Roadmap for Epigenomics (http://nihroadmap.nih.gov/epigenomics/) and the Alliance for the Human Epigenome And Disease (AHEAD) (Jones et al. 2008). With reference epigenomes from normal human cell types including studies of cytosine methylation, we will establish a basis for recognizing abnormal patterns in disease, and can design the Population assays described earlier to study the most informative CG dinucleotides in the genome.

There is major potential scope for the epigenome in general and cytosine methylation in particular to mediate part of the risk of human disease and phenotypic variability. With constantly improving technology platforms, reference epigenomes and carefully-selected and characterized cell samples from affected and control subjects, we can begin to explore whether epigenomic dysregulation plays a role in a disease of interest, and if it does define the loci that are affected, leading to biomarker discovery and insights into the biology of the disease. We have the potential to return the epigenome to normal with drugs targeting the regulatory enzymes, such as DNMT or histone deacetylase inhibitors (Hellebrekers 2007), but these are at present very blunt tools with genome-wide effects. With locus-specific approaches we can perform more targeted interventions, requiring that we have a component of our efforts focused on how cytosine methylation is targeted to specific regions with sparing of other loci. These are all increasingly studied areas of epigenomic research generating fascinating new insights, promising to transform how we think about even well-studied regulators of the epigenome such as cytosine methylation.

Acknowledgments The author acknowledges support from the National Institutes of Health (R01 HD044078, R01 HG004401, R21 CA122339), the High-Q Foundation and the Herschaft Foundation.

References

Allen, M.D., et al., *Solution structure of the nonmethyl-CpG-binding CXXC domain of the leukaemia-associated MLL histone methyltransferase.* EMBO J, 2006. **25**(19): 4503–12.
Barton, S.C., et al., *Genome-wide methylation patterns in normal and uniparental early mouse embryos.* Hum Mol Genet, 2001. **10**(26): 2983–7.
Bernstein, B.E., et al., *A bivalent chromatin structure marks key developmental genes in embryonic stem cells.* Cell, 2006. **125**: 315–26.
Bernstein, B.E., et al., *Genomic maps and comparative analysis of histone modifications in human and mouse.* Cell, 2005. **120**(2): 169–81.
Bestor, T.H., *The DNA methyltransferases of mammals.* Hum Mol Genet, 2000. **9**(16): 2395–402.
Bhasin, M., et al., *Prediction of methylated CpGs in DNA sequences using a support vector machine.* FEBS Lett, 2005. **579**(20): 4302–8.
Bird, A.P., *CpG-rich islands and the function of DNA methylation.* Nature, 1986. **321**(6067): 209–13.
Bird, A.P., et al., *Non-methylated CpG-rich islands at the human alpha-globin locus: implications for evolution of the alpha-globin pseudogene.* EMBO J, 1987. **6**(4): 999–1004.
Bock, C., et al., *CpG island methylation in human lymphocytes is highly correlated with DNA sequence, repeats, and predicted DNA structure.* PLoS Genet, 2006. **2**(3): e26.
Cao, R. and Y. Zhang, *The functions of E(Z)/EZH2-mediated methylation of lysine 27 in histone H3.* Curr Opin Genet Dev, 2004 **14**(2): 155–64.
Cheng, X. and R.M. Blumenthal, *Mammalian DNA methyltransferases: a structural perspective.* Structure, 2008. **16**(3): 341–50.
Clark, S.J., J. Harrison, and M. Frommer, *CpNpG methylation in mammalian cells.* Nature Genet, 1995. **10**(1): 20–7.
Cokus, S.J., et al., *Shotgun bisulphite sequencing of the Arabidopsis genome reveals DNA methylation patterning.* Nature, 2008. **452**(7184): 215–9.
Down, T.A., et al., *A Bayesian deconvolution strategy for immunoprecipitation-based DNA methylome analysis.* Nature Biotechnol, 2008. **26**(7): 779–85.
Dupont, J.M., et al., *De novo quantitative bisulfite sequencing using the pyrosequencing technology.* Anal Biochem, 2004. **333**(1): 119–27.
Eckhardt, F., et al., *DNA methylation profiling of human chromosomes 6, 20 and 22.* Nature Genet, 2006.
Ehrich, M., et al., *Quantitative high-throughput analysis of DNA methylation patterns by base-specific cleavage and mass spectrometry.* Proc Natl Acad Sci USA, 2005. **102**(44): 15785–90.
Esteller, M., *Epigenetics provides a new generation of oncogenes and tumour-suppressor genes.* Br J Cancer, 2007. **96 Suppl**: R26–30.
Esteve, P.O., et al., *Direct interaction between DNMT1 and G9a coordinates DNA and histone methylation during replication.* Genes Dev, 2006. **20**(22): 3089–103.
Fazzari, M.J. and J.M. Greally, *Epigenomics: beyond CpG islands.* Nature Rev Genet, 2004. **5**(6): 446–55.
Feinberg, A.P. and B. Tycko, *The history of cancer epigenetics.* Nature Rev Cancer, 2004. **4**(2): 143–53.
Feltus, F.A., et al., *Predicting aberrant CpG island methylation.* Proc Natl Acad Sci USA, 2003. **100**(21): 12253–8.
Filion, G.J., et al., *A family of human zinc finger proteins that bind methylated DNA and repress transcription.* Mol Cell Biol, 2006. **26**(1): 169–81.
Flanagan, J.M., et al., *Intra- and interindividual epigenetic variation in human germ cells.* Am J Hum Genet, 2006. **79**(1): 67–84.
Fraga, M.F., et al., *Epigenetic differences arise during the lifetime of monozygotic twins.* Proc Natl Acad Sci USA, 2005. **102**(30): 10604–9.
Gardiner-Garden, M. and M. Frommer, *CpG islands in vertebrate genomes.* J Mol Biol, 1987. **196**(2): 261–82.

Gebhard, C., et al., *Genome-wide profiling of CpG methylation identifies novel targets of aberrant hypermethylation in myeloid leukemia.* Cancer Res, 2006. **66**(12): 6118–28.

Glass, J.L., et al., *CG dinucleotide clustering is a species-specific property of the genome.* Nucleic Acids Res, 2007. **35**(20): 6798–807.

Gottlicher, M., et al., *Valproic acid defines a novel class of HDAC inhibitors inducing differentiation of transformed cells.* EMBO J, 2001. **20**(24): 6969–78.

Hatada, I., et al., *Genome-wide profiling of promoter methylation in human.* Oncogene, 2006. **25**(21): 3059–64.

Hatchwell, E. and J.M. Greally, *The potential role of epigenomic dysregulation in complex human disease.* Trends Genet, 2007. **23**(11): 588–95.

Hayashi, H., et al., *High-resolution mapping of DNA methylation in human genome using oligonucleotide tiling array.* Hum Genet, 2007. **120**(5): 701–11.

Heintzman, N.D., et al., *Distinct and predictive chromatin signatures of transcriptional promoters and enhancers in the human genome.* Nature Genet, 2007. **39**(3): 311–318.

Hellebrekers, D.M., A.W. Griffioen, and M. van Engeland, *Dual targeting of epigenetic therapy in cancer.* Biochim Biophys Acta, 2007. **1775**(1): 76–91.

Hendrich, B. and S. Tweedie, *The methyl-CpG binding domain and the evolving role of DNA methylation in animals.* Trends Genet, 2003 **19**(5): 269–77.

Herman, J.G., et al., *Methylation-specific PCR: a novel PCR assay for methylation status of CpG islands.* Proc Natl Acad Sci U S A, 1996. **93**(18): 9821–6.

Hoque, M.O., et al., *Genome-wide promoter analysis uncovers portions of the cancer methylome.* Cancer Res, 2008. **68**(8): 2661–70.

Issa, J.P., *CpG island methylator phenotype in cancer.* Nature Rev Cancer, 2004. **4**(12): 988–93.

Jia, D., et al., *Structure of Dnmt3a bound to Dnmt3L suggests a model for de novo DNA methylation.* Nature, 2007. **449**(7159): 248–51.

Jones P.A., et al. *Moving AHEAD with an International Human Epigenome Project.* Nature 2008. **454**(7205): 711–715.

Kangaspeska, S., et al., *Transient cyclical methylation of promoter DNA.* Nature, 2008. **452**(7183): 112–5.

Kerkel, K., et al., *Genomic surveys by methylation-sensitive SNP analysis identify sequence-dependent allele-specific DNA methylation.* Nature Genet, 2008. **40**(7): 904–8.

Khulan, B., et al., *Comparative isoschizomer profiling of cytosine methylation: the HELP assay.* Genome Res, 2006. **16**(8): 1046–55.

Kim, T.H., et al., *Analysis of the vertebrate insulator protein CTCF-binding sites in the human genome.* Cell, 2007. **128**(6): 1231–45.

Korshunova, Y., et al., *Massively parallel bisulphite pyrosequencing reveals the molecular complexity of breast cancer-associated cytosine-methylation patterns obtained from tissue and serum DNA.* Genome Res, 2008. **18**(1): 19–29.

Kremenskoy, M., et al., *Genome-wide analysis of DNA methylation status of CpG islands in embryoid bodies, teratomas, and fetuses.* Biochem Biophys Res Commun, 2003. **311**(4): 884–90.

Kuang, S.Q., et al., *Genome-wide identification of aberrantly methylated promoter associated CpG islands in acute lymphocytic leukemia.* Leukemia, 2008.

Laird, P.W., *The power and the promise of DNA methylation markers.* Nature Rev Cancer, 2003. **3**(4): 253–66.

Lippman, Z., et al., *Profiling DNA methylation patterns using genomic tiling microarrays.* Nature Methods, 2005. **2**(3): 219–24.

Maekita, T., et al., *High levels of aberrant DNA methylation in Helicobacter pylori-infected gastric mucosae and its possible association with gastric cancer risk.* Clin Cancer Res, 2006. **12**(3 Pt 1): 989–95.

Matzke, M., et al., *RNA-directed DNA methylation and Pol IVb in Arabidopsis.* Cold Spring Harb Symp Quant Biol, 2006. **71**: 449–59.

Meissner, A., et al., *Genome-scale DNA methylation maps of pluripotent and differentiated cells.* Nature, 2008.7;**454**(**7205**):766–70.

Meissner, A., et al., *Reduced representation bisulfite sequencing for comparative high-resolution DNA methylation analysis.* Nucleic Acids Res, 2005. **33**(18): 5868–77.

Metivier, R., et al., *Cyclical DNA methylation of a transcriptionally active promoter.* Nature, 2008. **452**(7183): 45–50.

Mikkelsen, T.S., et al., *Genome-wide maps of chromatin state in pluripotent and lineage-committed cells.* Nature, 2007. **448**(7153): 553–60.

Morris, K.V., et al., *Small interfering RNA-induced transcriptional gene silencing in human cells.* Science, 2004. **305**(5688): 1289–92.

Okitsu, C.Y. and C.L. Hsieh, *DNA methylation dictates histone H3K4 methylation.* Mol Cell Biol, 2007. **27**(7): 2746–57.

Ooi, S.K. and T.H. Bestor, *The colorful history of active DNA demethylation.* Cell, 2008. **133**(7): 1145–8.

Ooi, S.K., et al., *DNMT3L connects unmethylated lysine 4 of histone H3 to de novo methylation of DNA.* Nature, 2007. **448**(7154): 714–7.

Ordway, J.M., et al., *Identification of novel high-frequency DNA methylation changes in breast cancer.* PLoS ONE, 2007. **2**(12): e1314.

Pfeifer, G.P., et al., *In vivo footprint and methylation analysis by PCR-aided genomic sequencing: comparison of active and inactive X chromosomal DNA at the CpG island and promoter of human PGK-1.* Genes Dev, 1990. **4**(8): 1277–87.

Pikaard, C.S., *Cell biology of the Arabidopsis nuclear siRNA pathway for RNA-directed chromatin modification.* Cold Spring Harb Symp Quant Biol, 2006. **71**: 473–80.

Reinders, J., et al., *Genome-wide, high-resolution DNA methylation profiling using bisulfite-mediated cytosine conversion.* Genome Res, 2008. **18**(3): 469–76.

Sarter, B., et al., *Sex differential in methylation patterns of selected genes in Singapore Chinese.* Hum Genet, 2005. **117**(4): 402–3.

Schilling, E. and M. Rehli, *Global, comparative analysis of tissue-specific promoter CpG methylation.* Genomics, 2007 **90**(3): 314–23.

Selker, E.U., *Genome defense and DNA methylation in Neurospora.* Cold Spring Harb Symp Quant Biol, 2004. **69**: 119–24.

Shen, L., et al., *Genome-wide profiling of DNA methylation reveals a class of normally methylated CpG island promoters.* PLoS Genet, 2007. **3**(10): 2023–36.

Shiota, K., *DNA methylation profiles of CpG islands for cellular differentiation and development in mammals.* Cytogenet Genome Res, 2004. **105**(2–4): 325–34.

Smallwood, A., et al., *Functional cooperation between HP1 and DNMT1 mediates gene silencing.* Genes Dev, 2007. **21**(10): 1169–78.

Smith, J.F., et al., *Identification of DNA Methylation in 3' Genomic Regions that are Associated with Upregulation of Gene Expression in Colorectal Cancer.* Epigenetics, 2007. **2**(3).

Song, F., et al., *Association of tissue-specific differentially methylated regions (TDMs) with differential gene expression.* Proc Natl Acad Sci USA, 2005. **102**(9): 3336–41.

Spitz, F., F. Gonzalez, and D. Duboule, *A global control region defines a chromosomal regulatory landscape containing the HoxD cluster.* Cell, 2003. **113**(3): 405–17.

Srinivasan, P.R., *Kinetics of incorporation of 5-methylcytosine in HeLa cells.* Biochim Biophys Acta, 1962. **55**: 553–6.

Strahl, B.D. and C.D. Allis, *The language of covalent histone modifications.* Nature, 2000. **403**(6765): 41–5.

Suter, C.M., D.I. Martin, and R.L. Ward, *Germline epimutation of MLH1 in individuals with multiple cancers.* Nature Genet, 2004. **36**(5): 497–501.

Suzuki, M.M. and A. Bird, *DNA methylation landscapes: provocative insights from epigenomics.* Nature Rev Genet, 2008. **9**(6): 465–76.

Suzuki, M.M., et al., *CpG methylation is targeted to transcription units in an invertebrate genome.* Genome Res, 2007. **17**(5): 625–31.

Taylor, K.H., et al., *Ultradeep bisulfite sequencing analysis of DNA methylation patterns in multiple gene promoters by 454 sequencing.* Cancer Res, 2007. **67**(18): 8511–8.

The ENCODE Project Consortium, *Identification and analysis of functional elements in 1% of the human genome by the ENCODE pilot project.* Nature, 2007. **447**(7146): 799–816.

Trinh, B.N., T.I. Long, and P.W. Laird, *DNA methylation analysis by MethyLight technology.* Methods, 2001. **25**(4): 456–62.

Vire, E., et al., *The Polycomb group protein EZH2 directly controls DNA methylation.* Nature, 2006. **439**(7078): 871–4.

Walsh, C.P. and T.H. Bestor, *Cytosine methylation and mammalian development.* Genes Dev, 1999. **13**(1): 26–34.

Waterland, R.A. and R.L. Jirtle, *Transposable elements: targets for early nutritional effects on epigenetic gene regulation.* Mol Cell Biol, 2003. **23**(15): 5293–300.

Waterland, R.A., *Assessing the effects of high methionine intake on DNA methylation.* J Nutr, 2006. **136**(6 Suppl): 1706S-1710S.

Weber, M., et al., *Chromosome-wide and promoter-specific analyses identify sites of differential DNA methylation in normal and transformed human cells.* Nat Genet, 2005. **37**(8): 853–62.

Weber, M., et al., *Distribution, silencing potential and evolutionary impact of promoter DNA methylation in the human genome.* Nature Genet, 2007. **39**(4): 457–66.

Zilberman, D. and S. Henikoff, *Genome-wide analysis of DNA methylation patterns.* Development, 2007 **134**(22): 3959–65.

Zilberman, D., et al., *Genome-wide analysis of Arabidopsis thaliana DNA methylation uncovers an interdependence between methylation and transcription.* Nature Genet, 2007. **39**(1): 61–9.

Structural and Biochemical Advances in Mammalian DNA Methylation

Xiaodong Cheng and Robert M. Blumenthal

> *"'Form follows function' – that has been misunderstood. Form and function should be one, joined in a spiritual union."*
> ...Frank Lloyd Wright

Abstract The control of transcription initiation in mammalian cells can be very broadly divided into three categories: intrinsic promoter strength and availability of core transcription machinery (Dvir et al. 2001, Sandelin 2007), the actions of promoter- or regulon-specific transcription factors (positive and negative) (e.g., (Malik and Roeder 2005, Hoffmann et al. 2006)), and the control of DNA accessibility by altering chromatin structure (Li et al. 2007, Berger 2007). This latter category, including posttranslational modifications to histones and postreplicational modification of DNA, is in many ways less well-understood than the other two. Nucleosomes are the fundamental building blocks of eukaryotic chromatin, and consist of ~146 base pairs of DNA wrapped twice around a histone octamer (Luger et al. 1997). A variety of protein-modifying enzymes (including methyltransferases, MTases) is responsible for histone modification, primarily at their flexible N-termini (Shilatifard 2006, Shi 2007, Bhaumik et al. 2007). We will touch on the functional links between histone modification and that of DNA, but the purpose of this chapter is to summarize, from a structural perspective, the rapidly-growing body of information about the proteins that methylate mammalian DNA.

Keywords Structure and function · Mammalian DNA methyltransferases · Dnmt1 · Dnmt3a · Dnmt3b · Dnmt3L · Unmethylated histone H3 lysine 4 · CpG spacing

1 Introduction

In mammals and other vertebrates, DNA methylation occurs at the C5 position of cytosine (5mC), mostly within CpG dinucleotides (Fig. 1A), with the enzymes using a conserved mechanism (Jeltsch 2006a, b) that has been studied best in the bacterial

---

X. Cheng (✉)
Department of Biochemistry, Emory University School of Medicine, Atlanta, GA 30322
e-mail: xcheng@emory.edu

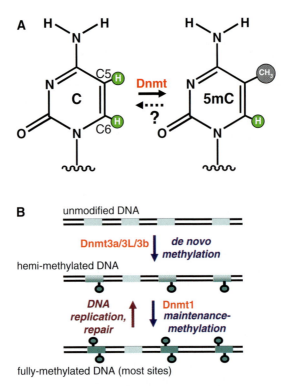

Fig. 1 DNA methylation. (**A**) DNA cytosine methylation at ring carbon C5. See text for a summary of the mechanism. The question mark indicates possible activity of DNA demethylases (Kress et al. 2006, Vairapandi 2004). (**B**) Maintenance *vs* de novo methylation. As described in the text, the roles of the Dnmts are not completely distinct in this respect. The boxed segments are substrate sequences (usually CpG), and the turquoise shapes represent methyl groups on the cytosines. Following replication or repair, the duplex is methylated on one strand only

5mC MTase M.HhaI (Klimasauskas et al. 1994, Sheikhnejad et al. 1999, Wu and Santi, 1987, Youngblood et al. 2007, Zhang and Bruice 2006). Briefly, this mechanism involves MTase binding to the DNA, eversion of the target nucleotide so that it projects out of the double helix ("base flipping"), covalent attack of a conserved Cys nucleophile on cytosine C6, transfer of the methyl group from AdoMet to the activated cytosine C5, and the various release steps. This methylation, together with histone modifications, plays an important role in modulating chromatin structure, thus controlling gene expression and many other chromatin-dependent processes (Kouzarides 2007). The resulting epigenetic effects maintain the various patterns of gene expression in different cell types (Turner 2007). Epigenetic processes include genomic imprinting (Hore et al. 2007), gene silencing (Miranda and Jones 2007, Lande-Diner et al. 2007), X chromosome inactivation (Yen et al. 2007), reprogramming in transferred nuclei (Yang et al. 2007, Reik 2007), and some elements of carcinogenesis (Gronbaek et al. 2007). DNA methylation is also associated with phenomena such as DNA repair (Walsh and Xu, 2006), initiation of sexual dimorphism (Schaefer et al. 2007), progression through cell division checkpoints (Unterberger et al. 2006), and suppression of the huge number of transposable and retroviral elements in the mammalian genome (Bird 1997, Howard et al. 2008, Yoder et al. 1997).

There are many recent reviews as well as other chapters in this volume on epigenetics and its associated histone modifications and DNA methylation (Goll and Bestor 2005, Malik and Roeder 2005, Hoffmann et al. 2006, Shilatifard 2006, Sandelin 2007, Li et al. 2007, Berger 2007, Shi 2007, Bhaumik et al. 2007, Allis et al. 2007). Here, we summarize the most recent structural and biochemical advances in the study of DNA methyltransferases.

2 Mammalian DNA Methyltransferases

In mammals, DNA nucleotide methyltransferases (Dnmts) include four members, in two families that are structurally and functionally distinct (Fig. 2). The Dnmt3 family establishes the initial CpG methylation pattern de novo, while Dnmt1 maintains this pattern during chromosome replication (Chen and Li 2006) and repair (Mortusewicz 2005) (Fig. 1B). As expected for a maintenance MTase, Dnmt1 has a 30–40-fold preference for hemimethylated sites (discussed in Jeltsch (2006a, b)). However, this division of labor is not so clear, as Dnmt1 activity is required for de novo methylation at non-CpG cytosines (Grandjean et al. 2007), and perhaps to an extent even in CpG islands (Feltus et al. 2003, Jair et al. 2006).

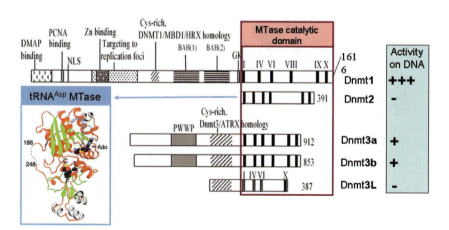

Fig. 2 Members of DNMT family. Schematic representation of Dnmt1 and Dnmt3. Dnmt2 is a tRNA^{Asp} MTase (Goll et al. 2006) (insert). Roman numerals refer to conserved motifs of DNA MTases (Kumar et al. 1994); motif IV includes the Cys nucleophile that forms a transient covalent bond to C6 of the target cytosine. Other details are explained in the text or in Goll and Bestor (2005)

The Dnmt3 family includes two active de novo Dnmts, Dnmt3a and Dnmt3b, and one regulatory factor, Dnmt3-Like protein (Dnmt3L) (Bestor 2000) (Fig. 2). Dnmt3a and Dnmt3b have similar domain arrangements: both contain a variable region at the N-terminus, followed by a PWWP domain that may be involved in nonspecific DNA binding (Lukasik et al. 2006, Qiu et al. 2002), a Cys-rich 3-Zn binding domain (six CXXC motifs), and a C-terminal catalytic domain. The amino acid sequence of Dnmt3L is very similar to that of Dnmt3a and Dnmt3b in the Cys-rich 3-Zn binding domain, but it lacks the conserved residues required for DNA MTase activity in the C-terminal domain. Dnmt2 appears to provide an example of divergent evolution: it was named based on its high sequence and structural similarity to known DNA MTases (Yoder and Bestor 1998, Okano et al. 1998, Dong et al. 2001), but actually methylates cytosine 38 in the anticodon loop of tRNA^{Asp} (Goll et al. 2006, Rai et al. 2007) (Fig. 2).

At the time of this writing, no structural information is available for any part of the large 183 kDa Dnmt1 protein. It was recently reported that the SRA protein/ubiquitin ligase Np95 (mouse) – ICBP90 (human) (Citterio et al. 2004, Muto

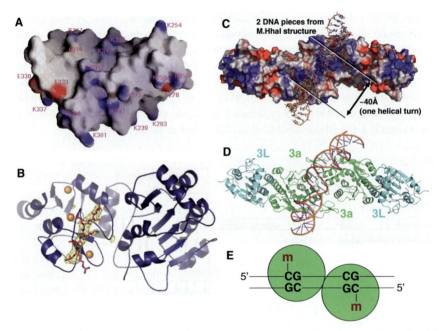

Fig. 3 Domain structures of Dnmt3 family. (**A**) The PWWP domain structure of Dnmt3b, rich in basic residues (Qiu et al. 2002). Selected charged, surface-exposed residues are indicated. (**B**) Structure of Dnmt3L with a bound histone H3 N-terminal tail (*orange*) (Ooi et al. 2007). (**C**) A surface representation of Dnmt3a-C/3L-C tetramer, with two short DNA molecules adopted by superimposition of the HhaI-DNA complex structure (Klimasauskas et al. 1994) onto individual Dnmt3a-C. (**D**) The Dnmt3a-C/3L-C tetramer with one contiguous curved DNA molecule covering two active sites. (**E**) The Dnmt3a dimer could in theory methylate two CpGs separated by one helical turn in one binding event

et al. 2002, Papait et al. 2007, Karagianni et al. 2008) targets Dnmt1 to hemimethylated replication forks (and presumably repair sites) (Sharif et al. 2007, Bostick et al. 2007, Achour et al. 2008). It appears that large conformational changes are involved in Dnmt1 transition to an active state, involving interactions between the amino-proximal and catalytic domains (Fatemi et al. 2001), modulated by phosphorylation of Ser515 (Goyal et al. 2007).

In contrast to Dnmt1, structures are available for the PWWP domain of Dnmt3b (Qiu et al. 2002) (Fig. 3A), intact Dnmt3L in complex with histone H3 amino-tail peptide (Ooi et al. 2007) (Fig. 3B), and a complex between the C-terminal domains of Dnmt3a and Dnmt3L (Jia et al. 2007) (Fig. 3C,D). We will discuss the implications of these structures.

3 Dnmt3L is a Regulatory Factor for De Novo DNA Methylation

The phenotype of Dnmt3L knockout mice is indistinguishable from that of a Dnmt3a conditional knockout, with both having altered sex-specific de novo methylation of DNA sequences in germ cells (Bourc'his et al. 2001, Bourc'his and Bestor 2004, Kaneda et al. 2004, Webster et al. 2005). These results indicate that Dnmt3a and Dnmt3L are both required for the methylation of most imprinted loci in germ cells. Dnmt3L co-localizes and co-immunoprecipitates with both Dnmt3a and Dnmt3b (Hata et al. 2002), and enhances de novo methylation by both of these MTases (Chedin et al. 2002, Suetake et al. 2004, Chen et al. 2005, Gowher et al. 2005, Kareta et al. 2006). The minimal regions required for interaction between Dnmt3L and Dnmt3a (or Dnmt3b), and for stimulated activity, are in the C-terminal domains of both proteins (Suetake et al. 2004, Chen et al. 2005, Gowher et al. 2005, Kareta et al. 2006, Margot et al. 2003), as illustrated by the structure of the complex between C-terminal domains (-C) of Dnmt3a and Dnmt3L (Jia et al. 2007) (Fig. 3C,D).

Both Dnmt3a-C and Dnmt3L-C have the characteristic fold of Class I, unpermuted, AdoMet-dependent MTases (Schubert et al. 2003). However, the methylation reaction product S-adenosyl-L-homocysteine (AdoHcy) was found only in Dnmt3a-C and not in Dnmt3L-C. This is consistent with Dnmt3a-C being the catalytic component of the complex, while Dnmt3L is inactive and unable to bind AdoMet (Gowher et al. 2005). The overall Dnmt3a-C / Dnmt3L-C complex is ~16 nm long, which is greater than the diameter of a 11-nm core nucleosome (Luger et al. 1997) (Fig. 4). This complex contains two monomers of Dnmt3a-C and two of Dnmt3L-C, and is a tetramer with two 3L-3a interfaces and one 3a-3a interface (3L-3a-3a-3L). Substituting key non-catalytic residues at the Dnmt3a-3L or Dnmt3a-3a interfaces eliminated enzymatic activity, indicating that both interfaces are essential for catalysis (Jia et al. 2007).

Dnmt3L appears to stabilize the conformation of the active-site loop of Dnmt3a, that contains the catalytic nucleophile (Cys706; Fig. 5), via interactions with the C-terminal portion of that loop (G718-L719-Y720; Fig. 5). Interestingly, point

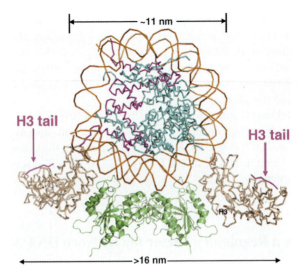

Fig. 4 A model of interaction of Dnmt3a-3L tetramer with nucleosome. A nucleosome is docked to a Dnmt3L-3a-3a-3L tetramer. The position of a peptide derived from the sequence of the histone H3 amino terminus is shown, taken from a cocrystal structure with this peptide bound to Dnmt3L (Ooi et al. 2007)

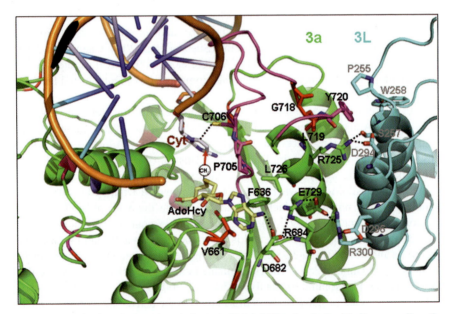

Fig. 5 The 3a-3L interface may contribute to the stability of cofactor binding as well as the active-site loop conformation. AdoHcy and residues involved in interactions are in stick model

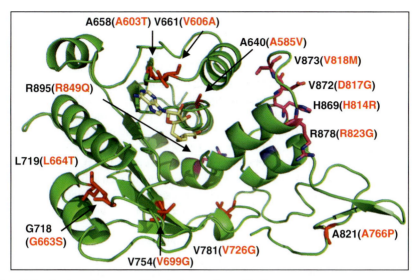

Fig. 6 Distribution of human ICF mutations on Dnmt3B-C. Assuming the Dnmt3b-C monomer has, as expected, a structure similar to that of Dnmt3a-C, the corresponding Dnmt3b residue number is in parenthesis. Adopted from supplementary of reference (Jia et al. 2007)

mutations of the codons corresponding to G718-L719 in human Dnmt3b are associated with the disease ICF (G663S and L664T; see below).

These loop-stabilizing interactions might explain the stimulation of Dnmt3a activity by Dnmt3L (Chedin et al. 2002, Suetake et al. 2004, Chen et al. 2005, Gowher et al. 2005, Kareta et al. 2006). The structure, docked to DNA with a flipped target Cyt (adopted from the HhaI-DNA structure), has the docked Cyt located between the nucleophile Cys706 and AdoMet (where a transferable methyl group was modeled onto the sulfur atom of AdoHcy; Fig. 5). The nucleophilic attack on Cyt C5 by Cys706 and the methyltransfer would occur from opposite directions, perpendicular to Cyt ring surface, as in M.HhaI.

The catalytic domain of Dnmt3b is ~80% identical to that of Dnmt3a, with no gaps or insertions. Point mutations in human Dnmt3b are responsible for a disorder called ICF syndrome (*I*mmunodeficiency, *C*entromere instability, and *F*acial anomalies), that results in death before adulthood (Okano et al. 1999, Xu et al. 1999). Most ICF mutations cluster in the C-terminal catalytic domain of Dnmt3b (Fig. 6). If the Dnmt3b monomer has, as expected, a structure similar to that of Dnmt3a, ICF mutations could reduce the enzymatic activity of Dnmt3b in several alternative ways: affecting overall stability (V699G, V726G, and A766P), altering conformation of the active-site loop (G663S, L664T) directly (or indirectly by affecting the interface with Dnmt3L), impairing interaction with the methyl donor AdoMet (A585V, V606A, and A603T), affecting the proposed 3b-3b interface (analogous to the 3a-3a interface; V818M, D817G, and H814R), or impairing its proposed interaction with DNA (R823G).

4 Dnmt3a Dimer Suggests that De Novo DNA Methylation Depends on CpG Spacing

Among known active DNA MTases, Dnmt3a and Dnmt3b have the smallest DNA binding domain (though it is absent altogether in Dnmt3L). This domain includes ~50 residues in Dnmt3a/b compared to, for example, ~85 residues in the bacterial GCGC MTase M.HhaI (Klimasauskas et al. 1994). However, dimerization via the 3a-3a interface brings two active sites together and effectively doubles the DNA-binding surface. Superimposing the Dnmt3a structure, onto that of M.HhaI complexed with a short oligonucleotide (Klimasauskas et al. 1994), yielded a model Dnmt3a-DNA complex with a short DNA duplex bound to each active site (Fig. 3C). The two DNA segments can be easily connected to form a contiguous DNA, such that the two active sites are located in the major groove about 40 Å apart (Fig. 3D).

This model suggests that dimeric Dnmt3a could methylate two CpGs separated by one helical turn in one binding event (Fig. 3E). A periodicity in the activity of Dnmt3a on long DNA substrates revealed a correlation of methylated CpG sites at distances of 8–10 base pairs, and the structural model of oligomeric Dnmt3a docked to DNA may explain this pattern (Jia et al. 2007). Similar periodicity is observed for the frequency of CpG sites in the differentially-methylated regions of 12 maternally-imprinted mouse genes (Jia et al. 2007). These results suggest a basis for the recognition and methylation of differentially-methylated regions in imprinted genes, involving detection of both CpG spacing and nucleosome modification (see below).

5 Dnmt3L Connects Unmethylated Lysine 4 of Histone H3 to De Novo DNA Methylation

DNA methylation and histone modifications are intricately connected with each other. Dnmt3a is fully active on nucleosomal DNA in vitro, unlike a bacterial CpG-specific DNA MTase (M.SssI) (Gowher et al. 2005). Mouse ES cells that lack the H3 lysine 9 (H3K9) MTases Suv39h1 and Suv39h2 show slight demethylation of satellite DNA (Lehnertz et al. 2003). Methylation of histone H3 lysine 4 (H3K4) has been suggested to protect gene promoters from de novo DNA methylation in somatic cells (Weber et al. 2007, Appanah et al. 2007). The mammalian de novo DNA methylation Dnmt3L-Dnmt3a machinery could translate patterns of H3K4 methylation, which are not themselves preserved during chromosome replication, into heritable patterns of DNA methylation that mediate transcriptional silencing of the affected sequences (Ooi et al. 2007).

Dnmt3a2 is a germ-cell-specific isoform of Dnmt3a that is also required for genomic imprinting (Chen et al. 2002). Dnmt3a2 and Dnmt3b, along with the four core histones, were identified as the main in vivo interaction partners of epitope-tagged Dnmt3L (Ooi et al. 2007). Peptide interaction assays showed that Dnmt3L specifically interacts with the extreme amino terminus of histone H3; this interaction was strongly inhibited by H3K4 methylation, but was insensitive to modifications at other positions (Ooi et al. 2007). Cocrystallization of Dnmt3L with the amino tail of H3 showed this tail bound to the Cys-rich 3-Zn binding domain of Dnmt3L (Fig. 3B), and substitution of key residues in the binding site eliminated the H3-Dnmt3L interaction. These data suggest that Dnmt3L is a probe of H3K4 methylation, and if the methylation is absent then Dnmt3L induces de novo DNA methylation by docking activated Dnmt3a2 to the nucleosome. There have been reports of an inverse relationship between H3K4 methylation and allele-specific DNA methylation at differentially methylated regions (Fournier et al. 2002, Vu et al. 2004, Yamasaki et al. 2005, Delaval et al. 2007).

6 Oligomerization by Dnmt3 Family

It is interesting that the sequences involved in the 3L-3a interface are highly conserved, represented by two pairs of phenylalanine, F728 and F768 of Dnmt3a and F261 and F301 of Dnmt3L (Fig. 7A). The 3a interface of Dnmt3L also supports formation of a Dnmt3L homodimer (Fig. 8A). Dnmt3a might use the same interface to form a Dnmt3a homo-oligomer, as suggested by analytical size exclusion chromatography of Dnmt3a2; this polypeptide has a theoretical mass of 78 kDa, but gave a broad peak of ~500 kDa (Fig. 8B). Furthermore, an F728A mutation of Dnmt3a2, that eliminates a hydrophobic interaction at the 3a-3L interface (Fig. 7A), disrupted the Dnmt3a2 homo-oligomer to yield a ~150 kDa dimer (Fig. 8B) and abolished MTase activity (Jia et al. 2007). The equivalent mutant in Dnmt3L, F261A, lost its ability to form a homodimer and, at the same time, its ability to stimulate wild type Dnmt3a2 activity (Jia et al. 2007). These data indicate that the two active members of Dnmt3 family, Dnmt3a and Dnmt3b, could form homo-oligomers (or even 3a-3b hetero-oligomers) via alternative interfaces involving the DNA binding domain and the phenylalanine stacking (the cartoon shown in Fig. 8B). The functions of Dnmt3 oligomers remain elusive (Li et al. 2007, Kato et al. 2007).

7 Perspective

The availability of human genome sequences, and those of other model research organisms, has provided answers to a wide range of questions that, in some cases, we did not even previously know to ask. Population studies of single-nucleotide polymorphism (SNP) haplotypes are yielding powerful insights into diseases such as cancer and diabetes. In combination with proteomics and transcriptomics, global analysis of genomic DNA methylation (Brown et al. 2007, Dunn et al. 2007, Schilling and Rehli 2007, Wu et al. 2007) is likely to play increasingly important roles in understanding normal and abnormal human development and physiology.

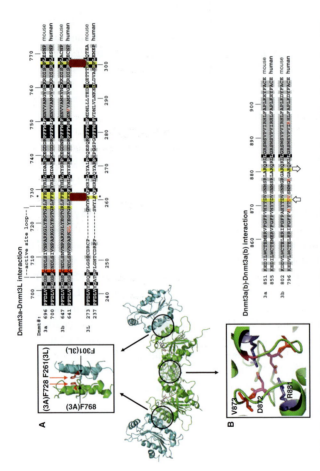

Fig. 7 Conserved Sequences of the 3a-3L and 3a-3a interfaces. (**A**) The Dnmt3a-3L interface is shown. Numbering above the sequences corresponds to the mouse ortholog. *White*-on-*black* residues are conserved in Dnmt3a, 3b, and 3L, while *gray*-highlighted positions are conserved (with ≤1 substitution) between 3a and 3b. Positions responsible for interactions between Dnmt3a and 3L are indicated by *lines*. The range of vertebrates with obvious Dnmt3L orthologs is much more restricted than that for 3a or 3b. The Dnmt3a-3a interface is shown, with the sequence highlighted as in (**A**). The *block arrows* underneath indicate reciprocal salt bridges between the conserved Arg and Asp, as shown at *left*

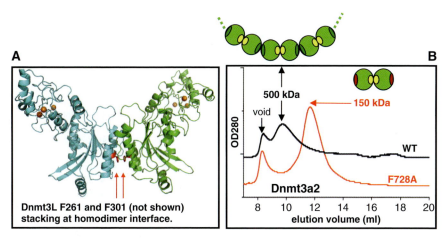

Fig. 8 Self-oligomerization (including dimerization) of Dnmt3. (**A**) Structure of the Dnmt3L-3L homo-dimer interface. (**B**) Size exclusion chromatography of wild-type Dnmt3a2 (*black trace*), or of an F728A mutant (*grey trace*) (adopted from supplementary of reference (Jia et al. 2007)). The cartoons indicate the interpretation of oligomerization

The experimental characterization of Dnmts is providing a rapidly-growing and convergent picture of the kinetic mechanisms, binding partners, chromatin recognition, and in some cases structures of these proteins. However, understanding the basis for establishing, maintaining, and disturbing DNA methylation patterns will require a much better understanding of the union between form and function in the Dnmt proteins than we currently possess.

Acknowledgments We thank most warmly our colleagues (Drs. Steen K.T. Ooi, Timothy H. Bestor, Emily Bernstein, C. David Allis, Renata Z. Jurkowska, and Albert Jeltsch) and coworkers (Drs. Da Jia, Zhe Yang, Keqin Li, Chen Qiu, Xing Zhang, and John R. Horton) whose hard work was responsible for much of the DNA methyltransferase work cited in this review. Work in the authors' laboratories is supported in part by grants (NIH GM049245 and GM068680 to XDC; NSF 0516692 to RMB) and the Georgia Research Alliance (to XDC).

References

Achour, M., Jacq, X., Ronde, P., Alhosin, M., Charlot, C., Chataigneau, T., Jeanblanc, M., Macaluso, M., Giordano, A., Hughes, A.D., Schini-Kerth, V.B., and Bronner, C. (2008). The interaction of the SRA domain of ICBP90 with a novel domain of DNMT1 is involved in the regulation of VEGF gene expression. Oncogene **27,** 2187–2197.

Allis, C.D., Jenuwein, T., and Reinberg, D. eds. (2007). Epigenetics (Cold Spring Harbor, NY: Cold Spring Harbor Laboratory Press).

Appanah, R., Dickerson, D.R., Goyal, P., Groudine, M., and Lorincz, M.C. (2007). An unmethylated 3' promoter-proximal region is required for efficient transcription initiation. PLoS Genet *3,* e27.

Berger, S.L. (2007). The complex language of chromatin regulation during transcription. Nature *447,* 407–412.

Bestor, T.H. (2000). The DNA methyltransferases of mammals. Hum Mol Genet *9*, 2395–2402.

Bhaumik, S.R., Smith, E., and Shilatifard, A. (2007). Covalent modifications of histones during development and disease pathogenesis. Nat Struct Mol Biol *14*, 1008–1016.

Bird, A. (1997). Does DNA methylation control transposition of selfish elements in the germline? Trends Genet *13*, 469–472.

Bostick, M., Kim, J.K., Esteve, P.O., Clark, A., Pradhan, S., and Jacobsen, S.E. (2007). UHRF1 plays a role in maintaining DNA methylation in mammalian cells. Science *317*, 1760–1764.

Bourc'his, D., and Bestor, T.H. (2004). Meiotic catastrophe and retrotransposon reactivation in male germ cells lacking Dnmt3L. Nature *431*, 96–99.

Bourc'his, D., Xu, G.L., Lin, C.S., Bollman, B., and Bestor, T.H. (2001). Dnmt3L and the establishment of maternal genomic imprints. Science *294*, 2536–2539.

Brown, S.E., Fraga, M.F., Weaver, I.C., Berdasco, M., and Szyf, M. (2007). Variations in DNA methylation patterns during the cell cycle of HeLa cells. Epigenetics *2*, 54–65.

Chedin, F., Lieber, M.R., and Hsieh, C.L. (2002). The DNA methyltransferase-like protein DNMT3L stimulates de novo methylation by Dnmt3a. Proc Natl Acad Sci USA *99*, 16916–16921.

Chen, T., and Li, E. (2006). Establishment and maintenance of DNA methylation patterns in mammals. Curr Top Microbiol Immunol *301*, 179–201.

Chen, T., Ueda, Y., Xie, S., and Li, E. (2002). A novel Dnmt3a isoform produced from an alternative promoter localizes to euchromatin and its expression correlates with active de novo methylation. J Biol Chem *277*, 38746–38754.

Chen, Z.X., Mann, J.R., Hsieh, C.L., Riggs, A.D., and Chedin, F. (2005). Physical and functional interactions between the human DNMT3L protein and members of the de novo methyltransferase family. J Cell Biochem *95*, 902–917.

Citterio, E., Papait, R., Nicassio, F., Vecchi, M., Gomiero, P., Mantovani, R., Di Fiore, P.P., and Bonapace, I.M. (2004). Np95 is a histone-binding protein endowed with ubiquitin ligase activity. Mol Cell Biol *24*, 2526–2535.

Delaval, K., Govin, J., Cerqueira, F., Rousseaux, S., Khochbin, S., and Feil, R. (2007). Differential histone modifications mark mouse imprinting control regions during spermatogenesis. EMBO J *26*, 720–729.

Dong, A., Yoder, J.A., Zhang, X., Zhou, L., Bestor, T.H., and Cheng, X. (2001). Structure of human DNMT2, an enigmatic DNA methyltransferase homolog that displays denaturant-resistant binding to DNA. Nucleic Acids Res *29*, 439–448.

Dunn, J.J., McCorkle, S.R., Everett, L., and Anderson, C.W. (2007). Paired-end genomic signature tags: a method for the functional analysis of genomes and epigenomes. Genet Eng (N Y) *28*, 159–173.

Dvir, A., Conaway, J.W., and Conaway, R.C. (2001). Mechanism of transcription initiation and promoter escape by RNA polymerase II. Curr Opin Genet Dev *11*, 209–214.

Fatemi, M., Hermann, A., Pradhan, S., and Jeltsch, A. (2001). The activity of the murine DNA methyltransferase Dnmt1 is controlled by interaction of the catalytic domain with the N-terminal part of the enzyme leading to an allosteric activation of the enzyme after binding to methylated DNA. J Mol Biol *309*, 1189–1199.

Feltus, F.A., Lee, E.K., Costello, J.F., Plass, C., and Vertino, P.M. (2003). Predicting aberrant CpG island methylation. Proc Natl Acad Sci USA *100*, 12253–12258.

Fournier, C., Goto, Y., Ballestar, E., Delaval, K., Hever, A.M., Esteller, M., and Feil, R. (2002). Allele-specific histone lysine methylation marks regulatory regions at imprinted mouse genes. EMBO J *21*, 6560–6570.

Goll, M.G., and Bestor, T.H. (2005). Eukaryotic cytosine methyltransferases. Annu Rev Biochem *74*, 481–514.

Goll, M.G., Kirpekar, F., Maggert, K.A., Yoder, J.A., Hsieh, C.L., Zhang, X., Golic, K.G., Jacobsen, S.E., and Bestor, T.H. (2006). Methylation of tRNAAsp by the DNA methyltransferase homolog Dnmt2. Science *311*, 395–398.

Gowher, H., Liebert, K., Hermann, A., Xu, G., and Jeltsch, A. (2005). Mechanism of stimulation of catalytic activity of Dnmt3A and Dnmt3B DNA-(cytosine-C5)-methyltransferases by Dnmt3L. J Biol Chem *280*, 13341–13348.

Gowher, H., Stockdale, C.J., Goyal, R., Ferreira, H., Owen-Hughes, T., and Jeltsch, A. (2005). De novo methylation of nucleosomal DNA by the mammalian Dnmt1 and Dnmt3A DNA methyltransferases. Biochemistry *44*, 9899–9904.

Goyal, R., Rathert, P., Laser, H., Gowher, H., and Jeltsch, A. (2007). Phosphorylation of serine-515 activates the Mammalian maintenance methyltransferase dnmt1. Epigenetics *2*, 155–160.

Grandjean, V., Yaman, R., Cuzin, F., and Rassoulzadegan, M. (2007). Inheritance of an Epigenetic Mark: The CpG DNA Methyltransferase 1 Is Required for De Novo Establishment of a Complex Pattern of Non-CpG Methylation. PLoS One *2*, e1136.

Gronbaek, K., Hother, C., and Jones, P.A. (2007). Epigenetic changes in cancer. APMIS *115*, 1039–1059.

Hata, K., Okano, M., Lei, H., and Li, E. (2002). Dnmt3L cooperates with the Dnmt3 family of de novo DNA methyltransferases to establish maternal imprints in mice. Development *129*, 1983–1993.

Hoffmann, A., Natoli, G., and Ghosh, G. (2006). Transcriptional regulation via the NF-kappaB signaling module. Oncogene *25*, 6706–6716.

Hore, T.A., Rapkins, R.W., and Graves, J.A. (2007). Construction and evolution of imprinted loci in mammals. Trends Genet *23*, 440–448.

Howard, G., Eiges, R., Gaudet, F., Jaenisch, R., and Eden, A. (2008). Activation and transposition of endogenous retroviral elements in hypomethylation induced tumors in mice. Oncogene *10;27*:404–408.

Jair, K.W., Bachman, K.E., Suzuki, H., Ting, A.H., Rhee, I., Yen, R.W., Baylin, S.B., and Schuebel, K.E. (2006). De novo CpG island methylation in human cancer cells. Cancer Res *66*, 682–692.

Jeltsch, A. (2006a). Molecular enzymology of mammalian DNA methyltransferases. Curr Top Microbiol Immunol *301*, 203–225.

Jeltsch, A. (2006b). On the enzymatic properties of Dnmt1: specificity, processivity, mechanism of linear diffusion and allosteric regulation of the enzyme. Epigenetics *1*, 63–66.

Jia, D., Jurkowska, R.Z., Zhang, X., Jeltsch, A., and Cheng, X. (2007). Structure of Dnmt3a bound to Dnmt3L suggests a model for de novo DNA methylation. Nature *449*, 248–251.

Kaneda, M., Okano, M., Hata, K., Sado, T., Tsujimoto, N., Li, E., and Sasaki, H. (2004). Essential role for de novo DNA methyltransferase Dnmt3a in paternal and maternal imprinting. Nature *429*, 900–903.

Karagianni, P., Amazit, L., Qin, J., and Wong, J. (2008). ICBP90, a novel methyl K9 H3 binding protein linking protein ubiquitination with heterochromatin formation. Mol Cell Biol *28*, 705–717.

Kareta, M.S., Botello, Z.M., Ennis, J.J., Chou, C., and Chedin, F. (2006). Reconstitution and mechanism of the stimulation of de novo methylation by human DNMT3L. J Biol Chem *281*, 25893–25902.

Kato, Y., Kaneda, M., Hata, K., Kumaki, K., Hisano, M., Kohara, Y., Okano, M., Li, E., Nozaki, M., and Sasaki, H. (2007). Role of the Dnmt3 family in de novo methylation of imprinted and repetitive sequences during male germ cell development in the mouse. Hum Mol Genet *16*, 2272–2280.

Klimasauskas, S., Kumar, S., Roberts, R.J., and Cheng, X. (1994). HhaI methyltransferase flips its target base out of the DNA helix. Cell *76*, 357–369.

Kouzarides, T. (2007). Chromatin modifications and their function. Cell *128*, 693–705.

Kress, C., Thomassin, H., and Grange, T. (2006). Active cytosine demethylation triggered by a nuclear receptor involves DNA strand breaks. Proc Natl Acad Sci USA *103*, 11112–11117.

Kumar, S., Cheng, X., Klimasauskas, S., Mi, S., Posfai, J., Roberts, R.J., and Wilson, G.G. (1994). The DNA (cytosine-5) methyltransferases. Nucleic Acids Res *22*, 1–10.

Lande-Diner, L., Zhang, J., Ben-Porath, I., Amariglio, N., Keshet, I., Hecht, M., Azuara, V., Fisher, A.G., Rechavi, G., and Cedar, H. (2007). Role of DNA methylation in stable gene repression. J Biol Chem *282*, 12194–12200.

Lehnertz, B., Ueda, Y., Derijck, A.A., Braunschweig, U., Perez-Burgos, L., Kubicek, S., Chen, T., Li, E., Jenuwein, T., and Peters, A.H. (2003). Suv39h-mediated histone H3 lysine 9 methylation directs DNA methylation to major satellite repeats at pericentric heterochromatin. Curr Biol *13*, 1192–1200.

Li, B., Carey, M., and Workman, J.L. (2007). The role of chromatin during transcription. Cell *128*, 707–719.

Li, J.Y., Pu, M.T., Hirasawa, R., Li, B.Z., Huang, Y.N., Zeng, R., Jing, N.H., Chen, T., Li, E., Sasaki, H., and Xu, G.L. (2007). Synergistic function of DNA methyltransferases Dnmt3a and Dnmt3b in the methylation of Oct4 and Nanog. Mol Cell Biol *27*, 8748–8759.

Luger, K., Mader, A.W., Richmond, R.K., Sargent, D.F., and Richmond, T.J. (1997). Crystal structure of the nucleosome core particle at 2.8 A resolution. Nature *389*, 251–260.

Lukasik, S.M., Cierpicki, T., Borloz, M., Grembecka, J., Everett, A., and Bushweller, J.H. (2006). High resolution structure of the HDGF PWWP domain: a potential DNA binding domain. Protein Sci *15*, 314–323.

Malik, S., and Roeder, R.G. (2005). Dynamic regulation of pol II transcription by the mammalian Mediator complex. Trends Biochem Sci *30*, 256–263.

Margot, J.B., Ehrenhofer-Murray, A.E., and Leonhardt, H. (2003). Interactions within the mammalian DNA methyltransferase family. BMC Mol Biol *4*, 7.

Miranda, T.B., and Jones, P.A. (2007). DNA methylation: the nuts and bolts of repression. J Cell Physiol *213*, 384–390.

Mortusewicz, O., Schermelleh, L., Walter, J., Cardoso, M.C., and Leonhardt, H. (2005). Recruitment of DNA methyltransferase I to DNA repair sites. Proc Natl Acad Sci USA *102*, 8905–8909.

Muto, M., Kanari, Y., Kubo, E., Takabe, T., Kurihara, T., Fujimori, A., and Tatsumi, K. (2002). Targeted disruption of Np95 gene renders murine embryonic stem cells hypersensitive to DNA damaging agents and DNA replication blocks. J Biol Chem *277*, 34549–34555.

Okano, M., Bell, D.W., Haber, D.A., and Li, E. (1999). DNA methyltransferases Dnmt3a and Dnmt3b are essential for de novo methylation and mammalian development. Cell *99*, 247–257.

Okano, M., Xie, S., and Li, E. (1998). Dnmt2 is not required for de novo and maintenance methylation of viral DNA in embryonic stem cells. Nucleic Acids Res *26*, 2536–2540.

Ooi, S.K., Qiu, C., Bernstein, E., Li, K., Jia, D., Yang, Z., Erdjument-Bromage, H., Tempst, P., Lin, S.P., Allis, C.D., Cheng, X., and Bestor, T.H. (2007). DNMT3L connects unmethylated lysine 4 of histone H3 to de novo methylation of DNA. Nature *448*, 714–717.

Papait, R., Pistore, C., Negri, D., Pecoraro, D., Cantarini, L., and Bonapace, I.M. (2007). Np95 is implicated in pericentromeric heterochromatin replication and in major satellite silencing. Mol Biol Cell *18*, 1098–1106.

Qiu, C., Sawada, K., Zhang, X., and Cheng, X. (2002). The PWWP domain of mammalian DNA methyltransferase Dnmt3b defines a new family of DNA-binding folds. Nat Struct Biol *9*, 217–224.

Rai, K., Chidester, S., Zavala, C.V., Manos, E.J., James, S.R., Karpf, A.R., Jones, D.A., and Cairns, B.R. (2007). Dnmt2 functions in the cytoplasm to promote liver, brain, and retina development in zebrafish. Genes Dev *21*, 261–266.

Reik, W. (2007). Stability and flexibility of epigenetic gene regulation in mammalian development. Nature *447*, 425–432.

Sandelin, A., Carninci, P., Lenhard, B., Ponjavic, J., Hayashizaki, Y., and Hume, D.A. (2007). Mammalian RNA polymerase II core promoters: insights from genome-wide studies. Nat Rev Genet *8*, 424–436.

Schaefer, C.B., Ooi, S.K., Bestor, T.H., and Bourc'his, D. (2007). Epigenetic decisions in mammalian germ cells. Science *316*, 398–399.

Schilling, E., and Rehli, M. (2007). Global, comparative analysis of tissue-specific promoter CpG methylation. Genomics *90*, 314–323.

Schubert, H.L., Blumenthal, R.M., and Cheng, X. (2003). Many paths to methyltransfer: a chronicle of convergence. Trends Biochem Sci 28, 329–335.

Sharif, J., Muto, M., Takebayashi, S.I., Suetake, I., Iwamatsu, A., Endo, T.A., Shinga, J., Mizutani-Koseki, Y., Toyoda, T., Okamura, K., Tajima, S., Mitsuya, K., Okano, M., and Koseki, H. (2007). The SRA protein Np95 mediates epigenetic inheritance by recruiting Dnmt1 to methylated DNA. Nature 450, 908-912.

Sheikhnejad, G., Brank, A., Christman, J.K., Goddard, A., Alvarez, E., Ford, H., Jr., Marquez, V.E., Marasco, C.J., Sufrin, J.R., O'Gara, M., and Cheng, X. (1999). Mechanism of inhibition of DNA (cytosine C5)-methyltransferases by oligodeoxyribonucleotides containing 5,6-dihydro-5-azacytosine. J Mol Biol 285, 2021–2034.

Shi, Y. (2007). Histone lysine demethylases: emerging roles in development, physiology and disease. Nat Rev Genet 8, 829–833.

Shilatifard, A. (2006). Chromatin modifications by methylation and ubiquitination: implications in the regulation of gene expression. Annu Rev Biochem 75, 243–269.

Suetake, I., Shinozaki, F., Miyagawa, J., Takeshima, H., and Tajima, S. (2004). DNMT3L stimulates the DNA methylation activity of Dnmt3a and Dnmt3b through a direct interaction. J Biol Chem 279, 27816–27823.

Turner, B.M. (2007). Defining an epigenetic code. Nat Cell Biol 9, 2–6.

Unterberger, A., Andrews, S.D., Weaver, I.C., and Szyf, M. (2006). DNA methyltransferase 1 knockdown activates a replication stress checkpoint. Mol Cell Biol 26, 7575–7586.

Vairapandi, M. (2004). Characterization of DNA demethylation in normal and cancerous cell lines and the regulatory role of cell cycle proteins in human DNA demethylase activity. J Cell Biochem 91, 572–583.

Vu, T.H., Li, T., and Hoffman, A.R. (2004). Promoter-restricted histone code, not the differentially methylated DNA regions or antisense transcripts, marks the imprinting status of IGF2R in human and mouse. Hum Mol Genet 13, 2233–2245.

Walsh, C.P., and Xu, G.L. (2006). Cytosine methylation and DNA repair. Curr Top Microbiol Immunol 301, 283–315.

Weber, M., Hellmann, I., Stadler, M.B., Ramos, L., Paabo, S., Rebhan, M., and Schubeler, D. (2007). Distribution, silencing potential and evolutionary impact of promoter DNA methylation in the human genome. Nat Genet 39, 457–466.

Webster, K.E., O'Bryan, M.K., Fletcher, S., Crewther, P.E., Aapola, U., Craig, J., Harrison, D.K., Aung, H., Phutikanit, N., Lyle, R., Meachem, S.J., Antonarakis, S.E., de Kretser, D.M., Hedger, M.P., Peterson, P., Carroll, B.J., and Scott, H.S. (2005). Meiotic and epigenetic defects in Dnmt3L-knockout mouse spermatogenesis. Proc Natl Acad Sci USA 102, 4068–4073.

Wu, J., Wang, S.H., Potter, D., Liu, J.C., Smith, L.T., Wu, Y.Z., Huang, T.H., and Plass, C. (2007). Diverse histone modifications on histone 3 lysine 9 and their relation to DNA methylation in specifying gene silencing. BMC Genomics 8, 131.

Wu, J.C., and Santi, D.V. (1987). Kinetic and catalytic mechanism of HhaI methyltransferase. J Biol Chem 262, 4778–4786.

Xu, G.L., Bestor, T.H., Bourc'his, D., Hsieh, C.L., Tommerup, N., Bugge, M., Hulten, M., Qu, X., Russo, J.J., and Viegas-Pequignot, E. (1999). Chromosome instability and immunodeficiency syndrome caused by mutations in a DNA methyltransferase gene. Nature 402, 187–191.

Yamasaki, Y., Kayashima, T., Soejima, H., Kinoshita, A., Yoshiura, K., Matsumoto, N., Ohta, T., Urano, T., Masuzaki, H., Ishimaru, T., Mukai, T., Niikawa, N., and Kishino, T. (2005). Neuron-specific relaxation of Igf2r imprinting is associated with neuron-specific histone modifications and lack of its antisense transcript Air. Hum Mol Genet 14, 2511–2520.

Yang, X., Smith, S.L., Tian, X.C., Lewin, H.A., Renard, J.P., and Wakayama, T. (2007). Nuclear reprogramming of cloned embryos and its implications for therapeutic cloning. Nat Genet 39, 295–302.

Yen, Z.C., Meyer, I.M., Karalic, S., and Brown, C.J. (2007). A cross-species comparison of X-chromosome inactivation in Eutheria. Genomics 90, 453–463.

Yoder, J.A., and Bestor, T.H. (1998). A candidate mammalian DNA methyltransferase related to pmt1p of fission yeast. Hum Mol Genet *7*, 279–284.

Yoder, J.A., Walsh, C.P., and Bestor, T.H. (1997). Cytosine methylation and the ecology of intragenomic parasites. Trends Genet *13*, 335–340.

Youngblood, B., Shieh, F.K., Buller, F., Bullock, T., and Reich, N.O. (2007). S-adenosyl-L-methionine-dependent methyl transfer: observable precatalytic intermediates during DNA cytosine methylation. Biochemistry *46*, 8766–8775.

Zhang, X., and Bruice, T.C. (2006). The mechanism of M.HhaI DNA C5 cytosine methyltransferase enzyme: a quantum mechanics/molecular mechanics approach. Proc Natl Acad Sci USA *103*, 6148–6153.

Epigenetic Profiling of Histone Variants

Steven Henikoff

Abstract Most histones are assembled into nucleosomes behind the replication fork to package newly synthesized DNA, but some histones are deposited independent of replication. Replication-independent histone variants of H3 and H2A have evolved to participate in gene regulation, transcriptional elongation, chromosome segregation and DNA repair in almost all eukaryotes. Because histone variants are deposited on a chromatinized template, they replace canonical replication-coupled histones in processes that involve partial or complete unravelling of nucleosomes. The recent application of high-resolution profiling to histone variants thus provides a genome-wide view of active processes that disrupt chromatin. Replacement of a canonical histone with a variant can profoundly alter chromatin properties and erase histone modifications. As such, the epigenomic profiling of histone variants and nucleosome positioning reveals both nucleosome dynamics and the basic organization of the epigenome.

Keywords ATP-dependent nucleosome remodelers · DNA microarrays · DNA sequencing · Histone chaperones · Nucleosomes

1 Introduction

The availability of large-scale sequence data, expression maps and functional annotations has resulted in a highly detailed characterization of genes and their expression in many genomes (Bevan et al. 2001; Wolfsberg et al. 2002; Celniker and Rubin 2003; Hillier et al. 2005). However, a description of genic features is insufficient for understanding the regulation of gene expression, especially in the context of development, where the same genomic sequence is responsible for vastly different cellular morphologies and behaviours (Allis et al. 2006). Furthermore, DNA sequence has been surprisingly ineffective in identifying the most basic features of

S. Henikoff (✉)
Howard Hughes Medical Institute, Fred Hutchinson Cancer Research Center, 1100 Fairview Ave. N., Seattle, Washington 98109, USA
e-mail: steveh@fhcrc.org

eukaryotic genomes, including genetic regulatory elements and replication origins (ENCODE 2007).

As a first step in addressing these limitations, a description of the epigenome is needed, namely the mapping of chromosomal proteins and their covalent modifications (Jones and Martienssen 2005). Fortunately, technological advances have more than kept pace with the need for epigenomic tools to provide high resolution maps of chromosomal features genome-wide. Whereas the most important genomic resources were created by large-scale sequencing centers during the genomics era, we are now witnessing a proliferation of powerful technologies that allow individual investigators to collect genome-wide datasets at high resolution. Epigenomic mapping is also cost-effective: whereas the $1000 genome remains a distant goal (Hutchison 2007), the $1000 epigenome for many complex eukaryotes has become a reality, and the cost per base continues to drop.

Unlike the genomic reference sequence for an organism, which is nearly invariant, the epigenome is rather a collection of diverse features that can differ radically between cell types (Jones and Martienssen 2005). The diversity of chromatin features has led to the concern that chromatin might be too complex for its properties to be well understood. For example, there are more possible combinations of histone covalent modifications than there are particles in the visible universe, and even if the effect of modifications is cumulative rather than combinatorial, there are still a very large number of potential chromatin features to catalog (Allis et al. 2006). Other chromatin features might be similarly complex, such as the many different nucleosome remodeling machines, which can have multiple interchangeable subunits (Varga-Weisz 2001). Most complex are the sequence-specific binding proteins, which probably number in the thousands for a multicellular eukaryote, with sometimes hundreds or thousands of genome-wide targets, only a handful of which are well-characterized (Berman et al. 2004). This epigenomic complexity presumably provides a suitably rich regulatory environment for specification of organismal complexity.

2 Chromatin Differentiation by Histone Variants

In contrast to the complexity of the machineries that modify, disrupt, bind to and bind in between nucleosomes, the histones themselves are relatively simple. Octamers consisting of two each of the four core histones, H2A, H2B, H3 and H4 wrap 147 bp of DNA centered around an H3-H3 four-helix bundle (Fig. 1). H3 and H2A have nearly universal variants, two each, and only a handful of clade-specific histone variants are known (Henikoff and Ahmad 2005). The CenH3 variant (CENP-A in mammals, Cse4 in budding yeast and Cid in flies) forms the foundation of centromeres in all eukaryotes examined (Amor et al. 2004), and a universal replacement variant, H3.3, is enriched in active chromatin (Ahmad and Henikoff 2002). H2A variants include H2A.X, which becomes serine-phosphorylated near its C-terminus as a signal to recruit the machinery for homology-based repair of broken DNA (Rogakou et al. 1998), and H2A.Z, whose precise biological function has been

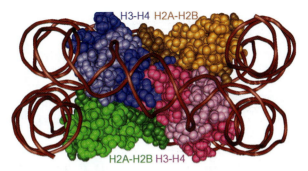

Fig. 1 A view of the nucleosome core particle looking down the pseudo-dyad axis, showing the eight histone-fold domains that comprise the core. Subunits of each heterodimer are differentially shaded. Partial unravelling of the nucleosome is required to release either of the H2A-H2B heterodimers, and much further unravelling would be needed to release an H3-H4 heterodimer. The two halves of the nucleosome are held together by an H3-H3 four-helix bundle (the blue-magenta interface), and a CenH3 hemisome (CenH3-H4-H2A-H2B) is predicted to appoximately align with either half (Dalal et al. 2007a)

a subject of considerable discussion (Henikoff and Ahmad 2005). MacroH2A and H2A[Bbd] are vertebrate-specific forms that have been implicated in gene-regulatory processes (Chadwick and Willard 2001; Angelov et al. 2003), and there are variants of H2A, H2B and H3 that are specialized for packaging sperm and pollen (Ueda et al. 2000; Govin et al. 2007). Variants of the H1 linker histone play roles in vertebrate early development, but because H1 is not a histone-fold protein, and it lies outside of the nucleosomal core, it is best classified together with other linker proteins such as the High Mobility Group (HMG) proteins (Catez et al. 2006).

Histone variants represent the first level of differentiation of chromatin on which all other chromatin-associated processes must act, and so provide a natural starting point for epigenomic profiling studies. This chapter will focus mainly on methods used for profiling histone variants that have been the subject of epigenomic studies (H3.3 and H2A.Z), and will highlight what has been learned about chromatin-associated processes from studying them.

3 Incorporation of Histone Variants into Nucleosomes

3.1 Replication-Coupled Nucleosome Assembly

Most histones are deposited behind the replication fork in a tightly cell-cycle regulated process that packages newly synthesized DNA into nucleosomes (Wolffe 1992) (Fig. 2 left). Pre-existing nucleosomes are retained, while new nucleosomes are deposited in gaps created by the semi-conservative replication of DNA. Despite a large number of studies performed for more than 30 years, there is no compelling evidence that nucleosomal octamers ever split at the H3-H3 dyad axis (Annunziato 2005). Rather, the H3-H4 tetramer is inherited intact and evidently at

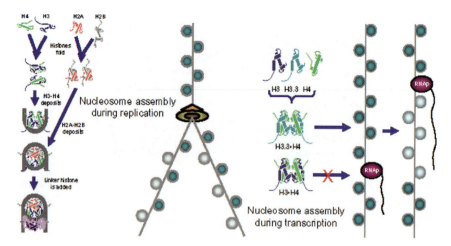

Fig. 2 Schematic diagrams of nucleosome assembly pathways. *Left*: Replication-coupled assembly is a step-wise process in which H3-H4 is first deposited as the DNA wraps around, followed by addition of H2A-H2B above and below the assembled (H3-H4)$_2$ tetramer. Assembly is completed with the addition of a linker histone, such as H1. Center: The result of de novo nucleosome assembly is a mixture of new and old nucleosomes on daughter strands. Right: Replication-independent assembly of H3.3-containing nucleosomes involves the deposition of H3.3-H4, but not H3-H4 during active processes such as transcription

random to either of the two daughter strands (Fig. 2 middle), and new (H3-H4)$_2$ tetramers are assembled by the CAF-1 nucleosome assembly complex (Smith and Stillman 1989). Other chaperones, such as FACT, facilitate the retention of H2A-H2B dimers during transcription (Belotserkovskaya et al. 2003), and new H2A-H2B dimers can be deposited on either old or new (H3-H4)$_2$ tetramers at replication (Jackson 1988).

3.2 Replication-Independent Nucleosome Assembly

In contrast to replication-coupled (RC) processes that assemble the major histones, histone variants are deposited outside of replication (Henikoff and Ahmad 2005) (Fig. 2 right). Deposition of histone variants on already chromatinized templates implies that new variant proteins are either exchanged with their counterparts in nucleosome cores or nucleosomes are first evicted and new nucleosomes deposited de novo. Either way, nucleosomes are unraveled, either partially to incorporate new H2A and H2B or almost completely to incorporate new H3 and H4 (see Fig. 1). Spontaneous unwrapping of nucleosomes in vivo is thought to allow for transient exposure of sequences (Polach and Widom 1995), and occasionally this process may result in exchange of H2A-H2B dimers (Thiriet and Hayes 2005). However, distinct ATP-driven processes are found to underlie the replacement of histones incorporated during replication with histone variants, as described below.

Upon synthesis, histones fold together as dimeric units of H2A-H2B and H3-H4 and associate with 'escort' proteins that have acidic patches to neutralize the highly basic charge of histones (Loyola and Almouzni 2004). For example, free H2A-H2B dimers are often associated with the NAP-1 protein, which *in vitro* can facilitate their exchange with H2A-H2B dimers present in nucleosomes (Park et al. 2005). Likewise, H3-H4 dimers are typically associated with the Asf1 protein in vivo (Loyola and Almouzni 2004). Asf1 is thought to present dimers to CAF-1 and other histone chaperones for rapid assembly into nucleosomes. Asf1 has also been shown to play an active role in nucleosome assembly and disassembly, because it can facilitate the formation or disassociation of $(H3-H4)_2$ tetramers (Adkins et al. 2004; English et al. 2006). These escort proteins do not discriminate between histone variants: NAP-1 has been found to be associated with H2A.Z-H2B and Asf1 with H3.3-H4 in vivo (Mizuguchi et al. 2004; Tagami et al. 2004). Rather, distinct complexes are found to discriminate between replication-independent (RI) variants and facilitate their incorporation in vivo.

3.3 Variant-Specific Assembly Complexes

Incorporation of H2A.Z-H2B dimers is catalyzed by the Swr1 SWI/SNF ATPase, which uses the energy of ATP hydrolysis to remove H2A-H2B and replace it with H2A.Z-H2B (Mizuguchi et al. 2004). In vivo, the soluble form of Swr1 is part of a large complex with some components that are shared with other SWI/SNF ATPases and that are conserved in evolution. H3.3-H4 dimers are assembled into nucleosomes by the HIRA assembly complex (Tagami et al. 2004), which includes Asf1, and this process is facilitated by the CHD1 ATP-dependent nucleosome remodeling protein (Konev et al. 2007). *Drosophila* CenH3-H4 dimers are not associated with Asf-1 in vivo, but rather with the RbAp48 chaperone protein (Furuyama et al. 2006), a highly abundant WD-40 protein that is also a stoichiometric component of the CAF-1 and HIRA complexes (Tagami et al. 2004). RbAp48 is necessary for replication-independent (RI) centromere assembly in *Schizosaccharomyces pombe* and human cells (Hayashi et al. 2004), and *Drosophila* RbAp48 (NURF p55) can assemble either H3-H4 or CenH3-H4 into nucleosome particles (Furuyama et al. 2006). CenH3 is packaged into 'hemisomes' of CenH3, H4, H2A and H2B (Dalal et al. 2007b), which implies that RbAp48 performs only one round of dimer assembly, in contrast to CAF-1/Asf1 which would need to perform two successive rounds to assemble new histone octamers (Loyola and Almouzni 2004).

The dynamics of histone replacement is not well understood. Repair of DNA damage is followed by CAF-1-mediated replacement with H3-H4 (Polo et al. 2006). The entire nucleosome might be replaced, because unravelling of the DNA gyres just beyond the dyad axis to release half of a nucleosome would be expected to destabilize the entire particle (See Fig. 1). Still, it is possible that nucleosomes are transiently split for replacement, perhaps with the involvement of Asf1 in 'prying' apart half-tetramers of $(H3-H4)_2$ in vitro (English et al. 2006; Natsume et al. 2007). There is similar uncertainty about the process of histone replacement during transcriptional elongation, which results in the deposition of H3.3-H4. It is not known whether histones are replaced a dimer at a time or involve eviction followed by immediate replacement.

Histone variants are mostly non-randomly distributed in the genome, and the basis for their localization remains unknown. The most distinctly localized variant is CenH3, which is confined to a single restricted location on each chromosome, and mislocalization causes neocentromere formation in *Drosophila* (Heun et al. 2006; Moreno-Moreno et al. 2006). Although it has been generally assumed that CenH3s are actively targeted to centromeres, there does not appear to be any specific DNA sequence requirements for localization (Warburton 2004), except for budding yeast. Alternatively, CenH3s might be promiscuously deposited and evicted from non-centromeric regions, and the utilization of the non-specific RbAp48 chaperone is consistent with this scenario (Furuyama et al. 2006). It is also unclear what causes the SWR1 complex to deposit H2A.Z to particular sites, or why H3.3 is localized to regions of active chromatin. In order to help understand the basis for localization and in vivo functions of histone variants, it is important to map their positions at high resolution in the genome.

4 Technologies for Profiling Histone Variants

The recent explosion of powerful epigenomic technologies have begun to be applied to histone variants. Landscapes for both H2A.Z and H3.3 have been determined in some organisms and compared with genetic landmarks and other chromatin-based patterns (Mito et al. 2005; Raisner et al. 2005; Albert et al. 2007; Barski et al. 2007; Mito et al. 2007). Both microarray-based and sequence-based approaches have been applied.

4.1 Microarray-Based Methods

The popularity of transcriptional profiling and single-nucleotide polymorphism genotyping on microarrays for the past decade has sparked the strong demand for better and denser array platforms (Hoheisel et al. 2006). Chips with enough probes to cover a transcriptome became common, and these high-density arrays could also be applied to large segments of genomes. Meanwhile, techniques that allowed for profiling of epigenomes began to appear in 2000 (van Steensel 2005). In the most common application, antibodies are used to separate chromatin that carries an epitope of interest, and the DNA is extracted, labeled and hybridized to microarrays (chromatin immunoprecipitation on a chip, or ChIP-chip) (Ren et al. 2000; Iyer et al. 2001). In DamID, a chimeric protein consisting of a chromatin protein of interest is fused to the *Escherichia coli* Dam DNA methyltransferase, which preferentially methylates DNA in its vicinity, and methylated DNA is targeted for enrichment by the use of modification-specific restriction enzymes (van Steensel et al. 2001). In the case of histone variants, chromatin affinity purification has been the preferred method, either by ChIP-chip (Raisner et al. 2005) or by using streptavidin to purify biotinylated histones (Mito et al. 2005). When coupled with high-density microarrays that tile large portions of the genome, these methods have provided some of our first glimpses into epigenomic landscapes.

4.2 Sequence-Based Methods

Affinity capture also lends itself to sequence-based approaches. Sequence-based transcriptional profiling began with concatemerized tags in the Serial Analysis of Gene Expression (SAGE) method (Velculescu et al. 1995), and this approach was later applied to chromatin subject to affinity capture (ChIP-seq) (Roh et al. 2004; Albert et al. 2007a; Robertson et al. 2007). An advantage of ChIP-seq is that counts of tags provide an absolute measure, as opposed to a ratio of pulled-down to input chromatin that is typically obtained using microarrays. In addition, sequence-based chromatin profiling does not require any prior choice, or even prior knowledge of genomic landmarks of interest because the tags themselves can provide that information, whereas the tiling of microarrays limits the portion of the genome that can be assayed. The expense of Sanger sequencing has been a serious limitation to the application of ChIP-seq, but with the recent availability of massively parallel sequencing technologies, this approach is becoming increasing popular (See Chapters "Strategies for Epigenome Analysis" and "Sequencing the Epigenome"). Unlike Sanger sequencing, in which polymerase addition products are resolved by size on gels or capillaries, these new sequencing methods perform single addition reactions on immobilized templates in parallel on the surface of a flow cell, and record the addition after each cycle. Both the 454 and Illumina Solexa machines have been applied to ChIP-seq of histone variants, with impressive results. The Solexa platform is especially well-suited to ChIP-seq, because it provides several millions of short mappable sequences, corresponding to multiple rounds of single-base addition by a DNA polymerase, at a cost that is comparable to the cost of a DNA microarray (Barski et al. 2007; Mikkelsen et al. 2007; Robertson et al. 2007). Sequencing-by-synthesis using 454, Solexa, ABI Solid (which performs additions using a DNA ligase), Helicos Heliscope and perhaps other technologies, are likely to become the platforms of choice for many chromatin profiling studies in the near future.

4.3 Which Method to Use?

Current microarray-based and sequence-based readouts are competitive for genome-wide profiling, but which to choose currently depends on the density of features being profiled. For example, each of the eight lanes of a Solexa flow cell can provide ~5 million mappable reads for ~$1000, which is the same approximate cost of a NimbleGen tiling array with 2.1 million 60 mer probes. Both are highly suitable for genome-wide chromatin profiling, but there are trade-offs. Consider a situation in which there are 10,000 sites throughout the genome, such as sites of transcription factor binding (Robertson et al. 2007). In this application, $1000 buys an average of 500 tags per site, which is more than enough to provide a quantitative map of factor binding that is limited in resolution only by the average size of fragments pulled down by the antibody. In practice the two approaches appear to yield comparable transcription factor profiles that provide technical validation of the alternative technologies (Robertson et al. 2007). The Solexa system also has the potential for 'barcoding' libraries, in which the first few rounds of sequencing-by-synthesis read off the identifier code for an individual, engineered during library preparation. By pooling barcoded libraries from multiple individuals, a single run can provide multiple profiles. ChIP-seq using sequencing-by-synthesis technologies is so new that it is difficult to judge how soon they will become as routine as ChIP-chip is now, but at least for mapping transcription factor binding sites, it appears that they have the edge.

Now consider a situation in which a chromatin feature occupies a large percentage of the genome. Nucleosomes are extreme examples, insofar as they package the entire genome, separated only by short linkers. The high abundance of nucleosome variants, in excess of 10% of the genome, means that it is not appropriate to think of variant profiles in terms of discrete sites, but rather broad landscapes, and the same goes for abundant histone modifications and DNA methylation. The high abundance and broad distribution of nucleosomes means that unlike transcription factors, an accurate map of nucleosomal features will require deep coverage of the entire single-copy genome in order to get quantitative data. In this case, the 2.1 million probes on the NimbleGen array, each able to provide a quantitative readout of nucleosome density, seems to have an advantage over the 5 million Solexa tags, which would be spread too thinly to provide robust statistics of nucleosome density. For example, the single-copy human genome ($\sim$1500 Mb) can be tiled at 700-bp resolution with 2.1 million 60mers, each of which provides a quantitative measure of hybridized fragments that averages over 3–4 nucleosomes, and a $\sim$100 Mb genome, such as those of *Drosophila*, *Caenorhabditis elegans* or *Arabidopsis* can be tiled with three probes per nucleosome, enough to provide single-nucleosome resolution. A Solexa lane devoted to a shotgun library would provide on average one read per 600 bp for the 3-Mb human genome and about one read per 30 bp for the model organism genomes. Converting counts of sequence reads to a quantitative measure requires a sufficient number of reads for robust statistics, and even averaging over a few nucleosomes will not provide that for the human genome, and for model genomes, the coverage is marginal. Therefore it seems that current microarrays have advantages over current deep sequencing platforms for variant profiling, and it is likely that both will be used in combination to obtain the most informative data for the near future.

An especially exciting recent development is the introduction of microarray capture strategies, in which genomic libraries are reduced in complexity by hybridization to programmable microarrays, followed by high-throughput sequencing (Albert et al. 2007b; Hodges et al. 2007; Okou et al. 2007). In this way, deeper sequence coverage can be obtained for genomic regions of interest, which greatly increases the potential of deep sequencing for routine profiling applications. For example, deep coverage of a ChIP-seq library derived from H2A.Z nucleosomes provided basepair resolution mapping of nucleosome positions, thus allowing for precise 'rotational' positioning of the H2A.Z nucleosome core particle (Albert et al. 2007a).

5 Profiling of H3 Variants

5.1 CenH3

The presence of highly repetitive satellite DNA sequences at the centromeres of most eukaryotes has thus far limited profiling of CenH3 to centromeres that lack repeats. In the case of budding yeast, single-nucleosome mapping indicates that there is only one CenH3 nucleosome at the genetically defined centromere (Furuyama and Biggins 2007). The 125-bp size of the functional yeast centromere, of which only the ∼80-bp CDE II region is available for CenH3 binding, is consistent with the presence of a single hemisome at the yeast centromere (Dalal et al. 2007a). Satellite repeats are absent on some spontaneously appearing human neocentromeres that maintain otherwise acentric fragments, which has allowed human CENP-A to be mapped by ChIP (Saffery et al. 2003; Alonso et al. 2007). Rice CenH3 has also been profiled at low resolution at the native centromere Chromosome 8 (cen8), which almost completely lacks satellite repeats (Nagaki et al. 2004). In these studies, arrays of CenH3 were found in the vicinity of active genes, although in the case of rice cen8, CenH3 is most abundant in gene-poor regions (Yan et al. 2005).

5.2 H3.3

Only four amino acid residues distinguish H3.3 from H3, of which the three that specify RI versus RC assembly are buried within the nucleosome (Ahmad and Henikoff 2002). As a result, there have been few antibodies that can distinguish the two forms, and nearly all studies on H3.3 properties have utilized chimeric proteins produced transgenically. To deal with this challenge, we have adopted a biotin-tagging approach, in which a 23-amino acid tag that was selected to be an excellent substrate for *E. coli* biotin ligase (BirA) is encoded at the N-terminus of the chromatin protein (de Boer et al. 2003). When both a tagged histone and BirA are produced in the same cell, the tag gets biotinylated and incorporated into chromatin, allowing for the extraordinarily high affinity of streptavidin for biotin to be used to pull down chromatin (Mito et al. 2005). Affinity capture is quantitative, so that there is essentially no risk of fractionation, which can complicate ChIP-based methods. Yields are very high using this method following the preparation of chromatin using a standard procedure of micrococcal nuclease digestion down to mostly mononucleosomes to solubilize chromatin and fragment the DNA. As a result, DNA extracted from affinity-purified chromatin can be labelled without the need for amplification.

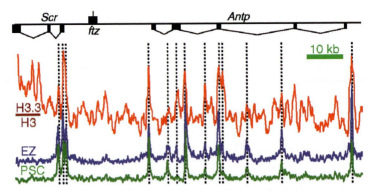

Fig. 3 Profile of histone replacement at the Antennapedia Complex (ANTP-C) in Drosophila S2 cells (Mito et al. 2007). Genes in the ANTP-C are regulated by proteins in the Polycomb and trithorax Groups. Histone replacement (H3.3/H3) profiles are shown in red. Chip-chip profiles of Polycomb Group protein for Enhancer-of-zeste (EZ, blue curve), and Posterior-sex-combs (PSC, green curve) (Schwartz et al. 2006) correspond to sharp local peaks of histone replacement (red curve). Reproduced from (Mito et al. 2007) with permission

Our application of this method to H3.3 and H3 to *Drosophila* S2 cells genome-wide has revealed characteristic H3.3 enrichment profiles for active genes, nucleosome depletion over promoters and conspicuous peaks of H3.3 enrichment over sites of binding of Polycomb Group and trithorax-Group proteins, which act at distinct sites to maintain developmental programs (Mito et al. 2005; Mito et al. 2007) (Fig. 3). H3.3 has also been found to be an essential component of epigenetic memory during early frog development (Ng and Gurdon 2008). The evident involvement of H3.3 in basic mechanisms that underlie epigenetic inheritance during development means that profiling of H3.3 deposition might provide a general map of epigenetic regulatory elements important for gene regulation.

5.3 Histone Turnover

Histone variant profiling using tags can potentially provide insights into histone dynamics, because incorporation of a variant requires nucleosome unraveling and replacement of endogenous histones with the tagged version. In the case of H3.3 profiling, the time-scale of incorporation was on the order of a day or so, which was insufficient to reveal replacement kinetics, but rather provided a snapshot of histone replacement in dividing cells (Mito et al. 2005). Nevertheless, the interpretation of the histone replacement process as revealing chromatin dynamics was strongly supported by studies in budding yeast, in which alternatively tagged versions of H3 were produced constitutively and in a pulse, and the ratio of the two tags used to calculate turnover rates (Dion et al. 2007; Jamai et al. 2007; Rufiange et al. 2007). Histone turnover was high in genetic regulatory elements, including promoters and boundaries (Dion et al. 2007). Because yeast have only one form of H3, and it is the ortholog of H3.3 (Ahmad and Henikoff 2002), the close correspondence between results of profiling H3.3 in *Drosophila* and H3 turnover in yeast indicates the action of a general process of histone replacement at epigenetic regulatory elements.

The realization that histones are replaced during the course of the cell cycle, and that high levels of turnover occur at regulatory regions, raises questions about the interpretation of histone modifications as static 'marks'. Histone modifications associated with active chromatin are turning over with their substrates and so intermediate forms will be lost (Dion et al. 2007). Therefore, for a full understanding of the epigenome, we will need to explore how it changes over time, a challenge for future epigenetic profiling efforts.

6 Profiling of H2A Variants

6.1 H2A.Z

H2A.Z is essential in animals, but not in yeast, a situation that has allowed the powerful tools of yeast genetics to be applied to its study. H2A.Z has been examined in yeast using both ChIP-chip and ChIP-seq (Raisner et al. 2005; Zhang et al. 2005; Albert et al. 2007a). These studies have revealed a remarkably stereotypic distribution of H2A.Z, in which nearly all genes show H2A.Z primarily localized over the first nucleosome downstream of the transcriptional start site (TSS), and a large fraction of genes also show just H2A.Z upstream of the TSS (Fig. 4). Because the TSS is in a region that appears to be free of nucleosomes, the flanking H2A.Z nucleosomes would seem to define the chromatin landscape of promoters (Fig. 4A–B). A ChIP-seq study of human H2A.Z chromatin shows a similar average profile (Barski et al. 2007) (Fig. 4C), which implies that H2A.Z plays a conserved role in defining the promoter landscape.

Although the localization of H2A.Z is intriguing, the non-essentiality of the variant in yeast (Santisteban et al. 2000) indicates that its function is unlike that of transcription factors, which specify and regulate promoter identity. Rather H2A.Z would seem to play a role in maintaining chromatin around promoters. Earlier work in yeast demonstrated that H2A.Z chromatin has properties of an insulator (Meneghini et al. 2003), and a comparable function at promoters would help to maintain their robustness, although the mechanism whereby H2A.Z nucleosomes insulate is unknown.

Whereas studies of H2A.Z in vertebrates suggest that nucleosomes that contain this variant are inherently more stable than those with H2A (Park et al. 2004), studies of yeast H2A.Z nucleosomes have led to the opposite conclusion (Zhang et al. 2005). An attractive resolution of this enigma is that nucleosome core particles containing both H2A.Z and H3.3 are unstable relative to those containing H2A and H3.3 (Jin and Felsenfeld 2007). Indeed there appears to be a hierarchy of nucleosome stability, with H2A.Z destabilizing H3.3-containing tetramers and stabilizing H3-containing tetramers. Because yeast H3 is actually an H3.3 (Malik and Henikoff 2003), yeast nucleosomes would be destabilized by H2A.Z, whereas studies in vertebrates were performed with the major H3 form. Just what properties

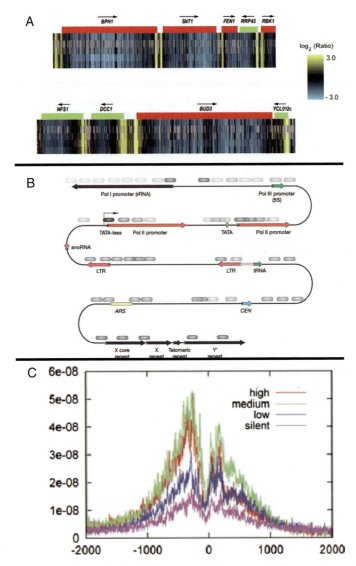

Fig. 4 H2A.Z nucleosome profiles in budding yeast and human cells illustrate the excellent correspondence between H2A.Z patterns around transcriptional start sites between yeast and humans and between ChIP-chip and ChIP-seq. (**A**) Heat map representation of H2A.Z densities in two representative regions of the yeast genome, where yellow represents enrichment and blue represents depletion relative to the genome-wide median using ChIP-chip (Raisner et al. 2005). (**B**) Generalized schematic summary of H2A.Z nucleosome positions using ChIP-seq, where the darkness of the ovals represents the relative level of H2A.Z (Albert et al. 2007a). (**C**) Genome-wide average profiles of H2A.Z nucleosomes aligned around transcription start sites (0 on the x-axis) in human T-cells using ChIP-seq, showing that highly expressed genes display the most conspicuous average pattern, although even silent genes show enrichment both upstream and downstream of transcriptional start sites. (Barski et al. 2007). Reproduced from (Raisner et al. 2005), (Albert et al. 2007a) and (Barski et al. 2007) with permission

of H3.3 nucleosomes makes them behave differently in vitro (Okuwaki et al. 2005; Jin and Felsenfeld 2007; Sun et al. 2007) and in vivo (Jin and Felsenfeld 2006; Ng and Gurdon 2008) is unknown; however active chromatin is specifically enriched in H3.3 that is phosphorylated on serine-28 (Sun et al. 2007). This modification would presumably interfere with the methylation of lysine-27, a key modification that is thought to help stabilize epigenetically silent chromatin (Cao et al. 2002; Bernstein et al. 2006).

6.2 Other H2A Variants

Vertebrate-specific histone variants are particularly interesting candidates for epigenomic profiling. Cytogenetic studies have revealed that macroH2A is enriched and H2A^{Bbd} is depleted from the inactivated mammalian X chromosome (Chadwick and Willard 2001, 2004). Both variants have distinct structural features. The macroH2A histone-fold domain is attached to a globular domain that binds an ADP-ribose metabolite (Kustatscher et al. 2005). Fine-structure cytological analysis shows that macroH2A binds to a subset of facultative heterochromatin on the inactive X chromosome. H2A^{Bbd} nucleosomes are structurally distinct from bulk nucleosomes in that they protect less DNA from nuclease digestion (Bao et al. 2004), and they facilitate the assembly and disassembly of core particles, especially those containing H3.3 (Okuwaki et al. 2005). As for H2A.X, its distribution is expected to be highly uniform, insofar as its role in DNA break repair would require it to be near to sites of DNA damage, that is, the entire genome (Malik and Henikoff 2003).

7 The Epigenomics Era

Ever since the completion of the draft human genome sequence in 2001, it has become common to refer to the beginning of the 21st century as marking the start of the 'post-genomic era' (Janitz 2007). However, like the term 'post-modernism', post-genomics is a conceptually vacuous term that leaves no room for naming the era that would presumably follow it. Fortunately, recent technological developments in genomics and progress in understanding epigenetic mechanisms have ushered in the 'epigenomics era', wherein new tools and strategies allow us to probe gene and chromosomal regulatory processes on a genomic scale.

Unlike the genomics era, where completion of the human genome sequence represented a clear goal, there is no single epigenome around which the troops can rally. Rather, we are presented with many epigenomes that differ from tissue to tissue, from cell to cell and perhaps from moment to moment. But the complexities of the epigenomic landscape evolved from common conserved components, and we can take advantage of this conservation in choosing what features of the landscape to examine. In this regard, histone variants represent a first level of differentiation of chromatin, with only a handful of players that are nearly universal among eukaryotes. As described in this chapter, histone variants are amenable to genome-wide profiling using increasingly powerful technologies. Better understanding of the processes responsible for the histone variant landscape and the relationship between variants, transcription factors, DNA methylation and histone modifications will put us in a better position to exploit this knowledge to improve the human condition.

Acknowledgments I thank past and present members of my laboratory for stimulating discussions and experiments that have made the study of histone variants so much fun.

References

Adkins, M.W., Howar, S.R., and Tyler, J.K. 2004. Chromatin disassembly mediated by the histone chaperone Asf1 is essential for transcriptional activation of the yeast PHO5 and PHO8 genes. Mol Cell **14**: 657–666.

Ahmad, K. and Henikoff, S. 2002. The histone variant H3.3 marks active chromatin by replication-independent nucleosome assembly. Mol Cell **9**: 1191–1200.

Albert, I., Mavrich, T.N., Tomsho, L.P., Qi, J., Zanton, S.J., Schuster, S.C., and Pugh, B.F. 2007a. Translational and rotational settings of H2A.Z nucleosomes across the Saccharomyces cerevisiae genome. Nature **446**: 572–576.

Albert, T.J., Molla, M.N., Muzny, D.M., Nazareth, L., Wheeler, D., Song, X., Richmond, T.A., Middle, C.M., Rodesch, M.J., Packard, C.J., Weinstock, G.M., and Gibbs, R.A. 2007b. Direct selection of human genomic loci by microarray hybridization. Nat Methods **4**: 903–905.

Allis, C.D., Jenuwein, T., and Reinberg, D. 2006. Epigenetics. Cold Spring Harbor Laboratory Press, Cold Spring Harbor.

Alonso, A., Fritz, B., Hasson, D., Abrusan, G., Cheung, F., Yoda, K., Radlwimmer, B., Ladurner, A.G., and Warburton, P.E. 2007. Co-localization of CENP-C and CENP-H to discontinuous domains of CENP-A chromatin at human neocentromeres. Genome Biol **8**: R148.

Amor, D.J., Kalitsis, P., Sumer, H., and Choo, K.H. 2004. Building the centromere: from foundation proteins to 3D organization. Trends Cell Biol **14**: 359–368.

Angelov, D., Molla, A., Perche, P.Y., Hans, F., Cote, J., Khochbin, S., Bouvet, P., and Dimitrov, S. 2003. The histone variant macroH2A interferes with transcription factor binding and SWI/SNF nucleosome remodeling. Mol Cell **11**: 1033–1041.

Annunziato, A.T. 2005. Split decision: What happens to nucleosomes during DNA replication? J Biol Chem **280**: 12065–12068.

Bao, Y., Konesky, K., Park, Y.J., Rosu, S., Dyer, P.N., Rangasamy, D., Tremethick, D.J., Laybourn, P.J., and Luger, K. 2004. Nucleosomes containing the histone variant H2A.Bbd organize only 118 base pairs of DNA. Embo J **23**: 3314–3324.

Barski, A., Cuddapah, S., Cui, K., Roh, T.Y., Schones, D.E., Wang, Z., Wei, G., Chepelev, I., and Zhao, K. 2007. High-resolution profiling of histone methylations in the human genome. Cell **129**: 823–837.

Belotserkovskaya, R., Oh, S., Bondarenko, V.A., Orphanides, G., Studitsky, V.M., and Reinberg, D. 2003. FACT facilitates transcription-dependent nucleosome alteration. Science **301**: 1090–1093.

Berman, B.P., Pfeiffer, B.D., Laverty, T.R., Salzberg, S.L., Rubin, G.M., Eisen, M.B., and Celniker, S.E. 2004. Computational identification of developmental enhancers: conservation and function of transcription factor binding-site clusters in Drosophila melanogaster and Drosophila pseudoobscura. Genome Biol **5**: R61.

Bernstein, B.E., Mikkelsen, T.S., Xie, X., Kamal, M., Huebert, D.J., Cuff, J., Fry, B., Meissner, A., Wernig, M., Plath, K., Jaenisch, R., Wagschal, A., Feil, R., Schreiber, S.L., and Lander, E.S.

2006. A bivalent chromatin structure marks key developmental genes in embryonic stem cells. Cell **125**: 315–326.
Bevan, M., Mayer, K., White, O., Eisen, J.A., Preuss, D., Bureau, T., Salzberg, S.L., and Mewes, H.-W. 2001. Sequence and analysis of the Arabidopsis genome. Current Opinions in Plant Biology **4**: 105–110.
Cao, R., Wang, L., Wang, H., Xia, L., Erdjument-Bromage, H., Tempst, P., Jones, R.S., and Zhang, Y. 2002. Role of histone H3 lysine 27 methylation in Polycomb-group silencing. Science **298**: 1039–1043.
Catez, F., Ueda, T., and Bustin, M. 2006. Determinants of histone H1 mobility and chromatin binding in living cells. Nat Struct Mol Biol **13**: 305–310.
Celniker, S.E. and Rubin, G.M. 2003. The Drosophila melanogaster genome. Annu Rev Genomics Hum Genet **4**: 89–117.
Chadwick, B.P. and Willard, H.F. 2001. A novel chromatin protein, distantly related to histone H2A, is largely excluded from the inactive X chromosome. J Cell Biol **152**: 375–384.
Chadwick, B.P. and Willard, H.F. 2004. Multiple spatially distinct types of facultative heterochromatin on the human inactive X chromosome. Proc Natl Acad Sci USA **101**: 17450–17455.
Dalal, Y., Furuyama, T., Vermaak, D., and Henikoff, S. 2007a. Structure, dynamics, and evolution of centromeric nucleosomes. Proc Natl Acad Sci USA **104**: 15974–15981.
Dalal, Y., Wang, H., Lindsay, S., and Henikoff, S. 2007b. Tetrameric structure of centromeric nucleosomes in Drosophila cells. PLoS Biol **5**: e218.
de Boer, E., Rodriguez, P., Bonte, E., Krijgsveld, J., Katsantoni, E., Heck, A., Grosveld, F., and Strouboulis, J. 2003. Efficient biotinylation and single-step purification of tagged transcription factors in mammalian cells and transgenic mice. Proc Natl Acad Sci USA **100**: 7480–7485.
Dion, M., Kaplan, T., Friedman, N., and Rando, O.J. 2007. Dynamics of replication-independent histone turnover in budding yeast. Science **315**: 1405–1408.
ENCODE project consortium et al. 2007. Identification and analysis of functional elements in 1% of the human genome by the ENCODE pilot project. Nature **447**: 799–816.
English, C.M., Adkins, M.W., Carson, J.J., Churchill, M.E., and Tyler, J.K. 2006. Structural basis for the histone chaperone activity of Asf1. Cell **127**: 495–508.
Furuyama, S. and Biggins, S. 2007. Centromere identity is specified by a single centromeric nucleosome in budding yeast. Proc Natl Acad Sci USA **104**: 14706–14711.
Furuyama, T., Dalal, Y., and Henikoff, S. 2006. Chaperone-mediated assembly of centromeric chromatin in vitro. Proc Natl Acad Sci U S A **103**: 6172–6177.
Govin, J., Escoffier, E., Rousseaux, S., Kuhn, L., Ferro, M., Thevenon, J., Catena, R., Davidson, I., Garin, J., Khochbin, S., and Caron, C. 2007. Pericentric heterochromatin reprogramming by new histone variants during mouse spermiogenesis. J Cell Biol **176**: 283–294.
Hayashi, T., Fujita, Y., Iwasaki, O., Adachi, Y., Takahashi, K., and Yanagida, M. 2004. Mis16 and Mis18 are required for CENP-A loading and histone deacetylation at centromeres. Cell **118**: 715–729.
Henikoff, S. and Ahmad, K. 2005. Assembly of variant histones into chromatin. Ann Rev Cell Dev Biol **21**: 133–153.
Heun, P., Erhardt, S., Blower, M.D., Weiss, S., Skora, A.D., and Karpen, G.H. 2006. Mislocalization of the Drosophila centromere-specific histone CID promotes formation of functional ectopic kinetochores. Dev Cell **10**: 303–315.
Hillier, L.W., Coulson, A., Murray, J.I., Bao, Z., Sulston, J.E., and Waterston, R.H. 2005. Genomics in C. elegans: so many genes, such a little worm. Genome Res **15**: 1651–1660.
Hodges, E., Xuan, Z., Balija, V., Kramer, M., Molla, M.N., Smith, S.W., Middle, C.M., Rodesch, M.J., Albert, T.J., Hannon, G.J., and McCombie, W.R. 2007. Genome-wide in situ exon capture for selective resequencing. Nat Genet **39**: 1522–1527.
Hoheisel, J.D. 2006. Microarray technology: beyond transcript profiling and genotype analysis. Nat Rev Genet **7**: 200–210.
Hutchison, C.A., 3rd. 2007. DNA sequencing: bench to bedside and beyond. Nucleic Acids Res **35**: 6227–6237.

Iyer, V.R., Horak, C.E., Scafe, C.S., Botstein, D., Snyder, M., and Brown, P.O. 2001. Genomic binding sites of the yeast cell-cycle transcription factors SBF and MBF. Nature **409**: 533–538.

Jackson, V. 1988. Deposition of newly synthesized histones: hybrid nucleosomes are not tandemly arranged on daughter DNA strands. Biochemistry (Mosc) **27**: 2109–2120.

Jamai, A., Imoberdorf, R.M., and Strubin, M. 2007. Continuous histone H2B and transcription-dependent histone H3 exchange in yeast cells outside of replication. Mol Cell **25**: 345–355.

Janitz, M. 2007. Assigning functions to genes–the main challenge of the post-genomics era. Rev Physiol Biochem Pharmacol **159**: 115–129.

Jin, C. and Felsenfeld, G. 2006. Distribution of histone H3.3 in hematopoietic cell lineages. Proc Natl Acad Sci U S A **103**: 574–579.

Jin, C. and Felsenfeld, G. 2007. Nucleosome stability mediated by histone variants H3.3 and H2A.Z. Genes Dev **21**: 1519–1529.

Jones, P.A. and Martienssen, R. 2005. A blueprint for a Human Epigenome Project: the AACR Human Epigenome Workshop. Cancer Res **65**: 11241–11246.

Konev, A.Y., Tribus, M., Park, S.Y., Podhraski, V., Lim, C.Y., Emelyanov, A.V., Vershilova, E., Pirrotta, V., Kadonaga, J.T., Lusser, A., and Fyodorov, D.V. 2007. CHD1 motor protein is required for deposition of histone variant H3.3 into chromatin in vivo. Science **317**: 1087–1090.

Kustatscher, G., Hothorn, M., Pugieux, C., Scheffzek, K., and Ladurner, A.G. 2005. Splicing regulates NAD metabolite binding to histone macroH2A. Nat Struct Mol Biol **12**: 624–625.

Loyola, A. and Almouzni, G. 2004. Histone chaperones, a supporting role in the limelight. Biochim Biophys Acta **1677**: 3–11.

Malik, H.S. and Henikoff, S. 2003. Phylogenomics of the nucleosome. Nat Struct Biol **10**: 882–891.

Meneghini, M.D., Wu, M., and Madhani, H.D. 2003. Conserved histone variant H2A.Z protects euchromatin from the ectopic spread of silent chromatin. Cell **112**: 725–736.

Mikkelsen, T.S., Ku, M., Jaffe, D.B., Issac, B., Lieberman, E., Giannoukos, G., Alvarez, P., Brockman, W., Kim, T.K., Koche, R.P., Lee, W., Mendenhall, E., O'Donovan, A., Presser, A., Russ, C., Xie, X., Meissner, A., Wernig, M., Jaenisch, R., Nusbaum, C., Lander, E.S., and Bernstein, B.E. 2007. Genome-wide maps of chromatin state in pluripotent and lineage-committed cells. Nature **448**: 553–560.

Mito, Y., Henikoff, J., and Henikoff, S. 2005. Genome-scale profiling of histone H3.3 replacement patterns. Nat Genet **37**: 1090–1097.

Mito, Y., Henikoff, J., and Henikoff, S. 2007. Histone replacement marks the boundaries of cis-regulatory domains. Science **315**: 1408–1411.

Mizuguchi, G., Shen, X., Landry, J., Wu, W.H., Sen, S., and Wu, C. 2004. ATP-driven exchange of histone H2AZ variant catalyzed by SWR1 chromatin remodeling complex. Science **303**: 343–348.

Moreno-Moreno, O., Torras-Llort, M., and Azorin, F. 2006. Proteolysis restricts localization of CID, the centromere-specific histone H3 variant of Drosophila, to centromeres. Nucleic Acids Res **34**: 6247–6255.

Nagaki, K., Cheng, Z., Ouyang, S., Talbert, P.B., Kim, M., Jones, K.M., Henikoff, S., Buell, C.R., and Jiang, J. 2004. Sequencing of a rice centromere uncovers active genes. Nat Genet **36**: 138–145.

Natsume, R., Eitoku, M., Akai, Y., Sano, N., Horikoshi, M., and Senda, T. 2007. Structure and function of the histone chaperone CIA/ASF1 complexed with histones H3 and H4. Nature **446**: 338–341.

Ng, R.K. and Gurdon, J.B. 2008. Epigenetic memory of an active gene state depends on histone H3.3 incorporation into chromatin in the absence of transcription. Nat Cell Biol **10**: 102–109.

Okou, D.T., Steinberg, K.M., Middle, C., Cutler, D.J., Albert, T.J., and Zwick, M.E. 2007. Microarray-based genomic selection for high-throughput resequencing. Nat Methods **4**: 907–909

Okuwaki, M., Kato, K., Shimahara, H., Tate, S., and Nagata, K. 2005. Assembly and disassembly of nucleosome core particles containing histone variants by human nucleosome assembly protein I. Mol Cell Biol **25**: 10639–10651.

Park, Y.J., Chodaparambil, J.V., Bao, Y., McBryant, S.J., and Luger, K. 2005. Nucleosome assembly protein 1 exchanges histone H2A-H2B dimers and assists nucleosome sliding. J Biol Chem **280**: 1817–1825.

Park, Y.J., Dyer, P.N., Tremethick, D.J., and Luger, K. 2004. A new fluorescence resonance energy transfer approach demonstrates that the histone variant H2AZ stabilizes the histone octamer within the nucleosome. J Biol Chem **279**: 24274–24282.

Polach, K.J. and Widom, J. 1995. Mechanism of protein access to specific DNA sequences in chromatin: a dynamic equilibrium model for gene regulation. J Mol Biol **254**: 130–149.

Polo, S.E., Roche, D., and Almouzni, G. 2006. New histone incorporation marks sites of UV repair in human cells. Cell **127**: 481–493.

Raisner, R.M., Hartley, P.D., Meneghini, M.D., Bao, M.Z., Liu, C.L., Schreiber, S.L., Rando, O.J., and Madhani, H.D. 2005. Histone variant H2A.Z marks the 5' ends of both active and inactive genes in euchromatin. Cell **123**: 233–248.

Ren, B., Robert, F., Wyrick, J.J., Aparicio, O., Jennings, E.G., Simon, I., Zeitlinger, J., Schreiber, J., Hannett, N., Kanin, E., Volkert, T.L., Wilson, C.J., Bell, S.P., and Young, R.A. 2000. Genome-wide location and function of DNA binding proteins. Science **290**: 2306–2309.

Robertson, G., Hirst, M., Bainbridge, M., Bilenky, M., Zhao, Y., Zeng, T., Euskirchen, G., Bernier, B., Varhol, R., Delaney, A., Thiessen, N., Griffith, O.L., He, A., Marra, M., Snyder, M., and Jones, S. 2007. Genome-wide profiles of STAT1 DNA association using chromatin immunoprecipitation and massively parallel sequencing. Nat Methods **4**: 651–657.

Rogakou, E.P., Pilch, D.R., Orr, A.H., Ivanova, V.S., and Bonner, W.M. 1998. DNA double-stranded breaks induce histone H2AX phosphorylation on serine 139. J Biol Chem **273**: 5858–5868.

Roh, T.Y., Ngau, W.C., Cui, K., Landsman, D., and Zhao, K. 2004. High-resolution genome-wide mapping of histone modifications. Nat Biotechnol **22**: 1013–1016.

Rufiange, A., Jacques, P.E., Bhat, W., Robert, F., and Nourani, A. 2007. Genome-wide replication-independent histone H3 exchange occurs predominantly at promoters and implicates H3 K56 acetylation and Asf1. Mol Cell **27**: 393–405.

Saffery, R., Sumer, H., Hassan, S., Wong, L.H., Craig, J.M., Todokoro, K., Ansderson, M., Stafford, A., and Andy Choo, K.H. 2003. Transcription within a functional human centromere. Mol Cell **12**: 509–516.

Santisteban, M.S., Kalashnikova, T., and Smith, M.M. 2000. Histone H2A.Z regulates transcription and is partially redundant with nucleosome remodeling complexes. Cell **103**: 411–422.

Schwartz, Y.B., Kahn, T.G., Nix, D.A., Li, X.Y., Bourgon, R., Biggin, M., and Pirrotta, V. 2006. Genome-wide analysis of Polycomb targets in Drosophila melanogaster. Nat Genet **38**: 700–705.

Smith, S. and Stillman, B. 1989. Purification and characterization of CAF-I, a human cell factor required for chromatin assembly during DNA replication in vitro. Cell **58**: 15–25.

Sun, J.M., Chen, H.Y., Espino, P.S., and Davie, J.R. 2007. Phosphorylated serine 28 of histone H3 is associated with destabilized nucleosomes in transcribed chromatin. Nucleic Acids Res **35**: 6640–6647.

Tagami, H., Ray-Gallet, D., Almouzni, G., and Nakatani, Y. 2004. Histone H3.1 and H3.3 complexes mediate nucleosome assembly pathways dependent or independent of DNA synthesis. Cell **116**: 51–61.

Thiriet, C. and Hayes, J.J. 2005. Replication-independent core histone dynamics at transcriptionally active loci in vivo. Genes Dev **19**: 677–682.

Ueda, K., Kinoshita, Y., Xu, Z.J., Ide, N., Ono, M., Akahori, Y., Tanaka, I., and Inoue, M. 2000. Unusual core histones specifically expressed in male gametic cells of Lilium longiflorum. Chromosoma **108**: 491–500.

van Steensel, B. 2005. Mapping of genetic and epigenetic regulatory networks using microarrays. Nat Genet **37 Suppl**: S18–24.

van Steensel, B., Delrow, J., and Henikoff, S. 2001. Chromatin profiling using targeted DNA adenine methyltransferase. Nat Genet **27**: 304–308.

Varga-Weisz, P.D. 2001. ATP-dependent chromatin remodeling factors: nucleosome shufflers with many missions. Oncogene **20**: 3076–3085.

Velculescu, V.E., Zhang, L., Vogelstein, B., and Kinzler, K.W. 1995. Serial analysis of gene expression. Science **270**: 484–487.

Warburton, P.E. 2004. Chromosomal dynamics of human neocentromere formation. Chromosome Res **12**: 617–626.

Wolffe, A.P. 1992. Chromatin: Structure and function. Academic Press, San Diego.

Wolfsberg, T.G., Wetterstrand, K.A., Guyer, M.S., Collins, F.S., and Baxevanis, A.D. 2002. A user's guide to the human genome. Nat Genet **32 Suppl**: 1–79.

Yan, H., Jin, W., Nagaki, K., Tian, S., Ouyang, S., Buell, C.R., Talbert, P.B., Henikoff, S., and Jiang, J. 2005. Transcription and histone modifications in the recombination-free region spanning a rice centromere. Plant Cell **17**: 3227–3238.

Zhang, H., Roberts, D.N., and Cairns, B.R. 2005. Genome-wide dynamics of Htz1, a histone H2A variant that poises repressed/basal promoters for activation through histone loss. Cell **123**: 219–231.

Epigenetic Phenomena and Epigenomics in Maize

Jay B. Hollick and Nathan Springer

Abstract Maize research has provided much of the initial documentation and characterization of epigenetic phenomena such as transposable element inactivation, paramutation and imprinting. Current efforts are beginning to yield an understanding of the molecular mechanisms responsible for these epigenetic behaviors. Complementary research in many organisms has now provided strong evidence for the role of repetitive DNA features in facilitating epigenetic control of genome functions. The repetitive and complex structure of the maize genome together with the high level of structural diversity between maize haplotypes suggests that maize research has a significant role to play in understanding the dynamic relationships between genome structure and function.

Keywords Paramutation · Imprinting · Transposons · Maize · Epigenomics

1 Introduction

As a result of over 100 years of active research and academic breeding, maize represents the best understood example of crop domestication. It is expected that, at some point, the remarkable improvements in plant growth and yield achieved by maize breeders would be limited by the extent of genetic variation present in cultivated germplasm as static alleles recombined in various combinations promise only so much potential. As our recognition and understanding of chromosome-based control systems has emerged, it seems possible that breeding programs might have tapped into, and indeed exploited, epigenetic sources of variation in creating present

---

J.B. Hollick (✉)
University of California, Department of Plant and Microbial Biology, 111 Koshland Hall #3102, Berkeley CA USA 94720-3102
e-mail: hollick@nature.berkeley.edu

N. Springer (✉)
University of Minnesota, Department of Plant Biology, 250 Biosciences center, 1445 Gortner Ave., Saint Paul MN 55105
e-mail: springer@umn.edu

day production hybrids. Knowledge regarding the extent and interaction of these epigenomic resources may, in fact, prove instructive to future plant improvement efforts. The purpose of this chapter is to provide an overview of the types of epigenomic variation known to exist in maize, along with our current understanding of the nuclear systems responsible for generating and maintaining this variation. This summary, together with our perspective, is offered for whatever predictive or experimental values it may afford to future research and breeding.

The research of Barbara McClintock and Alexander Brink provided some of the earliest and best studied examples of plant epigenetics (Fedoroff and Botstien 1992; Brink 1973). The discovery of epigenetic regulatory systems in maize primarily came from the detailed study of genetic features that present inheritance patterns, or instabilities, not adequately explained from Mendelian genetic principles. With its ease of manual pollination and with entire progeny sets borne on single ears, the diploid maize plant is ideally designed for these studies requiring genetic mapping and pedigree analyses. The majority of these investigated instabilities are manifest at loci responsible for visual and non-essential traits, especially within pigment pathways. Whether by human selection or experimental necessity, derivative alleles of the genes controlling red and purple flavanoid-based pigments have been relatively easy to obtain and culture. We will draw from the classic works of McClintock and Brink as well as the contemporary research focused on a set of these unstable pigment alleles to illustrate the various concepts of transposon control, paramutation, and parental imprinting that have emerged regarding the action of epigenetic regulatory mechanisms on specific genomic features. It is from these concepts and mechanisms that we will then consider the organization, diversity, and function of the maize epigenome.

1.1 Maize Flavanoid Genetics

The flavanone molecule can be differentially modified to produce either a phlobaphene or anthocyanin pigment. Biosynthesis of flavanone and anthocyanins requires the sequential action of enzymes encoded by genes such as *anthocyaninless1* (*a1*) that are transcriptionally stimulated by the combined action of myb- and basic helix-loop-helix (bHLH)-type proteins (see Dooner et al. 1991 for review). These myb transcriptional regulators are encoded by the functional homeologues *colored aleurone1* (*c1*) and *purple plant1* (*pl1*) while the bHLH transcriptional regulators are encoded the functional homeologues *colored1* (*r1*) and *colored plant1* (*b1*). It is the specific combination of *c1/pl1* and *r1/b1* alleles that determines the timing and tissue specificity of anthocyanin production, although, most alleles confer the following distribution patterns; seedling (R1 + PL1), plant (B1 + PL1), anthers (R1 + PL1) and seed (R1 + C1). In contrast, regulation of phlobaphene synthesis occurs primarily in maternal cob tissues and requires only the action a myb protein encoded by the *pericarp color1* (*p1*) locus. Unstable alleles have been described at nearly all the enzymatic and regulatory genes of the anthocyanin pathway. This observation suggests that nearly any maize gene can be subject to unstable behaviors. The operation and nature of these instabilities acting on experimentally tractable genes of the anthocyanin pathway are likely to reflect the general features operating within the maize genome.

2 Epigenetic Phenomena in Maize

There is on-going research into the genetic and molecular basis of several epigenetic phenomena in maize. We will attempt to summarize exciting new findings that have arisen from these research efforts. We will review the progress made towards understanding transposable element inactivation, imprinting and paramutation.

2.1 Transposable Element Inactivation

McClintock (1951) was the first to describe a nuclear system operating to suppress the action of transposons. Her discoveries arose from experiments designed to induce segmental deficiencies using a chromosome type breakage-fusion-bridge (BFB) cycle. BFB cycles are initiated when two chromatids with double strand breaks fuse and are subsequently fractured along the resulting chromatid bridge in the following anaphase. The BFB cycle continues in subsequent daughter cells until broken chromatids are "healed", presumably through addition of functional telomeres. McClintock found that BFB cycles occurring in early embryogenesis had two remarkable effects. The chromosome complement was frequently rearranged at sites not anticipated to be involved in the BFB cycle, and there was a burst of new unstable, or mutable, phenotypes found among self pollinated progeny. As the BFB-induced rearrangements were primarily focused at sites of conspicuous cytological heterochromatin, McClintock concluded that the origin of mutable loci was similarly related to induced alterations in the heterochromatin (McClintock 1951). This summation was prescient to our emerging molecular concept of "heterochromatin" and its general role in transposon control (Slotkin and Martienssen 2007). As McClintock's studies suggest, it was alterations of the heterochromatin that led to the novel sources of unstable phenotypic variations found in her cultures.

Transposons are generally classified by their mode of transposition as either Type I (retrotransposons) or Type II (DNA transposons) (Wicker et al. 2007). Among the Type II class is a newly discovered group of elements with a distinct mode of transposition known as helitrons (Kapitonov and Jurka 2001). We will describe each major group of transposable elements and discuss what is known about the epigenetic mechanisms that contribute to their regulation. In addition, we will consider how these transposable elements may contribute to the epigenetic control of nearby genes.

2.1.1 DNA Transposons

Maize research has played a leading role in our understanding of the behavior and nuclear control of DNA transposons. These elements encode a transposase protein that acts on terminal inverted repeat sequences (TIRs) to affect a cut-and-paste type of transposition of the DNA itself. There are at least six well-known DNA transposon families in maize (*Dotted, Dt*; *Mutator, Mu*; *Activator, Ac*; *Enhancer/Suppressor-mutator, En/Spm*; *P instability factor, PIF*; *Doppia, Dop*) and three of these (*Mu, Ac, En/Spm*) have received considerable attention regarding their mode of action and epigenetic control. Intact elements are referred to as "autonomous" as they encode a functional transposase enzyme and contain the TIRs necessary for mobilization. Derivative elements that lack the ability to encode a transposase yet retain the TIRs are referred to as "non-autonomous" as they can still transpose in the presence of an active autonomous element of a like family member. For example, Miniature Inverted repeat Transposable Elements (MITES) are no more than *PIF* TIRs themselves (Casa et al. 2000). Defective derivative elements are unable to excise due to loss or impairment of the TIRs. Study of these DNA transposons has been greatly facilitated by their occasional association with genes. It was McClintock's recognitions that (1) such associations could cause alterations in the patterns of gene expression and (2) that orderly mitotic segregation events affecting the dosage of genetically unlinked elements could alter these gene-controlling properties that led her to speculate that a conceptually similar system operated normally during the course of developmental differentiation (McClintock 1951).

TIR-type elements and their derivatives can control or interfere with normal modes of gene regulation in many different ways. In the simple case of a coding sequence insertion, the element serves to either interfere with mRNA maturation or produces an altered reading frame that disrupts typical protein function. For example, the fully recessive *anthocyaninless1* reference allele is due to the insertion of a non-autonomous *rDt* within the third exon. In the presence of an active autonomous *Dt* element, the *rDt* element in *a1* can excise and restore *a1* gene function. The resulting plant or kernel phenotype is described as mutable since there are individual somatic sectors containing anthocyanin. The position, sizes, and shapes of the pigmented sectors reflect the developmental timing of the excision event and the clonal relationships of the cells descended from that event. However, there are many other ways in which a transposon can control the expression of a gene either directly or though epigenetic modifications.

In some cases, the insertion of a TIR element controls gene expression in different ways depending on the presence or absence of *trans*-acting functions produced from an autonomous element (Fig. 1). The derivative *a1-m2* allele described by McClintock (1951) contains a non-autonomous *Spm* element inserted into the putative *a1* promoter (Masson et al. 1987; Schwarz-Sommer et al. 1987). Anthocyanin production — caused by A1 expression from the *a1-m2* allele — is dependent on the presence of an active, autonomous, *Spm* element. Not only is excision of the nonautonomous *Spm* element from *a1-m2* dependent on *Spm* transposase, but low levels of "leaky" uniform pigmentation is also dependent on autonomous *Spm* functions encoded in *trans*. This dependency is thought to be related to the binding of the major encoded non-transposase protein from *Spm* called TnpA to specific sequences found in *Spm* termini (Gierl et al. 1988). In contrast to *a1-m2*, weak A1 expression from the *a1-m1* derivative that contains a nonautonomous *Spm* element

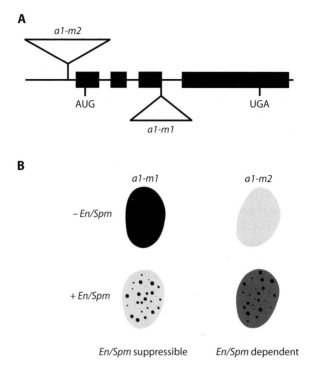

Fig. 1 *En/Spm* derivative alleles of *a1*. (**A**) Structural representations of the *En/Spm*-suppressible and *En/Spm*-dependent *a1* derivative alleles, *a1-m1* and *a1-m2*. The *a1* exons are represented by large blocks and positions of defective *En/Spm* transposons found in the respective alleles are indicated by the attendant triangles. Features are drawn to scale. (**B**) Kernel phenotypes typical of the respective genotypes illustrating the *En/Spm*-suppressible and *En/Spm*-dependent nature of kernel pigmentation. Spots of dark pigment seen with both *a1* alleles are indicative of somatic excision events of the respective defective *En/Spm* transposons occurring during kernel development that restore wild-type A1 expression

inserted near an exon-intron junction (Schwarz-Sommer et al. 1987) is suppressed by autonomous *Spm* functions. In this case, it could be that the nonautonomous *Spm* element is spliced out of a proportion of the *a1-m1* RNA transcripts but that the *a1-m1* transcription or RNA splicing is impaired when the autonomous *Spm* functions are present. These *Spm*-dependent and *Spm*-suppressible alleles can thus be used experimentally as visual "reporters" of autonomous *Spm* activity. Such reporters serve as exquisitely sensitive monitors of the nuclear system acting to modulate the behavior of these autonomous elements. The observations that modulations, or changes in epigenetic state, of a transposon family can control the expression of protein-coding genes that reside near autonomous or non-autonomous elements provide the basis for McClintock's description of transposons as "controlling elements" (McClintock 1951).

Most of the well-studied maize TIR-type transposons "cycle" between active and inactive states. These changes in state — whether measured directly via RNA production or indirectly via a reporter allele — are correlated with changes in the extent of cytosine methylation, especially in the TIRs (Chandler and Walbot 1986; Banks et al. 1988) *Ac* is not transcribed while in the inactive state (Kunze et al. 1988) and this inactive state is associated with methylation of *Ac* DNA near the transcriptional start site and leader sequence (Schwartz and Dennis 1986; Chomet et al. 1987). "Cryptic", or heritably inactive, *Spm* elements are heavily methylated at the TIRs, subterminal repeats, and a GC-rich region encompassing most of *TnpA* exon1 (Banks et al. 1988). In contrast, "active" *Spm* elements are extensively hypomethylated in these regions. An intermediate methylation state is associated with a "programmable" behavior (Banks et al. 1988). *Spm* reporter alleles such as *a1-m2* are not expressed, nor are excisions detected, in the presence of a programmable *Spm* allele unless it has been immediately segregated from an active *Spm* element in the prior generation. McClintock referred to this observation as presetting (McClintock 1964). The activity of certain *Spm* states (programmable) is preset in the prior generation through some form of interaction with an active *Spm* element. This behavior is similar, in certain respects, to paramutation in which allelic interactions lead to meiotically heritable changes in gene regulation. Given repeated exposures to an active *Spm* element, a cryptic element can be transformed through a programmable state to a fully active state (Fedoroff 1989). Given the origins of these mutable loci, these studies were among the first to highlight the epigenetic modification of cytosine methylation as a molecular hallmark of heterochromatin.

Suppressible alleles derived from *Mutator* transposon insertions have illustrated a developmental action of the nuclear system regulating transposon activity. The suppressible *high chlorophyll fluorescence106* (*hcf106*) allele contains a nonautonomous *Mu1* element at the beginning of a transcription unit encoding an essential chloroplast protein. When *MuDR* is active — that is when *MuDR* expresses its *trans*-acting functions from the *mudrA* and *mudrB* coding regions — *hcf106* fails to produce detectable mRNA (Barkan and Martienssen 1991) and the seedlings exhibit a chlorotic mutant phenotype. The normal phenotype is "suppressed" by active *MuDR* transposons. However, when epigenetic inactivation of *MuDR* occurs, the plants or clonal sectors exhibit a wild-type phenotype (Martienssen and Baron 1994) resulting from *hcf106* RNAs being intitiated from an outward reading promoter of the resident *Mu1* element (Barkan and Martienssen 1991). By monitoring multiple *Mu* suppressible alleles in the same plant it was found that the entire family of *Mu* elements is coordinately regulated (Martienssen and Baron 1994). The suppressible alleles provide an excellent example of epigenetic inheritance as plants or cells with identical DNA sequences will exhibit clearly distinct phenotypes. The suppressible alleles also illustrate that transposons can induce "cryptic" variation that is only revealed when the epigenetic states of the transposon is changed.

The suppressible *a1-mum2* allele is regulated similarly to *hcf106* and also contains a nonautonomous *Mu1* just upstream of the transcription unit (Pooma et al. 2002). This allele is weakly expressed in the seed, but is strongly suppressed in the plant when there are active *MuDR* elements present. Sectors of pigment occur in the plant as *MuDR* elements are lost in either post-replicative somatic segregations (Chomet et al. 1991) or are epigenetically silenced (Slotkin et al. 2005).

The *a1-mum2* allele was used by Slotkin et al. (2005) to identify and clone a naturally occurring inverted duplication of a *MuDR* element called *"MuKiller"* (*MuK*) that causes heritable epigenetic silencing of autonomous *MuDR* elements via a small RNA interference pathway (Slotkin et al. 2005). Suppressible alleles not only reflect the normal operation of endogenous nuclear control pathways on specific autonomous elements, but they can also be used as tools to dissect these pathways via either forward or reverse-genetics approaches.

The exact mechanisms involved in identifying and epigenetically modifying DNA transposons are still being elucidated. There is now evidence that epigenetic repression of *MuDR* activity is also correlated with the both increased TIR cytosine methylation and the presence of complementary small RNAs. The genetic action of *MuDR* elements that are inactivated and hypermethylated by *MuK* can be revived following passage through plants deficient for a putative RNA-dependent RNA polymerase encoded by the *mediator of paramutation1* (*mop1*) locus (Lisch et al. 2002; Woodhouse et al. 2006a, 2006b). MOP1 is the likely maize orthologue of *Arabidopsis* RDR2, which is required for the generation of 24nt small RNAs from primarily "heterochromatic" origins (Chan et al. 2004; Kasschau et al. 2007). Consistent with this idea, 24nt and 26nt small RNAs with complementarity to *MuDR* are absent in *mop1* mutants (Woodhouse et al. 2006b). Over the course of five generations in the absence of MOP1 function, cytosine methylation of the TIR adjacent to *mudrA* is progressively lost and the reference *MuDR* element regains the genetic functions reported by *a1-mum2* (Lisch et al. 2002; Woodhouse et al. 2006a). The MOP1-dependent small RNAs thus appear to represent a nuclear system that reinforces a repressive state characterized by increased levels of cytosine methylation. These observations suggest that some examples of maize heterochromatin are based on small RNAs, which specify particular epigenomic landscapes that can be meiotically heritable. This is fully consistent with mutational studies of *Arabidopsis* and rice showing that DNA methylation, histone modifications and 24nt small RNAs are intimately related to the epigenetic control of DNA transposons (Miura et al. 2001; Tompa et al. 2002; Zilberman et al. 2003; Kato et al. 2003; Lippman et al. 2003; Kato et al. 2004; Ebbs and Bender 2006; Ding et al. 2007; Kasschau et al. 2007). Involvement of *Mu* small RNAs in the maintenance of epigenetic states may underlie the coordinate regulation of *Mu* elements that are scattered throughout the genome.

2.1.2 Retrotransposons

Similar to other plants, the maize genome is predominated by repetitive sequences, primarily retrotransposons. Sequence surveys estimate that 60–70% of the maize genome is composed of recognized transposons (Meyers et al. 2001; Liu et al. 2007). Members of the *gypsy* and *copia* superfamilies of the long terminal repeat (LTR) class of retrotransposons are found in large nested arrangements (SanMiguel et al. 1996). By comparing the rates of nucleotide divergence in extant arrays of LTRs, there is evidence for several "bursts" of retrotransposon activity within the maize genome during the past three million years (SanMiguel et al. 1998). Based on initial sequencing information, the emerging maize genome landscape is one of relatively gene-rich regions flanked by large rafts of nested LTR transposons (Liu et al. 2007).

Although there are many different classes of maize type I transposons (LTR and non-LTR types that all accumulate via an RNA intermediate) (Kumar and Bennetzen 1999), there are several predominant families, such as *Huck*, *Ji* and *Opie*, that each contain >20,000 members (Vitte and Bennetzen 2006) and account for ~30% of the maize genome (Meyers et al. 2001). The apparent distributions of different transposons in the genome suggest some degree of functional specialization (Lamb et al. 2007). For example, Liu et al. (2007) found that *Ogre* elements are over represented in BAC clones devoid of genic sequences and that *Ji* elements are more represented in gene-rich regions. The functional significance of these trends is as yet unknown. It is anticipated that much of the nuclear heterochromatin is devoted to maintaining these type I transposons in both transcriptionally and recombinationally inert states.

In general, maize retrotransposons exist in a heterochromatic state reflected by high levels of cytosine methylation. Analyses using methyl-sensitive restriction enzymes (Bennetzen et al. 1994) or methyl-filtration sequencing (Rabinowicz et al. 1999; Meyers et al. 2001) have provided evidence that the majority of maize retrotransposons are heavily methylated. Analysis of a small family of LTR retrotransposons shows that these elements contain high levels of cytosine methylation, even when inserted into protein coding genes (N.M. Springer unpublished data). The high frequency of C to T transition mutations documented in nested LTR arrays also supports the idea that cytosines in type I transposons are typically methylated (Vitte and Bennetzen 2006) and epigenetically repressed. Indeed, studies of mutants in other plant species that are impaired in epigenetic repression finds evidence for retrotransposon reactivation (Hirochika et al. 2000; Lindroth et al. 2001; Ding et al. 2007; Huettel et al. 2007; Rangwala and Richards, 2007).

Although LTR retrotransposons comprise a significant portion of the maize genome they do not account for an equal portion of the maize transcriptome. Vicient et al. (2001) searched the public maize EST database and found that only .0249% of the ESTs represented LTR retrotransposons. It is possible that many of these sequences actually represent transcripts that do not originate from retrotransposons but instead represent read-through from adjacent promoters. The fact that relatively few retrotransposons are observed in EST databases, or by microarray hybridizations, may reflect low transcription rates for these elements or may be due to an efficient process of degradation for retrotransposon transcripts. While many plant LTR retrotransposons are not generally represented by large RNA species, some retrotransposon RNAs are specifically found in response to developmental or environmental stimuli. The maize *PREM-2* retrotransposon is only expressed in early microspores (Turcich et al. 1996) and the tobacco retrotransposon, *Tnt1*, is expressed at low levels in roots (Pouteau et al. 1991). One recent study found that retrotransposon RNAs are preferentially expressed in shoot apical meristem tissue (Ohtsu et al. 2007). The most common stimulus involved in expression of retrotransposons is tissue culture (Wessler 1996). The tobacco *Tnt1*, *Tto1*, and*Tto2* and rice

Tos10, Tos17 and *Tos19* retrotransposons are all activated by tissue culture and show increases in copy number in cell cultures (Hirochika 1993; Hirochika et al. 1996; Grandbastien, 2004).

2.1.3 Helitrons

Helitrons are a poorly understood type of DNA element that presumably replicates via a rolling-circle-type mechanism that have been recently described in several eukaryotes (Kapitonov and Jurka 2001). These elements can be quite large (>50 kb) and are defined by very few conserved structural features making their annotation from DNA sequence difficult (Kapitonov and Jurka 2001; Lai et al. 2005; Brunner et al. 2005a, b). Interestingly, it has been noted that *helitrons* often "capture" genes or gene fragments between the termini (Brunner et al. 2005a, b; Lai et al. 2005; Morgante et al. 2005). Virtually nothing is known regarding the regulation and action of *helitrons* but they appear to be very prevalent in the maize genome. Due to the fact that they can capture and move genic fragments these elements are a frequent source of copy number variation (CNV) between maize inbred lines (Brunner et al. 2005a, b; Lai et al. 2005; Morgante et al. 2005). In a modest survey of annotated maize BAC clones, roughly 20% of all the gene predictions were incomplete and it was proposed that many of these represent *helitron* insertions (Morgante et al. 2005).

Genes, or fragments of genes, amplified or mobilized by transposons could potentially lead to novel sources of phenotypic variation. Sequence analyses provide evidence that both *Mu* transposons and helitrons can "capture" fragments of genes and move these throughout the genome (*Mu*: Jin and Bennetzen 1994; Bureau et al. 1994; Jiang et al. 2004; Bennetzen 2005; *helitrons*: Lai et al. 2005; Morgante et al. 2005; Brunner et al. 2005a, b). Copy number variation is likely an important contributor to phenotypic variation in plant and animal species (Beckmann et al. 2007). In some cases, the movement of genes can result in exon shuffling or novel chimeric genes (Morgante et al. 2005). In other cases a full length gene may be moved to a genomic region that is subject to different regulatory mechanisms (Jiang et al. 2004). The duplication of genic sequences may have significant implications for both epigenetic and non-epigenetic regulatory control of gene expression and gene balance (Birchler and Veitia 2007).

Much of our understanding of DNA transposons has derived from the pioneering work of maize geneticists. The well pedigreed genetic materials of their legacies are archived and readily available for contemporary study. The extensive detail to which the behavior of these elements has been described makes these materials an unparalleled, and largely untapped, resource for understanding the nuclear system responsible for modulating transposon action. The extent to which this knowledge may relate to the developmental control of the epigenome is unknown, but certain molecular components have now been found through studies directed at the behavior known as paramutation that establish a mechanistic link between the system of transposon control and developmental gene regulation (Dorweiler et al. 2000, Woodhouse et al. 2006a, b; Lisch et al. 2002; Alleman et al. 2006). It is therefore anticipated that study of maize transposons will continue to contribute fundamental knowledge of epigenomic control in multicellular eukaryotes.

2.2 Imprinting

Imprinting occurs when two alleles exhibit differential expression in the same organism depending upon which parent they were inherited from; for example, when the allele inherited from the maternal parent is expressed but the allele inherited from the paternal parent is transcriptionally inactive. Phenotypic studies of gynogenetic (only maternal contributions) or androgenetic (only paternal contributions) organisms in placental mammals and some plants suggested the requirement for contributions of both the maternal and paternal genome. The restricted occurrence of imprinting to organisms whose offspring rely on maternal sources of nutrient acquisition has led to a universal parental conflict theory regarding its origins (Haig and Westoby 1989). Imprinting in plants was first documented at the maize *r1* locus (Kermicle 1970, 1978). Kermicle and colleagues demonstrated differences in the phenotype condition by some *r1* locus haplotypes depending upon whether they were maternally or paternally transmitted. The maternally transmitted haplotype provides solid kernel coloration while the paternally transmitted allele conditions a mottled pattern. This difference is due to parent-of-origin and not simply gene dosage effects (Kermicle 1970, 1978; Kermicle and Alleman 1990). Interestingly, while some *r1* haplotypes are subject to imprinting, the majority do not exhibit any evidence of imprinting (Kermicle and Alleman 1990).

The imprinting observed in plants occurs in the endosperm; a terminally differentiated tissue that results from the double fertilization in flowering plants. The triploid endosperm genome is the product of two maternal haploid genomes and a single paternal haploid genome. There is evidence that the endosperm exhibits unique epigenetic states relative to other plant tissues (Lauria et al. 2004; Baroux et al. 2007). Indeed the endosperm provides a ploidy barrier that restricts crosses between different ploidy levels and this ploidy barrier acts to restrict endosperm development (Lin 1984).

The analysis of imprinting in maize has revealed several different variations (reviewed by Springer and Gutierrez-Marcos 2008). There are imprinted genes, such as Zm*Fie1* and *Mez1*, that exhibit complete maternal imprinted expression throughout endosperm development (Danilevskaya et al. 2003; Gutierrez-Marcos et al. 2003; Haun et al. 2007). Expression is only detected from the maternal alleles of these genes and imprinting has been detected for all the genetically diverse alleles that have been tested. For other examples of imprinting, such as the *ZmFie2* gene, complete maternal imprinted expression is detected at early stages of endosperm development but the expression becomes bi-allelic at later stages of development. Several of the genes with imprinted expression show examples of differential imprinting (Guo et al. 2004; Stupar et al. 2007). Differential imprinting occurs when there is primarily expression from one allele but low levels of the other allele are still detected (Dilkes and Comai 2004). There is also evidence for paternal imprinted expression, preferential expression of the paternal allele, in maize (Gutierrez-Marcos et al. 2003). The variation in the different types of imprinting observed in maize suggests the potential for multiple imprinting mechanisms.

Imprinting results in differential levels of expression from two, nearly identical, alleles that are present within the same nucleus. In addition, the "imprint" is erased and reset each generation. These features imply that imprinting is the result of different epigenetic modifications on the maternal and paternal alleles. Imprinting results in biased expression of the maternal and paternal alleles. This could be achieved through allele-specific activation of one of the alleles from a default silent state or through allele-specific silencing from a default active state. There is evidence for the allele-specific activation model in both maize and *Arabidopsis*. Several imprinted genes, such as *FWA* and *ZmFie1*, are only expressed in endosperm tissue and only from the maternal allele in the endosperm (Kinoshita et al. 2004; Danilevskaya et al. 2003). This suggests a default silenced state from which the maternal allele is derepressed in the endosperm. The allele-specific activation model is also supported by several genetic studies in *Arabidopsis*. Mutations in the maintenance DNA methyltransferase, *MET1*, result in bi-allelic activation and a lack of imprinting for the *FWA*, *MEA* and *FIS2* genes (Xiao et al. 2003; Kinoshita et al. 2004; Jullien et al. 2006). This suggests that CpG methylation is required to maintain the default silenced states of this imprinted gene. Mutations in the *DEMETER* gene abolish imprinting of the *MEA* and *FWA* gene such that neither the maternal or paternal alleles are expressed in endosperm tissue (Choi et al. 2002; Kinoshita et al. 2004). *DEMETER* encodes a DNA glycosylase that is specifically expressed in the central cell of the female gametophyte. This protein then acts to remove cytosine methylation present at the maternal allele of the imprinted gene (Gehring et al. 2006). This action results in allele-specific activation of the maternal alleles of *FWA* and *MEA*.

Analyses of DNA methylation at several imprinted loci in maize suggest that a similar mechanism occurs at the *ZmFie1* and *Mez1* genes (Gutierrez-Marcos et al. 2006; Haun et al. 2007; Hermon et al. 2007). These two genes exhibit bi-allelic methylation in vegetative tissues but low levels of DNA methylation at the maternal allele in endosperm tissue. However, *ZmFie2* exhibits a different type of DNA methylation profile during development. This gene exhibits low levels of DNA methylation in vegetative tissue but higher levels of DNA methylation at the paternal allele during early stages of endosperm development. This may suggest that an allele-specific silencing mechanism is responsible for imprinting at this locus. A study by Lauria et al. (2004) demonstrated that many loci exhibit differential methylation of the maternal and paternal alleles during endosperm development.

There are several experimental hurdles that have impaired the progress of research on the mechanism for imprinting. In order to observe imprinting it is often necessary to generate heterozygous individuals. This severely restricts the options for genetic screens. One recessive mutation identifies the *maternal de-repression of r1* (*mdr1*) locus that encodes a function that affects imprinting at *r1* but the molecular nature and action of *mdr1* remains unknown (Kermicle 1978; Alleman and Doctor 2000). In addition, the tissue that exhibits imprinting, the endosperm, is a largely consumed during *Arabidopsis* embryogenesis. Maize provides several advantages for studying imprinting. The endosperm is persistent, relatively large and easily accessible. A single endosperm provides enough tissue for performing DNA methylation analyses and expression assays. In addition, it is quite easy to perform large numbers of controlled crosses in maize to analyze genetic factors that affect imprinting. The availability of dominant negative lines (McGinnis et al. 2007) is likely to facilitate genetic screens to identify the factors that are required to establish, maintain and interpret the epigenetic marks required for imprinting.

2.3 Paramutation

Paramutation describes a particular type of meiotically heritable change in gene regulation that is typically brought about by allelic interactions (Brink 1958; Chandler and Stam 2004). The term can be applied to describe the process or the end result similar to the ways in which "mutation" is used. Haplotype is used in place of "allele" for this discussion since some of the loci in question are actually multigenic. Examples of paramutation have been documented for specific haplotypes of the *r1*, *b1*, *p1* and *pl1* loci (Brink 1956, Coe 1966, Sidorenko and Peterson 2001, Hollick et al. 1995). The first example, noted by Brink (1956), was manifest as a reduction in the normal imprinted kernel pigmentation conferred by a specific *r1* haplotype (*R-r:standard*; *R-r*) following its paternal transmission from heterozygous condition with another *r1* haplotype known as *R-stippled* (*Rst*). *R-r* is invariably and heritably changed with regards to its imprinted pigmenting action in *Rst* / *R-r* heterozygotes. A later study by Mikula (1985) would show that the severity of this paramutation event occurring at *r1* can be influenced by environmental conditions during the seedling phase of growth. The apparent violation of Mendel's first law (that genetic factors remain unchanged in heterozygotes), together with Mikula's evidence that the process is capable of environmental perception, present important exceptions to the basic tenets of modern evolutionary biology and population genetics.

Two features distinguish paramutation from other described examples of gene silencing. First, paramutation can alter the regulatory properties of a given haplotype rather than simply silencing its action (Hollick et al. 2000). More similar to examples of heterochromatin-based position effect variegation (Weiler and Wakimoto 1995), paramutant states at *r1* and *pl1* are often manifested as variegated phenotypes (Brink 1956; Hollick et al. 1995). Second, the subsequent ability to facilitate paramutation on susceptible haplotypes is an outcome of the process itself. That is, for example, *R-r* transmitted from a *Rst*/*R-r* plant is able to facilitate paramutation to another *R-r* haplotype in subsequent generations. However, genetic mutations that affect the stability of haplotypes subject to paramutation have also been shown to similarly affect silenced transgenes (McGinnis et al. 2006) and repressed *MuDR* elements (Woodhouse et al. 2006a). Thus, paramutation appears to reflect a unique application of some of the same cellular machinery generally used to repress specific genomic features.

Examples of maize paramutation exhibit general behaviors that influence heritable phenotypic variation in non-Mendelian ways. Paramutation invariably occurs when a susceptible (paramutable) haplotype is combined in heterozygous condition with a facultative (paramutagenic) haplotype. Paramutable haplotypes are inherently unstable and can spontaneously change to a paramutant state (Styles and Brink 1969; Coe 1966; Das and Messing 1994; Hollick et al. 1995). The nature of this inherent instability is unknown but there is some indication it may be related to genetic background (Walbot 2001). Most paramutable haplotypes can also exist in variable states of phenotypic expression. In any one plant, or kernel, the haplotype can confer high levels of anthocyanin production, virtually undetectable levels, or intermediate levels. In experimentally tractable cases, pigmentation is found correlated with both RNA levels and transcription rates as measured using isolated nuclei (Patterson et al. 1993; Hollick et al. 2000). Levels of pigmentation conferred by the paramutable *pl1* haplotype are inversely related to its paramutagenic strength (Hollick et al. 1995). Thus single paramutable haplotypes are capable of displaying a range of both phenotypic and regulatory variation and the stability of the most active state is dependent on background modifiers and interactions between specific haplotype partners. Two general models, involving either direct homologue contact or a sequence-specific diffusible substance, have been proposed to account for these haplotype interactions but precise mechanisms that facilitate paramutation are still unknown. The latter concept finds some support in the observation that paramutation at the *b1* locus is impaired in *mop1* mutant plants (Dorweiler et al. 2000). *Mop1* encodes an RDR2-like protein that is likely involved in the generation of small RNAs (Alleman et al. 2006; Woodhouse et al. 2006b). Hence the action of an RDR2-like protein is needed to establish a meiotically heritable paramutagenic state. The mode of establishment is, however, intimately dependent on the mechanism acting to maintain these states (Hollick et al. 2005) so it remains to be seen if an RNA component truly serves as a facilitator of paramutation.

Studies of diverse *r1* and *pl1* haplotypes show that maintenance of paramutagenic states is also dependent on haplotype interactions (Styles and Brink 1966, 1969; Hollick and Chandler 1998; Gross and Hollick 2007); the paramutant state is reversible. Repressed *r1* and *pl1* haplotypes regain pigmenting function, and correspondingly lose paramutagenic action, when carried in the heterozygous condition with other haplotypes that do not undergo paramutation or when carried over a chromosome deficiency. This reactivation or reversal of state can occur within a single generation or over the course of several generations. Some *pl1* haplotypes that are not susceptible to paramutation themselves, nonetheless contain features that act to stablize a paramutagenic state carried on the alternate homologue (Gross and Hollick 2007). Thus with certain examples of paramutation, genetic action is variable and highly dependent on localized interchromosomal interactions. In specific cases, the level of pigment action displayed by certain heterozygotes exceeds that of either homozygote alone. These are examples of single locus heterosis, or overdominance, in which a type of epigenetic complementation occurs to maximize gene expression (Kermicle and Alleman 1990; Hollick and Chandler 1998; Gross and Hollick 2007). The extent to which this type of "epihybridity" contributes to the agronomically critical behavior of hybrid vigor remains to be determined.

Most of the haplotypes described at the *r1*, *b1*, *p1*, and *pl1* loci are not susceptible to paramutation. It is therefore assumed that those haplotypes that are subject to paramutation [*R-r*, *B1-Intense (B1-I)*, *P1-rr*, and *Pl1-Rhoades (Pl1-Rh)*],

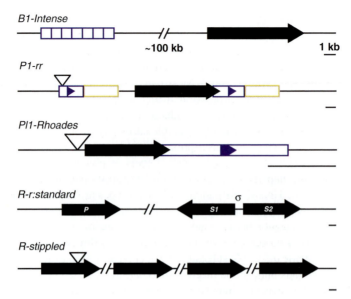

Fig. 2 Alleles and haplotypes with paramutation properties. Transcription units (*solid black arrows*), direct repeats (*colored*), and transposon features (*vertical triangles*) are highlighted for the respective alleles or haplotypes discussed in the text. Features are drawn to the scales indicated by the respective 1 kb intervals found below each drawing. Hash marks indicate intervening sequences of >10 kb or as indicated. Colored horizontal triangles in *P1-rr* and *Pl1-Rhoades* represent the respective 3′ regions of each transcription unit. Several features are labeled in the *R-r:standard* haplotype; the *P* transcription unit is expressed in plant tissues, *S1* and *S2* are expressed in the seed, and σ represents the small intervening region between *S1* and *S2*

have unique structural features that mediate the behavior. Many of these haplotypes are associated with complex arrangements of duplicated sequences and several of these unusual features have been functionally implicated in facilitating paramutation (Fig. 2). Within the multigenic *R-r* haplotype itself, paramutation only affects regulation of the seed-specific *r* genes (*S1* and *S2*); the centromere proximal, plant-specific, *r* gene (*P*) appears largely unaffected (Brown 1966). The two seed-specific *r* coding regions are arranged in inverted arrangement with a 400 bp of intervening sequence (referred to as σ) serving as the promoter region for both (Walker et al. 1995). The σ region contains a terminal fragment of a *doppia* transposon along with rearranged segments of the presumptive *P* promoter (Walker et al. 1995). *Doppia* belongs to the superfamily of CACTA-type elements that also includes *En/Spm* (Bercury et al. 2001) and it has been proposed that paramutation operates on this feature at *R-r* in ways conceptually similar to presetting (Martienssen 1996). A similar terminal *doppia* fragment is found immediately 5′ of the *Pl1-Rh* and *Pl1-Blotched* haplotypes (Cocciolone and Cone 1993; Hollick et al. 2000). Since only the *Pl1-Rh* haplotype is sensitive to paramutation (Hollick et al. 2000; Gross and Hollick 2007), a functional role of this *doppia* fragment in mediating paramutation is unclear.

Transgenic analyses, derivative haplotypes and forward genetic screens have helped define many of the *cis*-acting features required to facilitate paramutation in *trans*. Each example apparently has unique *cis*-linked features functionally involved with the process. Transgenic studies identified a 1.2 kb region of unique sequence found in a direct repeat arrangement both 5′ and 3′ of the *P1-rr* coding region that can facilitate paramutation in *trans* (Sidorenko and Peterson 2001). Recombination derivatives functionally identify the repeated nature of a region consisting of seven 853 bp tandemly duplicated sequences nearly 100 kb 5′ of the *B1-I* coding region (Stam et al. 2002a). Deletion derivatives identify the σ region of *R-r* as important (Kermicle 1996; Walker 1998). Recombinant derivatives and trisomic manipulations show that the repeated nature of paramutagenic *Rst* (4 tandem *r*-genes each separated by greater than 10 kb) is quantitatively responsible (Kermicle et al. 1995). A similar result was found with the paramutagenic *R-marbled* haplotype (3 tandem *r*-genes) (Panavas et al. 1999). Directed loss-of-function mutations that specifically interfere with *Pl1-Rhoades* RNA production also prohibit the *trans*-acting functions required to facilitate paramutation (Gross and Hollick 2007). The unifying feature underlying these apparently disparate *cis*-linked elements is that they all contain either experimentally described enhancers (Stam et al. 2002b; Cocciolone et al. 2000) or basal components presumably required for transcription (Kermicle 1996; Walker 1998; Gross and Hollick 2007). Thus functional interactions between these unique regulatory elements and the transcription unit in question, appears to be required to facilitate the paramutation process in *trans*.

Forward mutation screens for increased pigmentation in specific genetic backgrounds have helped identify many of the *trans*-acting components affecting paramutation. Maintenance of paramutagenic *Pl1-Rh* states requires at least 10 unique genetic components as defined by EMS-derived recessive mutations (Dorweiler et al. 2000; Hollick and Chandler 2001; Hollick et al. 2005; J.B.H., unpublished). The *mop1* and *required to maintain repression1* (*rmr1*) genes have been cloned by positional methods (Alleman et al. 2006; Woodhouse et al. 2006b; Hale et al. 2007) and the remaining eight *rmr* genes remain important targets for similar cloning projects. RMR1 is a novel protein with a Snf2 domain similar to the yeast Rad54p that facilitates Rad51p mediated single strand DNA invasion during homology searching in DNA recombination (Krogh and Symington 2004). The Snf2 motif is found in a large number of eukaryotic proteins characterized as having chromatin remodeling functions (Flaus et al. 2006). RMR1 is most closely related to the *Arabidopsis* CLASSY1 (CLSY1) and DEFECTIVE IN RNA-DEPENDENT DNA METHYLATION1 (DRD1) proteins (Hale et al. 2007).

Collectively, RMR1, CLSY1, and DRD1 define three monophyletic clades of a plant-specific group of proteins required for aspects of small RNA accumulation or function (Hale et al. 2007; Smith et al. 2007; Huettel et al. 2006). Both CLSY1 and the large subunit of RNA Pol IVa are needed for accumulation of 24nt small RNAs derived from repeated sequences (Smith et al. 2007). Both DRD1 and RMR1 are required to maintain *de novo* cytosine methylation patterns specifically in CNN contexts represented by small RNA populations (Kanno et al. 2004; 2005 Hale et al. 2007). RMR1 function is directed to the *doppia* fragment found in *Pl1-Rh* and is required for the accumulation of *doppia* related small RNAs (~26nt). Hence, a putative RNA-directed DNA methylation pathway operating through RMR1 — and presumably MOP1 — action maintains a heterochromatic-like chromatin state at the proximate *doppia* fragment of *Pl1-Rh*. Surprisingly, this RMR1-dependent heterochromatic feature centered on the *doppia* fragment is correlated with effects on *pl1* RNA stability but not transcription rates; leading to a model in which nascent *pl1* RNAs are subjected to a co-transcriptional processing similar to that seen in *S. pombe* (Hale et al. 2007; Buhler et al. 2007). Since, the *doppia* cytosine methylation patterns appear unaffected by paramutation, it has been proposed that paramutation alters properties of the molecular boundary found at the juxtaposition between heterochromatin and euchromatin domains (Hale et al. 2007). Despite the lack of evidence that paramutation at *b1* or *pl1* is associated with any changes in cytosine methylation patterns (Patterson et al. 1993; Hollick et al. 2000; Hale et al. 2007), cytosine methylation levels of the *S1* and *S2* genes of *R-r* are increased following exposure to *Rst* (Eggleston et al. 1995; Walker 1998) unless the complex contains deletions of the sigma region (Walker 1998). Paramutation of *P1-rr* is also strongly correlated with increased cytosine methylation levels (Sidorenko and Peterson 2001). Given that paramutation is meiotically heritable, it will be surprising — though not unprecedented (see Cavalli and Paro 1998; Nakayama et al. 2000) — if the heritable changes at functionally essential features are not due to reversible DNA modifications.

Mutant developmental phenotypes of both *mop1* and *rmr6* mutants indicate that expression patterns of specific developmental regulators are canalized during development by mechanisms similar to those employed in paramutation at *b1*, *pl1* and *r1* (Dorweiler et al. 2000; Hollick et al. 2005; Parkinson et al. 2007). Many of the mutant phenotypes appear similar to those seen in plants with specific microRNA-based mutations (Parkinson et al. 2007). mRNA profiles of *mop1* and *rmr6* mutants relative to wild-type siblings could be performed on highly defined tissues and/or developmental timepoints to identify important developmental regulators subject to MOP1/RMR6 epigenomic control. Comparative maize epigenome profiling based on specific DNA and/or other chromatin modifications that are dependent on MOP and RMR functions should likewise be informative.

The extent to which paramutation operates throughout the maize genome is currently unknown. One emerging concept from genetic analyses is that paramutation may correspond to alterations in boundary function between heterochromatic and euchromatic domains (Stam et al. 2002a; Hale et al. 2007). The detailed genetic characterizations of the different maize paramutation systems together with the promising application of biochemical and cytological approaches suggest that a detailed understanding of the molecular mechanism is imminent. Studies of the *mop* and *rmr* genes highlight mechanistic relationships between transgene silencing, transposon control, developmental canalization, and paramutation. It is anticipated that the entrées afforded by studies of *mop* and *rmr* functions will thus serve to characterize the sequence features and nuclear system responsible for specifying and modulating the maize epigenome.

3 Epigenomics in Maize

There is a rich history in the characterization and study of epigenetic phenomena in maize. However, there have been relatively few studies dedicated to a systematic study of the maize epigenome. Primarily, this is due to the large size and complicated structure of the maize genome. While these features have slowed epigenomic research efforts, it is likely that these factors provide a rich breeding ground for epigenetic regulation of maize genes and thus will make maize an important model system for the study of epigenomics. In this section we will describe the organization of the maize genome and the variation that exists between maize haplotypes. Then we will discuss why this organization is likely to spawn a high number of examples of epigenetic regulation and the evidence that this is occurring.

3.1 Maize Genome Organization and Variability

When considering the likely impact and prevalence of epigenetic regulation within an organism it is important to consider (a) the factors that condition epigenetic regulation, (b) the organization of the genome with respect to the genes and the factors conditioning epigenetic regulation, and (c) the variability for the factors that condition epigenetic regulation between different haplotypes. We will tackle each of these issues separately to generate a view of the current maize genome and how it is influenced by epigenetic regulation.

What are the factors that condition epigenetic regulation? This is a question that broadly applies to any organism or type of epigenetic regulation. The overwhelming trends that have emerged from the past decades of research into epigenetic phenomena have been the importance of repeats (direct and indirect) and transposable elements (which frequently contain direct or indirect repeats). There is evidence that many of the *Arabidopsis* genes that have become subject to epigenetic regulation reside in close proximity to transposons or retrotransposons (Lippman et al. 2003; Lippman et al. 2004; Kinoshita et al. 2007; Saze and Kakutani 2007; Yi and Richards 2007). There is strong evidence that epigenetic mechanisms are involved in the regulation of transposable elements (reviewed in Slotkin and Martienssen 2007). There is also evidence that changes in the epigenetic state of transposons can have effects on the expression of nearby genes that have not been directly targeted for epigenetic regulation (Barkan and Martienssen 1991; Morgan et al. 1999; Slotkin and Martienssen 2007; Hale et al. 2007). Given these findings, it is anticipated that the occurrence of transposable elements near genes and variation for the relative organization of transposable elements and genes will provide opportunities for epigenetic regulation and variation within a species.

What is the organization of the genome with respect to the genes and the factors conditioning epigenetic regulation? The maize genome is still a work in progress but there is sufficient data to provide a descriptive picture of its organization. The sequencing of several regions has revealed that, in general, genes exist alone or in small clusters that are separated by stretches of transposable elements (SanMiguel

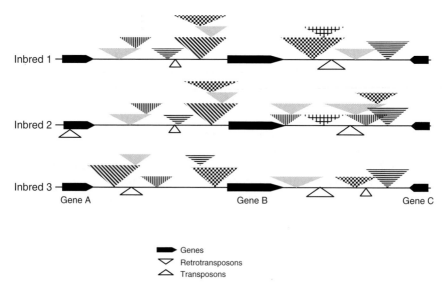

Fig. 3 The complex organization of the maize genome. This schematic provides an example of the complex organization of the maize genome. A region containing three genes (A, B and C) is sequenced in three different inbred lines (1, 2 and 3). The genes are illustrated using black solid arrows. The positions of retrotransposons are indicated by inverted triangles. Different classes of retrotransposon S are illustrated using different shading patterns. Note the differences in the retrotransposon content and organization between the different inbred lines. Several DNA transposons are also shown as triangles below the line. Similar to the retrotransposons, these elements exhibit variation in their localization between the different lines

et al. 1998; Fu et al. 2001; Brunner et al. 2005a, b; Messing et al. 2004; Messing, Dooner 2006; Wang and Dooner 2006; Wei et al. 2007). This organization has been referred to as gene "islands" in "seas" of transposable elements (illustrated in Fig. 3). It is quite rare to find five or more maize genes in a group without interruption by transposable elements. This organization is similar to that observed for the "heterochromatic knob" present on chromosome 4 in *Arabidopsis* (Lippman et al. 2004), which provides several examples of epigenetic regulation. However, it appears that this general organization predominates the maize genome. The majority of maize genes contain transposable elements located within 2 kb upstream of the transcription start site or 2 kb downstream of transcription termination (Haberer et al. 2005). Hence it has been suggested that maize transposons serve to divide and modularize the genome (Fedoroff 1999).

What is the variability for the factors that condition epigenetic regulation between different haplotypes? Based on extensive cytological studies, there is significant diversity in heterochromatin content and arrangement in various races of maize (McClintock et al. 1981; Kato et al. 2004). Some of the more conspicuous differences are known to affect general rates of recombination and chromosome segregation behaviors (Rhoades 1978). In addition, there is evidence from flow cytometry experiments that the size of the maize genome varies in different inbred lines (Laurie and Bennett 1985) and this variation is likely attributed to differences in repetitive sequences. The current maize genome sequencing effort is dedicated to producing a sequence for the B73 inbred genotype. However, several groups have performed sequencing of BAC clones from other maize genotypes. Aligning these chromosomal regions has allowed researchers to study the level of haplotype diversity (Fu and Dooner 2002; Brunner et al. 2005a, b; Wang and Dooner 2006). Fu and Dooner (2002) sequenced the region surrounding the *bz* locus from two different maize genotypes and found considerable variation for the content for low-copy genic sequences and for the amount, position and type of transposable elements between the two haplotypes (illustrated by the example in Fig. 3). The variation in the presence and position of low-copy genic sequences has been noted on a genome-wide scale (Morgante et al. 2005) and is likely due to the action of *helitron*-like transposable elements that have transposed fragments of the maize genome into non-allelic locations (Brunner et al. 2005a, b). A follow-up study by the Dooner group sequenced eight haplotypes at the *bz* locus and found that any two haplotypes shared 25–84% of the genomic DNA (Wang and Dooner 2006). The eight haplotypes demonstrate remarkable diversity for the content of transposable elements between genes. These results show the same gene being flanked by different transposable elements in different haplotypes. For example, a putative zinc-finger gene is flanked by five different types of elements in the eight haplotypes that were sequenced (Wang and Dooner 2006).

Together, the complex organization and structural variability of the maize genome are likely to provide ample opportunities for epigenetic regulation and variation. Since transposable elements can effect nearby genes by read-through transcription or chromatin effects (Whitelaw and Martin 2001), it is likely that many maize genes exhibit expression levels or patterns that are influenced by nearby transposable elements. If there is epigenetic variation regarding the state of transposable elements, then the nearby genes may also exhibit variation similar to the examples noted above. It has been suggested that large genomes themselves reflect the existence of a robust system of epigenetic control (Fedoroff 1999) since high levels of sequence redundancy threaten basic genomic integrity if recombination and transposition is left unchecked. Given this strong theoretical background for the existence of extensive epigenetic regulation and variation in maize what actual evidence is there to support this?

The first line of evidence to support the presence of high level of epigenetic variation in maize is based on the presence of more phenotypic variation than expected in certain populations (Rasmusson and Phillips 1997). For example, doubled haploids are expected to be 100% homozygous. However, there are a number of examples in which doubled haploid lines will exhibit heritable variation (Sprague et al. 1960; Rasmusson and Phillips 1997). This variation within a doubled haploid line is likely attributable to novel sequence rearrangements or epigenetic variation. Another example is the Illinois High Oil breeding experiment. This selection experiment has been on-going for over 100 years and there are still consistent gains being made (Moose et al. 2004). In addition, the gains, or loss, of oil production can be reversed when selection pressures are changed. This has been interpreted by some as an indication that at least a portion of the phenotypic variation is conditioned by epigenetic states (Moose et al. 2004).

The second line of evidence to support the high level of epigenetic variation in maize is based upon observations of DNA methylation patterns and the effects of DNA methylation. The DNA methylation patterns at specific loci or genome wide can vary in different maize lines (Kaeppler and Phillips 1993; Philips 1999). There is evidence for both genome-wide changes in DNA methylation levels between genotypes and for changes in the level of methylation at specific loci. In some instances these methylation states are highly heritable and in other cases they show instability. A recent study monitored gene expression changes that occurred in maize lines with a loss-of-function alleles for the chromomethylase *Zmet2* (Makarevitch et al. 2007). When the mutant allele was introgressed into the B73 genetic background, a set of ~70 loci exhibiting transcriptional alterations were identified. However, only 12 of these loci exhibited a similar response to a loss of CpNpG methylation in the Mo17 genetic background. A set of ~50 genes exhibit altered transcription levels only in the Mo17 genetic background. Further experiments revealed that many of these genes exhibit variable methylation levels in different maize inbreds that are correlated with their expression state. This study suggests that the targets of epigenetic regulation are highly variable between different maize inbred lines.

4 Perspective and Prospects of Maize Epigenomics

We are excited about the future prospects for epigenomics research in maize. Maize provides a strong model for epigenomics due to its high levels of natural variation, complex genome structure, cytogenetic, genetic and genomic resources and the fact that maize is an economically important crop. In order to realize the potential of maize as a useful model system it is critical to begin working towards a characterization of the maize epigenome. The maize genome represented by the B73 inbred line sequences will serve as the anchor scaffold for all subsequent comparative genome projects. Likewise, a representation of the B73 epigenome should stand as the reference for comparative epigenomics. The precision with which researchers could enrich diverse sources of developmental tissues and cell types for subsequent comparative epigenomics represents a significant strength of the maize system for future studies related to the epigenetic control of development and differentiation.

The high levels of natural variation within the maize species is an attractive feature of this system. As described above, maize varieties exhibit high levels of haplotype variation. In addition, maize varieties exhibit high levels of expression (Springer and Stupar 2007) and phenotypic variation (Flint-Garcia et al. 2005) as well. It is anticipated that a portion of the phenotypic diversity of maize is due to epigenetic variation between maize varieties. There are excellent resources that will allow researchers to address this issue. The existing global maize genetic diversity is largely represented in 25 inbred lines that are currently the subjects of a large public Nested-Association Mapping (NAM) project that has generated 5000 Recombinant Inbred Lines (RILs) for trait-to-gene identification (www.panzea.org; Zhao et al. 2006; Buckler et al. 2006). A high density SNP profile of the 25 inbreds, B73, and any RILs displaying a trait of interest can be compared to identify the cosegregating chromosome segment responsible for a given trait (Buckler et al. 2006). By studying these chromosomal segments researchers can assess whether the variation is epigenetic in nature. The NAM RIL platform holds great promise for its long-term use in dissecting and understanding the organization and dynamic operation of the maize epigenome.

The complex genome structure of maize also makes it an important model system. This genomic complexity has hampered efforts to completely sequence and assemble the maize genome. It will continue to cause difficulties in accurately studying the epigenome as it is quite difficult to study individual copies of the repetitive sequences. However, it is likely that as technologies advance we will identify appropriate tools to study specific regions. For example, high resolution cytogenetic studies or the use of microarrays for sequence capture of specific regions are likely to allow for more detailed evaluation of the complete maize epigenome. However, the same features that make maize technically difficult for these types of studies are what makes maize a biologically interesting species to study. The relatively simple structures of the *Arabidopsis* or rice genomes are unusual among plant species. Instead, most plant genomes exhibit complex structures more similar to that of maize. This complex structure provides ample opportunities for transposable elements to interact with genes and cause epigenetic regulation.

Aside from specific tests of individual epigenetic regulatory systems available from monitoring reporter alleles as discussed above, the broader types of epigenomic profiling available for evaluating B73 and the 25 diversity inbreds can consist of RNA profiling or genomic fractionations based on covalent modifications (i.e. cytosine methylation) or chromatin status (i.e. specific histone variants or modifications). In addition, as the number of immunocytochemical reagents expand, the protocols of RNA and DNA FISH are refined, and the imaging techniques such as structured illumination (Gustafsson et al. 2008) become more widely used, it is expected that the fine details of the maize chromosomes that made them the subject of choice for early cytogenetic studies will be diagnostic for profiling epigenomic variation and instructive for understanding the relationships between genome organization and epigenetic control.

Because of its importance to US agriculture, there is a wealth of data and archived germplasm related to corn improvement. We envision that these materials will be ripe for reevaluations focused on the structure and dynamic behaviors of their epigenomes. With a molecular understanding of maize epigenomic variation and the tools with which to quickly profile this variation, the epigenomic consequences of specific crosses and breeding schemes can be compared with historical field data to identify key interactions or epigenomic features related to specific morphometric results. These strategies hold the future promise of directing the mining of epigenomic variation in global maize accessions and providing predictive information to aid marker-assisted selection breeding programs.

The potential for understanding the cellular and molecular mechanisms at work in maize epigenomic control is significant. As previously mentioned, there are outstanding pedigreed materials available for studies of transposon control and paramutation, and there is now an expanding collection of maize mutants defective in various aspects of normal epigenetic control. Because position-based cloning in maize is now straight-forward and routine (Bortiri et al. 2006), the molecular identification of remaining *mop* and *rmr* genes should occur quickly. Epigenomic profiling using these mutants should expand the list of genomic targets under epigenetic control. Combined with the highly defined behaviors of known epigenomic targets, knowledge of MOP and RMR actions together with specific immunological reagents should help motivate a rich set of experiments to understand the molecular interface between specific genomic features and the nuclear system acting to modulate their expression.

Aside from the architecture of the maize epigenome and the nuclear machinery controlling its function, principle information is needed in understanding its perception of the external environment. In her Nobel lecture, McClintock (1984) described the dynamic potential of genomes to respond to shocks of various types. Her own work showed that BFB cycles resulted in alterations to the heterochromatin that produced novel sources of epigenetic-based variation detected by transposon insertions into or nearby normal Pol II genes. Mikula (1985) found that the paramutation process at *r1* was enhanced under conditions of relatively high temperature during a phenocritical time during seedling development. Clearly, the maize epigenome can perceive and respond in heritable ways to stressful conditions, but the mode of this perception is completely unknown. It is anticipated that further understanding of the maize epigenome and its control system will eventually illuminate this connection between environmental perception and heritable "genetic" changes.

References

Alleman M, Doctor J (2000) Genomic imprinting in plants: observations and evolutionary implications. Plant Mol Biol 43: 147–161

Alleman M, Sidorenko L, McGinnis K, Seshadri V, Dorweiler JE, White J, Sikkink K, Chandler VL (2006) An RNA-dependent RNA polymerase is required for paramutation in maize. Nature 442: 295–298

Banks J, Masson P, Fedoroff N (1988) Molecular mechanisms in the developmental regulation of the maize *Suppressor-mutator* transposable element. Genes Dev 2: 1364–1380

Barkan A, Martienssen R (1991) Inactivation of maize transposon *mu* suppresses a mutant phenotype by activating an outward-reading promoter near the end of *mu1*. Proc Natl Acad Sci U S A 88: 3502–3506

Baroux C, Pecinka A, Fuchs J, Schubert I, Grossniklaus U (2007) The triploid endosperm genome of *Arabidopsis* adopts a peculiar, parental-dosage-dependent chromatin organization. Plant Cell 19: 1782–1794

Beckmann JS, Estivill X, Antonarakis SE (2007) Copy number variants and genetic traits: closer to the resolution of phenotypic to genotypic variability. Nat Rev Genet 8: 639–646

Bennetzen JL, Schrick K, Springer PS, Brown WE, SanMiguel P (1994) Active maize genes are unmodified and flanked by diverse classes of modified, highly repetitive DNA. Genome 37: 565–576

Bennetzen J (2005) Transposable elements, gene creation and genome rearrangement in flowering plants. Curr Opin Genet Dev 15: 621–627

Bercury SD, Panavas T, Irenze K, Walker EL (2001) Molecular analysis of the *Doppia* transposable element of maize. Plant Mol Biol 47: 341–351

Birchler J, Veitia R (2007) The gene balance hypothesis: From classical genetics to modern genomics. Plant Cell 19: 395–402
Bortiri E, Jackson D, Hake S (2006) Advances in maize genomics: the emergence of positional cloning. Curr Opin Plant Biol 9: 164–171
Brink RA (1973) Paramutation. Annu Rev Genet 7: 129–152
Brink RA (1958) Paramutation at the R locus in maize. Cold Spring Harb Symp Quant Biol 23: 379–391
Brink RA (1956) A Genetic change associated with the R locus in maize which is directed and potentially reversible. Genetics 41: 872–889
Brown DF (1966) Paramutability of R and r mutant genes derived from an R Allele in maize. Genetics 54: 899–910
Brunner S, Fengler K, Morgante M, Tingey S, Rafalski A (2005a) Evolution of DNA sequence nonhomologies among maize inbreds. Plant Cell 17: 343–360
Brunner S, Pea G, Rafalski A (2005b) Origins, genetic organization and transcription of a family of non-autonomous helitron elements in maize. Plant J 43: 799–810
Buckler E, Gaut B, McMullen M (2006) Molecular and functional diversity of maize. Curr Opin Plant Biol 9: 172–176
Buhler M, Haas W, Gygi SP, Moazed D (2007) RNAi-dependent and -independent RNA turnover mechanisms contribute to heterochromatic gene silencing. Cell 129: 707–721
Bureau T, White S, Wessler S (1994) Transduction of a cellular gene by a plant retroelement. Cell 77: 479–480
Casa AM, Brouwer C, Nagel A, Wang L, Zhang Q, Kresovich S, Wessler SR (2000) Inaugural article: the MITE family heartbreaker (Hbr): molecular markers in maize. Proc Natl Acad Sci U S A 97: 10083–10089
Cavalli G, Paro R (1998) Chromo-domain proteins: linking chromatin structure to epigenetic regulation. Curr Opin Cell Biol 10: 354–360
Chan SW, Zilberman D, Xie Z, Johansen LK, Carrington JC, Jacobsen SE (2004) RNA silencing genes control de novo DNA methylation. Science 303: 1336
Chandler VL, Stam M (2004) Chromatin conversations: mechanisms and implications of paramutation. Nat Rev Genet 5: 532–54
Chandler VL, Walbot V (1986) DNA modification of a maize transposable element correlates with loss of activity. Proc Natl Acad Sci U S A 83: 1767–1771
Choi Y, Gehring M, Johnson L, Hannon M, Harada JJ, Goldberg RB, Jacobsen SE, Fischer RL (2002) DEMETER, a DNA glycosylase domain protein, is required for endosperm gene imprinting and seed viability in *Arabidopsis*. Cell 110: 33–42
Chomet P, Lisch D, Hardeman KJ, Chandler VL, Freeling M (1991) Identification of a regulatory transposon that controls the *Mutator* transposable element system in maize. Genetics 129: 261–270
Chomet PS, Wessler S, Dellaporta SL (1987) Inactivation of the maize transposable element *Activator (Ac)* is associated with its DNA modification. EMBO J 6: 295–302
Cocciolone SM, Cone KC (1993) *Pl-Bh*, an anthocyanin regulatory gene of maize that leads to variegated pigmentation. Genetics 135: 575–588
Cocciolone SM, Sidorenko LV, Chopra S, Dixon PM, Peterson T (2000) Hierarchical patterns of transgene expression indicate involvement of developmental mechanisms in the regulation of the maize *P1-rr* promoter. Genetics 156: 839–846
Coe EH (1966) The properties, origin, and mechanism of conversion-type inheritance at the *B* locus in maize. Genetics 53: 1035–1063
Danilevskaya ON, Hermon P, Hantke S, Muszynski MG, Kollipara K, Ananiev EV (2003) Duplicated *fie* genes in maize: expression pattern and imprinting suggest distinct functions. Plant Cell 15: 425–438
Das OP, Messing J (1994) Variegated phenotype and developmental methylation changes of a maize allele originating from epimutation. Genetics 136: 1121–1141
Dilkes BP, Comai L (2004) A differential dosage hypothesis for parental effects in seed development. Plant Cell 16: 3174–3180

Ding Y, Wang X, Su L, Zhai J, Cao S, Zhang D, Liu C, Bi Y, Qian Q, Cheng Z, Chu C, Cao X (2007) SDG714, a histone H3K9 methyltransferase, is involved in Tos17 DNA methylation and transposition in rice. Plant Cell 19: 9–22

Dooner HK, Robbins TP, Jorgensen RA (1991) Genetic and developmental control of anthocyanin biosynthesis. Annu Rev Genet 25: 173–199

Dorweiler JE, Carey CC, Kubo KM, Hollick JB, Kermicle JL, Chandler VL (2000) *Mediator of paramutation1* is required for establishment and maintenance of paramutation at multiple maize loci. Plant Cell 12: 2101–2118

Ebbs ML, Bender J (2006) Locus-specific control of DNA methylation by the *Arabidopsis* SUVH5 histone methyltransferase. Plant Cell 18: 1166–1176

Eggleston WB, Alleman M, Kermicle JL (1995) Molecular organization and germinal instability of *R*-stippled maize. Genetics 141: 347–360

Fedoroff N, Botstien D (1992) The dynamic genome. Cold Spring Harbor Laboratory Press, New York

Fedoroff N (1989) The heritable activation of cryptic *Suppressor-mutator* elements by an active element. Genetics 121: 591–608

Fedoroff NV (1999) Transposable elements as a molecular evolutionary force. Ann N Y Acad Sci 870: 251–264

Flaus A, Martin DM, Barton GJ, Owen-Hughes T (2006) Identification of multiple distinct Snf2 subfamilies with conserved structural motifs. Nucleic Acids Res 34: 2887–2905

Flint-Garcia SA, Thuillet AC, Yu J, Pressoir G, Romero SM, Mitchell SE, Doebley J, Kresovich S, Goodman MM, Buckler ES (2005) Maize association population: a high-resolution platform for quantitative trait locus dissection. Plant J 44: 1054–1064

Fu H, Dooner HK (2002) Intraspecific violation of genetic colinearity and its implications in maize. Proc Natl Acad Sci U S A 99: 9573–9578

Fu H, Park W, Yan X, Zheng Z, Shen B, Dooner HK (2001) The highly recombinogenic *bz* locus lies in an unusually gene-rich region of the maize genome. Proc Natl Acad Sci U S A 98: 8903–8908

Gehring M, Huh JH, Hsieh TF, Penterman J, Choi Y, Harada JJ, Goldberg RB, Fischer RL (2006) DEMETER DNA glycosylase establishes MEDEA polycomb gene self-imprinting by allele-specific demethylation. Cell 124: 495–506

Gierl A, Lutticke S, Saedler H (1988) TnpA product encoded by the transposable element *En-1* of *Zea mays* is a DNA binding protein. EMBO J 7: 4045–4053

Grandbastien MA (2004) Stress activation and genomic impact of plant retrotransposons. J Soc Biol 198: 425–432

Gross SM, Hollick JB (2007) Multiple *trans*-sensing interactions affect meiotically heritable epigenetic states at the maize *pl1* locus. Genetics 176: 829–839

Guo M, Rupe MA, Zinselmeier C, Habben J, Bowen BA, Smith OS (2004) Allelic variation of gene expression in maize hybrids. Plant Cell 16: 1707–1716

Gustafsson MGL, Shao L, Carlton PM, Wang CJR, Golubovskaya IN, Cande WZ, Agard DA, Sedat JW. (2008) Three-dimensional resolution doubling in wide-field fluorescence microscopy by structured illumination. Biophys J 94(12) 4957–4970

Gutierrez-Marcos JF, Costa LM, Dal Pra M, Scholten S, Kranz E, Perez P, Dickinson HG (2006) Epigenetic asymmetry of imprinted genes in plant gametes. Nat Genet 38: 876–878

Gutierrez-Marcos JF, Pennington PD, Costa LM, Dickinson HG (2003) Imprinting in the endosperm: a possible role in preventing wide hybridization. Philos Trans R Soc Lond B Biol Sci 358: 1105–1111

Haberer G, Young S, Bharti AK, Gundlach H, Raymond C, Fuks G, Butler E, Wing RA, Rounsley S, Birren B, Nusbaum C, Mayer KF, Messing J (2005) Structure and architecture of the maize genome. Plant Physiol 139: 1612–1624

Haig D, Westoby M (1989) Parent-specific gene-expression and the triploid endosperm. Am Nat 134: 147–155

Hale CJ, Stonaker JL, Gross SM, Hollick JB (2007) A novel Snf2 protein maintains *trans*-generational regulatory states established by paramutation in maize. PLoS Biol 5: 2156–2165

Haun WJ, Laoueille-Duprat S, O'connell MJ, Spillane C, Grossniklaus U, Phillips AR, Kaeppler SM, Springer NM (2007) Genomic imprinting, methylation and molecular evolution of maize Enhancer of zeste (Mez) homologs. Plant J 49: 325–337

Hermon P, Srilunchang KO, Zou J, Dresselhaus T, Danilevskaya ON (2007) Activation of the imprinted Polycomb Group *Fie1* gene in maize endosperm requires demethylation of the maternal allele. Plant Mol Biol 64: 387–395

Hirochika H (1993) Activation of tobacco retrotransposons during tissue culture. EMBO J 12: 2521–2528

Hirochika H, Okamoto H, Kakutani T (2000) Silencing of retrotransposons in *Arabidopsis* and reactivation by the *ddm1* mutation. Plant Cell 12: 357–369

Hirochika H, Sugimoto K, Otsuki Y, Tsugawa H, Kanda M (1996) Retrotransposons of rice involved in mutations induced by tissue culture. Proc Natl Acad Sci U S A 93: 7783–7788

Hollick JB, Chandler VL (2001) Genetic factors required to maintain repression of a paramutagenic maize *pl1* allele. Genetics 157: 369–378

Hollick JB, Chandler VL (1998) Epigenetic allelic states of a maize transcriptional regulatory locus exhibit overdominant gene action. Genetics 150: 891–897

Hollick JB, Kermicle JL, Parkinson SE (2005) *Rmr6* maintains meiotic inheritance of paramutant states in *Zea mays*. Genetics 171: 725–740

Hollick JB, Patterson GI, Asmundsson IM, Chandler VL (2000) Paramutation alters regulatory control of the maize *pl1* locus. Genetics 154: 1827–1838

Hollick JB, Patterson GI, Coe EH,Jr, Cone KC, Chandler VL (1995) Allelic interactions heritably alter the activity of a metastable maize *pl* allele. Genetics 141: 709–719

Huettel B, Kanno T, Daxinger L, Aufsatz W, Matzke AJM, Matzke M (2006) Endogenous targets of RNA-directed DNA methylation and Pol IV in *Arabidopsis*. ENBO J. 25: 2828–2836

Huettel B, Kanno T, Daxinger L, Bucher E, van der Winden J, Matzke AJ, Matzke M (2007) RNA-directed DNA methylation mediated by DRD1 and Pol IVb: a versatile pathway for transcriptional gene silencing in plants. Biochim Biophys Acta 1769: 358–374

Jiang N, Bao Z, Zhang X, Eddy SR, Wessler SR (2004) Pack-MULE transposable elements mediate gene evolution in plants. Nature 431: 569–573

Jin YK, Bennetzen JL (1994) Integration and nonrandom mutation of a plasma membrane proton ATPase gene fragment within the Bs1 retroelement of maize. Plant Cell 6: 1177–1186

Jullien PE, Kinoshita T, Ohad N, Berger F (2006) Maintenance of DNA methylation during the *Arabidopsis* life cycle is essential for parental imprinting. Plant Cell 18: 1360–1372

Kaeppler SM, Phillips RL (1993) Tissue culture-induced DNA methylation variation in maize. Proc Natl Acad Sci U S A 90: 8773–8776

Kanno T, Aufsatz W, Jaligot E, Mette MF, Matzke M, Matzke AJ (2005) A SNF2-like protein facilitates dynamic control of DNA methylation. EMBO Rep 6: 649–655

Kanno T, Mette MF, Kreil DP, Aufsatz W, Matzke M, Matzke AJ (2004) Involvement of putative SNF2 chromatin remodeling protein DRD1 in RNA-directed DNA methylation. Curr Biol 14: 801–805

Kapitonov VV, Jurka J (2001) Rolling-circle transposons in eukaryotes. Proc Natl Acad Sci U S A 98: 8714–8719

Kasschau KD, Fahlgren N, Chapman EJ, Sullivan CM, Cumbie JS, Givan SA, Carrington JC (2007) Genome-wide profiling and analysis of *Arabidopsis* siRNAs. PLoS Biol 5: e57

Kato A, Lamb JC, Birchler JA (2004) Chromosome painting using repetitive DNA sequences as probes for somatic chromosome identification in maize. Proc Natl Acad Sci U S A 101: 13554–13559

Kato M, Miura A, Bender J, Jacobsen SE, Kakutani T (2003) Role of CG and non-CG methylation in immobilization of transposons in *Arabidopsis*. Curr Biol 13: 421–426

Kermicle JL (1996) Epigenetic silencing and activation of a maize *r* gene. In VEA Russo, RA Martienssen, AD Riggs, eds, Epigenetic mechanisms of gene regulation. Cold Spring Harbor Laboratory Press, New York, pp 267–287

Kermicle JL (1978) Imprinting of gene action in maize endosperm. Maize breeding and genetics. Wiley, New York, pp 357–371

Kermicle JL (1970) Dependence of the *R-mottled* aleurone phenotype in maize on mode of sexual transmission. Genetics 66: 69–85

Kermicle JL, Alleman M (1990) Gametic imprinting in maize in relation to the angiosperm life cycle. Dev Suppl 9–14

Kermicle JL, Eggleston WB, Alleman M (1995) Organization of paramutagenicity in *R-stippled* maize. Genetics 141: 361–372

Kinoshita T, Miura A, Choi Y, Kinoshita Y, Cao X, Jacobsen SE, Fischer RL, Kakutani T (2004) One-way control of *FWA* imprinting in *Arabidopsis* endosperm by DNA methylation. Science 303: 521–523

Kinoshita Y, Saze H, Kinoshita T, Miura A, Soppe WJ, Koornneef M, Kakutani T (2007) Control of *FWA* gene silencing in *Arabidopsis thaliana* by SINE-related direct repeats. Plant J 49: 38–45

Krogh BO, Symington LS (2004) Recombination proteins in yeast. Annu Rev Genet 38: 233–271

Kumar A, Bennetzen JL (1999) Plant retrotransposons. Annu Rev Genet 33: 479–532

Kunze R, Starlinger P, Schwartz D (1988) DNA methylation of the maize transposable element *Ac* interferes with its transcription. Mol Gen Genet 214: 325–327

Lai J, Li Y, Messing J, Dooner HK (2005) Gene movement by Helitron transposons contributes to the haplotype variability of maize. Proc Natl Acad Sci U S A 102: 9068–9073

Lamb JC, Meyer JM, Corcoran B, Kato A, Han F, Birchler JA (2007) Distinct chromosomal distributions of highly repetitive sequences in maize. Chromosome Res 15: 33–49

Lauria M, Rupe M, Guo M, Kranz E, Pirona R, Viotti A, Lund G (2004) Extensive maternal DNA hypomethylation in the endosperm of *Zea mays*. Plant Cell 16: 510–522

Laurie DA, Bennett MD (1985) Nuclear DNA content in the genera *Zea* and Sorghum. Intergeneric, interspecific and intraspecific variation. Heredity 55: 307–313

Lee EA, Ahmadzadeh A, Tollenaar M (2005) Quantitative genetic analysis of the physiological processes underlying maize grain yield. Crop Sci 45: 981–987

Lin BY (1984) Ploidy barrier to endosperm development in maize. Genetics 107: 103–115

Lindroth AM, Cao X, Jackson JP, Zilberman D, McCallum CM, Henikoff S, Jacobsen SE (2001) Requirement of CHROMOMETHYLASE3 for maintenance of CpXpG methylation. Science 292: 2077–2080

Lippman Z, Gendrel AV, Black M, Vaughn MW, Dedhia N, McCombie WR, Lavine K, Mittal V, May B, Kasschau KD, Carrington JC, Doerge RW, Colot V, Martienssen R (2004) Role of transposable elements in heterochromatin and epigenetic control. Nature 430: 471–476

Lippman Z, May B, Yordan C, Singer T, Martienssen R (2003) Distinct mechanisms determine transposon inheritance and methylation via small interfering RNA and histone modification. PLoS Biol 1: E67

Lisch D, Carey CC, Dorweiler JE, Chandler VL (2002) A mutation that prevents paramutation in maize also reverses *Mutator* transposon methylation and silencing. Proc Natl Acad Sci U S A 99: 6130–6135

Liu R, Vitte C, Ma J, Mahama AA, Dhliwayo T, Lee M, Bennetzen JL (2007) A GeneTrek analysis of the maize genome. Proc Natl Acad Sci U S A 104: 11844–11849

Makarevitch I, Stupar RM, Iniguez AL, Haun WJ, Barbazuk WB, Kaeppler SM, Springer NM (2007) Natural variation for alleles under epigenetic control by the maize chromomethylase *Zmet2*. Genetics 177: 749–760

Martienssen R (1996) Epigenetic phenomena: paramutation and gene silencing in plants. Curr Biol 6: 810–813

Martienssen R, Baron A (1994) Coordinate suppression of mutations caused by Robertson's mutator transposons in maize. Genetics 136: 1157–1170

Masson P, Surosky R, Kingsbury JA, Fedoroff NV (1987) Genetic and molecular analysis of the *Spm*-dependent *a-m2* alleles of the maize *a* locus. Genetics 117: 117–137

McClintock B (1964) Aspects of gene regulation in maize. Carnegie Inst Wash Year Book 63: 592–602

McClintock B, Kato A, Blumenschein A (1981) Chromosome constitution of races of maize. Its significance in the interpretation of relationships between races and varieties in the Americas. Colegio de Postgraduados, Mexico

McClintock B (1984) The significance of responses of the genome to challenge. Science 226: 792–801
McClintock B (1951) Chromosome organization and genic expression. Cold Spring Harb Symp Quant Biol 16: 13–47
McGinnis KM, Springer C, Lin Y, Carey CC, Chandler V (2006) Transcriptionally silenced transgenes in maize are activated by three mutations defective in paramutation. Genetics 173: 1637–1647
McGinnis K, Murphy N, Carlson AR, Akula A, Akula C, Basinger H, Carlson M, Hermanson P, Kovacevic N, McGill MA, Seshadri V, Yoyokie J, Cone K, Kaeppler HF, Kaeppler SM, Springer NM (2007) Assessing the Efficiency of RNA Interference for Maize Functional Genomics. Plant Physiol 143: 1441–1451
Messing J, Bharti AK, Karlowski WM, Gundlach H, Kim HR, Yu Y, Wei F, Fuks G, Soderlund CA, Mayer KF, Wing RA (2004) Sequence composition and genome organization of maize. Proc Natl Acad Sci U S A 101: 14349–14354
Messing J, Dooner H (2006) Organization and variability of the maize genome. Curr Opin Plant Biol 9: 157–163
Meyers B, Tingey S, Morgante M (2001) Abundance, distribution, and transcriptional activity of repetitive elements in the maize genome. Genome Res 11: 1660–1676
Mikula BC (1995) Environmental programming of heritable epigenetic changes in paramutant *r*-gene expression using temperature and light at a specific stage of early development in maize seedlings. Genetics 140: 1379–1387
Miura A, Yonebayashi S, Watanabe K, Toyama T, Shimada H, Kakutani T (2001) Mobilization of transposons by a mutation abolishing full DNA methylation in *Arabidopsis*. Nature 411: 212–214
Moose SP, Dudley JW, Rocheford TR (2004) Maize selection passes the century mark: a unique resource for 21st century genomics. Trends Plant Sci 9: 358–364
Morgan HD, Sutherland HG, Martin DI, Whitelaw E (1999) Epigenetic inheritance at the *agouti* locus in the mouse. Nat Genet 23: 314–318
Morgante M, Brunner S, Pea G, Fengler K, Zuccolo A, Rafalski A (2005) Gene duplication and exon shuffling by helitron-like transposons generate intraspecies diversity in maize. Nat Genet 37: 997–1002
Nakayama J, Klar AJ, Grewal SI (2000) A chromodomain protein, Swi6, performs imprinting functions in fission yeast during mitosis and meiosis. Cell 101: 307–317
Ohtsu K, Smith MB, Emrich SJ, Borsuk LA, Zhou R, Chen T, Zhang X, Timmermans MC, Beck J, Buckner B, Janick-Buckner D, Nettleton D, Scanlon MJ, Schnable PS (2007) Global gene expression analysis of the shoot apical meristem of maize (*Zea mays* L.). Plant J 52: 391–404
Panavas T, Weir J, Walker EL (1999) The structure and paramutagenicity of the *R-marbled* haplotype of *Zea mays*. Genetics 153: 979–991
Parkinson SE, Gross SM, Hollick JB (2007) Maize sex determination and abaxial leaf fates are canalized by a factor that maintains repressed epigenetic states. Dev Biol 308: 462–473
Patterson GI, Thorpe CJ, Chandler VL (1993) Paramutation, an allelic interaction, is associated with a stable and heritable reduction of transcription of the maize *b* regulatory gene. Genetics 135: 881–894
Philips RL (1999) Research needs in heterosis. The genetics and exploitation of heterosis in crops. Crop Science Society of America, Madison, WI, pp 501–508
Pooma W, Gersos C, Grotewold E (2002) Transposon insertions in the promoter of the *Zea mays a1* gene differentially affect transcription by the Myb factors P and C1. Genetics 161: 793–801
Pouteau S, Spielmann A, Meyer C, Grandbastien MA, Caboche M (1991) Effects of Tnt1 tobacco retrotransposon insertion on target gene transcription. Mol Gen Genet 228: 233–239
Rabinowicz PD, Schutz K, Dedhia N, Yordan C, Parnell LD, Stein L, McCombie WR, Martienssen RA (1999) Differential methylation of genes and retrotransposons facilitates shotgun sequencing of the maize genome. Nat Genet 23: 305–308
Rangwala SH, Richards EJ (2007) Differential epigenetic regulation within an *Arabidopsis* retroposon family. Genetics 176: 151–160

Rasmusson DC, Phillips RL (1997) Plant breeding progress and genetic diversity from de novo variation and elevated epistasis. Crop Sci 37: 303–310

Rhoades MM (1978) Genetic effects of heterochromatin in maize. Maize breeding and genetics., Ed Walden, J.B. John Wiley and Sons, Toronto, pp 641–671

SanMiguel P, Gaut BS, Tikhonov A, Nakajima Y, Bennetzen JL (1998) The paleontology of intergene retrotransposons of maize. Nat Genet 20: 43–45

SanMiguel P, Tikhonov A, Jin YK, Motchoulskaia N, Zakharov D, Melake-Berhan A, Springer PS, Edwards KJ, Lee M, Avramova Z, Bennetzen JL (1996) Nested retrotransposons in the intergenic regions of the maize genome. Science 274: 765–768

Saze H, Kakutani T (2007) Heritable epigenetic mutation of a transposon-flanked *Arabidopsis* gene due to lack of the chromatin-remodeling factor DDM1. EMBO J 26: 3641–3652

Schwartz D, Dennis E (1986) Transposase activity of the *Ac* controlling element in maize is regulated by its degree of methylation. Mol Gen Genet 205: 476–482

Schwarz-Sommer Z, Shepherd N, Tacke E, Gierl A, Rohde W, Leclercq L, Mattes M, Berndtgen R, Peterson PA, Saedler H (1987) Influence of transposable elements on the structure and function of the *A1* gene of *Zea mays*. EMBO J 6: 287–294

Sidorenko LV, Peterson T (2001) Transgene-induced silencing identifies sequences involved in the establishment of paramutation of the maize *p1* gene. Plant Cell 13: 319–335

Slotkin RK, Freeling M, Lisch D (2005) Heritable transposon silencing initiated by a naturally occurring transposon inverted duplication. Nat Genet 37: 641–644

Slotkin RK, Martienssen R (2007) Transposable elements and the epigenetic regulation of the genome. Nat Rev Genet 8: 272–285

Smith LM, Pontes O, Searle I, Yelina N, Yousafzai FK, Herr AJ, Pikaard CS, Baulcombe DC (2007) An SNF2 protein associated with nuclear RNA silencing and the spread of a silencing signal between cells in *Arabidopsis*. Plant Cell 19: 1507–1521

Sprague GF, Russell WA, Penny LH (1960) Mutations affecting quantitative traits in the selfed progeny of doubled monoploid maize stocks. Genetics 45: 855–866

Springer NM, Gutierrez-Marcos J (2008) Imprinting in maize. The maize handbook. Springer, New York

Springer NM, Stupar RM (2007) Allelic variation and heterosis in maize: how do two halves make more than a whole? Genome Res 17: 264–275

Stam M, Belele C, Dorweiler JE, Chandler VL (2002a) Differential chromatin structure within a tandem array 100 kb upstream of the maize *b1* locus is associated with paramutation. Genes Dev 16: 1906–1918

Stam M, Belele C, Ramakrishna W, Dorweiler JE, Bennetzen JL, Chandler VL (2002b) The regulatory regions required for *B'* paramutation and expression are located far upstream of the maize *b1* transcribed sequences. Genetics 162: 917–930

Stupar RM, Hermanson PJ, Springer NM (2007) Nonadditive expression and parent-of-origin effects identified by microarray and allele-specific expression profiling of maize endosperm. Plant Physiol 145: 411–425

Styles ED, Brink RA (1969) The metastable nature of paramutable *R* alleles in maize. IV. Parallel enhancement of *R* action in heterozygotes with *r* and in hemizygotes. Genetics 61: 801–811

Styles ED, Brink RA (1966) The metastable nature of paramutable *R* alleles in maize. I. Heritable enhancement in level of standard *R* action. Genetics 54: 433–439

Tompa R, McCallum CM, Delrow J, Henikoff JG, van Steensel B, Henikoff S (2002) Genome-wide profiling of DNA methylation reveals transposon targets of CHROMOMETHYLASE3. Curr Biol 12: 65–68

Turcich M, Bokhari-Riza A, Hamilton, He C, Messier W, Stewart C (1996) PREM-2, a copia-type retroelement in maize is expressed preferentially in early microspores. Sex Plant Reprod 9: 65–74

Vicient CM, Jaaskelainen MJ, Kalendar R, Schulman AH (2001) Active retrotransposons are a common feature of grass genomes. Plant Physiol 125: 1283–1292

Vitte C, Bennetzen JL (2006) Analysis of retrotransposon structural diversity uncovers properties and propensities in angiosperm genome evolution. Proc Natl Acad Sci U S A 103: 17638–17643

Walbot V (2001) Imprinting of *R-r*, paramutation of *B-I* and *Pl*, and epigenetic silencing of *MuDR/Mu* transposons in *Zea mays L.* are coordinately affected by inbred background. Genet Res 77: 219–226

Walker EL (1998) Paramutation of the *r1* locus of maize is associated with increased cytosine methylation. Genetics 148: 1973–1981

Walker EL, Robbins TP, Bureau TE, Kermicle J, Dellaporta SL (1995) Transposon-mediated chromosomal rearrangements and gene duplications in the formation of the maize *R-r* complex. EMBO J 14: 2350–2363

Wang Q, Dooner HK (2006) Remarkable variation in maize genome structure inferred from haplotype diversity at the *bz* locus. Proc Natl Acad Sci U S A 103: 17644–17649

Wei F, Coe E, Nelson W, Bharti AK, Engler F, Butler E, Kim H, Goicoechea JL, Chen M, Lee S, Fuks G, Sanchez-Villeda H, Schroeder S, Fang Z, McMullen M, Davis G, Bowers JE, Paterson AH, Schaeffer M, Gardiner J, Cone K, Messing J, Soderlund C, Wing RA (2007) Physical and genetic structure of the maize genome reflects its complex evolutionary history. PLoS Genet 3: e123

Weiler KS, Wakimoto BT (1995) Heterochromatin and gene expression in Drosophila. Annu Rev Genet 29: 577–605

Wessler SR (1996) Turned on by stress. Plant retrotransposons. Curr Biol 6: 959–961

Whitelaw E, Martin DI (2001) Retrotransposons as epigenetic mediators of phenotypic variation in mammals. Nat Genet 27: 361–365

Wicker T, Sabot F, Hua-Van A, Bennetzen JL, Capy P, Chalhoub B, Flavell A, Leroy P, Morgante M, Panaud O, Paux E, SanMiguel P, Schulman AH (2007) A unified classification system for eukaryotic transposable elements. Nat Rev Genet 8: 973–982

Woodhouse MR, Freeling M, Lisch D (2006a) Initiation, establishment, and maintenance of heritable *MuDR* transposon silencing in maize are mediated by distinct factors. PLoS Biol : e339

Woodhouse MR, Freeling M, Lisch D (2006b) The *mop1* (*mediator of paramutation1*) mutant progressively reactivates one of the two genes encoded by the *MuDR* transposon in maize. Genetics 172: 579–592

Xiao W, Gehring M, Choi Y, Margossian L, Pu H, Harada JJ, Goldberg RB, Pennell RI, Fischer RL (2003) Imprinting of the *MEA* Polycomb gene is controlled by antagonism between MET1 methyltransferase and DME glycosylase. Dev Cell 5: 891–901

Yi H, Richards EJ (2007) A cluster of disease resistance genes in *Arabidopsis* is coordinately regulated by transcriptional activation and RNA silencing. Plant Cell 19: 2929–2939

Zhao W, Canaran P, Jurkuta R, Fulton T, Glaubitz J, Buckler E, Doebley J, Gaut B, Goodman M, Holland J, Kresovich S, McMullen M, Stein L, Ware D (2006) Panzea: a database and resource for molecular and functional diversity in the maize genome. Nucleic Acids Res 34: D752–7

Zilberman D, Cao X, Jacobsen SE (2003) ARGONAUTE4 control of locus-specific siRNA accumulation and DNA and histone methylation. Science 299: 716–719

Epigenetic Silencing of Pericentromeric Heterochromatin by RNA Interference in *Schizosaccharomyces pombe*

Sarahjane Locke and Robert Martienssen

Abstract The formation and spreading of heterochromatin by both RNA interference (RNAi) dependent and independent mechanisms is important for chromosome organization and cohesion, proper centromere function, and silencing. Schizosaccharomyces pombe is a useful model organism for the study of initiation, maintenance, and inheritance of epigenetic marks. Recent publications in the field have helped to explain the mechanism and functional consequences of programing the epigenome with specific focus on identifying effector complexes, gene silencing and position effect variegation, the cell cycle, and function of conserved regions of heterochromain.

Keywords *S. pombe*, · RNAi · Heterochromatin · Position effect variegation · Silencing · Centromeres

Schizosaccharomyces pombe, also known as fission yeast, is a unicellular, haploid, eukaryote. Its small, fully sequenced genome, roughly 12.5 Mb, comprises three chromosomes (Wood et al. 2002). Aside from its role in beer making in sub-Saharan Africa, fission yeast has gained popularity as a model organism because, like higher eukaryotes, its centromeres are large and organized in tandem repeats and it has an RNA interference (RNAi) pathway; neither of which are found in the budding yeast *Saccharomyces cerevisiae*.

1 Higher Order Chromatin Structure and PEV

Post translational modification of histone tails and interaction with various effector proteins packages chromosomal material into two distinct domains: euchromatin and heterochromatin. Heterochromatin is highly condensed, perturbing transcription, and is often associated with repetitive elements (Richards and Elgin 2002).

S. Locke (✉)
Cold Spring Harbor Laboratory, 1 Bungtown Road, Cold Spring Harbor NY 11724
e-mail: locke@cshl.edu

In *S. pombe*, centromeres, telomeres, and the mating type locus are packaged into heterochromatin, characterized by hypoacetylated histones, and histone H3 lysine 9 methylation (H3K9me). Conversely, hyperacetylated histones and H3K4me are marks of euchromatin, a less densely packaged form of chromatin associated with active transcription. Position effect variegation (PEV), first described in the complex eye of *Drosophila melanogaster*, demonstrates that the position of a gene relative to heterochromatin can affect its expression (Fig. 1) (Ekwall et al. 1997; Schotta et al. 2003; Talbert and Henikoff 2006). In other words PEV results from the "spreading" of silent heterochromatin into neighboring genes. *S. pombe* heterochomatin can also confer silencing from centromeric repeats, for example, into

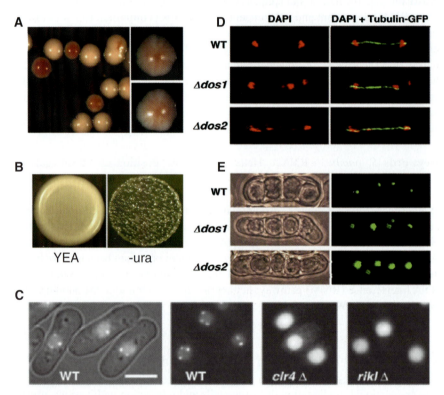

Fig. 1 Heterochromatic Effects in *S. pombe* (A) Colonies grown up from a single wild type cell showing position effect variegation of an $ade6^+$ reporter gene inserted within pericentromeric repeats. Silenced $ade6^+$ results in red colonies. (B) Growth of 10^5 cells in each spot, showing position effect variegation of an $ura4^+$ reporter gene inserted within pericentromeric repeats. Silenced $ura4^+$ results in no growth on media lacking uracil. (C) Dislocalization of the heterochromatic protein Swi6 fused with GFP indicates a loss of heterochromatin in *clr4* and *rik1* (Pidoux et al. 2000). (D) Lagging chromosomes are observed during late mitotic anaphase with DAPI staining in *dos1* and *dos2* (Li et al. 2005). (E) Aberrant number of nuclei per spore in *dos1* and *dos2* asci as seen by GFP-Swi6 (Li et al. 2005)

reporter genes inserted within them (Allshire 1994). This silencing depends on RNAi (Volpe et al. 2002).

The signature epigenetic mark of heterochromatin in *S. pombe* is H3K9me. H3K9 can be mono, di, or tri-methylated by Clr4, the only histone methyl transferase (HMT) responsible for depositing this mark in *S. pombe* (Nakayama et al. 2001). A *Su(var)3-9* family homolog, Clr4 contains a catalytic SET and chromo domain (CD) (Ivanova et al. 1998). It has recently been determined that some H3K9 methylation can be reversed by demethylases like Lsd1, resulting in a dynamic chromatin state that acts to regulate transcription and determine chromatin boundaries (Lan et al. 2007). Similarly, reversible acetylation plays an important part in regulating chromatin state. For example, the hypoacetylation observed in heterochromatin is a direct result of the activity of multiple histone deacetylases (HDACs) like Clr3 and Clr6 which deacetylate H3K14 and H3K9, respectively (Ekwall 2005). Treatment with an HDAC inhibitor like trichostatin-A (TSA), results in the heritable loss of heterochromatin and the dissociation of the heterochromatic protein Swi6 (Ekwall et al. 1997).

2 Centromeres

S. pombe centromeres are 35-110kb, and are made up of numerous heterochromatic tandem repeats flanking a central core region of specialized chromatin structure associated with the histone H3 homolog CENH3/CENP-A (Chikashige et al. 1989; Clarke and Baum 1990; Murakami et al. 1991; Polizzi and Clarke 1991; Wood et al. 2002). Both the central core and the heterochromatic flanking repeats are required for centromere function in kinetochore attachment, chromosome segregation and sister chromatid cohesion (Clarke and Baum1990; Hahnenberger et al. 1991; Allshire et al. 1995) (Fig. 1). The central core and heterochromatic repeats are distinct domains that differ in sequence and chromatin state, specifying the binding of different effector proteins to each domain: the chromodomain containing proteins Swi6 and Chp1 coat the pericentromeric repeats and are distinctly separated by tRNA boundary elements from Mis6 which binds the central regions (Partridge et al. 2000).

The heterochromatic repetitive sequences bordering the central core consist of innermost (*imr*) and outermost (*otr*) repeats. The *otr* is further classified into *dg* and *dh* repeats that are juxtaposed in various orientations and orders differing between the three centromeres (Chikashige et al. 1989; Clarke and Baum 1990; Murakami et al. 1991).

Though promoters are contained within these heterochromatic repetitive elements (Djupedal et al. 2005) the repeats themselves are transcriptionally and post-transcriptionally silenced by RNAi. The insertion of $ura4^+$ and/or $ade6^+$ reporter genes within pericentromeric repeats results in PEV in a wildtype background (Fig. 1) (Allshire 1994). RNAi mutants lose the ability to silence such reporter genes, indicating an essential role for RNAi in the spreading of heterochromatin (Volpe et al. 2002). Despite its importance for proper centromere function and the ability to confer silencing on reporter genes, RNAi plays only a minor role at the heterochromatic mating type locus and telomeres, despite these regions containing similar repeats.

3 RNAi-Mediated Epigenetic Silencing in *S. pombe*

S. pombe is unique in that it only has one copy of each of the major components of the RNAi machinery; an RNaseH-like Argonaute (Ago1), an RNaseIII-like Dicer (Dcr1), and an RNA directed RNA Polymerase (Rdp1). RNAi mutants, namely Δ*ago1*, Δ*dcr1*, or Δ*rdp1*, accumulate centromeric transcripts and lose small interfering RNAs (siRNAs) mapping to those transcripts (Volpe et al. 2002; Li et al. 2005). This indicates that siRNAs are produced by transcription and processing of heterochromatic repeats by RNAi. These mutants also lack the ability to silence reporter genes inserted within heterochromatic regions and exhibit lagging chromosomes at anaphase, resembling mutants in *clr4*, *swi6* and cohesin (Fig. 1). ChIP data suggest these phenotypes are a direct result of the disturbance of RNAi-mediated formation and maintenance of heterochromatin at the centromere (Volpe et al. 2002; Hall et al. 2003; Volpe et al. 2003).

Unlike RNAi mutants in which both forward and reverse repeat transcripts accumulate, mutants lacking the heterochromatic protein Swi6 have an intact RNAi pathway and accumulate only forward transcripts (Volpe et al. 2002). This suggests that forward transcripts are transcriptionally silenced through repressive heterochromatin formation, which requires Swi6, while reverse transcripts are post-transcriptionally silenced by rapid processing into siRNA. Thus RNAi mediates both transcriptional (TGS) and post transcriptional (PTGS) gene silencing (Cerutti and Casas-Mollano 2006).

Paradoxically, then, RNAi-mediated heterochromatin formation and maintenance at the centromere requires the transcription of heterochromatic repeats (Fig. 2). The pericentromeric repeats are transcribed from heterochromatic promoters by RNA Polymerase II (polII) (Djupedal et al. 2005). These transcripts are then quickly processed by the RNA Dependent RNA Polymerase Complex (RDRC). This complex is comprised of Rdp1, the RNA helicase Hrr1, and a member of the polyA polymerase family Cid12 (Motamedi et al. 2004). Processing by RDRC results in a double stranded RNA substrate for Dcr1, which produces siRNAs. siRNAs are loaded into the PAZ domain of Ago1 in the RNA Induced Initiation of Transcriptional Silencing complex, RITS (Verdel et al. 2004). The CD containing protein Chp1 brings the RITS complex to heterochromatin through binding of H3K9me2, thus RITS association with chromatin is dependent on Clr4 (Partridge et al. 2002). RITS and RDRC physically interact in a Dcr1 and Clr4 dependent manner and localize to the *otr* (Motamedi et al. 2004). RITS is guided by the bound siRNA to a target complementary message (Verdel et al. 2004; Irvine et al. 2006). The slicing activity of Ago1 is necessary for not just heterochromatin formation, but also for proper recruitment of RDRC, suggesting that RDRC acts on sliced transcripts (Irvine et al. 2006).

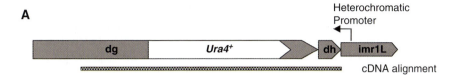

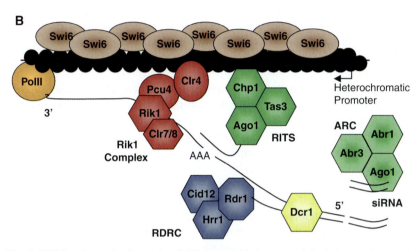

Fig. 2 RNAi pathway in *S. pombe* (**A**) Cartoon depicting part of the left arm of centromere I, with a *ura4+* reporter gene inserted within the pericentromeric repeats. An alignment of the cDNA coming from this region shows cotranscription of the reporter gene. (**B**) Cartoon depicting the RNAi pathway. Black circles are histones methylated on H3K9

The RNAi pathway recruits the chromatin modification machinery, including Clr4 (Fig. 2). Clr4 is recruited to chromatin in complex with the cullin E3 ubiquitin ligase, Pcu4, and Rik1, a protein that shares homology to DNA damage binding protein Ddb1 as well as the cleavage and polyadenylation specificity factor CPSF (Sadaie et al. 2004; Horn et al. 2005; Jia et al. 2005). The Rik1 complex also includes two novel proteins required for the localization of Swi6 to heterochromatin, Clr8 and Clr7 also known as Dos1/Raf1 and Dos2/Raf2 respectively (Horn et al. 2005; Li et al. 2005; Thon et al. 2005), as well as the 14-3-3 protein Rad24 (Moazed et al. 2006ch09:moazed2006). Noncoding RNAs from *dg* repeats accumulate in mutants in each of these components, and H3K9 methylation is completely lost, resembling Δ*clr4* (Fig. 1) (Li et al. 2005).

4 Investigations into the RNAi Pathway

Though *S. pombe* has only one copy of the three main components of the RNAi machinery, the pathway consists of multiple players and sophisticated mechanisms about which we still have much to learn.

Buker et al. have identified a new *S. pombe* Argonaute complex, independent of RITS. ARC for Argonaute siRNA chaperone complex, contains Ago1 and two argonaute binding proteins, Arb1 and Arb2 (Buker et al. 2007). Like other RNAi components Arb1/2 are required for spreading of silencing into reporter genes, heterochromatin formation, and siRNA generation at centromeres, and do not seem to be required at the mating type locus. Predominantly duplex siRNAs were identified in purified ARC suggesting that siRNAs produced by Dcr1 are first loaded on Ago1 in ARC. Arb1 inhibits the slicer activity of Ago1 (Fig. 2). Once Ago1 dissociates from ARC, slicing activity is restored and releases the passenger strand of siRNA, resulting in a catalytically active RITS containing only Ago1 loaded with single stranded siRNA.

Irvine et al. have shown *S. pombe* Argonaute to be an RNaseH-like siRNA-dependent slicer of target messages, similar to the Argonautes found in animals and plants (Irvine et al. 2006). The magnesium-dependent catalytic activity requires a conserved D-D-H motif. In slicing mutants the levels of Rdp1 and H3K9me at centromeric repeats decrease, accompanied by a de-repression of pericentromeric repeat transcription and a dramatic loss of spreading of heterochromatin into a $ura4^+$ reporter gene inserted within these repeats. Buker et al. confirm that slicer activity by single stranded siRNA-bound Ago1 is required for its association with and the spreading of heterochromatin (Buker et al. 2007). Because significant levels of H3K9me2 remain associated with the repeats of slicer mutants, but not with the reporter genes, slicing seems to be predominantly required for spreading of heterochromatin, perhaps via co-transcription from the repeats.

Tas3 bridges the association of Ago1 with Chp1 as a member of the RITS complex. Disrupting the association between Tas3 and Ago1, in $tas3_{WG}$ cells, did not seem to result in any of the usual RNAi mutant phenotypes (Partridge et al. 2007). However, a Tas3 mutant, that doesn't bind Chp1 but still binds Ago1, $tas3_{10-24}$, does show a loss of centromeric heterochromatin formation (H3K9me2), an accumulation of centromeric transcripts and the disruption of RITS and RDRC association with centromeres (DeBeauchamp et al. 2008). In agreement with the model proposed by Buhler et al. and Irvine et al. in which siRNAs basepair with nascent synthesizing transcript, Ago1 in a $tas3_{10-24}$ was able to associate with and slice centromeric transcripts (DeBeauchamp et al. 2008). Combining mutants inhibiting Ago1's ability to efficiently bind siRNA with $tas3_{WG}$ results in an $\Delta ago1$-like phenotype (Partridge et al. 2007). These results suggest that the interaction between Tas3 and Chp1 is required for RITS assembly, and that both Tas3 and siRNA can recruit Ago1.

H3K9me2 is lost entirely in $\Delta clr4$ mutants, but upon reintroduction of Clr4, these levels are restored at centromeres. In contrast significant levels of H3K9me2 are retained over centromeric repeats in $\Delta chp1$ strains. However, restoration of repeat associated H3K9me2 fails to occur in $\Delta clr4 \Delta chp1$ (Sadaie et al. 2004) or in $\Delta clr4$ $tas3_{WG}$ double mutant strains (Partridge et al. 2007) when Clr4 is reintroduced. Interestingly, reconstituted Dcr1 in a $tas3_{WG} \Delta dcr1$ strain was able to efficiently silence centromeric transcripts and restore siRNA. This work suggests RITS is required for restoration of H3K9me2, and may initially be recruited via Chp1, Tas3, and then Ago1. RITS then recruits RDRC so that siRNA can be synthesized and loaded onto Ago1. Spreading of heterochromatin from repeats into reporter genes requires RITS and RNAi (Irvine et al. 2006), and perhaps this spreading stabilizes H3K9me2 after it is established *de novo*.

5 Co-transcriptional Gene Silencing and the Cell Cycle

Establishment and maintenance of centromeric heterochromatin depend on the transcription of *dg* and *dh* repeats, indicating an essential interaction between RNAi and transcription machinery. Studies of the cell cycle reveal some clues as to how "silent" chromatin can be transcribed to maintain a heterochromatic state.

Buhler et al. have shown that tethering Tas3 to a nascent transcript from endogenous, euchromatic *ura4*, via the fusion protein Tas3-λN, is sufficient for RNAi-dependent (and HDAC-dependent) silencing in *cis* as assayed by growth on FOA, ChIP with antibodies to H3K9me2 and Swi6, and a loss of *ura4* mRNA (Bühler et al. 2006). Tas3-λN results in the RNAi-dependent production of siRNAs and the recruitment of Chp1 at and around the *ura4* locus. However, tethering of other members of RITS or RDRC did not result in silencing. The repressive chromatin at *ura4* in Tas3-λN was not able to be maintained and inherited upon replacement with Tas3. Importantly, the transcription of *ura4* by polII is required for silencing, suggesting that Tas3-λN is localizing and binding the RITS complex directly to the transcript and not to the DNA; similar to the importance of transcription in spreading and silencing at the centromere (Irvine et al. 2006). PolII levels were unchanged in the presence or absence of RNAi machinery, either at the endogenous *ura4* with or without Tas3-λN or at a *ura4$^+$* within pericentromeric *dh* repeats (Bühler et al. 2006). Similarly, there was no increase in polII levels at centromeric repeats in Δ*dcr1* and Δ*clr4* mutants as compared to wildtype. These results agree with previous run-on transcription experiments, in which levels of nascent reverse-strand pre-siRNA are unchanged in RNAi mutants and in Δ*swi6* (Volpe et al. 2002), along with levels of association of *dh* repeats with polII (Kato et al. 2005). In contrast, the less abundant forward strand transcripts are transcriptionally silenced (Volpe et al. 2002), and recruit polII in RNAi mutants (Djupedal et al. 2005). This suggests a *co*-transcriptional gene silencing (CTGS) model in which siRNAs basepair with pre-mRNA as it is being synthesized by polII; this accounts for why tethering Tas3-λN is enough to silence *ura4*.

The siRNAs produced from Tas3-λN are only able to silence in *cis* (Bühler et al. 2006), and have no effect on a second unlinked locus. Bühler et al. show that the *cis* restriction is ensured by the exoribonuclease activity of Eri1, named for the enhanced RNAi phenotype of its mutants. Eri1 is an RNase T exonuclease that negatively regulates RNAi through the degradation of the 3' end of double stranded siRNA and is also involved in the processing of rRNA (Gabel and Ruvkun 2008). This further supports Tas3-λN acting on local, nascent transcript and not on mature transcripts. Though initiation was inefficient, siRNAs could act in *trans* to promote heterochromatin formation at a euchromatic loci in Δ*eri1* and once initiated heterochromatin could be efficiently maintained (Bühler et al. 2006).

Heterochromatin is classically characterized as highly condensed chromosomal material and has been thought of as transcriptionally inert. However, with the discovery of RNAi-dependent silencing it became clear that the heterochromatic repeats of *S. pombe* centromeres must be transcribed. Kloc et al. helped put to rest the apparent paradox (Kloc et al. 2008). Upon investigating RNAi regulation during the cell cycle, they observed that *dg* and *dh* transcripts followed by siRNAs appear predominantly in S phase. Interestingly, forward strand transcripts appear first, at low levels and initiate close to origins of replication. Reverse transcripts appear shortly thereafter and are processed into siRNA. During this time, H3S10ph appears at centromeric repeats, resulting in destabilization of heterochromatin via the "phosphomethyl switch" by which Swi6 is inhibited or displaced from H3K9me by phosphorylation of the neighboring Serine-10 (Chen et al. 2008; Kloc et al. 2008). The RNAi machinery, however, does not seem to be cell cycle regulated. Thus transient production of pre-siRNA and siRNA during S phase, because of the phopshomethyl switch, can guide recovery of H3K9me2 levels which fall after replication. Importantly, this work not only explains transcription of heterochromatic regions, but also provides a mechanism for the epigenetic inheritance of histone modifications during replication.

6 Mating Type Locus and Subtelomeric Regions

In addition to the centromeres, *S. pombe* has two other main regions of heterochromatin; the mating type locus and telomeres. These regions, though they contain similar heterochromatic repeats as those found at the centromeres, do not rely as heavily on the RNAi pathway for silencing. It appears, however, that some proteins involved in RNAi act independently at these locations.

The *tlh* genes encode a telomere-linked helicase and are found at the ends of each chromosome. They are closely related to non-coding *dh* and *dg* centromeric repeats. RNAi plays a role in *tlh* silencing (Mandell et al. 2005) but Chp1 has a stronger effect on silencing than Ago1, while Dcr1 and Rdp1 are not required, suggesting Chp1 might function in a separate pathway at telomeres (Hansen et al. 2006). In addition to Δ*chp1*, Δ*clr4*, *clr6-1*Δ*clr3*, Δ*pcu4*, Δ*dos1*, Δ*dos2*, and Δ*taz1* result in a high accumulation of *tlh* transcripts. As with centromeric and mating type silencing, treatment with the HDAC inhibitor TSA leads to an accumulation of *tlh* transcripts, however the treatment has much longer lasting effects at telomeres than at centromeres; recovery time is 72hrs and 12hrs respectively, indicating the importance of histone deacetylation for heterochromatin formation at telomeres.

At the mating type locus where RNAi plays little role in silencing, $tas3_{10-24}$, which does not bind Chp1, did nothing to de-repress *mat2* and *mat3* (DeBeauchamp et al. 2008). However, once heterochromatin is lost from the mating type locus in Δ*clr4* $tas3_{10-24}$ double mutants, it is difficult to reestablish by reintroduction of Clr4 (DeBeauchamp et al. 2008). Chp1 is also required for heterochromatic establishment at the *cenH* repeat found between the silent cassettes (Sadaie et al. 2004).

In contrast, Tas3 and Chp1 may play independent roles at telomeres. Deletion of either gene results in accumulation of subtelomeric *tlh* transcripts, but as seen at the mating type locus, H3K9me2 levels are maintained in $tas3_{10-24}$ despite loss of Chp1 association. Double mutants have similar levels of *tlh* transcripts as single mutants, however, indicating they play independent roles in similar or redundant pathways.

7 RNAi-Independent Heterochromatin Formation

RNAi is not the only pathway responsible for methylation of H3K9 by Clr4.

Mutations in Clr3 HDAC activity decrease H3K9me2 at *mat2* and *mat3*, relieving silencing (Nakayama et al. 2001). When both Dcr1 and Clr3 are deleted, Clr4 is no longer able to localize to centromeric repeats suggesting that these are the only two pathways through which H3K9 is methylated by Clr4 (Yamada et al. 2005). The activity of HDACs Clr3 and Clr6 on H3K14 and H3K9 respectively is necessary for a stepwise methylation of H3K9 by Clr4 (Ekwall 2005). Though they are redundant, RNAi has a much more prevalent role at the centromere (Volpe et al. 2002) while Clr3 has a stronger effect on the mating type locus, where inhibition of HDAC activity leads to an inherited loss of heterochromatin (Ekwall et al. 1997; Yamada et al. 2005).

Recently Sugiyama et al. (Sugiyama et al. 2007) reported the existence of a multienzyme complex through which Clr3 mediates transcriptional gene silencing, termed SHREC (Snf2/HDAC-containing repressor complex). Purification of Clr3-FLAG pulled down Clr1 and Clr2, factors involved in heterochromatic silencing at the mating type locus, as well as Ccq1 which acts on telomeres, and Mit1 a hitherto uncharacterized SNF2 ATPase homolog. Ccq1 is localized only at telomeres suggesting it acts with Taz1 to help recruit SHREC. The rest of the SHREC components were found at all heterochromatic regions. Interestingly, Clr2 was also seen at the central core domain of centromeres. Though SHREC can be recruited to chromatin independent of Swi6, it is necessary for SHREC's maintained association with heterochromatin and for establishing association with telomeres. In the absence of SHREC, H3K14ac and polII occupancy increase at pericentromeric heterochromatin and centromeric reporter genes. Under these conditions, H3K9 methylation at centromeric repeats becomes entirely dependent on RNAi. Interestingly, SHREC seems to play a role in heterochromatin formation through nucleosomal positioning in addition to its HDAC and ATPase properties.

8 Reprogramming the *S. pombe* Epigenome

In addition to histone methylation, histone demethylation also plays an important role, especially when silencing and H3K9 methylation extend beyond constitutive heterochromatin to encompass euchromatic genes. In these cases, reversibility of histone modification can be utilized to reprogram gene expression, as well as chromosomal organization. Genome-wide mapping of histone modifications in *S. pombe* has greatly advanced our understanding of these events (Lan et al. 2007; Opel et al. 2007; Zhang et al. 2008).

At first thought to be histone H3 lysine-4 demethylases (Gordon et al. 2007), the Lysine-Specific Demethylase (LSD) homologs in *S. pombe* act on histone H3 lysine-9 (Lan et al. 2007). In complex with two additional PHD domain proteins that presumably recognize H3K9me, LSDs act as co-activators of transcription of a subset of euchromatic genes. In *lsd1* mutants, this subset of genes is down-regulated due to the presence of H3K9me3 at promoters. Δ*lsd1* mutants are slow growing while Δ*lsd2* mutants are lethal. These growth defects are partially suppressed in a Δ*clr4* mutant background, directly implicating K9 methylation. LSD proteins can also have a repressive function, which is less well understood but helps to limit the boundaries of heterochromatin both at the centromere and at the mating type locus, where these proteins are also found (Lan et al. 2007). Genome-wide association studies suggest that this repressive function is mediated by Clr6, a histone deacetylase, reminiscent of LSD1 histone deacetylase association in mammalian cells (Opel et al. 2007).

RNAi also appears to play a role in euchromatic H3K9 methylation. Gullerova and Proudfoot report that transcriptional readthrough of a small subset of convergently transcribed genes in the *S. pombe* genome results in the generation of double stranded RNA, followed by the production of RNAi-dependent heterochromatin at the 3′ end of these genes (Gullerova and Proudfoot 2008). Transcriptional readthrough, RNAi and heterochromatin formation at euchromatic loci occurs transiently during the G1 phase of the cell cycle, earlier than pericentromeric heterochromatin which is only transcribed during S phase (Kloc et al. 2008). This allows retention of cohesin during the following G2, premature termination of transcription and abolition of readthrough for the rest of the cell cycle. The role of histone demethylation during the cell cycle has not been examined, but promises to shed light on the reprogramming of both heterochromatic and euchromatic marks to regulate both gene expression and chromatin organization during cell proliferation.

9 Functional Consequences of RNAi-Mediated Heterochromatin Formation

Heterochromatin plays other roles in fission yeast biology, in addition to the retention of cohesin and proper chromosome segregation. These roles have been recently brought to light, and involve establishment of the kinetochore and targeting of transposable elements.

CENP-A replaces histone H3 at the central core region of centromeres and is necessary for kinetochore assembly. Though the central core and *otr* are distinct regions of varying chromatin and protein composition, centromeric heterochromatin, namely H3K9me, is necessary for the establishment of CENP-A at the central region (Folco et al. 2008). A centromeric epiallele without CENP-A can switch to a fully functional centromere in the presence of Clr4. Maintenance of CENP-A, however, is not heterochromatin-dependent. This work implicates RNAi, as the main source of heterochromatin formation and maintenance at the *otr*, in the establishment of a unique chromatin at the central core.

Some mobile elements in *S. cerevisiae* encode chromodomains and integrate preferentially in heterochomatic silent regions of the genome (Zou et al. 1996). Chromo domain containing retrotransposons (CR retrotransposons) associate clearly with heterochromatic centromeric repeats (Miller et al. 1998; Cheng et al. 2002). Gao et al. have determined the integration preference for repeat-rich regions of five different representatives of retrotransposons from chromoviruses. They further show that the chromodomain of the fungal element MAGGY interacts with H3K9me in *S. pombe* (Gao et al. 2008). Targeting to heterochromatin may help to maintain and propagate these elements while the elements themselves help to maintain and propagate heterochromatin.

10 Summary

Heterochromatin is critical for chromosome organization, chromosome cohesion, centromere function and transposon silencing. It is the quintessential epigenetic material, remaining condensed from interphase to interphase, but capable of being lost and re-established without changes in the nucleotide sequence. Mechanisms that maintain heterochromatin during chromosomal replication, that spread heterochromatin to neighboring genes, and that initiate its formation, are rapidly being uncovered in fission yeast and other model organisms. These mechanisms include RNA interference, which has the important property of sequence specificity for heterochromatic repeats, as well as RNAi-independent histone modification, for example via deacetylation. The interplay between these mechanisms will contribute to our understanding of the epigenome of higher as well as lower eukaryotic organisms.

Acknowledgments We thank our colleagues M.Zaratiegui, D. Irvine, K. Hansen, A. Chang and A. Kloc for creative and helpful discussions. SL is a graduate student with the Watson School of Biological Sciences. Work in the authors' laboratory is supported by a grant from the National Institutes of Health (GM076396), and by grants from the National Science Foundation to RAM.

References

Allshire, R.C., Javerzat, J.P., Redhead, N.J., and Cranston, G. 1994. Position effect variegation at fission yeast centromeres. *Cell* **76**(1): 157–169.

Allshire, R.C., Nimmo, E.R., Ekwall, K., Javerzat, J.P., and Cranston, G. 1995. Mutations derepressing silent centromeric domains in fission yeast disrupt chromosome segregation. *Genes Dev* **9**(2): 218–233.

Bühler, M., Verdel, A., and Moazed, D. 2006. Tethering RITS to a nascent transcript initiates RNAi- and heterochromatin-dependent gene silencing. *Cell* **125**(5): 873–886.

Buker, S.M., Iida, T., Bühler, M., Villén, J., Gygi, S.P., Nakayama, J., and Moazed, D. 2007. Two different Argonaute complexes are required for siRNA generation and heterochromatin assembly in fission yeast. *Nat Struct Mol Biol* **14**(3): 200–207.

Cerutti, H. and Casas-Mollano, J.A. 2006. On the origin and functions of RNA-mediated silencing: from protists to man. *Curr Genet* **50**(2): 81–99.

Chen, E.S., Zhang, K., Nicolas, E., Cam, H.P., Zofall, M., and Grewal, S.I. 2008. Cell cycle control of centromeric repeat transcription and heterochromatin assembly. *Nature* **451**(7179): 734–737.

Cheng, Z., Dong, F., Langdon, T., Ouyang, S., Buell, C.R., Gu, M., Blattner, F.R., and Jiang, J. 2002. Functional rice centromeres are marked by a satellite repeat and a centromere-specific retrotransposon. *Plant Cell* **14**(8): 1691–1704.

Chikashige, Y., Kinoshita, N., Nakaseko, Y., Matsumoto, T., Murakami, S., Niwa, O., and Yanagida, M. 1989. Composite motifs and repeat symmetry in S. pombe centromeres: direct analysis by integration of NotI restriction sites. *Cell* **57**(5): 739–751.

Clarke and Baum, M.P. 1990. Functional analysis of a centromere from fission yeast: a role for centromere-specific repeated DNA sequences. *Mol Cell Biol* **10**(5): 1863–1872.

DeBeauchamp, J.L., Moses, A., Noffsinger, V.J., Ulrich, D.L., Job, G., Kosinski, A.M., and Partridge, J.F. 2008. Chp1-Tas3 interaction is required to recruit RITS to fission yeast centromeres and for maintenance of centromeric heterochromatin. *Mol Cell Biol* **28**(7): 2154–2166.

Djupedal, I., Portoso, M., Spåhr, H., Bonilla, C., Gustafsson, C.M., Allshire, R.C., and Ekwall, K. 2005. RNA Pol II subunit Rpb7 promotes centromeric transcription and RNAi-directed chromatin silencing. *Genes Dev* **19**(19): 2301–2306.

Ekwall, K. 2005. Genome-wide analysis of HDAC function. *Trends Genet* **21**(11): 608–615.

Ekwall, K., Olsson, T., Turner, B.M., Cranston, G., and Allshire, R.C. 1997. Transient inhibition of histone deacetylation alters the structural and functional imprint at fission yeast centromeres. *Cell* **91**(7): 1021–1032.

Folco, H.D., Pidoux, A.L., Urano, T., and Allshire, R.C. 2008. Heterochromatin and RNAi are required to establish CENP-A chromatin at centromeres. *Science* **319**(5859): 94–97.

Gabel, H.W. and Ruvkun, G. 2008. The exonuclease ERI-1 has a conserved dual role in 5.8S rRNA processing and RNAi. *Nat Struct Mol Biol* **15**(5): 531–533.

Gao, X., Hou, Y., Ebina, H., Levin, H.L., and Voytas, D.F. 2008. Chromodomains direct integration of retrotransposons to heterochromatin. *Genome Res* **18**(3): 359–369.

Gordon, M., Holt, D.G., Panigrahi, A., Wilhelm, B.T., Erdjument-Bromage, H., Tempst, P., Bähler, J., and Cairns, B.R. 2007. Genome-wide dynamics of SAPHIRE, an essential complex for gene activation and chromatin boundaries. *Mol Cell Biol* **27**(11): 4058–4069.

Gullerova, M. and Proudfoot, N.J. 2008. Cohesin complex promotes transcriptional termination between convergent genes in S. pombe. *Cell* **132**(6): 983–995.

Hahnenberger, K.M., Carbon, J., and Clarke, L. 1991. Identification of DNA regions required for mitotic and meiotic functions within the centromere of Schizosaccharomyces pombe chromosome I. *Mol Cell Biol* **11**(4): 2206–2215.

Hall, I.M., Noma, K., and Grewal, S.I. 2003. RNA interference machinery regulates chromosome dynamics during mitosis and meiosis in fission yeast. *Proc Natl Acad Sci USA* **100**(1): 193–198.

Hansen, K.R., Ibarra, P.T., and Thon, G. 2006. Evolutionary-conserved telomere-linked helicase genes of fission yeast are repressed by silencing factors, RNAi components and the telomere-binding protein Taz1. *Nucleic Acids Res* **34**(1): 78–88.

Horn, P.J., Bastie, J.N., and Peterson, C.L. 2005. A Rik1-associated, cullin-dependent E3 ubiquitin ligase is essential for heterochromatin formation. *Genes Dev* **19**(14): 1705–1714.

Irvine, D.V., Zaratiegui, M., Tolia, N.H., Goto, D.B., Chitwood, D.H., Vaughn, M.W., Joshua-Tor, L., and Martienssen, R.A. 2006. Argonaute slicing is required for heterochromatic silencing and spreading. *Science* **313**(5790): 1134–1137.

Ivanova, A.V., Bonaduce, M.J., Ivanov, S.V., and Klar, A.J. 1998. The chromo and SET domains of the Clr4 protein are essential for silencing in fission yeast. *Nat Genet* **19**(2): 192–195.

Jia, S., Kobayashi, R., and Grewal, S.I. 2005. Ubiquitin ligase component Cul4 associates with Clr4 histone methyltransferase to assemble heterochromatin. *Nat Cell Biol* **7**(10): 1007–1013.

Kato, H., Goto, D.B., Martienssen, R.A., Urano, T., Furukawa, K., and Murakami, Y. 2005. RNA polymerase II is required for RNAi-dependent heterochromatin assembly. *Science* **309**(5733): 467–469.

Kloc, A., Zaratiegui, M., Nora, E., and Martienssen, R. 2008. RNA Interference guides histone modification during the S phase of chromosomal replication. *Curr Biol* **18**(7): 490–495.

Lan, F., Zaratiegui, M., Villén, J., Vaughn, M.W., Verdel, A., Huarte, M., Shi, Y., Gygi, S.P., Moazed, D., Martienssen, R.A., and Shi, Y. 2007. S. pombe LSD1 homologs regulate heterochromatin propagation and euchromatic gene transcription. *Mol Cell* **26**(1): 89–101.

Li, F., Goto, D.B., Zaratiegui, M., Tang, X., Martienssen, R., and Cande, W.Z. 2005. Two novel proteins, dos1 and dos2, interact with rik1 to regulate heterochromatic RNA interference and histone modification. *Curr Biol* **15**(16): 1448–1457.

Mandell, J.G., Bähler, J., Volpe, T.A., Martienssen, R.A., and Cech, T.R. 2005. Global expression changes resulting from loss of telomeric DNA in fission yeast. *Genome Biol* **6**(1): R1.

Miller, J.T., Dong, F., Jackson, S.A., Song, J., and Jiang, J. 1998. Retrotransposon-related DNA sequences in the centromeres of grass chromosomes. *Genetics* **150**(4): 1615–1623.

Moazed, D., Buhler, M., Buker, S.M., Colmenares, S.U., Gerace, E.L., Gerber, S.A., Hong, E.J., Motamedi, M.R., Verdel, A., Villen, J., and Gygi, S.P. 2006. Studies on the mechanism of RNAi-dependent heterochromatin assembly. *Cold Spring Harb Symp Quant Biol* **71**: 461–471.

Motamedi, M.R., Verdel, A., Colmenares, S.U., Gerber, S.A., Gygi, S.P., and Moazed, D. 2004. Two RNAi complexes, RITS and RDRC, physically interact and localize to noncoding centromeric RNAs. *Cell* **119**(6): 789–802.

Murakami, S., Matsumoto, T., Niwa, O., and Yanagida, M. 1991. Structure of the fission yeast centromere cen3: direct analysis of the reiterated inverted region. *Chromosoma* **101**(4): 214–221.

Nakayama, J., Rice, J.C., Strahl, B.D., Allis, C.D., and Grewal, S.I. 2001. Role of histone H3 lysine 9 methylation in epigenetic control of heterochromatin assembly. *Science* **292**(5514): 110–113.

Opel, M., Lando, D., Bonilla, C., Trewick, S.C., Boukaba, A., Walfridsson, J., Cauwood, J., Werler, P.J., Carr, A.M., Kouzarides, T., Murzina, N.V., Allshire, R.C., Ekwall, K., and Laue, E.D. 2007. Genome-wide studies of histone demethylation catalysed by the fission yeast homologues of mammalian LSD1. *PLoS ONE* **2**(4): e386.

Partridge, J.F., Borgstrøm, B., and Allshire, R.C. 2000. Distinct protein interaction domains and protein spreading in a complex centromere. *Genes Dev* **14**(7): 783–791.

Partridge, J.F., DeBeauchamp, J.L., Kosinski, A.M., Ulrich, D.L., Hadler, M.J., and Noffsinger, V.J. 2007. Functional separation of the requirements for establishment and maintenance of centromeric heterochromatin. *Mol Cell* **26**(4): 593–602.

Partridge, J.F., Scott, K.S., Bannister, A.J., Kouzarides, T., and Allshire, R.C. 2002. cis-acting DNA from fission yeast centromeres mediates histone H3 methylation and recruitment of silencing factors and cohesin to an ectopic site. *Curr Biol* **12**(19): 1652–1660.

Pidoux, A.L., Uzawa, S., Perry, P.E., Cande, W.Z., and Allshire, R.C. 2000. Live analysis of lagging chromosomes during anaphase and their effect on spindle elongation rate in fission yeast. *J Cell Sci* **113 Pt 23**: 4177–4191.

Polizzi, C. and Clarke, L. 1991. The chromatin structure of centromeres from fission yeast: differentiation of the central core that correlates with function. *J Cell Biol* **112**(2): 191–201.

Richards, E.J. and Elgin, S.C. 2002. Epigenetic codes for heterochromatin formation and silencing: rounding up the usual suspects. *Cell* **108**(4): 489–500.

Sadaie, M., Iida, T., Urano, T., and Nakayama, J. 2004. A chromodomain protein, Chp1, is required for the establishment of heterochromatin in fission yeast. *EMBO J* **23**(19): 3825–3835.

Schotta, G., Ebert, A., Dorn, R., and Reuter, G. 2003. Position-effect variegation and the genetic dissection of chromatin regulation in Drosophila. *Semin Cell Dev Biol* **14**(1): 67–75.

Sugiyama, T., Cam, H.P., Sugiyama, R., Noma, K., Zofall, M., Kobayashi, R., and Grewal, S.I. 2007. SHREC, an effector complex for heterochromatic transcriptional silencing. *Cell* **128**(3): 491–504.

Talbert, P.B. and Henikoff, S. 2006. Spreading of silent chromatin: inaction at a distance. *Nat Rev Genet* **7**(10): 793–803.

Thon, G., Hansen, K.R., Altes, S.P., Sidhu, D., Singh, G., Verhein-Hansen, J., Bonaduce, M.J., and Klar, A.J. 2005. The Clr7 and Clr8 directionality factors and the Pcu4 cullin mediate heterochromatin formation in the fission yeast Schizosaccharomyces pombe. *Genetics* **171**(4): 1583–1595.

Verdel, A., Jia, S., Gerber, S., Sugiyama, T., Gygi, S., Grewal, S.I., and Moazed, D. 2004. RNAi-mediated targeting of heterochromatin by the RITS complex. *Science* **303**(5658): 672–676.

Volpe, T., Schramke, V., Hamilton, G.L., White, S.A., Teng, G., Martienssen, R.A., and Allshire, R.C. 2003. RNA interference is required for normal centromere function in fission yeast. *Chromosome Res* **11**(2): 137–146.

Volpe, T.A., Kidner, C., Hall, I.M., Teng, G., Grewal, S.I., and Martienssen, R.A. 2002. Regulation of heterochromatic silencing and histone H3 lysine-9 methylation by RNAi. *Science* **297**(5588): 1833–1837.

Wood, V. Gwilliam, R. Rajandream, M.A. Lyne, M. Lyne, R. Stewart, A. Sgouros, J. Peat, N. Hayles, J. Baker, S. Basham, D. Bowman, S. Brooks, K. Brown, D. Brown, S. Chillingworth, T. Churcher, C. Collins, M. Connor, R. Cronin, A. Davis, P. Feltwell, T. Fraser, A. Gentles, S. Goble, A. Hamlin, N. Harris, D. Hidalgo, J. Hodgson, G. Holroyd, S. Hornsby, T. Howarth, S. Huckle, E.J. Hunt, S. Jagels, K. James, K. Jones, L. Jones, M. Leather, S. McDonald, S. McLean, J. Mooney, P. Moule, S. Mungall, K. Murphy, L. Niblett, D. Odell, C. Oliver, K. O'Neil, S. Pearson, D. Quail, M.A. Rabbinowitsch, E. Rutherford, K. Rutter, S. Saunders, D. Seeger, K. Sharp, S. Skelton, J. Simmonds, M. Squares, R. Squares, S. Stevens, K. Taylor, K. Taylor, R.G. Tivey, A. Walsh, S. Warren, T. Whitehead, S. Woodward, J. Volckaert, G. Aert, R. Robben, J. Grymonprez, B. Weltjens, I. Vanstreels, E. Rieger, M. Schäfer, M. Müller-Auer, S. Gabel, C. Fuchs, M. Düsterhöft, A. Fritzc, C. Holzer, E. Moestl, D. Hilbert, H. Borzym, K. Langer, I. Beck, A. Lehrach, H. Reinhardt, R. Pohl, T.M. Eger, P. Zimmermann, W. Wedler, H. Wambutt, R. Purnelle, B. Goffeau, A. Cadieu, E. Dréano, S. Gloux, S. Lelaure, V. Mottier, S. Galibert, F. Aves, S.J. Xiang, Z. Hunt, C. Moore, K. Hurst, S.M. Lucas, M. Rochet, M. Gaillardin, C. Tallada, V.A. Garzon, A. Thode, G. Daga, R.R. Cruzado, L. Jimenez, J. Sánchez, M. del Rey, F. Benito, J. Domínguez, A. Revuelta, J.L. Moreno, S. Armstrong, J. Forsburg, S.L. Cerutti, L. Lowe, T. McCombie, W.R. Paulsen, I. Potashkin, J. Shpakovski, G.V. Ussery, D. Barrell, B.G. Nurse, P. and Cerrutti, L. 2002. The genome sequence of Schizosaccharomyces pombe. *Nature* **415**(6874): 871–880.

Yamada, T., Fischle, W., Sugiyama, T., Allis, C.D., and Grewal, S.I. 2005. The nucleation and maintenance of heterochromatin by a histone deacetylase in fission yeast. *Mol Cell* **20**(2): 173–185.

Zhang, K., Mosch, K., Fischle, W., and Grewal, S.I. 2008. Roles of the Clr4 methyltransferase complex in nucleation, spreading and maintenance of heterochromatin. *Nat Struct Mol Biol* **15**(4): 381–388.

Zou, S., Ke, N., Kim, J.M., and Voytas, D.F. 1996. The Saccharomyces retrotransposon Ty5 integrates preferentially into regions of silent chromatin at the telomeres and mating loci. *Genes Dev* **10**(5): 634–645.

Describing Epigenomic Information in Arabidopsis

Ian R. Henderson

Abstract Epigenetic modifications of the DNA and histones serve as heritable marks that can influence gene expression states. Genetic and genomic approaches are being used in the model plant *Arabidopsis thaliana* to understand how plants use epigenetic information. Tiling microarrays and high throughput sequencing have mapped the distribution of DNA methylation, histone methylation and small RNAs at a genome-wide scale. This has refined our models for genome organization and gene regulation in *A.thaliana* and revealed a number of unexpected patterns, such as DNA methylation within the body of genes. Integrating these large datasets and understanding the relationships between these marks will be an exciting challenge for the future.

Keywords Arabidopsis · Genomics · Epigenetics · Chromatin · RNAi

1 Introduction

The term, epigenetic, is used to describe heritable changes in expression state that are not due to changes in the primary DNA sequence (Fig. 1A). Epigenetic states are typically maintained in the absence of the signal that initiates them. Inheritance of epigenetic states is associated with covalent modifications of the DNA and histones, and these marks can be required for silent or active transcription. Plants have provided a rich source for the study of epigenetic inheritance and notable discoveries include transposable elements (Comfort 2001), paramutation (Chandler and Stam 2004), small RNAs (Hamilton and Baulcombe 1999), RNA-directed DNA methylation (RdDM) (Wassenegger, Heimes et al. 1994) and a mechanism for active DNA demethylation (Choi et al. 2002; Gong et al. 2002; Gehring et al. 2006; Morales-Ruiz et al. 2006). Plants are also distinguished from animals by a number of characteristics that may be of interest from an epigenetic point of view; for example,

---

I.R. Henderson (✉)
Department of Plant Sciences, Downing Street, University of Cambridge, CB2 3EA, UK
e-mail: irh25@cam.ac.uk

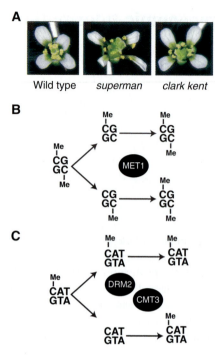

Fig. 1 A: Epigenetic silencing of *SUPERMAN* (*SUP*) by DNA methylation. Wild type *A.thaliana* possesses flowers with 6 stamens (the male reproductive structures). Classical genetic mutations in the *SUP* gene cause a homeotic increase in the number of stamens. The *clark kent* alleles are epi-mutations of *SUP* caused by DNA cytosine hypermethylation. **B**: Schematic diagram illustrating how MET1 uses hemi-methylated CG dinucleotides to maintain cytosine methylation through DNA replication. **C**: Schematic diagram illustrating maintenance of DNA methylation at an asymmetric (CAT) site through DNA replication. This type of methylation is redundantly maintained mainly by DRM2 and CMT3. As one CAT site is unmethylated after DNA replication, an active signal must be used to maintain this type of methylation

their propensity to undergo polyploidization (Otto 2007) and their developmental plasticity (Xu et al. 2006).

The ephemeral crucifer *Arabidopsis thaliana*, is currently the best developed model plant, though many other species have rapidly growing molecular resources (Somerville and Meyerowitz 2002; Bowman et al. 2007). The characteristics that lead to the selection of *A.thaliana* for study include its rapid life cycle (6 weeks in laboratory strains), diploid genetics, relatively compact genome (125 megabases over 5 chromosomes) and self-fertility (allowing homozygous strains to be easily maintained) (Somerville and Meyerowitz, 2002). Since its widespread adoption, a range of tools have been developed for *A.thaliana*; including a complete genome sequence (AGI 2000), a facile method for transformation using *Agrobacterium tumefaciens* (Clough 2005) and the generation of large databases of sequence-indexed Transfer-DNA (T-DNA) insertions (Alonso et al. 2003). In addition to being an excellent model for plant biology, *A.thaliana* also possesses features that make it an attractive system for the study of epigenetic inheritance. First, *A.thaliana* uses the majority of known epigenetic marks conserved in other eukaryotes; for example DNA cytosine methylation and covalent modification of the histones. Plants also generate small RNAs through the RNA interference (RNAi) pathway, which are capable of directing DNA methylation (Wassenegger et al. 1994; Matzke and Birchler 2005). A major advantage of *A.thaliana* is that it tolerates genomic changes than would cause lethality in most mammalian species. For example, viable mutant backgrounds with dramatically reduced DNA can be generated (Zhang and Yazaki 2006; Cokus et al. 2008) and ploidy can be manipulated (Scott et al. 1998; Chen et al. 2004). In this review I will highlight how epigenetic mechanisms have been studied on a genome-wide scale in *A.thaliana*, and what these approaches have taught us about epigenetic inheritance in plants.

2 Mapping DNA Cytosine Methylation

5-methyl cytosine is a modification of DNA typically associated with transcriptional silencing in eukaryotes (Suzuki and Bird 2008). Animals most frequently possess DNA methylation in the symmetrical CG sequence context (Suzuki and Bird 2008). The palindromic nature of CG dinucleotides provides a mechanism for epigenetic maintenance of cytosine methylation. DNA replication of a fully methylated (both strands) CG site will generate two hemi-methylated daughter chromosomes. The Dnmt1-class of methyltransferases (*METHYLTRANSFERASE1*, *MET1* in *A.thaliana*) preferentially recognizes hemi-methylated CG sites and adds a methyl-group to the opposite strand, maintaining this mark efficiently following DNA replication (Cheng 1995) (Fig. 1B). Plants also show DNA methylation in non-CG sequence contexts (CHG and CHH, where H is anything apart from G) (Chan, Henderson et al. 2005). Non-CG methylation is maintained redundantly by DOMAINS REARRANGED METHYLASE2 (DRM2, a homolog of the mammalian Dnmt3 methyltransferases) and CHROMOMETHYLASE3 (CMT3, a plant specific methyltransferase) at most loci (Cao and Jacobsen 2002a, b; Cokus et al. 2008; Lister et al. 2008) (Fig. 1C). As asymmetric (CHH) sites lack cytosine on one strand, a different mechanism must maintain this type of DNA methylation through DNA replication (Fig. 1C).

Mapping DNA cytosine methylation on a genome-wide scale requires two main advances; techniques to distinguish methylated and unmethylated DNA and a high throughput method to describe the isolated DNA (Zilberman and Henikoff 2007). Genome-wide mapping has been made possible in *A.thaliana* by the availability of tiling microarrays (Zhang et al. 2006; Vaughn et al. 2007; Zilberman et al. 2007). More recently, advances in high throughput sequencing technology have provided the means to map deeply at single base-pair resolution (Cokus et al. 2008; Lister et al. 2008). As tiling arrays often lack highly repeated components of the genome, sequencing technologies carry an advantage in this regard. Currently there are several means to specifically detect methylated DNA, including (i) treatment with methyl-sensitive restriction endonucleases, (ii) purification using recombinant methyl-C binding domains, (iii) immuno-purification using methyl-C antibodies and (iv) sodium bisulfite conversion (Zilberman and Henikoff 2007).

Restriction endonucleases vary widely in enzymatic sensitivity to cytosine methylation. For example, *Hpa*II and *Msp*I both cut at CCGG sites but the former is inhibited by methylation of either cytosine, while the latter only if the first cytosine is methylated (Zilberman and Henikoff 2007). In contrast, McrBC will cleave at sites (G/A-methyl-C) located between two methylated cytosines, which can be up to 3 kilobases apart (Zilberman and Henikoff 2007). Treatment with the appropriate enzyme can thus be used to enrich or remove methylated sequences, which can then be mapped to the genome (Tompa et al. 2002; Lippman et al. 2004; Vaughn et al. 2007). A disadvantage to using restriction enzymes is that they limit analysis to cytosine bases within their target recognition sites. Alternatively, methyl-cytosine DNA can be directly purified using either methyl-binding domains or methyl-C antibodies (Zhang et al. 2006; Zilberman et al. 2007). Prior to purification of methyl-cytosine DNA the sample is usually fragmented by sonication, meaning that the average fragment size is a major determinant of mapping resolution (Zhang et al. 2006; Zilberman et al. 2007). One limitation to affinity purification is that is not possible to know the sequence context of the methylated cytosines in the purified fragments. Knowledge of sequence context is important as loci vary in their silencing dependence on CG versus non-CG DNA. For example, silencing at the tandem repeats upstream of *FWA* depends mainly on CG methylation, while those at *SDC* depend on non-CG methylation (Soppe et al. 2000; Saze et al. 2003; Henderson and Jacobsen 2008). To determine sequence context information sodium bisulfite conversion can be used, which causes cytosine deamination to uracil, while methylated cytosine is not modified. Following bisulfite treatment the DNA is subjected to high throughput sequencing (BS-seq) where unmethylated cytosines will be present as thymine, while methylated sites are indicated by cytosine (Cokus et al. 2008; Lister et al. 2008). Conversion of unmethylated cytosines to thymines leads to a reduction in sample sequence complexity, meaning specialized analytical methods are required to accurately map the sequencing reads (Cokus et al. 2008; Lister et al. 2008). Good sequencing depth is also required to reliably detect CHH methylation, which is present at low levels ($\sim$1–15%) (Cokus et al. 2008; Lister et al. 2008). In addition to providing sequence context information, BS-seq also appears to have greater sensitivity than microarray based methods and is better able to analyze repetitive sequences (Cokus et al. 2008; Lister et al. 2008). For example, BS-Seq detected methylation within the telomeric and rDNA repeats, which are not represented on the available tiling arrays (Cokus et al. 2008).

The genome-wide maps of *A.thaliana* DNA methylation have shown that it strongly correlates with repeated sequences, transposons and siRNAs, which are abundant in the peri-centromeric regions (Tompa et al. 2002; Lippman et al. 2004; Zhang et al. 2006; Zilberman et al. 2007; Cokus et al. 2008; Lister et al. 2008). This likely reflects a type of genome-defense, as loss of DNA methylation can cause transposon transcription and movement (Miura et al. 2001; Singer et al. 2001; Kato et al. 2003). Fewer expressed genes have been found to be promoter-methylated, though a large class of genes shows CG methylation within their open reading frames (body methylation) (Tran et al. 2005; Zhang et al. 2006; Zilberman et al. 2007; Cokus et al. 2008). The function of this methylation is unclear but was found to anti-correlate with silent expression, indicating that it does not block transcription (Zhang et al. 2006; Zilberman et al. 2007). This is consistent with studies showing that RdDM targeting to a transgene promoter, but not open reading frame, causes transcriptional silencing (Jones et al. 1999). Interestingly, comparison of two laboratory strains of *A.thaliana* indicates that body methylation within genes can be polymorphic between populations (Vaughn et al. 2007).

The discovery of unexpected distributions of epigenetic information, such as genic CG methylation, highlights the advantages of unbiased genomic approaches. By combining BS-seq techniques with combinations of DNA methyltransferase mutations, the genetic requirements for methylation in different sequence contexts can be assayed on a genome-wide scale (Cokus et al. 2008; Lister et al. 2008). For example, although non-CG methylation is dramatically reduced in *drm1 drm2 cmt3*, residual amounts were found to remain in this triple mutant, particularly in the densely methylated peri-centromeric regions, (Cokus et al. 2008; Lister et al. 2008). This supports previous observations that a methyltransferase in addition to DRM2 and CMT3, perhaps MET1, is able to methylate non-CG sequences (Henderson et al. 2006; Henderson and Jacobsen 2008). Interestingly, both *drm1 drm2 cmt3* and *met1 cmt3* show an equal loss of CHH DNA methylation, suggesting that maintenance of CHH methylation may be influenced by both CG and CHG methylation (Cokus et al. 2008). A further surprising observation is that *met1 drm1 drm2* gene bodies show ectopic CHG methylation (in a similar pattern to the absent CG body methylation), again suggestive of redundant and compensatory interactions between the DNA methyltransferases (Cokus et al. 2008; Lister et al. 2008).

3 Mapping Histone Modifications

Histones are modified by a wide-range of covalent modifications, including methyl-, acetyl-, phosphoryl- and ubiquityl- groups, each with specific genomic distributions and functions (Mendenhall and Bernstein et al. 2008). These modifications can be stably inherited through mitosis, though mechanisms by which specific histone modifications are copied through DNA replication are currently unclear. Genome-wide mapping of histone modifications relies upon the availability of specific antibodies. These antibodies can then be used to purify chromatin associated with the mark of interest, using techniques such as chromatin immunoprecipitation (ChIP). Once purified, the associated DNA can be mapped to the genome by hybridization to tiling microarrays (ChIP-chip) or through high throughput sequencing (ChIP-Seq). These approaches have been used to define histone modification maps of a large number of marks in animal systems (Mendenhall and Bernstein et al. 2008).

The first marks to be profiled in this way in *A.thaliana* were trimethylation of histone H3 at lysine 27 (H3K27m3) and dimethylation of H3K9 (H3K9m2) using ChIP-chip (Turck et al. 2007; Zhang et al. 2007a). Consistent with previous studies that used ChIP to analyze single loci, H3K9m2 was found with the repeated sequences (Turck et al. 2007). Plants and mammals use the conserved Polycomb Response Complex2 (PRC2) to mark genes with H3K27m3 and to stably silence them during development (Kohler and Villar 2008). Although this mark is required for gene silencing, it shows a markedly different genomic distribution to both DNA cytosine methylation and siRNAs. The latter are most dense over peri-centromeric, repeated sequences, while H3K27m3 is found with genes in the chromosome arms (Turck et al. 2007; Zhang et al. 2007a). A large number of genes ($\sim$18%), many of which were transcription factors, overlapped with H3K27m3 in seedlings, indicating that this mark may be frequently used to regulate gene expression and development (Turck et al. 2007; Zhang et al. 2007a). In *Drosophila melanogaster* polycomb response elements (PREs) recruit polycomb proteins and H3K27m3, which can then spread into broad (hundreds of kilobases) domains (Kohler and Villar 2008). This type of spreading was not observed in *A.thaliana*, where it was generally confined to individual genes, suggesting that the mechanism of H3K27m3 spreading may differ between these systems (Turck, Roudier et al. 2007; Zhang et al. 2007a). As Polycomb-type mechanisms are generally involved in developmental silencing, it will be interesting to describe tissue-specific maps of H3K27m3 throughout the *A.thaliana* life-cycle.

Genome-wide maps of non-histone chromatin proteins have also been generated, specifically for LIKE-HETEROCHROMATIN PROTEIN1 (LHP1) (Turck et al. 2007; Zhang et al. 2007b). LHP1 resembles two animal chromodomain proteins, HETEROCHROMATIN PROTEIN1 (HP1) and POLYCOMB (Pc), which are known to bind H3K9m3 and H3K27m3 respectively (Fischle et al. 2005; Grewal and Jia 2007; Schwartz and Pirrotta 2008). Binding of HP1 and Pc to histone methyl-lysines is also important for the function, maintenance and spreading of these chromatin marks (Grewal and Jia 2007; Schwartz and Pirrotta 2008). Although LHP1 has close homology to HP1 several lines of evidence suggested that it is unlikely to play a role in silencing mediated by H3K9 methylation; immunofluorescence of LHP1 showed a euchromatic staining pattern and *lhp1* mutants exhibit developmental phenotypes associated with mis-expression of genes (Gaudin et al. 2001; Libault et al. 2005; Nakahigashi et al. 2005). *LHP1* has also been shown to be required for silencing of *FLC* by vernalization, a process that involves H3K27m3 and a PRC2 complex (Mylne et al. 2006; Sung et al. 2006). To map genome-binding sites for LHP1 two techniques have been used; ChIP-chip of an epitope-tagged line (Turck et al. 2007) and DamID (Zhang et al. 2007b). Dam-ID tethers the protein of interest to the bacterial Dam adenine-methyltransferase. As adenine methylation is not generally found in eukaryotic genomes, the presence of this DNA modification is used to indicate localization of Dam fusion proteins (van Steensel et al. 2001). Consistent with genetic analysis of *lhp1* function, the LHP1 genomic binding sites were found to closely coincide with H3K27m3 (Turck et al. 2007; Zhang et al. 2007b). Hence, although LHP1 was originally identified as being related to HP1, it appears that it plays a functional role closer to animal Pc (Turck et al. 2007; Zhang et al. 2007b). This serves as an additional demonstration for how the definition of chromosomal distributions can help assign a function to histone modifications and chromatin proteins.

4 Mapping Small RNAs

Since their discovery, 21–25 nucleotide small RNAs generated by the RNAi pathway have emerged as widespread regulators of gene expression and genome function (Hamilton and Baulcombe 1999; Ruvkun 2008). Generally, they are generated from double-stranded RNA (dsRNA) substrates through the action of DICER riboendonucleases (Farazi et al. 2008). Plant small RNAs are bound by members of the ARGONAUTE (AGO) family, which mediate their activity in gene regulation (Farazi et al. 2008). Small RNAs can act post-transcriptionally to suppress expression of mRNAs with which they share sequence complementarity, via endonucleolytic cleavage or translational suppression (Farazi et al. 2008). Effects of small RNAs on transcription and chromatin structure have also been discovered in several eukaryotic species (Matzke and Birchler 2005). In plants the expression of dsRNA and small RNAs is capable of targeting DNA methylation and transcriptional silencing to homologous DNA sequences (Wassenegger et al. 1994; Aufsatz et al. 2002). *A.thaliana* has a highly duplicated RNAi system with functionally distinct DICER-LIKE (DCL) (4) and AGO proteins (10) (Xie et al. 2004). The DCL enzymes are known to process dsRNA into siRNAs of distinct sizes; DCL1 generates 21nt miRNAs, DCL2 generates 22nt siRNAs, DCL3 generates 24nt siRNAs and DCL4 generates 21nt siRNAs (Kurihara and Watanabe 2004; Xie et al. 2004; Gasciolli et al. 2005; Xie et al. 2005; Blevins et al. 2006; Deleris et al. 2006; Henderson et al. 2006). DCL3 has been shown genetically to be the major enzyme required for transcriptional silencing and RdDM (Chan 2004; Xie et al. 2004; Zilberman et al. 2004; Henderson et al. 2006). However, there is also evidence for hierarchical processing redundancy between the DCL enzymes (Gasciolli et al. 2005; Blevins et al. 2006; Deleris et al. 2006; Henderson et al. 2006). One explanation for DCL redundancy may be to make viral silencing suppressors less effective (Ding and Voinnet 2007).

To determine which regions of the *A.thaliana* genome generate small RNAs high throughput sequencing technologies have been employed (Lu et al. 2005; Henderson et al. 2006; Rajagopalan et al. 2006; Kasschau et al. 2007; Zhang et al. 2007c; Lister et al. 2008; Mosher et al. 2008). Several technologies are available to purify, clone and sequence large numbers of small RNAs. An advantage to certain techniques is the ability to determine the exact size of the cloned small RNAs, as this can provide information on which DCL likely generated them. It has been found that all size classes of siRNAs show a strong correlation with repeated sequences and DNA methylation (Zhang et al. 2006; Cokus et al. 2008; Lister et al. 2008). This is consistent with the known function of siRNA in guiding DNA methylation to transformed repeated sequences (Soppe et al. 2000; Cao and Jacobsen 2002a, b; Chan 2004; Zilberman et al. 2004; Henderson and Jacobsen 2008). Although repeats are commonly associated with siRNA, the mechanism by which this pattern emerges is not yet clear. An exciting finding has been the involvement of plant specific DNA-dependent RNA polymerase complexes in RdDM, which are termed NRPD or PolIV (Herr et al. 2005; Kanno et al. 2005; Onodera et al. 2005; Pontier et al. 2005). One variant of this complex, containing the NRPD1a subunit, appears to be generally required for all repeat-associated siRNAs, apart from those derived from inverted-repeat sequences (Zhang et al. 2007c; Mosher et al. 2008). Repeat siRNAs also generally require RNA-DEPENDENT RNA POLYMERASE2 (RDR2) for their accumulation (Xie et al. 2004; Lu et al. 2006). This leads to a model whereby RDR2 and the NRPD1a complex act together to generate substrate dsRNA for siRNA production. A key unanswered question is what targets the activity of these proteins to repeated sequences in the first instance?

The role for DNA methylation in targeting of siRNA biogenesis has been tested by sequencing small RNAs from methyltransferase mutants (Lister et al. 2008). Many siRNA clusters were found to be reduced in *met1* and *drm1 drm2 cmt3* and interestingly these mutants also showed novel clusters of siRNA not observed in wild type (Lister et al. 2008). This influence of DNA methylation on siRNA accumulation is consistent with previous observations that siRNAs homologous to the 5S rDNA repeats are dependent upon *DRM2* (Zilberman et al. 2004). Simultaneous, integrated analysis of several types of epigenetic information can thus reveal unexpected effects.

A further way to analyze siRNA function is to characterize the populations bound by specific AGOs, the siRNA effector proteins (Farazi et al. 2008). Several AGO proteins have been immuno-precipitated and the associated siRNAs sequenced (Baumberger and Baulcombe 2005; Qi et al. 2006; Mi et al. 2008; Montgomery et al. 2008). As one example, this demonstrated that AGO1 tends to associate with 21nt miRNAs and 21nt siRNAs, while AGO4 is predominantly associated with 24nt siRNA, consistent with genetic analysis of their functions (Zilberman et al. 2003; Vaucheret et al. 2004; Baumberger and Baulcombe 2005; Qi et al. 2006). Interestingly, certain AGO proteins have been shown to preferentially associate with siRNAs sharing the same 5′-nucleotide (Lam et al. 2005; Lister et al. 2008; Mi et al. 2008; Montgomery et al. 2008). Although the siRNAs bound by AGO4 are required to target DRM2 cytosine methyltransferase activity to homologous DNA (Cao and Jacobsen 2002a, b; Chan 2004), many mechanistic questions remain. For example, whether RNA::DNA or RNA::RNA hybridization events are involved during homology recognition?

5 Prospects

As technology advances it will become cheaper and easier to obtain comprehensive maps of many epigenomic features. Integrating these types of epigenomic maps will be an exciting and revealing task. However, these maps remain purely descriptive until we combine them with genetics and experiment. A key question to address will be the mechanism by which these distinctive patterns of epigenetic information are established and maintained? For example, what determines the boundaries of different types of information? A strong correlation is observed between siRNAs, repeated sequences and DNA methylation in *A.thaliana*, but generally silencing does not spread into adjacent non-repeated sequences. However, this generality is violated at loci such as *SDC*, where methylation and siRNAs spread over 1 kb upstream of seven tandem repeats (Henderson and Jacobsen 2008). What determines whether spreading occurs or not is still poorly understood in plants, however exciting work suggests that this may involve histone demethylation (Saze and Kakutani 2007; Saze et al. 2008). In wild type, the *BONSAI* (*BNS*) gene is expressed, but in the absence of the INCREASED BONSAI METHYLATION1 (IBM1) JmJ-C class histone demethylase, methylation and siRNAs spread from an adjacent retrotransposon and silence *BNS* expression (Saze and Kakutani 2007; Saze et al. 2008). This strongly suggests that some aspect of boundary function involves histone demethylation in *A.thaliana*. There are also multiple DNA demethylases in this species (Choi et al. 2002; Gong et al. 2002; Gehring et al. 2006; Morales-Ruiz et al. 2006) and mutants in these genes show altered distributions of DNA methylation at gene boundaries (Lister et al. 2008). Understanding what targets these demethylases may advance our models for how epigenetic information is patterned in plants.

The Col accession of *A.thaliana* is the most commonly used wild type background for genomic studies. However, widespread natural populations of *A.thaliana* have been collected and analyzed for sequence polymorphisms (Borevitz et al. 2007; Clark et al. 2007). Natural variation in epigenetic information has also begun to be analyzed (Rangwala et al. 2006; Shindo et al. 2006; Vaughn et al. 2007; Zhai et al. 2008; Zhang et al. 2008). For example, stable and divergent patterns of gene body CG DNA methylation were observed between the Col and L.*er* accessions (Vaughn et al. 2007). Genomic resources are also increasingly available in species closely related to *A.thaliana*, which will allow periods of greater divergence to be addressed and a means to test the role of epigenetic information in chromosome evolution (Schranz et al. 2006). Indeed, epigenetic changes have been observed following ploidy manipulation in *Arabidopsis*, which is thought to occur commonly during plant speciation events (Pontes et al. 2004; Wang et al. 2004; Madlung et al. 2005; Wang et al. 2006). It will also be important to extend study of epigenetic information into plant species with more complex, repeat rich genomes. For example, the 17,000 megabase, hexaploid wheat genome is several times larger than the human genome. Knowledge of the epigenetic organization of plant genomes will likely be useful to successfully breed and manipulate these essential agricultural species.

Acknowledgments I.R.H. is supported by a Royal Society University Research Fellowship. Thank you to Suhua Feng for comments and apologies to authors whose work I did not have space to cite.

References

Arabidopsis genome initiative (A.G.I.) (2000). "Analysis of the genome sequence of the flowering plant Arabidopsis thaliana." Nature **408**(6814): 796–815.
Alonso, J. M., A. N. Stepanova, et al. (2003). "Genome-wide insertional mutagenesis of Arabidopsis thaliana." Science **301**(5633): 653–7.
Aufsatz, W., M. F. Mette, et al. (2002). "RNA-directed DNA methylation in Arabidopsis." Proc Natl Acad Sci U S A **99 Suppl 4**: 16499–506.

Baumberger, N. and D. C. Baulcombe (2005). "Arabidopsis ARGONAUTE1 is an RNA Slicer that selectively recruits microRNAs and short interfering RNAs." Proc Natl Acad Sci U S A **102**(33): 11928–33.

Blevins, T., R. Rajeswaran, et al. (2006). "Four plant Dicers mediate viral small RNA biogenesis and DNA virus induced silencing." Nucleic Acids Res **34**(21): 6233–46.

Borevitz, J. O., S. P. Hazen, et al. (2007). "Genome-wide patterns of single-feature polymorphism in Arabidopsis thaliana." Proc Natl Acad Sci U S A **104**(29): 12057–62.

Bowman, J. L., S. K. Floyd, et al. (2007). "Green genes-comparative genomics of the green branch of life." Cell **129**(2): 229–34.

Cao, X. and S. E. Jacobsen (2002a). "Locus-specific control of asymmetric and CpNpG methylation by the DRM and CMT3 methyltransferase genes." Proc Natl Acad Sci U S A **99 Suppl 4**: 16491–8.

Cao, X. and S. E. Jacobsen (2002b). "Role of the arabidopsis DRM methyltransferases in de novo DNA methylation and gene silencing." Curr Biol **12**(13): 1138–44.

Chan, S. W., I. R. Henderson, et al. (2005). "Gardening the genome: DNA methylation in Arabidopsis thaliana." Nat Rev Genet **6**(5): 351–60.

Chan, S. W., D. Zilberman, et al. (2004). "RNA silencing genes control de novo DNA methylation." Science **303**(5662): 1336.

Chandler, V. L. and M. Stam (2004). "Chromatin conversations: mechanisms and implications of paramutation." Nat Rev Genet **5**(7): 532–44.

Chen, J. Z., J. Wang, et al. (2004). "The development of an Arabidopsis model system for genome-wide analysis of polyploidy effects." Biol J Linn Soc Lond **82**(4): 689–700.

Cheng, X. (1995). "Structure and function of DNA methyltransferases." Annu Rev Biophys Biomol Struct **24**: 293–318.

Choi, Y., M. Gehring, et al. (2002). "DEMETER, a DNA glycosylase domain protein, is required for endosperm gene imprinting and seed viability in arabidopsis." Cell **110**(1): 33–42.

Clark, R. M., G. Schweikert, et al. (2007). "Common sequence polymorphisms shaping genetic diversity in Arabidopsis thaliana." Science **317**(5836): 338–42.

Clough, S. J. (2005). "Floral dip: agrobacterium-mediated germ line transformation." Methods Mol Biol **286**: 91–102.

Cokus, S. J., S. Feng, et al. (2008). "Shotgun bisulphite sequencing of the Arabidopsis genome reveals DNA methylation patterning." Nature **452**(7184): 215–9.

Comfort, N. C. (2001). "From controlling elements to transposons: Barbara McClintock and the Nobel Prize." Trends Biochem Sci **26**: 454–457.

Deleris, A., J. Gallego-Bartolome, et al. (2006). "Hierarchical action and inhibition of plant Dicer-like proteins in antiviral defense." Science **313**(5783): 68–71.

Ding, S. W. and O. Voinnet (2007). "Antiviral immunity directed by small RNAs." Cell **130**(3): 413–26.

Farazi, T. A., S. A. Juranek, et al. (2008). "The growing catalog of small RNAs and their association with distinct Argonaute/Piwi family members." Development **135**(7): 1201–14.

Fischle, W., B. S. Tseng, et al. (2005). "Regulation of HP1-chromatin binding by histone H3 methylation and phosphorylation." Nature **438**(7071): 1116–22.

Gasciolli, V., A. C. Mallory, et al. (2005). "Partially redundant functions of Arabidopsis DICER-like enzymes and a role for DCL4 in producing trans-acting siRNAs." Curr Biol **15**(16): 1494–500.

Gaudin, V., M. Libault, et al. (2001). "Mutations in LIKE HETEROCHROMATIN PROTEIN 1 affect flowering time and plant architecture in Arabidopsis." Development **128**: 4847–4858.

Gehring, M., J. H. Huh, et al. (2006). "DEMETER DNA glycosylase establishes MEDEA polycomb gene self-imprinting by allele-specific demethylation." Cell **124**(3): 495–506.

Gong, Z., T. Morales-Ruiz, et al. (2002). "ROS1, a repressor of transcriptional gene silencing in Arabidopsis, encodes a DNA glycosylase/lyase." Cell **111**(6): 803–14.

Grewal, S. I. and S. Jia (2007). "Heterochromatin revisited." Nat Rev Genet **8**(1): 35–46.

Hamilton, A. J. and D. C. Baulcombe (1999). "A species of small antisense RNA in posttranscriptional gene silencing in plants." Science **286**(5441): 950–2.

Henderson, I. R. and S. E. Jacobsen (2008). "Tandem repeats upstream of the Arabidopsis endogene SDC recruit non-CG DNA methylation and initiate siRNA spreading." Genes Dev **22**(12): 1597–606.

Henderson, I. R., X. Zhang, et al. (2006). "Dissecting Arabidopsis thaliana DICER function in small RNA processing, gene silencing and DNA methylation patterning." Nat Genet **38**(6): 721–5.

Herr, A. J., M. B. Jensen, et al. (2005). "RNA polymerase IV directs silencing of endogenous DNA." Science **308**(5718): 118–20.

Jones, L., A. J. Hamilton, et al. (1999). "RNA-DNA interactions and DNA methylation in post-transcriptional gene silencing." Plant Cell **11**(12): 2291–301.

Kanno, T., B. Huettel, et al. (2005). "Atypical RNA polymerase subunits required for RNA-directed DNA methylation." Nat Genet **37**(7): 761–5.

Kasschau, K. D., N. Fahlgren, et al. (2007). "Genome-wide profiling and analysis of Arabidopsis siRNAs." PLoS Biol **5**(3): e57.

Kato, M., A. Miura, et al. (2003). "Role of CG and non-CG methylation in immobilization of transposons in Arabidopsis." Curr Biol **13**(5): 421–6.

Kohler, C. and C. B. Villar (2008). "Programming of gene expression by Polycomb group proteins." Trends Cell Biol **18**(5): 236–43.

Kurihara, Y. and Y. Watanabe (2004). "Arabidopsis micro-RNA biogenesis through Dicer-like 1 protein functions." Proc Natl Acad Sci U S A **101**(34): 12753–8.

Lam, S. Y., S. R. Horn, et al. (2005). "Crossover interference on nucleolus organizing region-bearing chromosomes in Arabidopsis." Genetics **170**(2): 807–12.

Libault, M., F. Tessadori, et al. (2005). "The Arabidopsis LHP1 protein is a component of euchromatin." Planta **222**(5): 910–25.

Lippman, Z., A. V. Gendrel, et al. (2004). "Role of transposable elements in heterochromatin and epigenetic control." Nature **430**(6998): 471–6.

Lister, R., R. C. O'Malley, et al. (2008). "Highly integrated single-base resolution maps of the epigenome in Arabidopsis." Cell **133**(3): 523–36.

Lu, C., K. Kulkarni, et al. (2006). "MicroRNAs and other small RNAs enriched in the Arabidopsis RNA-dependent RNA polymerase-2 mutant." Genome Res **16**(10): 1276–88.

Lu, C., S. S. Tej, et al. (2005). "Elucidation of the small RNA component of the transcriptome." Science **309**(5740): 1567–9.

Madlung, A., A. P. Tyagi, et al. (2005). "Genomic changes in synthetic Arabidopsis polyploids." Plant J **41**(2): 221–30.

Matzke, M. A. and J. A. Birchler (2005). "RNAi-mediated pathways in the nucleus." Nat Rev Genet **6**(1): 24–35.

Mendenhall, E. M. and B. E. Bernstein (2008). "Chromatin state maps: new technologies, new insights." Curr Opin Genet Dev **18**(2): 109–15.

Mi, S., T. Cai, et al. (2008). "Sorting of small RNAs into Arabidopsis argonaute complexes is directed by the 5' terminal nucleotide." Cell **133**(1): 116–27.

Miura, A., S. Yonebayashi, et al. (2001). "Mobilization of transposons by a mutation abolishing full DNA methylation in Arabidopsis." Nature **411**(6834): 212–4.

Montgomery, T. A., M. D. Howell, et al. (2008). "Specificity of ARGONAUTE7-miR390 interaction and dual functionality in TAS3 trans-acting siRNA formation." Cell **133**(1): 128–41.

Morales-Ruiz, T., A. P. Ortega-Galisteo, et al. (2006). "DEMETER and REPRESSOR OF SILENCING 1 encode 5-methylcytosine DNA glycosylases." Proc Natl Acad Sci U S A **103**(18): 6853–8.

Mosher, R. A., F. Schwach, et al. (2008). "PolIVb influences RNA-directed DNA methylation independently of its role in siRNA biogenesis." Proc Natl Acad Sci U S A **105**(8): 3145–50.

Mylne, J. S., L. Barrett, et al. (2006). "LHP1, the Arabidopsis homologue of HETEROCHROMATIN PROTEIN1, is required for epigenetic silencing of FLC." Proc Natl Acad Sci U S A **103**(13): 5012–7.

Nakahigashi, K., Z. Jasencakova, et al. (2005). "The Arabidopsis heterochromatin protein1 homolog (TERMINAL FLOWER2) silences genes within the euchromatic region but not genes positioned in heterochromatin." Plant Cell Physiol **46**(11): 1747–56.

Onodera, Y., J. R. Haag, et al. (2005). "Plant nuclear RNA polymerase IV mediates siRNA and DNA methylation-dependent heterochromatin formation." Cell **120**(5): 613–22.

Otto, S. P. (2007). "The evolutionary consequences of polyploidy." Cell **131**(3): 452–62.

Pontes, O., N. Neves, et al. (2004). "Chromosomal locus rearrangements are a rapid response to formation of the allotetraploid Arabidopsis suecica genome." Proc Natl Acad Sci U S A **101**(52): 18240–5.

Pontier, D., G. Yahubyan, et al. (2005). "Reinforcement of silencing at transposons and highly repeated sequences requires the concerted action of two distinct RNA polymerases IV in Arabidopsis." Genes Dev **19**(17): 2030–40.

Qi, Y., X. He, et al. (2006). "Distinct catalytic and non-catalytic roles of ARGONAUTE4 in RNA-directed DNA methylation." Nature **443**(7114): 1008–12.

Rajagopalan, R., H. Vaucheret, et al. (2006). "A diverse and evolutionarily fluid set of microRNAs in Arabidopsis thaliana." Genes Dev **20**(24): 3407–25.

Rangwala, S. H., R. Elumalai, et al. (2006). "Meiotically stable natural epialleles of Sadhu, a novel Arabidopsis retroposon." PLoS Genet **2**(3): e36.

Ruvkun, G. (2008). "Tiny RNA: Where do we come from? What are we? Where are we going?" Trends Plant Sci **13**(7): 313–6.

Saze, H. and T. Kakutani (2007). "Heritable epigenetic mutation of a transposon-flanked Arabidopsis gene due to lack of the chromatin-remodeling factor DDM1." Embo J **26**(15): 3641–52.

Saze, H., O. Mittelsten Scheid, et al. (2003). "Maintenance of CpG methylation is essential for epigenetic inheritance during plant gametogenesis." Nat Genet **34**(1): 65–9.

Saze, H., A. Shiraishi, et al. (2008). "Control of genic DNA methylation by a jmjC domain-containing protein in Arabidopsis thaliana." Science **319**(5862): 462–5.

Schranz, M. E., M. A. Lysak, et al. (2006). "The ABC's of comparative genomics in the Brassicaceae: building blocks of crucifer genomes." Trends Plant Sci **11**(11): 535–42.

Schwartz, Y. B. and V. Pirrotta (2008). "Polycomb complexes and epigenetic states." Curr Opin Cell Biol **20**(3): 266–73.

Scott, R. J., M. Spielman, et al. (1998). "Parent-of-origin effects on seed development in Arabidopsis thaliana." Development **125**(17): 3329–41.

Shindo, C., C. Lister, et al. (2006). "Variation in the epigenetic silencing of FLC contributes to natural variation in Arabidopsis vernalization response." Genes Dev **20**(22): 3079–83.

Singer, T., C. Yordan, et al. (2001). "Robertson's Mutator transposons in A. thaliana are regulated by the chromatin-remodeling gene Decrease in DNA Methylation (DDM1)." Genes Dev **15**(5): 591–602.

Soppe, W. J., S. E. Jacobsen, et al. (2000). "The late flowering phenotype of fwa mutants is caused by gain-of-function epigenetic alleles of a homeodomain gene." Mol Cell **6**(4): 791–802.

Somerville, C.R. and Meyerowitz, E.E. eds. (2002). The Arabidopsis Book. Rockville, MD, American Society of Plant Biologists.

Sung, S., Y. He, et al. (2006). "Epigenetic maintenance of the vernalized state in Arabidopsis thaliana requires LIKE HETEROCHROMATIN PROTEIN 1." Nat Genet **38**(6): 706–10.

Suzuki, M. M. and A. Bird (2008). "DNA methylation landscapes: provocative insights from epigenomics." Nat Rev Genet **9**(6): 465–76.

Tompa, R., C. M. McCallum, et al. (2002). "Genome-wide profiling of DNA methylation reveals transposon targets of CHROMOMETHYLASE3." Curr. Biol. **12**: 65–68.

Tran, R. K., J. G. Henikoff, et al. (2005). "DNA methylation profiling identifies CG methylation clusters in Arabidopsis genes." Curr Biol **15**(2): 154–9.

Turck, F., F. Roudier, et al. (2007). "Arabidopsis TFL2/LHP1 specifically associates with genes marked by trimethylation of histone H3 lysine 27." PLoS Genet **3**(6): e86.

van Steensel, B., J. Delrow, et al. (2001). "Chromatin profiling using targeted DNA adenine methyltransferase." Nat Genet **27**(3): 304–8.

Vaucheret, H., F. Vazquez, et al. (2004). "The action of ARGONAUTE1 in the miRNA pathway and its regulation by the miRNA pathway are crucial for plant development." Genes Dev **18**(10): 1187–97.

Vaughn, M. W., M. Tanurd Ic, et al. (2007). "Epigenetic Natural Variation in Arabidopsis thaliana." PLoS Biol **5**(7): e174.

Wang, J., L. Tian, et al. (2006). "Genomewide nonadditive gene regulation in Arabidopsis allotetraploids." Genetics **172**(1): 507–17.

Wang, J., L. Tian, et al. (2004). "Stochastic and epigenetic changes of gene expression in Arabidopsis polyploids." Genetics **167**(4): 1961–73.

Wassenegger, M., S. Heimes, et al. (1994). "RNA-directed de novo methylation of genomic sequences in plants." Cell **76**(3): 567–76.

Xie, Z., E. Allen, et al. (2005). "DICER-LIKE 4 functions in trans-acting small interfering RNA biogenesis and vegetative phase change in Arabidopsis thaliana." Proc Natl Acad Sci U S A **102**(36): 12984–9.

Xie, Z., L. K. Johansen, et al. (2004). "Genetic and functional diversification of small RNA pathways in plants." PLoS Biol **2**(5): E104.

Xu, J., H. Hofhuis, et al. (2006). "A molecular framework for plant regeneration." Science **311**(5759): 385–8.

Zhai, J., J. Liu, et al. (2008). "Small RNA-directed epigenetic natural variation in Arabidopsis thaliana." PLoS Genet **4**(4): e1000056.

Zhang, X., O. Clarenz, et al. (2007a). "Whole-genome analysis of histone H3 lysine 27 trimethylation in Arabidopsis." PLoS Biol **5**(5): e129.

Zhang, X., S. Germann, et al. (2007b). "The Arabidopsis LHP1 protein colocalizes with histone H3 Lys27 trimethylation." Nat Struct Mol Biol **14**(9): 869–71.

Zhang, X., I. R. Henderson, et al. (2007c). "Role of RNA polymerase IV in plant small RNA metabolism." Proc Natl Acad Sci U S A **104**(11): 4536–41.

Zhang, X. and S. E. Jacobsen (2006). "Genetic analyses of DNA methyltransferases in Arabidopsis thaliana." Cold Spring Harb Symp Quant Biol **71**: 439–47.

Zhang, X., S. Shiu, et al. (2008). "Global analysis of genetic, epigenetic and transcriptional polymorphisms in Arabidopsis thaliana using whole genome tiling arrays." PLoS Genet **4**(3): e1000032.

Zhang, X., J. Yazaki, et al. (2006). "Genome-wide high-resolution mapping and functional analysis of DNA methylation in arabidopsis." Cell **126**(6): 1189–201.

Zilberman, D., X. Cao, et al. (2003). "ARGONAUTE4 control of locus-specific siRNA accumulation and DNA and histone methylation." Science **299**(5607): 716–9.

Zilberman, D., X. Cao, et al. (2004). "Role of Arabidopsis ARGONAUTE4 in RNA-directed DNA methylation triggered by inverted repeats." Curr Biol **14**(13): 1214–20.

Zilberman, D., M. Gehring, et al. (2007). "Genome-wide analysis of Arabidopsis thaliana DNA methylation uncovers an interdependence between methylation and transcription." Nat Genet **39**(1): 61–9.

Zilberman, D. and S. Henikoff (2007). "Genome-wide analysis of DNA methylation patterns." Development **134**(22): 3959–65.

Role of Small RNAs in Establishing Chromosomal Architecture in Drosophila

James A. Birchler

Abstract The role of small RNA silencing is well established for its action in post-transcriptional activity as a defense against viruses and as an experimental tool. However, evidence from many organisms indicates a role of small RNAs in establishing chromatin domains in the nucleus. Here, the role of RNA silencing components in chromatin modifications in Drosophila is reviewed. Mutations in genes involved with the production of both short interfering RNA (siRNA) and piwi interacting RNA (piRNA) affect the chromatin configuration involved with transgene silencing, pairing sensitive silencing, heterochromatin, centomeres and telomeres. The small RNA pathways are also involved with the integrity of chromatin insulators and the nucleolus.

Keywords RNAi · siRNA · Transgene silencing · Telomeres · Chromatin insulators · Heterochromatin · Pairing sensitive silencing · Centromeres · piRNA

The role of small RNAs in chromosomal architecture traces back to the discovery of transgene silencing in plants. The first such case involved a transcriptional silencing in which promoters shared homology with each other (Matzke et al. 1989). When combined in the same plant, the two different transgenes were inactive, but would regain activity when segregated away from each other in meiosis. In parallel, attempts to transform petunia with chalcone synthase transgenes to make them darker resulted in the opposite effect, namely white flowers (Napoli et al. 1990; van der Krol et al. 1990). The basis of this silencing was revealed to be post-transcriptional and was termed cosuppression. A large literature developed on the two types of transgene silencing in plants in the early 1990s. The phenomenon of RNA interference was discovered in nematodes (Guo and Kemphues, 1995). RNA interference as a biological technique refers to the use of double stranded RNAs to target the posttranscriptional destruction of the homologous messenger

J.A. Birchler (✉)
Division of Biological Sciences, Tucker Hall, University of Missouri, Columbia, MO 65211
e-mail: BirchlerJ@Missouri.edu

RNA (Fire et al. 1998). This is accomplished by the cleavage of the dsRNA to small RNAs in the range of 21–25 bp in length (Hamilton and Baulcombe, 1999). However, the small RNAs and the accompanying machinery are also implicated in transcriptional silencing, for example, by producing short RNAs homologous to promoter sequences that are then capable of causing transcriptional silencing (Mette et al. 2000) as well as in other transcriptional silencing (Pal Bhadra et al. 2002; Volpe et al. 2002). Recent data has provided evidence that small RNAs are involved in establishing various chromatin domains across the chromosome. This review will summarize the evidence that has accumulated in Drosophila for the involvement of small RNAs in the establishment of chromatin configurations in different parts of the chromosome. (See also Chapters "Epigenetic Silencing of Pericentromeric Heterochromatin by RNA Interference in *Schizosaccharomyces pombe*" and "Describing Epigenomic Information in Arabidopsis" for additional background on the small RNA machinery derived from studies in *Schizosaccharomyces pombe* and *Arabidopsis*).

1 Genes Involved with "RNAi" in Drosophila

The metabolism of double stranded RNAs in Drosophila to produce siRNAs is catalyzed by the product of the *dicer-2* gene (Lee et al. 2004). The Argonaute2 (*Ago2*) gene product is the "slicer" function in this pathway and associates with the RNAi induced silencing complex (RISC). The endogenous microRNAs are metabolized primarily by *dicer-1* (Lee et al. 2004) and the "slicer" function in this case is *Ago1*. Another clade of the argonaute family in flies involves the *piwi*, *aubergine* (*aub*) and *Argonaute3* genes (Gunawardane et al. 2007; Brennecke et al. 2007). These gene products all likely possess a "slicer" activity and are involved with the generation of repeat associated small interfering RNAs (rasiRNA) that are slightly larger than the canonical siRNAs. The rasiRNAs in the germline are generated by a dicer independent mechanism based on their larger size and distinct termini that are inconsistent with dicer enzymatic activity (Vagin et al. 2006; Gunawardane et al. 2007; Brennecke et al. 2007). While these gene products are involved with the destruction of transposable element transcripts in the germline, there is also evidence that they exhibit somatic functions that involve both posttranscriptional and transcriptional silencing as well as gene activation activities (Kennerdell et al. 2002; Pal Bhadra et al. 2002; 2004b; Brower-Toland et al. 2007; Yin and Lin, 2007). Two other gene products, both with predicted double stranded RNA helicase activity, have been demonstrated to be required for RNAi and have been used extensively in studies of the effects on the RNAi machinery on various chromosomal processes. These are *spindle-E* or *homeless* (*hls*) (Kennerdell et al. 2002) and *Lighten-up* (*Lip*) (Csink et al. 1994; Ishizuka et al. 2002; Kavi et al. 2005) or *Rm62*. The precise function of these helicases in RNAi is unknown. Other gene products are involved in small RNA metabolism (Kavi et al. 2005), but have been used infrequently in studies of silencing and chromosomal architecture.

2 Transgene Silencing in Drosophila

A similar phenomena in animal species to cosuppession described in plants involved the silencing of a hybrid transgene involving the *white* eye color gene promoter fused to the structural portion of the *Alcohol dehydrogenase* gene (Pal Bhadra et al. 1997; 1999). With increasing copy number, the total amount of messenger RNA declined and the endogenous *Adh* gene was also brought into the silencing pool. The multiple silenced transgenes but not a single active copy showed the accumulation of the Polycomb repressive chromatin complex and the silencing was modulated by mutations in Polycomb group genes (for further details on the mechanisms of Polycomb complex action see Chapter "Polycomb Complexes and the Role of Epigenetic Memory in Development" by Schwartz and Pirrotta).

This type of silencing operates at the transcriptional level. Run on transcription assays showed a similar profile to the steady state level of RNA from the transgenes (Pal Bhadra et al. 2002). The argonaute family genes, *piwi* and *aubergine*, would ameliorate the silencing to varying degrees (Pal Bhadra et al. 2002; Birchler et al. 2003). The *piwi* mutation would also block posttranscriptional silencing of an *Adh* transgene, suggesting that this gene product is involved with both transcriptional and posttranscriptional effects (Pal Bhadra et al. 2002). In the latter case, the production of small interfering RNAs was eliminated and thus these results provided evidence for a connection between the "RNAi" machinery and transcriptional silencing.

The *w-Adh* transgenes exhibit the phenomenon of pairing sensitive silencing (Pal Bhadra et al. 1997). In other words, when homologous copies are present in the genome, the total expression is less than when a single copy is present. In Drosophila, one should recall, there is pairing of homologues in somatic cells. Pairing sensitive silencing was first defined with *engrailed-white* (*en-w*) transgenes (Kassis et al. 1991). Studies of multiple copies of *en-w* indicated that this transgene also exhibits cosuppression across the genome and raised the possibility of a connection between the two types of silencing. Indeed, mutations in the RNAi machinery do impact pairing sensitive silencing although the effect is not always a suppression response (Pal Bhadra et al. 2004a; Grimaud et al. 2006).

The pursuit of pairing sensitive silencing eventually led to the discovery of the involvement of the small RNA pathway in "chromosome kissing" (Grimaud et al. 2006). The Fab-7 Polycomb Response Element (PRE) from the *bithorax* locus has been transformed to a number of sites in the genome. At any one site, it exhibits pairing sensitive silencing. This silencing can spread to adjacent genes. In one notable case on the X chromosome, the transgene was inserted near the *scalloped* wing shape gene (*sd*) (Bantignies et al. 2003). This silencing, however, requires the presence of the endogenous *Abd-B* sequence of the *bithorax* locus. These interactions again suggest similarities between pairing sensitive silencing and cosuppression of homologous endogenous genes and their derived transgenes. FISH of the transgenes and the endogenous locus indicate that they associate ("chromosome kissing") and were dependent on full expression of the Polycomb complex gene products.

The silencing by *Fab-7* is diminished in mutant flies for *dicer-2*, *aubergine* and *piwi*, suggesting a role of small RNAs in the process (Grimaud et al. 2006). Indeed, siRNAs homologous to the transgene can be found in flies carrying multiple copies and their quantities are diminished in the mutants. Furthermore, the protein products of *dicer-2* and *piwi* colocalize with Polycomb complex nuclear bodies. Homeotic genes such as *Antennapedia* and *Bithorax-C*, both carry PREs and will normally associate with each other during development. These associations are disrupted in *dicer-2* and *piwi* mutants, although the latter mutations do not produce homeotic phenotypes suggesting that the function of the homeotic genes is not impaired. Nevertheless, these results suggest a role of small RNAs in nuclear architecture and organization.

3 Heterochromatin

The Drosophila chromosomes are organized in such a fashion that most of the genes are located distally. The regions around the centromere encompassing from one-third to one-half of each chromosome arm is composed of heterochromatin. There are few genes located in this heterochromatin and it does not polytenize in larval tissues in which the euchromatin does. The heterochromatic regions remain adhered to each other in what is referred to as the chromocenter. Chromosomal rearrangements that place euchromatin next to heterochromatin will result in position effect variegation (PEV) in which the euchromatic genes will be silenced in a mosaic fashion. The heterochromatin is typically associated with chromatin marks that are characteristic of silenced regions such are H3-K9me2. Heterochromatin Protein 1 (HP1) is heavily concentrated in the heterchromatin and has an affinity for the dimethyl H3-K9 modification.

Mutations in the small RNA pathway genes lead to suppression of heterochromatic silencing and reduction but not elimination of the methylation of H3K9 consequent with a slight redistribution of HP1 to euchromatic sites of apparent lesser affinity (Pal Bhadra et al. 2004b). Repeat induced silencing of a *mini-white* array on chromosome 2 was also suppressed by *piwi*, *aubergine* and *homeless*. The PIWI protein interacts physically with HP1 (Brower-Toland et al. 2007) and binds repeat associated small interfering (rasi) RNAs (Saito et al. 2006). Later it was understood that the *Lighten-up* (*Lip*) gene encoded a double stranded RNA helicase that was required for RNAi (Ishizuka et al. 2002; Kavi et al. 2005). Earlier studies had demonstrated that mutations in this gene were strong suppressors of position effect variegation and cause up-regulation of several retrotransposons (Csink et al. 1994), thus providing further evidence for an involvement of the RNAi machinery in heterochromatin formation.

The tiny fourth chromosome of Drosophila consists of an interspersion of heterochromatin and euchromatin. One potential target for the establishment of the heterochromatic domains is the 1360 transposable element (Haynes et al. 2006).

This element contributes to the small RNA pool. Using knockdowns of *dicer-1* and *dicer-2* in Kc tissue culture cells showed that this element was upregulated under these circumstances. It is thus potentially the case that the structure of chromosome 4 is shaped at least in part by the targeting of chromatin marks by the small RNA machinery.

4 Centromeres

The centromere is the part of the chromosome that underlies the kinetochore, which attaches to the spindle apparatus for chromosome movement. The basal protein is a variant of histone H3 that anchors the kinetochore to the chromosome. In Drosophila, this protein is referred to as CID (centromere identifier). In mutants of *Ago2*, the quantity of CID on the chromosomes of early embryos was reduced relative to normal cells and chromosomes showed abnormal anaphase movements (Deshpande et al. 2005). Also, the magnitude of H3-K9me2 was reduced in heterochromatic regions and HP1 was redistributed in the embryonic nuclei to a more uniform configuration.

A satellite array known as 1.688 is present on the X chromosome in the centromeric region. This array is transcribed in the germline of males and females and produces sense and antisense siRNAs. In the *homeless* mutants, these arrays are up-regulated (Usakin et al. 2007) providing further evidence for a relationship between centromere functions and small RNA metabolism.

5 Telomeres

The telomeres in Drosophila are distinct from those of most other multicellular eukaryotes in that they are composed of specific retrotransposons. These elements, including TART and HeT-A, insert only into telomeric regions and thus continue to add material to prevent the gradual destruction of the chromosome with continued replications. The small RNA machinery affects these elements (see below) but obviously they escape silencing at sufficient levels to maintain the integrity of the telomeres.

The expression of TART and HeT-A has been studied in the germline. In mutants for *hls* and *aub*, there are differential effects of transpositions of either TART or HeT-A to the ends of chromosomes (Savitsky et al. 2006). The mutations also affect the amount of siRNAs homologous to the telomeric elements. Another element, TAHRE, is also present at the telomeres and under the control of the RNAi genes (Shpiz et al. 2007). The reasons why the various mutations affect the different elements in distinct manners, and what are the distinguishing features of the elements that condition a unique response, is unknown.

Another aspect of telomere biology that is affected by the small RNA machinery is trans-silencing of P elements that are inserted into telomere associated sequences (TAS) (Ronsseray et al. 1996). P element vectors inserted into these locations show variegation that is affected by the dosage of the HP1 gene (Ronsseray et al. 1996; Haley et al. 2005; Josse et al. 2007). These insertions can also silence other transgenes in the genome that carry homology to the TAS inserted elements (Ronsseray et al. 2003) and can act to silence all copies of P elements present in the genome. This type of silencing is only effective if the transgenes is inserted into a heterochromatic location of the TAS and not when the same transgene is present in euchromatin. This trans-acting effect is modulated by mutations in *aub* (Reiss et al. 2004), *homeless*, *piwi* and *armitage* (Josse et al. 2007) indicating an involvement of small RNAs.

6 Chromatin Insulators

Chromatin insulators function to block enhancer activity. In Drosophila, the most studied one is the gypsy insulator first found in the retrotransposon, gypsy. Three previously identified proteins are integral components of this insulator, which are encoded by *Suppressor of Hairy wing*, *mod(mdg4)* and *CP190*. In studies of these proteins, *Lip* was identified as an interactor, which led to the study of other RNAi components (Lei and Corces, 2006). *Lip* mutations actually cause an improvement of insulator function, whereas *piwi* and *aub* have a detrimental effect. The interaction of *Lip* with the other insulator proteins is RNA dependent. The source and function of these RNAs is yet to be determined.

7 Nucleolus

The nucleolus is the site of synthesis of the larger ribosomal RNAs. The RNAi genes including *dcr-2*, *Ago2*, *aub*, *piwi* and *hls* are required in their normal form in order for the proper functioning of the nucleolus (Peng and Karpen, 2007). When any of them are mutant, multiple nucleoli are generated and the methylation of H3K9 associated with ribosomal DNA is reduced. Thus, small RNAs are implicated in the normal functioning of the nucleolus as an additional involvement with chromosomal architecture.

8 Concluding Remarks

The major focus of RNAi research over the past decade has emphasized an understanding of the nature of the technical aspects and the mechanism of the post-transcriptional action. The usual rationalization for the presence of small RNA metabolism is as a defense against viruses and as a protection of the integrity of the genome against transposable elements. While these are certainly the case and important, the involvement of small RNAs in transcriptional processes and the establishment of chromosomal architecture is certainly pervasive as the above narrative illustrates. Given the involvement of RNA polymerase in transcriptional processes for the establishment of chromatin domains in fission yeast (Kato et al. 2005) and the role of RNA polymerase IV (Till and Ladurner, 2007) for silencing in the plant kingdom, it is likely that the RNAi machinery associates with PolII in some manner as a surveillance mechanism of nascent RNAs. With the recognition of certain secondary and tertiary structures of RNA, the appropriate enzymes are recruited for modification of the underlying chromatin to establish active or inactive gene expression. If additional evidence supports this view, then the so-called "RNAi machinery" will be recognized as having a much more fundamental role than previously realized in establishing patterns of gene expression and chromosomal architecture.

References

Bantignies F, Grimaud C, Lavrov S. Gabut M, Cavalli G (2003) Inheritance of Polycomb-dependent chromosomal interactions in Drosophila. Genes and Development 17: 2406–2420

Birchler J, Pal Bhadra M, Bhadra U (2003) Transgene cosuppression in animals. IN: RNAi: a guide to gene silencing. Edited by G. Hannon. Cold Spring Harbor Press, Cold Spring Harbor, New York, pp 23–42

Brennecke J, Aravin AA, Stark A, Dus M, Kellis M, Sachidanandam R, Hannon GJ (2007) Discrete small RNA-generating loci as master regulators of transposon activity in Drosophila. Cell 128: 1089–1103

Brower-Toland B, Findley SD, Jiang L, Liu L, Yin H, Dus M, Zhou P, Elgin SCR, Lin H (2007) Drosophila PIWI assocites with chromatin and interacts directly with HP1alpha. Genes and Development 21: 2300–2311

Csink AK, Linsk R, Birchler JA (1994) The *Lighten up* (*Lip*) gene of *Drosophila melanogaster*, a modifier of retroelement expression, position effect variegation and white locus insertion alleles. Genetics 138: 153–163

Deshpande G, Calhoun G, Schedl P (2005) Drosophila *argonaute-2* is required early in embryogenesis for the assembly of centric/centromeric heterochromatin, nuclear division, nuclear migration, and germ-cell formation. Genes and Development 19: 1680–1685

Fire A, Xu S, Montgomery MK, Kostas SA, Driver SE, Mello CC (1998) Potent and specific genetic interference by double-stranded RNA in *Caenorhabditis elegans*. Nature 391: 806–811

Grimaud C, Bantignies F, Pal-Bhadra M, Bhadra U, Cavalli G (2006) RNAi components are required for nuclear clustering of Polycomb Group Response Elements. Cell 124: 957–971

Gunawardane LS, Saito K, Nishida KM, Miyoshi K, Kawamura Y, Nagami T, Siomi H, Siomi MC (2007) A slicer-mediated mechanisms for repeat-associated siRNA 5' end formation in Drosophila. Science 315: 1587–1590

Guo S, Kemphues KJ (1995) pari-1, a gene required for establishing polarity in C. elegans embryos, encodes a putative Ser/Thr kinase that is asymmetrically distributed. Cell 81: 611–620

Haley KJ, Stuart JR, Raymond JD, Niemi JB, Simmons MJ (2005) Impairment of cytotype regulation of P-element activity in *Drosophila melanogaster* by mutations in the *Su(var)205* gene. Genetics 171(2): 583–595

Hamilton AJ, Baulcombe DC (1999) A species of small antisense RNA in posttranscriptional gene silencing in plants. Science 286: 950–952

Haynes KA, Caudy AA, Collins L, Elgin SCR (2006) Element 1360 and RNAi components contribute to HP1-dependent silencing of a pericentric reporter. Current Biology 16: 2222–2227

Ishizuka A, Siomi MC, Siomi H (2002) A Drosophila fragile X protein interacts with components of RNAi and ribosomal proteins. Genes and Development 16: 2497–2508

Josse T, Teysset T, Todeschini AL, Sidor CM, Anxolahere D, Ronsseray S (2007) Telomeric trans-silencing: an epigenetic repression combining RNA silencing and heterochromatin formation. PloS Genetics 3: 1633–1643

Kassis JA, VanSickle EP, Sensabaugh SM (1991) A fragment of *engrailed* regulatory DNA can mediate transvection of the *white* gene in Drosophila. Genetics 128: 751–761

Kato H, Goto DB, Martienssen RA, Urano T, Furukawa K, Murakami Y (2005) RNA polymerase II is required for RNAi-dependent heterochromatin assembly. Science 309: 467–469

Kavi HH, Fernandez HR, Xie W, Birchler JA (2005) RNA silencing in Drosophila. FEBS Lett. 579: 5940–5949

Kennerdell JR, Yamaguchi S, Carthew RW (2002) RNAi is activated during Drosophila oocyte maturation in a manner dependent on *aubergine* and *spindle-E*. Genes and Development 16: 1884–1889

Lee YS, Nakahara K, Pham JW, Kim K, He Z, Sontheimer EJ, Carthew RW (2004) Distinct roles for Drosophila Dicer-1 and Dicer-2 in the siRNA/miRNA silencing pathways. Cell 117: 69–81

Lei EP, Corces VG (2006) RNA interference machinery influences the nuclear organization of a chromatin insulator. Nature Genetics 38: 936–941

Matzke MA, Primig M, Trnovsky J, Matzke AJM (1989) Reversible methylation and inactivation of marker genes in sequentially transformed tobacco plants. EMBO J 8: 643–649

Mette MF, Aufsatz W, van der Winden J, Matzke MA, Matzke AJ (2000) Transcriptional silencing and promoter methylation triggered by double-stranded RNA. EMBO J 19: 5194–5201

Napoli C, Lemieux C, Jorgenson R (1990) Introduction of a chimeric chalcone synthase gene in Petunia results in reversible co-suppression of homologous genes in trans. The Plant Cell 2: 279–289

Pal-Bhadra M, Bhadra U, Birchler JA (1997) Cosuppression in Drosophila: gene silencing of *Alcohol dehydrogenase* by *white-Adh* transgenes is Polycomb dependent. Cell 90; 479–490

Pal-Bhadra M, Bhadra U, Birchler JA (1999) Cosuppression of nonhomologous transgenes in Drosophila involves mutually related endogenous sequences. Cell 99: 35–46

Pal Bhadra M, Bhadra U, Birchler JA (2002) RNAi related mechanisms affect both transcriptional and post-transcriptional transgene silencing in Drosophila. Molecular Cell 9: 315–327

Pal-Bhadra M, Bhadra U, Birchler JA (2004a) Interrelationship of RNA interference and transcriptional gene silencing in Drosophila. Cold Spring Harbor Symposia on Quantitative Biology 69: 433–438

Pal-Bhadra M, Leibovitch BA, Gandhi SG, Rao M, Bhadra U, Birchler JA, Elgin SC (2004b) Heterochromatic silencing and HP1 localization in Drosophila are dependent on the RNAi machinery. Science 303: 669–672

Peng JC, Karpen GH (2007) H3K9 methylation and RNA interference regulate nucleolar organization and repeated DNA stability. Nature Cell Biology 9: 25–35

Reiss D, Josse T, Anxolabehere D, Ronsseray S (2004) *aubergine* mutations in *Drosophila melanogaster* impair P cytotype determination by telomeric P elements inserted in heterochromatin. Molecular Genetics and Genomics 272: 336–43

Ronsseray S, Josse T, Boivin A, Anxolabehere D (2003) Telomeric transgenes and trans-silencing in Drosophila. Genetica 117: 327–35

Ronsseray S, Lehmann M, Nouaud D, Anxolabehere D (1996) The regulatory properties of autonomous subtelomeric P elements are sensitive to a suppressor of variegation in *Drosophila melanogaster*. Genetics 143: 1663–74

Saito K, Nishida KM, Mori T, Kawamura Y, Miyoshi K, Nagami T, Siomi H, Siomi MC (2006) Specific association of Piwi with rasiRNAs derived from retrotransposon and heterochromatic regions in the Drosophila genome. Genes and Development 20: 2214–2222.

Savitsky M, Kwon D, Georgiev P, Kalmykova A, Gvozdev V (2006) Telomere elongation is under the control of the RNAi-based mechanism in the Drosophila germline. Genes and Development 20: 345–354

Shpiz S, Kwon D, Uneva A, Kim M, Klenov M, Rozovsky Y, Georgiev P, Savitsky M, Kalmykova A (2007) Characterization of Drosophila telomeric retroelement TAHRE: transcription, transpositions and RNAi-based regulation of expression. Molecular Biology and Evolution 24: 2535–2545

Till S, Ladurner AG (2007) RNA PolIV plays catch with Argonaute 4. Cell 131: 643–645

Usakin L, Abad J, Vagin VV, de Pablos B, Villasante A, Gvozdov VA (2007) Transcription of the 1.688 satellite DNA family is under the control of RNA interference machinery in *Drosophila melanogaster* ovaries. Genetics 176: 1343–1349

Vagin VV, Sigova A, Li C, Seitz H, Gvozdev V, Zamore P (2006) A distinct small RNA pathway silences selfish genetic elements in the germline. Science 313: 320–324

van der Krol AR, Mur LA, Beld M, Mol JNM, Stuitje AR (1990) Flavanoid genes in Petunia: Addition of a limited number of gene copies may lead to a suppression of gene expression. Plant Cell 2: 291–299

Volpe TA, Kidner C, Hall IM, Ten G, Grewal SI, Martienssen RA (2002). Regulation of heterochromatic silencing and histone H3 lysine-9 methylation by RNAi. Science 297: 1833–1837.

Yin H, Lin H (2007) An epigenetic activation role of Piwi and a Piwi-associated piRNA in Drosophila melanogaster. Nature 450: 3173–3179

MacroRNAs in the Epigenetic Control of X-Chromosome Inactivation

Shinwa Shibata and Jeannie T. Lee

Abstract Sex chromosome dosage compensation in mammals is achieved by X-chromosome inactivation (XCI) in the female sex. In the mammalian female cells, only one X-chromosome is transcribed, while the other is permanently silenced. As a quintessential example of epigenetic control, XCI has been the subject of intense investigation. This process is regulated by complex interplay between multiple *cis*-acting non-coding genes, including *Xist*, *Tsix*, *Xite*, and *DXPas34*. All make large noncoding RNAs – so-called 'macroRNAs' – and together orchestrate the cascade of events involved in X-chromosome counting, choice, and the initiation of silencing. In addition to their well-established roles in cis, some of the non-coding loci also play roles *in trans*. This chapter will first summarize the current state of knowledge and focus on recent developments.

Keywords *Xist* · *Tsix* · *Xite* · *DXPas34* · X-chromosome inactivation · noncoding RNA · antisense genes · heterochromatin · CpG-methylation · histone modification · chromatin structure

1 Dosage Compensation Through X-Chromosome Inactivation

In many metazoans, sex is determined by a pair of heteromorphic chromosomes. Because the XX female and XY male have different sex chromosome constitutions, females have twice the dosage of X-linked genes when compared to males. To achieve sex chromosome dosage compensation between the sexes, various organisms have taken different strategies over evolutionary time (Lucchesi et al. 2005). Fruitflies (*Drosophila melanogaster*) increase transcription from the male single X by approximately two-fold (reviewed in (Oh et al. 2004)), whereas round worms

S. Shibata (✉)
Department of Stem Cell Biology, Graduate School of Medical Sciences, Kanazawa University, 13-1 Takara-machi, Kanazawa, Ishikawa 920-8640, Japan
e-mail: shinwa@med.kanazawa-u.ac.jp

(*Caenorhabditis elegans*) take the opposite strategy of reducing transcription twofold from both X-chromosomes in the XX hermaphrodite (reviewed in (Meyer et al. 2004)). For the mammal, whose sex chromosomes evolved entirely separately from those of the fruitfly and nematode, dosage compensation employs a third mechanism in which one of two Xs in the female is transcriptionally inactivated (Lyon, 1961). Intriguingly, although all three mechanisms achieve the same result – dosage equivalence of the X-chromosome in XX and XY individuals – the underlying mechanisms and molecular players are completely different. The fruitfly utilizes a complex of MSL proteins and roX RNAs to achieve X-upregulation. The round worm uses an entirely distinct protein complex which includes SMC proteins and condensins to turn down X-linked gene expression. This chapter will discuss the mammalian mechanism known as 'X-chromosome inactivation' (XCI).

Two forms of XCI have been described; random and imprinted. XCI choice occurs randomly in the embryo proper in all eutherian mammals studied to date (Lyon, 1961). In mouse embryos, random XCI occurs shortly after uterine implantation between 4.5 and 6.5 days post coitum (dpc) (Monk and Harper, 1979). Mouse embryonic stem (ES) cells derived from inner cell mass of blastocysts carry two active Xs (Xa) and are subject to random XCI when the ES cells are differentiated in culture (Kay et al. 1993; Norris et al. 1994). Because ES cells recapitulate XCI, they have provided an extremely useful model system to study XCI *ex vivo*.

Conceptually, random XCI can be divided into four steps (reviewed in (Lyon, 1999; Avner and Heard, 2001; Boumil and Lee, 2001)). Shortly after implantation, cells of the epiblast determine how many Xs they have relative to autosomes in a process we commonly refer to as 'counting'. If a cell has more than two Xs, it randomly selects one of its two Xs to become active X (Xa) and inactive X (Xi) in a step we call 'choice'. The 'silencing' step occurs only on the X chosen to become inactive and involves not only the initiation of silencing from a master X-linked locus but also the outward spread of silencing from the site of initiation. Once established, the Xi remains silent in all later cell divisions in the 'maintenance' phase. By this mechanism, all diploid cells carry only one Xa and inactivate all Xs in excess of it. Thus, XY and XO cells do not inactivate any X, XX cells inactivate one, and XXX cells inactivate two. As will be discussed below, each of these steps requires the action of non-coding genes.

In the second form of XCI, the paternally inherited X is preferentially inactivated. The imprinted form was likely the first mechanism to evolve in mammals, utilized by the marsupials some 150–200 million years ago (Sharman, 1971; Graves, 1996). The proposed evolutionary progression is reflected in the early development of the mouse, a eutherian mammal (Huynh and Lee, 2005; Huynh and Lee, 2003; Okamoto et al. 2004): The first form of dosage compensation evident in the mouse pre-implantation embryo is imprinted and this form persists into the extraembryonic lineages; however, following a reactivation event in the epiblast lineage of the inner cell mass, the embryo proper re-initiates dosage compensation using the random form of XCI. Thus, the adult female eutherian is a mosaic of cells that express only one of two X-chromosomes. Whether it occurs in the human remains unclear (reviewed in Brown and Robinson 2000) (Migeon et al. 1989).

Over the past several years, it has become increasingly evident that the mechanisms underlying imprinted and random XCI may not be entirely shared, as indeed elements required for random XCI in the eutherian do not seem to be present in the marsupial at all (Duret et al. 2006; Davidow et al. 2007; Hore et al. 2007; Shevchenko et al. 2007). Random XCI depends strictly on a cluster of noncoding elements at the 'X-inactivation center' (*Xic*), an X-linked region that controls the initiation, spread, and maintenance of silencing along the X-chromosome. Each of these noncoding elements makes at least one 'macroRNA', large noncoding transcripts so called to distinguish them from the small RNAs (microRNAs, siRNAs, and piRNAs) that have attracted much recent attention. Various groups have shown that there is broken synteny between eutherians and marsupials within this macroRNA locus (Davidow et al. 2007; Hore et al. 2007; Shevchenko et al. 2007) and that at least one of the essential noncoding genes originated as an apparently unrelated protein-coding element in the marsupial (Duret et al. 2006). Yet, the difference between random and imprinted XCI may not be as simple as whether there is dependence on macroRNA function. Although marsupial XCI may not require the *Xic*, imprinted XCI in the eutherian clearly does to some extent. In this chapter, we will summarize the state of the art in our understanding of how macroRNAs control XCI in general.

2 The X-Inactivation Center and Its MacroRNAs

The existence of a single X-linked region controlling XCI became progressively evident from work done during the period between 1970 and 1990 (Brown et al. 1991b; Cattanach and Isaacson, 1967; Rastan and Robinson, 1990b). X-autosome translocation chromosomes were found to retain silencing potential only when they possessed the region syntenic to human Xq13. Studies in the mouse later refined the core elements of the mouse *Xic* to a region of 100–450 kb region (Lee et al. 1996, 1999a; Heard et al. 1999; Migeon et al. 1999), an X-linked domain encodes many macroRNAs, including those made from *Xist*, *Tsix*, *Xite*, and *DXPas34* (Fig. 1, their functions are described later). Intriguingly, although the ancestral region might have once carried many protein-coding genes (Duret et al. 2006), the eutherian locus of today appears to be devoid of any conserved open reading frames (ORFs), suggesting that the *Xic* functions primarily as a noncoding locus. Given evidence in recent years of widespread noncoding transcription in the mammalian genome (Pheasant and Mattick, 2007), there appears to be much to learn from the *Xic*. The macroRNAs of the *Xic* are unique. They may be overlapping, antisense, very large or relatively small. Some are spliced but their function may not necessarily depend on splicing. All appear to be transcribed by RNA polymerase II and, though splicing can occur in vivo, they are not exported out of the nucleus.

The first hints of functional significance came out of transgenic work indicating that inserting *Xic* sequences into autosomes can induce silencing in cis of genes at

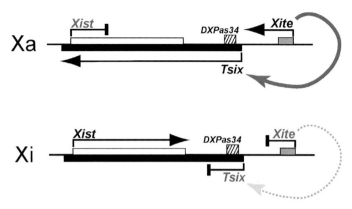

Fig. 1 Relationship of *Xist, Tsix, DXPas34*, and *Xite*

long range (Lee et al. 1996, 1999a; Heard et al. 1999; Migeon et al. 1999). This observation demonstrated that the *Xic* is sufficient to initiate XCI and formed the basis of the popular transgene assays that have been used in subsequent years to identify and characterize candidate elements within the *Xic*. On the other hand, it has also been observed that the *Xic* transgenes work more effectively when they are inserted in multicopy (Heard et al. 1999). This observation suggests that having multiple copies of an *Xic* element may help initiate or propagate silencing and may therefore make up for a deficiency of a critical factor on single copy transgenes. One such factor may be the long-hypothesized 'way stations' and 'booster elements' (Gartler and Riggs, 1983) which help the outward spread of the silencing complex from the *Xic* (see below). While the booster elements remain to be identified, the function of the *Xic* is clear. Some aspects of its function are rather surprising and all depend on the numerous noncoding RNA elements therein.

2.1 Xist

The *Xist* gene was firstly described as an unusual transcript expressed exclusively from the female Xi in humans (Brown et al. 1991a) and in mice (Borsani et al. 1991; Brockdorff et al. 1991). Dubbed the 'Xi-specific transcript', *Xist* RNA consists of multiple exons which together make a 17-kb transcript with several intriguing conserved repetitive motifs but no conserved ORF (Brockdorff et al. 1992; Brown et al. 1992). Its expression from the future Xi leads to accumulation along the entire X-chromosome in a distinctive pattern (Clemson et al. 1996; Chadwick and Willard, 2004; Duthie et al. 1999). It is generally believed that the spread of *Xist* RNA and its distribution along the Xi are central to the Xi's conversion to silent heterochromatin.

For random XCI, *Xist*'s functional significance has been clearly demonstrated by targeted mutagenesis in ES cells (Penny et al. 1996) and, for imprinted paternal XCI in the mouse placenta, by the inability to transmit an *Xist* mutation through the

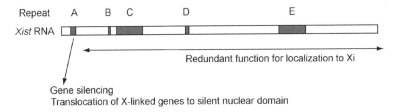

Fig. 2 Functional domains of *Xist* RNA

paternal germline (Marahrens et al. 1997). These studies showed that *Xist* is necessary to induce silencing in both forms of XCI. Conversely, ectopic expression of the *Xist* cDNA from an autosomal transgene also induces long-range gene silencing in cis (Wutz and Jaenisch, 2000). As is the case on the Xi, expression of *Xist* RNA on the autosome leads to the formation of an *Xist* RNA 'cloud' around the autosome (Wutz and Jaenisch, 2000; Lee and Jaenisch, 1997). Therefore, *Xist* expression is both necessary and sufficient for XCI silencing.

How does *Xist* RNA induce silencing? While the exact mechanism remains mysterious, some things seem clear. The *Xist* gene contains a number of notable conserved repeats, designated 'A' to 'E' (Fig. 2) (Brockdorff et al. 1992; Brown et al. 1992). The function of these repeats has been partially elucidated by extensive mutagenesis of the *Xist* cDNA on a transgene in the mouse system (Wutz et al. 2002). Intriguingly, the silencing function of *Xist* RNA depends strictly on repeat A. While other sequences and repeats B to E seem to be dispensable for silencing, it is thought that these elements might be important for localizing *Xist* RNA to the Xi. Human *XIST* RNA appears to have similar functional motifs (Chow et al. 2007). To elucidate the mechanism of RNA-induced silencing, much effort has been devoted to identifying factors that bind *Xist* RNA. However, these factors have remained elusive to date.

The importance of *Xist* for imprinted XCI in the mouse placental lineages contrasts sharply with its apparent dispensability in total-body XCI in the marsupial (Duret et al. 2006; Davidow et al. 2007; Hore et al. 2007; Shevchenko et al. 2007). However, it is currently not known whether *Xist* is required for the pre-implantation form of imprinted XCI in the mouse (Huynh and Lee, 2003, 2005; Okamoto et al. 2004). This developmentally early form of XCI may in fact be more similar to the evolutionarily ancestral form. The absence of *XIST* in the marsupial begs the obvious question of how XCI can be achieved without the silencer that is so critical to eutherians. It has been proposed that marsupial XCI may rely instead on germline events in the male (Cooper et al. 1993; Huynh and Lee, 2001; Lyon, 1999; McCarrey et al. 2002). The sex chromosomes are known to be inactivated during the pachytene stage of meiosis I ('meiotic sex chromosome inactivation', MSCI)(Lifschytz and Lindsley, 1972), and several recent report indicates that the X remains transcriptionally suppressed after meiosis I and through spermiogenesis in eutherians and marsupials (Greaves et al. 2006; Turner et al. 2006; Namekawa et al. 2006, 2007) (however see Chapter "Meiotic Silencing, Infertility and X Chromosome Evolution" by Turner). Thus, the imprinted paternal X of the marsupial female embryo may derive its silence from the previously inactivated status of the X in the paternal germline. While this hypothesis remains to be tested in the marsupial, the data so far are clear with respect to the mechanism of XCI and *Xist*: The noncoding *Xist* RNA is a relatively recent invention, occurring some 80–100 million years ago.

2.2 *Tsix*

Several years after the discovery of *Xist*, a large transcript complementary to *Xist* was found in undifferentiated mouse ES cells (Lee et al. 1999b). Its pattern of expression is reciprocal to that of *Xist* in ES cells and during XCI. Before XCI, the antisense gene is expressed from both Xs at a time when *Xist* expression is very low. Upon cell differentiation and the onset of XCI, the antisense gene is turned off on the future Xi, where *Xist* is then upregulated. On the future Xa, the persistence of the antisense transcript correlates with the repression of *Xist*. Named *"Tsix"* in reference to its antisense orientation, the gene was therefore suspected to play a role in the regulation of *Xist* since the time of its discovery (Lee et al. 1999b). To date, more than a dozen mutations (some described below) have been made in *Tsix*, each of which indeed demonstrates a role in repressing *Xist* expression (Lee and Lu, 1999; Sado et al. 2001).

Tsix initiates 12 kb downstream of *Xist* and encompasses the entire *Xist* gene (Lee et al. 1999b). One isoform of *Tsix* RNA has also been reported to initiate 15 kb upstream of its major promoter (Sado et al. 2001) and overlap with another noncoding gene, *Xite* (Ogawa and Lee, 2003). However, detailed analyses revealed that the upstream start site is minor and most *Tsix* transcription starts from the previously characterized major promoter (Shibata and Lee, 2003), yielding an unspliced transcript of 40 kb. A pol-II transcript (Sun et al. 2006), *Tsix* RNA is highly heterogeneous and has multiple splicing variants (Lee et al. 1999b; Sado et al. 2001, 2006; Shibata and Lee, 2003). However, splicing does not appear to be necessary for its function (Sado et al. 2006).

There is ongoing debate over whether *Tsix* function is conserved throughout Eutheria. Several groups have reported that human *TSIX* transcription is truncated and does not extend across the whole of *XIST* (Chow et al. 2003; Migeon, 2003; Migeon et al. 2002). It apparently also lacks a CpG-island (Migeon et al. 2002), which by contrast is very prominent in the 5′-portion of mouse *Tsix* (Lee et al. 1999b). More surprisingly, unlike mouse *Tsix*, human *TSIX* can apparently be expressed from Xi together with *XIST*, possibly suggesting species-specific differences in the way XCI is regulated (Chow et al. 2003; Migeon 2003; Migeon et al. 2002). Thus, while the role of *Tsix* in regulating mouse *Xist* seems clear, the mechanism of *XIST* regulation in humans has yet to be elucidated and the role of *TSIX* is currently an open question. However, the low degree of cross-species conservation in the region downstream of *Xist* (Migeon et al. 2002) may not serve as evidence against functional conservation of *Tsix* (Lee, 2003). Indeed, noncoding elements – free of the constraints posed by the amino acid code – may work as a noncoding RNA or binding sites for transcription factors and other chromatin-associated factors, in which case their function may depend more on secondary structures or discrete contact points rather than the linear sequence.

2.3 DXPas34

DXPas34 locus is a GC-rich 34-mer repeat element residing at the 5′-portion of *Tsix* gene in mice (Courtier et al. 1995; Avner et al. 1998; Debrand et al. 1999). CpG-methylation at the *DXPas34* locus was initially thought to be involved in X-chromosome imprint and/or choice of Xi because of its selective hypermethylation on the Xa (Courtier et al. 1995). Consistent with this interpretation, differentially methylated domains (DMD) have been found around *DXPas34* in gametes in a manner consistent with the expression pattern of *Tsix* (Boumil and Lee, 2001). Arguing against the idea, however, is a different study which does not find differential methylation of *DXPas34* (Prissette et al, 2001).

Regardless of whether differential methylation occurs on this repeat, the importance of *DXPas34* to XCI seems clear. Through targeted mutagenesis in ES cells, it was recently shown that, surprisingly, the *Tsix* promoter is dispensable for regulating *Xist* (Cohen et al. 2007). The transcription and function of *Tsix* were apparently rescued by inherent promoter activity within *DXPas34*. Indeed, the mutant ES cells showed no alteration in XCI choice despite the partial expression reduction and truncation of *Tsix*. By contrast, deletions of *DXPas34* do have effects. A deletion on a transgene in male ES cells (Vigneau et al. 2006) as well as targeted deletions of *DXPas34* in ES cells and mice (Cohen et al. 2007) demonstrated its unequivocal role in *Tsix* expression and X-chromosome choice. Furthermore, the transmission pattern of the *DXPas34* deletion in mice showed that the repeat is essential for imprinted XCI as well (Cohen et al. 2007). Recent findings suggest that differential binding of two transcription factors, Ctcf and Yy1, to the DMD in the *DXPas34* locus may be responsible for the monoallelic expression pattern of *Tsix* (Chao et al. 2002; Donohoe et al. 2007). *DXPas34* is also known to have inherent enhancer activity for *Tsix* (Stavropoulos et al. 2005).

Most intriguingly, *DXPas34* may have descended from an ERV retrotransposable element (Cohen et al. 2007). Although a tandem repeat of the 34mer element is not conserved in the human, remnants of the ERV can still be seen in human *TSIX* at approximately the same location. In the rat, *DXPas34* is recognizable in its entirety. Consistent with its being a retrotransposable element, the mouse repeat has pol-II activity and can drive expression of a luciferase reporter (Cohen et al. 2007). Furthermore, the endogenous element in mice produces bidirectional noncoding transcripts (Cohen et al. 2007), which therefore means that the 5′ end of *Tsix* makes both forward and reverse noncoding RNAs. Without the transcription elements within *DXPas34*, there is a surprising loss of *Tsix* repression during the maintenance stage of XCI (when the *Tsix* promoter is normally silent). One possible explanation is that noncoding transcription in *DXPas34* in the antisense orientation to *Tsix* may be important for repressing *Tsix* after establishment of XCI. Based on the phenotype of a *DXPas34* knockout in ES cells and mice, it is proposed that the transcription of *DXPas34* may both positively and negatively regulate *Tsix* (Cohen et al. 2007).

2.4 Xite

A large region upstream of *Tsix* is also known to be transcribed (Debrand et al. 1999). Several specific transcripts were subsequently identified as either an alternative splice form of *Tsix* (Sado et al. 2001) or as an independent transcript originating from the enhancer element for *Tsix* (Ogawa and Lee, 2003). In the latter case, the transcript was named *Xite* for "X-inactivation intergenic transcription elements" and shown to play an important role in XCI choice by a discrete knockout of *Xite* in ES cells (Ogawa and Lee, 2003). The locus contains developmentally-specific DNase-I-hypersensitive sites (DHS) and a *Tsix*-specific enhancer required for the persistence of *Tsix* expression during the XCI process (Ogawa and Lee, 2003; Stavropoulos et al. 2005). By promoting the expression of *Tsix*, the *Xite* locus regulates the choice decision and controls the likelihood with which the linked X-chromosome will be chosen for silencing in a nucleus with two or more X-chromosomes.

This region is included in a previously targeted 65-kb region 3' of *Xist* thought to be required for counting (Clerc and Avner, 1998; Morey et al. 2001, 2004). Its deletion on one X-chromosome in females results in nonrandom inactivation of the mutated X, consistent with the idea that a choice element resides in this region. In males, the deletion seems to cause upregulation of the *Xist* gene at least in a subset of cells, suggesting that a counting element also resides in this region. These ideas are in agreement with the occurrence of *Tsix, DXPas34*, and *Xite* in this region and their known regulatory roles, although a deletion of *Tsix, DXPas34*, or *Xite* individually does not have any phenotype in male ES cells or mice (Cohen et al. 2007; Lee, 2002; Lee and Lu, 1999; Ogawa and Lee, 2003). It seems likely that the more severe phenotype of the 65-kb deletion as compared to that of a deletion of *Tsix, DXPas34, or Xite* alone could be explained by its inclusion of all three elements, as well as portions of *Xist, Tsx*, and *Chic1*.

3 Coordinate Regulation of XCI by the Noncoding RNAs

3.1 Counting

X-chromosome counting occurs once during eutherian development, most likely shortly after implantation between 4.5 and 5.5 dpc when random XCI is first evident in the epiblast lineage (Monk and Harper, 1979). It is clear that embryos do not merely sense the number of X-chromosomes but also the relative number of autosome sets. Indeed, as in the fruitfly and round worm, the counting step actually measures the X-to-autosome ratio (X/A) (Avner and Heard, 2001; Lee, 2005; Meyer et al. 2004). Thus, the counting mechanism must involve both X-linked "numerator" elements and autosomally produced "denominator" elements made in precise and limited quantities. The act of counting must then represent the titration of numerators against denominators to calculate the X/A ratio (see (Lee and Lu, 1999; Lee, 2005) for full discussion). In its simplest rendition, numerators and denominators bind to each other in precise stoichiometric ratios; the complex then binds to one *Xic* and prevents the activation of *Xist* ("blocking factor"). The remaining *Xic* is 'unblocked' by the complex and, by default, is upregulated for *Xist* RNA. This is the so-called Blocking Factor Hypothesis (Lyon, 1999).

A second model proposes that two factors are required (Lee, 2005; Lee and Lu, 1999) and that the remaining X is not transactivated at *Xist* "by default". This model proposes that a second factor, comprising of untitrated denominators (autosomal) must bind to the remaining *Xic* and purposefully induce *Xist*. The second, so-called "competence factor" has been proposed to explain why male ES cells and embryos with a *Tsix* mutation can maintain *Xist* repression even though *Tsix* can no longer block *Xist* expression (Lee and Lu, 1999; Ohhata et al. 2006). The competence factor is thought to be required to induce *Xist* transcription and occurs only in cells bearing two or more X-chromosomes. The fact that, in some *Tsix* mutations, a small degree of *Xist* activation can be observed has been used to argue against a requirement for a competence factor (Clerc and Avner, 1998; Vigneau et al. 2006; Morey et al. 2004), suggesting that a competence factor may not be required. However, in these cases, *Xist* upregulation is only seen in a fraction of cells and may not lead to XCI (Ohhata et al. 2006). Clearly, *Tsix*-deficient male mice can be generated (Lee, 2000, 2002; Ohhata et al. 2006; Sado et al. 2001). Thus, it is unclear if the *Xist* clouds seen in these *Tsix* mutants represent true loss of counting or errant *Xist* expression in the context of low *Tsix* expression.

Not a single denominator has been identified in mammals. On the other hand, some of the numerator elements have been attributed to a broader region within the *Xic*, specifically within the region encompassing *Xite* and *Tsix* (Clerc and Avner, 1998; Lee, 2005; Lee and Lu, 1999; Morey et al. 2004) (Fig. 3). In principle, a mutation that changes the dosage of either the numerator or the denominator would have major effects on the initiation of XCI in female cells or on the blockage of XCI

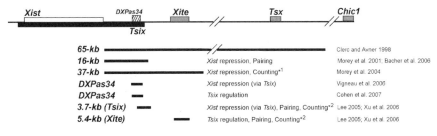

Fig. 3 DNA elements 3' to *Xist*

in male cells. Using the readout of aberrant Xi number, several studies have begun to shed light on the nature of the elements.

Deleting a 65 kb region downstream of *Xist* apparently results in the upregulation of *Xist* with evidence of XCI in some male cells (Clerc and Avner, 1998; Morey et al. 2004; Vigneau et al. 2006), suggesting that counting elements may lie within this region. Genetic manipulation of this region that includes *Tsx, Xite, Tsix, DXPas34*, and the 3' terminus of *Xist* has added to our knowledge of where some of the dosage-sensitive elements might lie. Specifically, a 3.7 kb deletion of the 5' end of *Tsix* causes the appearance of cells that display an aberrant number of Xi: Female ES cells homozygous for the *Tsix* deletion can possess 0, 1, or 2 Xi (Lee, 2005). Strangely, when sequences from *Tsix* and *Xite* are placed ectopically in multiple copies on an autosome, XCI is completely arrested in female cells, whereas they had no effect in male cells (Lee, 2005). A deletion of *DXPas34*, which lies within the critical region in *Tsix*, resulted in ectopic XCI upon differentiation in a fraction of male cells, consistent with the idea that *DXPas34* might be a part of the counting mechanism (Vigneau et al. 2006). Together, these data suggested that the 5' end of *Tsix* and the *Xite* region contain elements which govern the number of Xi in male and female cells: When deleted, an excess number of Xi can be the outcome; when introduced in supernumerary numbers, XCI is blocked. Thus, a dosage-sensitive element resides within a 15-kb region encompassing the 5' end of *Tsix* and *Xite* – a region that likely functions as an X-linked numerator for the assessment of the X/A ratio. Whether autosomally linked denominators bind to this region is currently under investigation.

3.2 Choice

In diploid cells with more than one X-chromosome, XCI is initiated and can occur randomly on any of the Xs present. A "choice" mechanism stochastically determines which will become Xa and which will become Xi. Many elements have been shown to affect choice, either by completely biasing the decision or only influencing it by causing a slight skew of the XCI pattern. At one extreme is imprinted XCI, in which the paternal X is invariably inactivated. At the other is the effect of the "*Xce*" or X-controlling element, a genetically defined X-linked but as yet unmapped locus that leads to slightly skewed XCI patterns (Cattanach and Isaacson, 1967; Cattanach and Williams, 1972). The skewing is apparent in offspring of parents from different strain backgrounds. For example, the *Mus castaneus* strain carries a relatively strong *Xce* allele and, when crossed to the 129 strain, will yield female offspring in which XCI takes place on the 129 X-chromosome in approximately 80% of cells (rather than in 50%, as would be expected if XCI were purely random). Linkage analyses have suggested that the *Xce* is closely linked to the X-inactivation center (Simmler et al. 1993; Avner et al. 1998).

In the interest of identifying novel regulators of XCI, much effort has been placed in finding elements that skew XCI. The 65 kb deletion made clear that a broad region downstream of *Xist* plays a major role in influencing choice: Female cells carrying the 65 kb deletion on one X show exclusive inactivation of the X with the deletion

(Clerc and Avner, 1998). It is now known that the elements responsible for determining choice reside within the three noncoding transcribed elements, *Tsix, Xite*, and *DXPas34* (Lee, 2000; Lee and Lu, 1999; Luikenhuis et al. 2001; Ogawa and Lee, 2003; Sado et al. 2001; Stavropoulos et al. 2001; Cohen et al. 2007). Whether *Xist* on a given female X chromosome is transactivated depends on whether *Tsix* expression persists on that X during the critical time window during which XCI can take place: When *Tsix* expression persists, *Xist* cannot be upregulated; when *Tsix* is downregulated, *Xist* can be induced in the female cell. The monoallelic accumulation of *Xist* RNA over the Xi is therefore the result of monoallelic persistence of *Tsix* on the future Xa and monoallelic repression on the future Xi.

Thus, any genetic element that regulates *Tsix* expression can theoretically affect XCI choice. Targeted mutagenesis and transcription assays have shown that *Xite* and *DXPas34* promote *Tsix* transcription. Two enhancer elements influence *Tsix* expression (Stavropoulos et al. 2005). One lies within a 1.2 kb region of *Xite* and has been shown to determine whether *Tsix* persists on the linked X chromosome at the onset of cell differentiation and XCI. Deleting the 1.2 kb enhancer in female ES cells leads to immediate repression of *Tsix* in cis upon cell differentiation, causing skewing of XCI to favor inactivation of the mutated X (Ogawa and Lee, 2003). The degree of skewing could be mild to severe. The second is a bipartite enhancer element located at the 5′ end of *Tsix* and includes *DXPas34* (Stavropoulos et al. 2005). There are developmentally specific DNase I hypersensitive sites within both enhancers, consistent with their regulation of XCI. Two groups have mutated *DXPas34* and surrounding sequences and, though the exact details are slightly different, both found that the level of *Tsix* expression is inversely correlated with the efficiency of XCI (Vigneau et al. 2006; Cohen et al. 2007). A deletion of *DXPas34* alone resulted in skewing of random XCI to favor silencing of the mutant X. These experiments demonstrate that *Tsix, Xite*, and *DXPas34* together designate the choice of future Xa and Xi.

XCI choice is also known to be influenced by elements within *Xist*. In humans, mutations within the *XIST* promoter have been shown to affect choice, as originally deduced from the occasional familial clustering of skewed XCI patterns in otherwise normal females (Plenge et al. 1997). Interestingly, one mutation occurs within a CTCF binding site (Pugacheva, 2005), believed to be a positive regulator of *XIST*, and seems to increase the strength of CTCF binding, thereby promoting the inactivation of the linked X-chromosome. On the basis of familial clustering and linkage analysis, an *XCE*-like region has also been postulated in humans (Naumova et al. 1998; Naumova et al. 1996). In mice, a mutation within the *Xist* gene body has also been shown to cause a primary defect in choice (Marahrens et al. 1998).

Imprinted XCI may be viewed as the most extreme case of skewed choice. While the elements responsible for imprinting are not yet known in marsupials, both *Xist* and *Tsix* play a role in imprinted XCI in the eutherian placenta (Lee, 2000; Marahrens et al. 1997; Sado et al. 2001). In the extraembryonic tissues, maternal-specific *Tsix* expression leads to paternal-specific *Xist* expression. These stereotyped expression patterns of the two noncoding genes are fundamental for establishing imprinted XCI. How is monoallelic *Tsix/Xist* expression adopted? In autosomally imprinted loci, allele-specific DNA methylation patterns established in the germline play a key role, often together with allele-specific binding of a chromatin insulator known as "Ctcf" (Bell et al. 1999; Hark et al. 2000; Kanduri et al. 2000a, 2000b; Lobanenkov et al. 1990; Ohlsson et al. 2001; Fedoriw et al.2004; Thorvaldsen et al. 2006; Szabo et al. 2000). Ctcf binds preferentially to an imprint control region when it is unmethylated and blocks enhancer-promoter interactions in cis. The absence of binding on the reciprocal allele enables transactivation of the linked allele. Therefore, DNA methylation and Ctcf binding patterns can together set up parent-specific expression of genes within some autosomally imprinted domains.

Whether DNA methylation and Ctcf also play a role in imprinted XCI remains to be seen. Mutations in the Dnmt1 maintenance methyltransferase, the de novo Dnmt3a/3b methyltransferases, and the germline Dnmt3L methyltransferase do not have obvious effects on imprinted XCI (Beard et al. 1995; Panning and Jaenisch, 1996; Sado et al. 2000, 2004; Bourc'his, 2001). However, there does appear to be germline-specific methylation patterns in *Xist* and *Tsix* (Zuccotti and Monk, 1995; Boumil et al. 2006; Ariel et al. 1995). Ctcf has been shown to bind both *Tsix* and *Xite* (Chao et al. 2002; Xu et al. 2007). In *Tsix*, many potential sites are found within the *DXPas34* locus. In ES cells, Yy1 appears to be a cofactor of Ctcf (Donohoe et al. 2007). It is proposed that the interaction between Yy1 and Ctcf transactivates *Tsix* in ES cells, as $Yy1^{+/-}$ male ES cells showed impaired *Tsix* and elevated *Xist* RNA levels in undifferentiated and early differentiating conditions. Some effects may also be evident in imprinted XCI, although a more thorough analysis needs to be undertaken. Together, these observations suggest that differential methylation at the DMD around the *DXPas34* locus and differential Ctcf-Yy1 binding might provide the foundation for imprinted XCI as well as random XCI. These possibilities remain to be investigated.

3.3 X–X Pairing

Intriguingly, the two female X-chromosomes pair transiently at the onset of XCI (Xu et al. 2006; Bacher et al. 2006). Because mammalian chromosomes were not thought to pair outside of meiosis, this discovery was somewhat surprising. Pairing occurs exclusively at the *Xic* – not elsewhere on the X – and occurs only upon cell differentiation primarily between days 1 and 4 when XCI takes place. *Tsix* and *Xite* are required for the pairing process, as deletions of either or both elements eliminate or severely retard pairing. Significantly, inserting fragments of *Tsix* and *Xite* into autosomes induce the autosomes to pair ectopically with the X, indicating that *Tsix* and *Xite* are also sufficient for pairing (Xu et al. 2006). As little as 1–2 kb of either noncoding gene appears to be sufficient for pairing and, in fact, the 1.6 kb *DXPas34* motif alone enables an autosome carrying the repeat element to pair with the X-linked *Xic* (Xu et al. 2007). The role of noncoding RNA in pairing is implied by the observation that blocking transcription by RNA polymerase II prevents formation of new pairs. The chromatin insulator Ctcf, which binds both *Tsix* and *Xite* within the critical pairing region, is apparently required for the process as well (Xu et al. 2007).

These findings led to a model in which a complex of RNA (possibly *Tsix* and *Xite* RNA themselves) and protein (such as Ctcf) serve to identify and then bind the two homologous *Xic*'s to each other at the onset of cell differentiation. Because *Tsix* and *Xite* are both expressed even prior to cell differentiation and Ctcf is also at least partially bound, additional factors must control the developmentally timed pairing event.

What could be the purpose of pairing? Several clues may hint at its purpose. Pairing coincides with the window of XCI and seems to occur just prior to the upregulation of *Xist* (Xu et al. 2006; Bacher et al. 2006). In the absence of pairing, XCI does not occur properly. Indeed, female ES cells carrying a homozygous deletion of *Tsix* shows very delayed pairing and a failure to count and choose Xs, as cells with 0, 1, or 2 Xi could be observed during differentiation (Xu et al. 2006; Lee, 2005). Furthermore, female ES cells carrying ectopic *Tsix* or *Xite* fragments showed ectopic pairing between the transgene-bearing autosome and one X chromosome, precluding normal pairing between the two Xs. Interestingly, the inhibition of pairing between the true Xs seemed to block the initiation of XCI completely. Collectively, these results led to the hypothesis that pairing enables a cell to count Xs and then choose between them for inactivation. Although the details are entirely mysterious, pairing may provide a mechanism of 'crosstalk' between the Xs to ensure that Xa and Xi are chosen in a mutually exclusive way (Xu et al. 2006).

3.4 Tsix Regulation of Xist

Differential *Tsix* expression between the two female X alleles provides the molecular basis for *Xist* allelic choice. By RNA-FISH analyses, one can observe that *Tsix* transcription is monoallelically terminated upon differentiation and *Xist* is monoallelically upregulated on the future Xi, while the opposite occurs on the future Xa (Lee et al. 1999b). The concept that *Tsix* negatively regulates *Xist* in cis has been confirmed through many experiments involving targeted mutagenesis of *Tsix*, all of which leads to nonrandom XCI of the mutated X in female cells (Lee and Lu, 1999; Sado et al. 2001; Lee, 2000; Luikenhuis et al. 2001; Shibata and Lee, 2004; Stavropoulos et al. 2001; Morey et al. 2001).

How does *Tsix* regulate *Xist*? *Tsix* could operate at several distinct levels – via specific DNA elements (such as *DXPas34*), through the non-coding *Tsix* RNA, via the act of antisense transcription, or through any combination of the above. The results of the initial *Tsix* knockout left open several possibilities. Because the $Tsix^{\Delta CpG}$ mutation deletes both the *Tsix* promoter and *DXPas34* (Lee and Lu, 1999), the critical aspect of *Tsix* function could reside in its transcriptional activity, the RNA, or critical DNA motifs such as *DXPas34*. *Tsix* mutations made subsequently have provided further clues. Forced expression of *Tsix* through either a constitutive promoter or an inducible promoter results in a gain-of-function in which the linked *Xist* allele cannot be upregulated and the linked X-chromosome is constitutively active (Luikenhuis et al. 2001; Stavropoulos et al. 2001). These experiments demonstrated that *Tsix* transcription is functional and that *Tsix* does not repress *Xist* merely through DNA motifs.

To test whether *Tsix* must be transcribed through its entire length, several groups created alleles that prematurely terminate the RNA by inserting a poly-A signal in the middle of its sequence without removing any DNA element (Luikenhuis et al. 2001; Shibata and Lee, 2004). These mutant cell lines also showed non-random XCI of the mutated X, indicating that *Tsix* transcription complementary to *Xist* is necessary for repression. If transcription is needed, does *Tsix* act as an RNA entity or is antisense transcription itself sufficient without requirement for specific RNA motifs? To begin to address this question, a *Tsix* knock-in was generated in female ES cells, in which a minigene (cDNA) expressing a major *Tsix* splice variant was inserted next to the *Xist* locus in the context of a *Tsix* truncation mutation (Shibata and Lee, 2004). This arrangement enabled one to test whether *Tsix* RNA could 'rescue' the *Tsix* truncation mutation. Significantly, the *Tsix* truncation was not rescued by the cDNA, suggesting that *Tsix* function requires more than the spliced antisense RNA.

However, these experiments do not rule out a role for the full-length RNA transcribed in the context of the endogenous locus. Indeed, a significant fraction of *Tsix* RNA is not spliced (Shibata and Lee, 2003). Evidence that the full-length RNA may be more critical than splice variants comes from yet another *Tsix* mutation in which a splice acceptor of exon 4 is destroyed in ES cells allowing investigation of the contribution of splicing (Sado et al. 2006). Disruption of exon 4 splice acceptor resulted in loss of spliced *Tsix* species and a relative increase of the full-length RNA, but the *Xist* locus remained stably repressed at the splicing-defective *Tsix* allele. Taken together, these many mutations show that transcription through all of the *Tsix* locus or the full-length RNA product itself provides the critical function in repressing *Xist*.

A breakthrough in understanding the mechanism of antisense regulation came from the recent work of several groups, which concluded that *Tsix* regulates *Xist* via co-transcriptionally directed chromatin changes (Sun et al. 2006; Navarro et al. 2006; Sado et al. 2005). The act of transcription through *Xist* in the antisense orientation brings with it a series of changes to the underlying histones including H4 acetylation, H3-K27 methylation, and H3-K4 methylation. The direction of chromatin change is currently under dispute. Through mutational analysis, Sado et al. reported that, in developing embryos, loss of *Tsix* on the future Xa results in open chromatin structure at the *Xist* promoter and exon 1, which includes vanishing loss of CpG-methylation, augmented acetyl-histone H4, elevated histone H3-dimethyl lysine 4 (H3K4m2), and emergence of additional DHS (Sado et al. 2005). This implies that *Tsix* transcription normally creates a more heterochromatic state in the *Xist* locus. In agreement, Navarro et al. argued that *Tsix* induces a heterochromatic state through modification of H3K4m2 over the *Xist/Tsix* region (Navarro et al. 2005) and suggested that Ctcf sites flanking both sides of the *Xist* promoter may be involved in maintaining heterochromatic structures therein (Navarro et al. 2006).

By contrast, Sun et al. reported that *Tsix*'s effect is quite the opposite (Sun et al. 2006): By allele-specific chromatin immunoprecipitations, they showed that

Tsix expression is accompanied by euchromatic modifications across the *Tsix/Xist* locus on the future Xa. Downregulation of *Tsix* on the future Xi induces a transient heterochromatic state in *Xist*, most eminently represented by histone H3-trimethyl lysine 27 (H3K27m3) modification. Thus, it is proposed that *Xist* is paradoxically upregulated in the context of "repressive" chromatin marks and is turned off in the context of "activating" chromatin marks. While these are significantly contrasting models, all three models agree on the point that *Tsix* transcription through the *Xist* locus controls sense RNA expression by inducing specific chromatin modifications.

Tsix has also been shown to control *Xist* through DNA methylation. Previously, differential CpG-methylation at the *Xist* locus was thought to preemptively dictate *Xist* transcription (Norris et al. 1994). However, loss of CpG-methylation by deleting the maintenance DNA methyltransferase, *Dnmt1*, only partially activated *Xist* expression in somatic cells and in ES cells (Beard et al. 1995; Panning and Jaenisch, 1996; Sado et al. 2000). Similarly, initiation and propagation of XCI was not grossly affected in ES cells devoid of both *Dnmt3a* and*Dnmt3b* de novo DNA methyltransferases, although mild derepression of *Xist* could be observed (Sado et al. 2004). These reports indicate that *Xist* is regulated properly without CpG-methylation during the initiation phase of XCI but left open the possibility that DNA methylation may play a role in maintenance of random XCI and imprinted XCI. Indeed, differential methylation of the *Xist* promoter has been reported in gametes and correlate with repression on the maternal allele and activity of the paternal allele (Ariel et al. 1995; Zuccotti and Monk, 1995). Differential methylation of *Tsix* and *Xite* has also been reported in gametes (Boumil et al. 2006). For random XCI, *Tsix* appears to directly affect the DNA methylation status of *Xist* but only after the XCI choice decision has been made (Sado et al. 2005; Sun et al. 2006). *Tsix* RNA forms a complex with Dnmt3a protein in the *Xist* promoter region and is hypothesized to recruit Dnmt3a activity to methylate the *Xist* promoter and permanently repress it on the future Xa (Sun et al. 2006). Thus, DNA methylation seems to be an important regulator of *Xist* but is a relatively late event.

Collectively, the broad array of data indicates that *Tsix* transcription has versatile effects on *Xist* chromatin structure (summarized in Table 1). *Tsix* controls *Xist* expression through transcription-coupled chromatin change by both directing or repelling specific histone modifications during the first phase and by controlling DNA methylation of the *Xist* promoter in the second phase. Still, our present knowledge is not yet complete and differences among the models need to be reconciled before a fully orchestrated model of *Xist* regulation by *Tsix* can be realized.

3.5 Initiation of Silencing

During the process of XCI, the earliest events observed on the future Xi are downregulation of *Tsix* RNA and upregulation of *Xist* RNA. The accumulation of *Xist* RNA on the X is quickly followed by recruitment of Ezh2-Eed complex (Plath et al. 2003; Silva et al. 2003), hypomethylation of H3K4m2 (Boggs et al. 2002), methylation of histone H3 lysine 9 (H3K9) (Boggs et al. 2002; Heard et al. 2001; Mermoud et al. 2002; Peters et al. 2002) and H3 lysine 27 (H3K27) (Plath

Table 1 Regulation of *Xist* chromatin structure by *Tsix*

Conferred chromatin feature by *Tsix*	Position	Cells	Reference
(+)H3K4m2	*Xist* gene body	male ES cells	Morey et al. (2004)
(+)H3K4m2	*Xist* gene body	male ES cells	Navarro et al. (2005)
(−)H3K4m2	*Xist* promoter / 5' of exon 1	male ES cells	Navarro et al. (2005)
(+)CpG-methylation	*Xist* promoter / 5' of exon 1	female and male embryos / extraembryonic tissues	Sado et al. (2005)
(−)DNase-I-hypersensitive sites	*Xist* promoter / 5' of exon 1	female and male embryos	Sado et al. (2005)
(−)H3K4m2	*Xist* promoter / 5' of exon 1	male embryonic mouse fibroblasts (MEF)	Sado et al. (2005)
(−)Acetyl-histone H4	*Xist* promoter / 5' of exon 1	male MEF	Sado et al. (2005)
(−)H3K4m2	*Xist* promoter	female embryoid bodies (EB)	Sun et al. (2006)
(+)H3K4m2	*Xist* gene body	female EB	Sun et al. (2006)
(−)H3K27m3	*Xist* promoter / gene body	female ES / EB	Sun et al. (2006)
(−)RNA pol II	*Xist* promoter	male ES cells	Navarro et al. (2006)
(−)TFIIB	*Xist* promoter	male ES cells	Navarro et al. (2006)
(+)H3K4m2	*Xist* gene body	male ES cells	Navarro et al. (2006)
(−)H3K4m2	5' of *Xist* exon 1 (CTCF)*	male ES cells	Navarro et al. (2006)
(−)H3K27m3	*Xist* gene body	male ES cells	Navarro et al. (2006)
(−)H3K4m3	5' of *Xist* exon 1 (CTCF)*	male ES cells	Navarro et al. (2006)
(+)H3K9m3	5' of *Xist* exon 1 (CTCF)*	male ES cells	Navarro et al. (2006)
(−)Acetyl-H3K9	5' of *Xist* exon 1 (CTCF)*	male ES cells	Navarro et al. (2006)
(+)CpG-methylation	5' of *Xist* exon 1 (CTCF)*	male ES cells	Navarro et al. (2006)

*CTCF-flanked 3-kb region including *Xist* P1 promoter and exon 1

et al. 2003; Silva et al. 2003), and late replication of the Xi (Keohane et al. 1996). Gene silencing becomes evident through exclusion of the transcription machinery (e.g., pol-II) and exclusion of hnRNA (Hall et al. 2002; Huynh and Lee, 2003; Chaumeil et al. 2006). How *Xist* RNA brings on these changes is not currently known, as interacting factors for the transcript have yet to be identified. However, genetic analyses have shown that developmentally timed expression of *Xist* RNA and the integrity of its silencing domain (Repeat A) are crucial for these changes (Wutz et al. 2002).

The histone methyltransferase (HMTase) catalyzing H3K9 methylation on Xi is not yet determined. On the other hand, the polycomb repressor complex 2 (PRC2) consisting of Ezh2, Eed, and Suz12, is known to catalyze H3K27 trimethylation on the future Xi (Plath et al. 2003; Silva et al. 2003). However, recent reports indicated that Eed is dispensable for random XCI (Kalantry and Magnuson, 2006) and its function can be replaced by the other polycomb complex, PRC1 (Schoeftner et al. 2006).

PRC1 proteins have in fact been shown to be recruited to Xi during the initiation and establishment phases (de Naploles et al. 2004; Fang et al. 2004; Hernandez-Munoz et al. 2005; Plath et al. 2004; Schoeftner et al. 2006). The Ring1B subunit catalyzes monoubiquitination of histone H2A at lysine 119 (H2AK119ub1) and the H2AK119ub1 modification is enriched on Xi shortly after *Xist* RNA accumulates on the X. However, even Ring1B is dispensable for the initiation and maintenance of XCI (Leeb and Wutz, 2007). These findings suggest functional redundancy of PRC1 and PRC2 in the initiation of XCI. Taken together, initiation and establishment of XCI are achieved by multiple redundant pathways which are based on repressive histone modifications placed by the Polycomb group (PcG) proteins (Table 2). These changes are soon followed by hypoacetylation of histone H4 (Keohane et al. 1996),

Table 2 Changes in chromatin factors associated with Xi formation

Chromatin factors	Timing	Reference
Histone H3-dimethyl lysine 9	Early	Heard et al. (2001) and Mermoud et al. (2002)
Hypoacetylation of histone H3 lysine 9	Early	Heard et al. (2001)
Hypomethylation of histone H3 lysine 4	Early	Heard et al. (2001) and Chaumeil et al. (2006)
Exclusion of RNA polymerase II	Early	Chaumei et al. (2006)
Histone H3-trimethyl lysine 27	Early, transient (?)	Silva et al. (2003) and Plath et al. (2003)
Eed-Ezh2	Early, transient	Mak et al. (2002); Silva et al. (2003) and Plath et al. (2003)
Suz12	Early, transient	de La Cruz et al. (2005) and Schoeftner et al. (2006)
Histone H4-monomethyl lysine 20	Early	Kohlmaier (2004) and Schoeftner et al. (2006)
Histone H2A-ubiquityl lysine 119	Early	de Naploles et al. (2004); Fang et al. (2004); Schoeftner et al. (2006) and Leeb and Wutz (2007)
Ring1B	Early	de Naploles et al. (2004); Fang et al. (2004); Schoeftner et al. (2006); Leeb and Wutz (2007)
Mel18, Mph1 (Phc1)	Early	de Naploles et al. 2004; Plath et al. 2004
Bmi-1, Cbx2, Phc2	Middle	Plath et al. 2004
Histone H4 hypoacetylation	Middle	Jeppesen and Turner 1993; Keohane et al. 1996; O'neill 2003
Histone macroH2A1	Middle	Costanzi and Pehrson 1998; Mermoud et al. 1999
Methylated CpG sequences	Late	Mohandas 1981; Keohane et al. 1996
HP1, histone H1, high mobility group protein (HMG-I/Y)	?	Chadwick and Willard 2003

deposition of the variant histone macroH2A1 (Mermoud et al. 1999; Costanzi and Pehrson, 1998), and methylation of promoter-associated CpG dinucleotides (Keohane et al. 1996). Thus, the Xi undergoes a series of dramatic changes during XCI.

3.6 Spreading of Silencing Along the X

How silencing spreads from the *Xic* and whether *Xist* RNA is involved is very poorly understood. Gartler and Riggs proposed the concept of "way stations" or "booster elements" which promote spreading of X-inactivation (Gartler and Riggs, 1983). Clearly, these elements are not X-chromosome specific, as autosomal segments translocated into the X-chromosome (Rastan and Brown, 1990a) and autosomes carrying insertion of the *Xic* can be silenced by XCI (Chow et al. 2007; Heard et al. 1999; Lee et al. 1996, 1999a; Migeon et al. 1999). However, autosomal silencing may not be as effective in X-autosomal translocations (White et al. 1998; Sharp et al. 2002; Hall et al. 2002; Popova et al. 2006) and in some cases of *Xic* trangenesis – in fact, multiple copies of *Xic* transgenes are required to induce silencing, as single-copy transgenes do not seem to be able to initiate random XCI at all (Heard et al. 1999).

These findings support the concept that the X carries booster elements that are either quantitatively or qualitatively different from those on autosomes. Such elements have not yet been identified, but Lyon has suggested LINE-1 repeats as "way stations" for the spreading of silencing along the X-chromosome (Lyon, 2000). LINE elements are some of the most abundant noncoding elements in the mammalian genome. Interestingly, genome-wide sequencing revealed that the X-chromosome is two-fold enriched for LINE-1 elements compared to autosomes (Bailey et al. 2000). It has also been noted that the concentration of LINE-1 elements is inversely correlated with the proportion of genes that escape XCI; moreover, in the context of X-autosome translocations, autosomal regions that are relatively depleted of LINE-1 elements have attenuated spread of XCI in mouse ES cells (Lyon, 2000; Carrel and Willard, 2005; Popova et al. 2006). However, whether LINEs are in fact the way stations remains to be tested.

Insight into how silencing spreads may be gained from studying how some regions of the X-chromosome block the advancement of silencing and thereby escape the XCI process. In humans, some 15–25% of the X-chromosome, particularly in the evolutionarily youngest strata of the X (short arm), escape silencing (Carrel and Willard, 2005). In mice, the mechanism of escape may not be as simple as having flanking chromatin insulators, as transgenesis work has shown that insertion of Ctcf binding sites cannot prevent silencing of a linked reporter gene on the Xi (Ciavatta et al. 2006).

The spreading function of *XIST/Xist* and silencing may be even more complex than is currently appreciated. Sub-chromosomal domains play an important role as well. Intriguingly, human Xi has been reported to be packaged into two non-overlapping types of heterochromatin – one defined by *XIST* RNA, histone macroH2A, and H3K27m3, and the other by H3K9m3, HP1 and H4K20m3 (Chadwick and Willard, 2004), implying that the Xi has two classes of heterochromatin of potentially different function. Other reports suggest that the Xi can be divided into an inner and outer domain. Recruitment of genes into the inner "*Xist* RNA compartment" depends on Repeat A of *Xist* and occurs during the early stage of XCI (Chaumeil et al. 2006; Clemson et al. 2006). This compartment lacks transcriptional machinery and harbors silent elements such as repetitive noncoding sequences (e.g., centromeric repeats, retrotransposable elements) and repressed X-linked genes. Genes that escape XCI tend to reside in the outer edge or outer domain of the Xi, where the genes presumably have greater access to the transcriptional and splicing machineries.

3.7 Maintenance of the Xa and Xi

It is customary to separate the maintenance phase of XCI from initiation and establishment, as genetic analyses have shown that molecular requirements for the two are only partially overlapping. The maintenance phase of XCI involves two processes in principle: one to maintain the repressed state of genes on Xi, and the other to prevent activation of silenced *Xist* gene on Xa.

Although *Xist* is absolutely essential for the initiation of silencing, it seems to be partially dispensable for the maintenance of Xi in mature cells, as deleting *Xist* after XCI has already taken place does not result in overt X-reactivation (Brown and Willard, 1994; Csankovszki et al. 1999). These findings showed that, once the silent configuration is established, repressive chromatin factors can be propagated – at least for several divisions in culture – in the absence of the noncoding RNA. This is consistent with the finding of an "XCI window" in undifferentiated cells or in early differentiating stages in which an Xi can be formed efficiently (Wutz and Jaenisch, 2000). After the window of up to 72 h into the in vitro differentiation period, cells become resistant to *Xist*-mediated silencing. Conversely, after this time window, the Xi state is stably "locked-in" and becomes resistant to reactivation even when *Xist* expression is removed. These observations indicate that the epigenetic machinery functioning in inducing silencing is primarily restricted to a particular developmental time window and that, once the critical period of XCI has passed, the Xa and Xi are very stable.

While the Xa and Xi are clearly very stable, several recent studies suggest that the Xs may be somewhat more plastic than previously thought. Indeed, the Xi continues to maintain an important relationship with *Xist* after the critical period has passed. Notably, *Xist* continues to be expressed throughout adult female life and loss of *Xist* expression on the Xi once silencing is established can lead to partial X-reactivation in some contexts (Csankovszki et al. 2001; Zhang et al. 2007). One study reports that the Xi is targeted to a perinucleolar compartment following homologous X–X pairing (Zhang et al. 2007). This perinucleolar targeting of Xi occurs once during the cell cycle, specifically during mid-late S phase when the Xi is replicated. Deleting

Xist on Xi leads to immediate dissociation from the perinucleolar compartment and this dissociation correlates with loss of H3K27m3 enrichment and partial reactivation of X-linked genes. It was proposed that the perinucleolar space comprises a functional compartment to which heterochromatin visits during S phase to be replicated.

The apparent stability of the Xi after *Xist* is deleted for several cell divisions may be explained by synergistic action of *Xist* RNA, CpG-methylation, and histone hypoacetylation. While deleting *Xist* in mature cells had little effect after a few cell divisions (Csankovszki et al. 1999), deleting *Xist* together with losing CpG methylation and histone deacetylation has a more pronounced effect (Csankovszki et al. 2001). Consistent with this observation, Atm (ataxia telangiectasia mutated) and Atr (ATM and Rad3 related) protein kinases, which exist in complexes with histone deacetylases and are key components in DNA damage response, may be involved in the maintenance of Xi (Ouyang et al. 2005). In addition, Atrx (alpha thalassemia mental retardation, X-linked), the SNF2 family of ATPase/helicase protein that is suggested to interact with Dnmts via its ATRX domain, was shown to play a role in imprinted XCI (Garrick et al. 2006). Taken together, these observations demonstrate that the repression of X-linked genes is mediated by highly redundant pathways, explaining why deleting *Xist* alone does not result in an immediate reactivation of X-linked genes. Clearly, however, losing *Xist* expression does gradually erode the Xi heterochromatin.

Studies have also shown that the Xa requires maintenance and depends on continued silence of *Xist*. Forced *Xist* expression in immature hematopoietic precursor cells of adult mice can lead to de novo silencing, although this was not the case in hematopoietic stem or mature blood cells (Savarese et al. 2006). Moreover, the human *XIST* gene could induce signs of silencing in somatic cells when ectopically expressed in a transgene-based system (Chow et al. 2007). In the endogenous context, the repressed state of *Xist* on Xa is maintained by CpG-methylation (Beard et al. 1995; Panning and Jaenisch, 1996; Sado et al. 2005; Sun et al. 2006) in conjunction with methylated DNA binding protein Mbd2 and histone hypoacetylation at the *Xist* promoter (Barr et al. 2007). Similar to the repression of X-linked genes, these factors have a synergistic effect on *Xist* repression, suggesting recruitment of repressor complex consisting of Mbd2 and histone deacetylases and/or Dnmts. Therefore, the active state of Xa is faithfully maintained by stable *Xist* silencing on that X. Should *Xist* become activated ectopically, at least some aspects of XCI can still take place in an *Xist*-dependent manner even after the original critical time window of XCI.

4 Concluding Remarks

These examples serve to illustrate the tremendous versatility of noncoding RNA in gene regulation and the pervasive importance of noncoding RNA elements for the control of XCI. Although good progress has been made in the past few years towards understanding XCI, much more remains mysterious. For example, how does X-X pairing take place and what message is transmitted by the Xs to each other? Are *Tsix* and *Xite* RNAs involved in the process? How does *Xist* RNA initiate the cascade of molecular changes on the future Xi? Equally important are the questions of how genes escape silencing and how the Xi is maintained in the inactive state. Finally, with the knowledge that imprinted XCI in marsupials does not involve macroRNAs of the *Xic*, how do we explain the mechanism of silencing in our close mammalian relatives? The paternal germline may hold part of the answer. It would not be surprising if more macroRNAs emerge as regulatory factors.

References

Ariel, M., Robinson, E., McCarrey, J. R., and Cedar, H. (1995). Gamete-specific methylation correlates with imprinting of the murine *Xist* gene. Nat Genet 9, 312–315.
Avner, P., and Heard, E. (2001). X-chromosome inactivation: counting, choice, and initiation. Nat Rev Genet 2, 59–67.
Avner, P., Prissette, M., Arnaud, D., Courtier, B., Cecchi, C., and Heard, E. (1998). Molecular correlates of the murine *Xce* locus. Genet Res, Camb 72, 217–224.
Bacher, C. P., Guggiari, M., Brors, B., Augui, S., Clerc, P., Avner, P., Eils, R., and Heard, E. (2006). Transient colocalization of X-inactivation centres accompanies the initiation of X inactivation. Nat Cell Biol 8, 293–299.
Bailey, J. A., Carrel, L., Chakravarti, A., and Eichler, E. E. (2000). Molecular evidence for a relationship between LINE-1 elements and X chromosome inactivation: the Lyon repeat hypothesis. Proc Natl Acad Sci U S A 97, 6634–6639.
Barr, H., Hermann, A., Berger, J., Tsai, H. H., Adie, K., Prokhortchouk, A., Hendrich, B., and Bird, A. (2007). Mbd2 contributes to DNA methylation-directed repression of the *Xist* gene. Mol Cell Biol 27, 3750–3757.
Beard, C., Li, E., and Jaenisch, R. (1995). Loss of methylation activates *Xist* in somatic but not in embryonic cells. Genes Dev 9, 2325–2334.
Bell, A. C., West, A. G., and Felsenfeld, G. (1999). The protein CTCF is required for the enhancer blocking activity of vertebrate insulators. Cell 98, 387–396.
Boggs, B. A., Cheung, P., Heard, E., Spector, D. L., Chinault, A. C., and Allis, C. D. (2002). Differentially methylated forms of histone H3 show unique association patterns with inactive human X chromosomes. Nat Genet 30, 73–76.
Borsani, G., Tonlorenzi, R., Simmler, M. C., Dandolo, L., Arnaud, D., Capra, V., Grompe, M., Pizzuti, A., Muzny, D., Lawrence, C., et al. (1991). Characterization of a murine gene expressed from the inactive X chromosome. Nature 351, 325–329.
Boumil, R. M., and Lee, J. T. (2001). 40 years of decoding the silence in X-chromosome inactivation. Hum Mol Genet 10, 2225–2232.
Boumil, R. M., Ogawa, Y., Sun, B. K., Huynh, K. D., and Lee, J. T. (2006). Differential methylation of *Xite* and CTCF sites in *Tsix* mirrors the pattern of X-inactivation choice in mice. Mol Cell Biol 26, 2109–2117.
Bourc'his, D., Xu, G. L., Lin, C. S., Bollman, B., and Bestor, T. H. (2001). Dnmt3L and the establishment of maternal genomic imprints. Science 294, 2536–2539.
Brockdorff, N., Ashworth, A., Kay, G. F., Cooper, P., Smith, S., McCabe, V. M., Norris, D. P., Penny, G. D., Patel, D., and Rastan, S. (1991). Conservation of position and exclusive expression of mouse *Xist* from the inactive X chromosome. Nature 351, 329–331.
Brockdorff, N., Ashworth, A., Kay, G. F., McCabe, V. M., Norris, D. P., Cooper, P. J., Swift, S., and Rastan, S. (1992). The product of the mouse *Xist* gene is a 15 kb inactive X-specific transcript containing no conserved ORF and located in the nucleus. Cell 71, 515–526.

Brown, C. J., Ballabio, A., Rupert, J. L., Lafreniere, R. G., Grompe, M., Tonlorenzi, R., and Willard, H. F. (1991a). A gene from the region of the human X inactivation centre is expressed exclusively from the inactive X chromosome. Nature 349, 38–44.

Brown, C. J., Hendrich, B. D., Rupert, J. L., Lafreniere, R. G., Xing, Y., Lawrence, J., and Willard, H. F. (1992). The human XIST gene: analysis of a 17 kb inactive X-specific RNA that contains conserved repeats and is highly localized within the nucleus. Cell 71, 527–542.

Brown, C. J., Lafreniere, R. G., Powers, V. E., Sebastio, G., Ballabio, A., Pettigrew, A. L., Ledbetter, D. H., Levy, E., Craig, I. W., and Willard, H. F. (1991b). Localization of the X inactivation centre on the human X chromosome in Xq13. Nature 349, 82–84.

Brown, C. J., and Robinson, W. P. (2000). The causes and consequences of random and non-random X chromosome inactivation in humans. Clin Genet 58, 353–363.

Brown, C. J., and Willard, H. F. (1994). The human X-inactivation centre is not required for maintenance of X-chromosome inactivation. Nature 368, 154–156.

Carrel, L., and Willard, H. F. (2005). X-inactivation profile reveals extensive variability in X-linked gene expression in females. Nature 434, 400–404.

Cattanach and Isaacson, J. H. (1967). Controlling elements in the mouse X chromosome. Genetics 57, 331–346.

Cattanach and Williams, C. E. (1972). Evidence of non-random X chromosome activity in the mouse. Genet Res 19, 229–240.

Chadwick, B. P., and Willard, H. F. (2004). Multiple spatially distinct types of facultative heterochromatin on the human inactive X chromosome. Proc Natl Acad Sci U S A 101, 17450–17455.

Chao, W., Huynh, K. D., Spencer, R. J., Davidow, L. S., and Lee, J. T. (2002). CTCF, a candidate trans-acting factor for X-inactivation choice. Science 295, 345–347. Epub 2001 Dec 2006.

Chaumeil, J., Le Baccon, P., Wutz, A., and Heard, E. (2006). A novel role for *Xist* RNA in the formation of a repressive nuclear compartment into which genes are recruited when silenced. Genes Dev 20, 2223–2237.

Chow, J. C., Hall, L. L., Baldry, S. E., Thorogood, N. P., Lawrence, J. B., and Brown, C. J. (2007). Inducible XIST-dependent X-chromosome inactivation in human somatic cells is reversible. Proc Natl Acad Sci U S A 104, 10104–10109.

Chow, J. C., Hall, L. L., Clemson, C. M., Lawrence, J. B., and Brown, C. J. (2003). Characterization of expression at the human XIST locus in somatic, embryonal carcinoma, and transgenic cell lines. Genomics 82, 309–322.

Ciavatta, D., Kalantry, S., Magnuson, T., and Smithies, O. (2006). A DNA insulator prevents repression of a targeted X-linked transgene but not its random or imprinted X inactivation. Proc Natl Acad Sci U S A 103, 9958–9963.

Clemson, C. M., Hall, L. L., Byron, M., McNeil, J., and Lawrence, J. B. (2006). The X chromosome is organized into a gene-rich outer rim and an internal core containing silenced nongenic sequences. Proc Natl Acad Sci U S A 103, 7688–7693.

Clemson, C. M., McNeil, J. A., Willard, H. F., and Lawrence, J. B. (1996). XIST RNA paints the inactive X chromosome at interphase: evidence for a novel RNA involved in nuclear/chromosome structure. J Cell Biol 132, 259–275.

Clerc, P., and Avner, P. (1998). Role of the region 3' to *Xist* exon 6 in the counting process of X-chromosome inactivation. Nat Genet 19, 249–253.

Cohen, D. E., Davidow, L. S., Erwin, J. A., Xu, N., Warshawsky, D., and Lee, J. T. (2007). The *DXPas34* repeat regulates random and imprinted X inactivation. Dev Cell 12, 57–71.

Cooper, D. W., Johnston., P. G., Watson, J. M., and Graves, J. A. M. (1993). X-inactivation in marsupials and monotremes. Seminars Dev Biol 4, 117–128.

Costanzi, C., and Pehrson, J. R. (1998). MacroH2A1 is concentrated in the inactive X chromosome of female mammals. Nature 393, 599–601.

Courtier, B., Heard, E., and Avner, P. (1995). *Xce* haplotypes show modified methylation in a region of the active X chromosome lying 3' to *Xist*. Proc Natl Acad Sci U S A 92, 3531–3535.

Csankovszki, G., Nagy, A., and Jaenisch, R. (2001). Synergism of *Xist* RNA, DNA methylation, and histone hypoacetylation in maintaining X chromosome inactivation. J Cell Biol *153*, 773–784.
Csankovszki, G., Panning, B., Bates, B., Pehrson, J. R., and Jaenisch, R. (1999). Conditional deletion of *Xist* disrupts histone macroH2A localization but not maintenance of X inactivation. Nat Genet *22*, 323–324.
Davidow, L. S., Breen, M., Duke, S. E., Samollow, P. B., McCarrey, J. R., and Lee, J. T. (2007). The search for a marsupial XIC reveals a break with vertebrate synteny. Chromosome Res *15*, 137–146.
de Napoles, M., Mermoud, J. E., Wakao, R., Tang, Y. A., Endoh, M., Appanah, R., Nesterova, T. B., Silva, J., Otte, A. P., Vidal, M., et al. (2004). Polycomb group proteins Ring1A/B link ubiquitylation of histone H2A to heritable gene silencing and X inactivation. Dev Cell *7*, 663–676.
Debrand, E., Chureau, C., Arnaud, D., Avner, P., and Heard, E. (1999). Functional analysis of the *DXPas34* locus, a 3' regulator of *Xist* expression. Mol Cell Biol *19*, 8513–8525.
Donohoe, M. E., Zhang, L. F., Xu, N., Shi, Y., and Lee, J. T. (2007). Identification of a Ctcf cofactor, Yy1, for the X chromosome binary switch. Mol Cell *25*, 43–56.
Duret, L., Chureau, C., Samain, S., Weissenbach, J., and Avner, P. (2006). The *Xist* RNA gene evolved in eutherians by pseudogenization of a protein-coding gene. Science *312*, 1653–1655.
Duthie, S. M., Nesterova, T. B., Formstone, E. J., Keohane, A. M., Turner, B. M., Zakian, S. M., and Brockdorff, N. (1999). *Xist* RNA exhibits a banded localization on the inactive X chromosome and is excluded from autosomal material in cis. Hum Mol Genet *8*, 195–204.
Fang, J., Chen, T., Chadwick, B., Li, E., and Zhang, Y. (2004). Ring1b-mediated H2A ubiquitination associates with inactive X chromosomes and is involved in initiation of X inactivation. J Biol Chem *279*, 52812–52815. Epub 52004 Oct 52826.
Fedoriw, A. M., Stein, P., Svoboda, P., Schultz, R. M., and Bartolomei, M. S. (2004). Transgenic RNAi reveals essential function for CTCF in H19 gene imprinting. Science *303*, 238–240.
Garrick, D., Sharpe, J. A., Arkell, R., Dobbie, L., Smith, A. J., Wood, W. G., Higgs, D. R., and Gibbons, R. J. (2006). Loss of Atrx affects trophoblast development and the pattern of X-inactivation in extraembryonic tissues. PLoS Genet *2*, e58.
Gartler, S. M., and Riggs, A. D. (1983). Mammalian X-chromosome inactivation. Annu Rev Genet *17*, 155–190.
Graves, J. A. M. (1996). Mammals that break the rules: Genetics of marsupials and monotremes. Annu Rev Genet *30*, 233–260.
Greaves, I. K., Rangasamy, D., Devoy, M., Marshall Graves, J. A., and Tremethick, D. J. (2006). The X and Y chromosomes assemble into H2A.Z-containing [corrected] facultative heterochromatin [corrected] following meiosis. Mol Cell Biol *26*, 5394–5405.
Hall, L. L., Byron, M., Sakai, K., Carrel, L., Willard, H. F., and Lawrence, J. B. (2002). An ectopic human XIST gene can induce chromosome inactivation in postdifferentiation human HT-1080 cells. Proc Natl Acad Sci U S A *99*, 8677–8682.
Hark, A. T., Schoenherr, C. J., Katz, D. J., Ingram, R. S., Levorse, J. M., and Tilghman, S. M. (2000). CTCF mediates methylation-sensitive enhancer-blocking activity at the H19/Igf2 locus. Nature *405*, 486–489.
Heard, E., Mongelard, F., Arnaud, D., and Avner, P. (1999). *Xist* yeast artificial chromosome transgenes function as X-inactivation centers only in multicopy arrays and not as single copies. Mol Cell Biol *19*, 3156–3166.
Heard, E., Rougeulle, C., Arnaud, D., Avner, P., Allis, C. D., and Spector, D. L. (2001). Methylation of histone H3 at Lys-9 is an early mark on the X chromosome during X inactivation. Cell *107*, 727–738.
Hernandez-Munoz, I., Lund, A. H., van der Stoop, P., Boutsma, E., Muijrers, I., Verhoeven, E., Nusinow, D. A., Panning, B., Marahrens, Y., and van Lohuizen, M. (2005). Stable X chromosome inactivation involves the PRC1 Polycomb complex and requires histone MACROH2A1 and the CULLIN3/SPOP ubiquitin E3 ligase. Proc Natl Acad Sci U S A *102*, 7635–7640.

Hore, T. A., Koina, E., Wakefield, M. J., and Graves, J. A. M. (2007). The region homologous to the X-chromosome inactivation centre has been disrupted in marsupial and monotreme mammals. Chromosome Res *15*, 147–161.

Huynh, K. D., and Lee, J. T. (2001). Imprinted X inactivation in eutherians: a model of gametic execution and zygotic relaxation. Curr Opin Cell Biol *13*, 690–697.

Huynh, K. D., and Lee, J. T. (2003). Inheritance of a pre-inactivated paternal X-chromosome in early mouse embryos. Nature *426*, 857–862.

Huynh, K. D., and Lee, J. T. (2005). X-chromosome inactivation: Linking ontogeny and phylogeny. Nat Rev Genet *6*, 410–418.

Kalantry, S., and Magnuson, T. (2006). The Polycomb group protein EED is dispensable for the initiation of random X-chromosome inactivation. PLoS Genet *2*, e66.

Kanduri, C., Holmgren, C., Pilartz, M., Franklin, G., Kanduri, M., Liu, L., Ginjala, V., Ulleras, E., Mattsson, R., and Ohlsson, R. (2000a). The 5′ flank of mouse H19 is an unusual chromatin conformation unidirectionally blocks enhancer-promoter communication. Curr Biol *10*, 449–457.

Kanduri, C., Pant, V., Loukinov, D., Pugacheva, E., Qi, C. F., Wolffe, A., Ohlsson, R., and Lobanenkov, V. V. (2000b). Functional association of CTCF with the insulator upstream of the H19 gene is parent of origin-specific and methylation-sensitive. Curr Biol *10*, 853–856.

Kay, G. F., Penny, G. D., Patel, D., Ashworth, A., Brockdorff, N., and Rastan, S. (1993). Expression of *Xist* during mouse development suggests a role in the initiation of X chromosome inactivation. Cell *72*, 171–182.

Keohane, A. M., O'Neill L, P., Belyaev, N. D., Lavender, J. S., and Turner, B. M. (1996). X-Inactivation and histone H4 acetylation in embryonic stem cells. Dev Biol *180*, 618–630.

Lee, J. T. (2000). Disruption of imprinted X inactivation by parent-of-origin effects at *Tsix*. Cell *103*, 17–27.

Lee, J. T. (2002). Homozygous *Tsix* mutant mice reveal a sex-ratio distortion and revert to random X-inactivation. Nat Genet *32*, 195–200.

Lee, J. T. (2003). Author reply to "Is *Tsix* repression of *Xist* specific to mouse?" Nat Genet *33*, 337–338.

Lee, J. T. (2005). Regulation of X-chromosome counting by *Tsix* and *Xite* sequences. Science *309*, 768–771.

Lee, J. T., Davidow, L. S., and Warshawsky, D. (1999b). *Tsix*, a gene antisense to *Xist* at the X-inactivation centre. Nat Genet *21*, 400–404.

Lee, J. T., and Jaenisch, R. (1997). Long-range cis effects of ectopic X-inactivation centres on a mouse autosome. Nature *386*, 275–279.

Lee, J. T., and Lu, N. (1999). Targeted mutagenesis of *Tsix* leads to nonrandom X inactivation. Cell *99*, 47–57.

Lee, J. T., Lu, N., and Han, Y. (1999a). Genetic analysis of the mouse X inactivation center defines an 80-kb multifunction domain. Proc Natl Acad Sci U S A *96*, 3836–3841.

Lee, J. T., Strauss, W. M., Dausman, J. A., and Jaenisch, R. (1996). A 450 kb transgene displays properties of the mammalian X-inactivation center. Cell *86*, 83–94.

Leeb, M., and Wutz, A. (2007). Ring1B is crucial for the regulation of developmental control genes and PRC1 proteins but not X inactivation in embryonic cells. J Cell Biol *178*, 219–229.

Lifschytz, E., and Lindsley, D. L. (1972). The role of X-chromosome inactivation during spermatogenesis. Proc Natl Acad Sci U S A *69*, 182–186.

Lobanenkov, V. V., Nicolas, R. H., Adler, V. V., Paterson, H., Klenova, E. M., Polotskaja, A. V., and Goodwin, G. H. (1990). A novel sequence-specific DNA binding protein which interacts with three regularly spaced direct repeats of the CCCTC-motif in the 5′ flaking sequence of the chicken c-myc gene. Oncogene *5*, 1743–1753.

Lucchesi, J. C., Kelly, W. G., and Panning, B. (2005). Chromatin remodeling in dosage compensation. Annu Rev Genet *39*, 615–651.

Luikenhuis, S., Wutz, A., and Jaenisch, R. (2001). Antisense transcription through the *Xist* locus mediates *Tsix* function in embryonic stem cells. Mol Cell Biol *21*, 8512–8520.

Lyon, M. F. (1961). Gene action in the X-chromosome of the mouse (Mus musculus L.). Nature *190*, 372–373.
Lyon, M. F. (1999). Imprinting and X chromosome inactivation, In Results and problems in cell differentiation, R. Ohlsson, ed. (Heidelberg: Springer-Verlag), pp. 73–90.
Lyon, M. F. (2000). LINE-1 elements and X chromosome inactivation: a function for "junk" DNA? Proc Natl Acad Sci U S A *97*, 6248–6249.
Marahrens, Y., Loring, J., and Jaenisch, R. (1998). Role of the *Xist* gene in X chromosome choosing. Cell *92*, 657–664.
Marahrens, Y., Panning, B., Dausman, J., Strauss, W., and Jaenisch, R. (1997). *Xist*-deficient mice are defective in dosage compensation but not spermatogenesis. Genes Dev *11*, 156–166.
McCarrey, J. D., Watson, C., Atencio, J., Ostermeier, G. C., Marahrens, Y., Jaenisch, R., and Krawetz, S. A. (2002). X-chromosome inactivation during spermatogenesis is regulated by an *Xist- Tsix*-independent mechanism in the mouse. Genesis *34*, 257–266.
Mermoud, J. E., Costanzi, C., Pehrson, J. R., and Brockdorff, N. (1999). Histone macroH2A1.2 relocates to the inactive X chromosome after initiation and propagation of X-inactivation. J Cell Biol *147*, 1399–1408.
Mermoud, J. E., Popova, B., Peters, A. H., Jenuwein, T., and Brockdorff, N. (2002). Histone H3 lysine 9 methylation occurs rapidly at the onset of random X chromosome inactivation. Curr Biol *12*, 247–251.
Meyer, B. J., McDonel, P., Csankovszki, G., and Ralston, E. (2004). Sex and X-chromosome-wide repression in Caenorhabditis elegans. Cold Spring Harb Symp Quant Biol *69*, 71–79.
Migeon, B. R. (2003). Is *Tsix* repression of *Xist* specific to mouse? Nat Genet *33*, 337; author reply 337–338.
Migeon, B. R., Beu, S. J. d., and Axelman, J. (1989). Frequent derepression of G6PD and HPRT on the marsupial inactive X chromosome associated with cell proliferation in vitro. Exp Cell Res *182*, 597–609.
Migeon, B. R., Kazi, E., Haisley-Royster, C., Hu, J., Reeves, R., Call, L., Lawler, A., Moore, C. S., Morrison, H., and Jeppesen, P. (1999). Human X inactivation center induces random X chromsome inactivation in male transgenic mice. Genomics *59*, 113–121.
Migeon, B. R., Lee, C. H., Chowdhury, A. K., and Carpenter, H. (2002). Species differences in *TSIX/ Tsix* reveal the roles of these genes in X-chromosome inactivation. Am J Hum Genet *71*, 286–293.
Monk, M., and Harper, M. I. (1979). Sequential X chromosome inactivation coupled with cellular differentiation in early mouse embryos. Nature *281*, 311–313.
Morey, C., Arnaud, D., Avner, P., and Clerc, P. (2001). *Tsix*-mediated repression of *Xist* accumulation is not sufficient for normal random X inactivation. Hum Mol Genet *10*, 1403–1411.
Morey, C., Navarro, P., Debrand, E., Avner, P., Rougeulle, C., and Clerc, P. (2004). The region 3' to *Xist* mediates X chromosome counting and H3 Lys-4 dimethylation within the *Xist* gene. EMBO J*23*, 594–604.
Namekawa, S., Park, P. J., Zhang, L. F., Shima, J., McCarrey, J. R., Griswold, M., and Lee, J. T. (2006). Post-meiotic sex chromatin in the male germline of mice. Curr Biol *16*, 660–667.
Namekawa, S. H., VandeBerg, J. L., McCarrey, J. R., and Lee, J. T. (2007). Sex chromosome silencing in the marsupial male germ line. Proc Natl Acad Sci U S A *104*, 9730–9735.
Naumova, A. K., Olien, L., Bird, L. M., Simth, M., Verner, A. E., Leppert, M., Morgan, K., and Sapienza, C. (1998). Genetic maping of X-linked loci involved in skewing of X chromosome inactivation in the human. Eur J Hum Genet *6*, 552–562.
Naumova, A. K., Plenge, R. M., Bird, L. M., Leppert, M., Morgan, K., Willard, H. F., and Sapienza, C. (1996). Heritability of X chromosome-inactivation phenotype in a large family. Am J Hum Genet *58*, 1111–1119.
Navarro, P., Page, D. R., Avner, P., and Rougeulle, C. (2006). *Tsix*-mediated epigenetic switch of a CTCF-flanked region of the *Xist* promoter determines the *Xist* transcription program. Genes Dev *20*, 2787–2792.

Navarro, P., Pichard, S., Ciaudo, C., Avner, P., and Rougeulle, C. (2005). *Tsix* transcription across the *Xist* gene alters chromatin conformation without affecting *Xist* transcription: implications for X-chromosome inactivation. Genes Dev *19*, 1474–1484.

Norris, D. P., Patel, D., Kay, G. F., Penny, G. D., Brockdorff, N., Sheardown, S. A., and Rastan, S. (1994). Evidence that random and imprinted *Xist* expression is controlled by preemptive methylation. Cell *77*, 41–51.

Ogawa, Y., and Lee, J. T. (2003). *Xite*, X-inactivation intergenic transcription elements that regulate the probability of choice. Mol Cell *11*, 731–743.

Oh, H., Bai, X., Park, Y., Bone, J. R., and Kuroda, M. I. (2004). Targeting dosage compensation to the X chromosome of Drosophila males. Cold Spring Harb Symp Quant Biol *69*, 81–88.

Ohhata, T., Hoki, Y., Sasaki, H., and Sado, T. (2006). *Tsix*-deficient X chromosome does not undergo inactivation in the embryonic lineage in males: implications for *Tsix*-independent silencing of *Xist*. Cytogenet Genome Res *113*, 345–349.

Ohlsson, R., Renkawitz, R., and Lobanenkov, V. V. (2001). CTCF is a uniquely versatile transcription regulator linked to epigenetics and disease. Trends Genet *7*, 520–527.

Okamoto, I., Otte, A. P., Allis, C. D., Reinberg, D., and Heard, E. (2004). Epigenetic dynamics of imprinted X inactivation during early mouse development. Science *303*, 633–644.

Ouyang, Y., Salstrom, J., Diaz-Perez, S., Nahas, S., Matsuno, Y., Dawson, D., Teitell, M. A., Horvath, S., Riggs, A. D., Gatti, R. A., and Marahrens, Y. (2005). Inhibition of Atm and/or Atr disrupts gene silencing on the inactive X chromosome. Biochem Biophys Res Commun *337*, 875–880.

Panning, B., and Jaenisch, R. (1996). DNA hypomethylation can activate *Xist* expression and silence X-linked genes. Genes Dev *10*, 1991–2002.

Penny, G. D., Kay, G. F., Sheardown, S. A., Rastan, S., and Brockdorff, N. (1996). Requirement for *Xist* in X chromosome inactivation. Nature *379*, 131–137.

Peters, A. H. F. M., Mermoud, J. E., O'Carroll, D., Pagani, M., Schweizer, D., Brockdorff, N., and Jenuwein, T. (2002). Histone H3 lysine 9 methylation is an epigenetic imprint of facultative heterochromatin. Nat Genet *30*, 77–80.

Pheasant, M., and Mattick, J. S. (2007). Raising the estimate of functional human sequences. Genome Res *17*, 1245–1253.

Plath, K., Fang, J., Mlynarczyk-Evans, S. K., Cao, R., Worringer, K. A., Wang, H., de la Cruz, C. C., Otte, A. P., Panning, B., and Zhang, Y. (2003). Role of histone H3 lysine 27 methylation in X inactivation. Science *300*, 131–135. Epub 2003 Mar 2020.

Plath, K., Talbot, D., Hamer, K. M., Otte, A. P., Yang, T. P., Jaenisch, R., and Panning, B. (2004). Developmentally regulated alterations in Polycomb repressive complex 1 proteins on the inactive X chromosome. J Cell Biol *167*, 1025–1035. Epub 2004 Dec 1020.

Plenge, R. M., Hendrich, B. D., Schwartz, C., Arena, J. F., Naumova, A., Sapienza, C., Winter, R. M., and Willard, H. F. (1997). A promoter mutation in the XIST gene in two unrelated families with skewed X-chromosome inactivation. Nat Genet *17*, 353–356.

Popova, B. C., Tada, T., Takagi, N., Brockdorff, N., and Nesterova, T. B. (2006). Attenuated spread of X-inactivation in an X;autosome translocation. Proc Natl Acad Sci U S A *103*, 7706–7711.

Prissette, M., El-Maarri, O., Arnaud, D., Walter, J., and Avner, P. (2001). Methylation profiles of *DXPas34* during the onset of X-inactivation. Hum Mol Genet *10*, 31–38.

Pugacheva, E. M., Tiwari, V. K., Abdullaev, Z., Vostrov, A. A., Flanagan, P. T., Quitschke, W. W., Loukinov, D. I., Ohlsson, R., and Lobanenkov, V. V. (2005). Familial cases of point mutations in the XIST promoter reveal a correlation between CTCF binding and pre-emptive choices of X chromosome inactivation. Hum Mol Genet *14*, 953–965.

Rastan, S., and Brown, S. D. (1990a). The search for the mouse X-chromosome inactivation centre. Genet Res *56*, 99–106.

Rastan, S., and Brown, S. D. M. (1990b). The search for the mouse X-chromosome inactivation centre. Genet Res, Camb *56*, 99–106.

Sado, T., Fenner, M. H., Tan, S. S., Tam, P., Shioda, T., and Li, E. (2000). X inactivation in the mouse embryo deficient for Dnmt1: distinct effect of hypomethylation on imprinted and random X inactivation. Dev Biol 225, 294–303.

Sado, T., Hoki, Y., and Sasaki, H. (2005). Tsix silences Xist through modification of chromatin structure. Dev Cell 9, 159–165.

Sado, T., Hoki, Y., and Sasaki, H. (2006). Tsix defective in splicing is competent to establish Xist silencing. Development (Cambridge, UK) 133, 4925–4931.

Sado, T., Okano, M., Li, E., and Sasaki, H. (2004). De novo DNA methylation is dispensable for the initiation and propagation of X chromosome inactivation. Development (Cambridge, UK) 131, 975–982.

Sado, T., Wang, Z., Sasaki, H., and Li, E. (2001). Regulation of imprinted X-chromosome inactivation in mice by Tsix. Development (Cambridge, UK) 128, 1275–1286.

Savarese, F., Flahndorfer, K., Jaenisch, R., Busslinger, M., and Wutz, A. (2006). Hematopoietic precursor cells transiently reestablish permissiveness for X inactivation. Mol Cell Biol 26, 7167–7177.

Schoeftner, S., Sengupta, A. K., Kubicek, S., Mechtler, K., Spahn, L., Koseki, H., Jenuwein, T., and Wutz, A. (2006). Recruitment of PRC1 function at the initiation of X inactivation independent of PRC2 and silencing. EMBO J 25, 3110–3122.

Sharman, G. B. (1971). Late DNA replication in the paternally derived X chromosome of female kangaroos. Nature 230, 231–232.

Sharp, A. J., Spotswood, H. T., Robinson, D. O., Turner, B. M., and Jacobs, P. A. (2002). Molecular and cytogenetic analysis of the spreading of X inactivation in X; autosome translocations. Hum Mol Genet 11, 3145–3156.

Shevchenko, A. I., Zakharova, I. S., Elisaphenko, E. A., Kolesnikov, N. N., Whitehead, S., Bird, C., Ross, M., Weidman, J. R., Jirtle, R. L., Karamysheva, T. V., et al. (2007). Genes flanking Xist in mouse and human are separated on the X chromosome in American marsupials. Chromosome Res 15, 127–136.

Shibata, S., and Lee, J. T. (2003). Characterization and quantitation of differential Tsix transcripts: implications for Tsix function. Hum Mol Genet 12, 125–136.

Shibata, S., and Lee, J. T. (2004). Tsix transcription- versus RNA-based mechanisms in Xist repression and epigenetic choice. Curr Biol 14, 1747–1754.

Silva, J., Mak, W., Zvetkova, I., Appanah, R., Nesterova, T. B., Webster, Z., Peters, A. H., Jenuwein, T., Otte, A. P., and Brockdorff, N. (2003). Establishment of histone h3 methylation on the inactive X chromosome requires transient recruitment of Eed-Enx1 polycomb group complexes. Dev Cell 4, 481–495.

Simmler, M.-C., Cattanach, B. M., Rasberry, C., Rougeulle, C., and Avner, P. (1993). Mapping the murine Xce locus with (CA)n repeats. Mamm Genome 4, 523–530.

Stavropoulos, N., Lu, N., and Lee, J. T. (2001). A functional role for Tsix transcription in blocking Xist RNA accumulation but not in X-chromosome choice. Proc Natl Acad Sci USA 98, 10232–10237.

Stavropoulos, N., Rowntree, R. K., and Lee, J. T. (2005). Identification of developmentally specific enhancers for Tsix in the regulation of X chromosome inactivation. Mol Cell Biol 25, 2757–2769.

Sun, B. K., Deaton, A. M., and Lee, J. T. (2006). A transient heterochromatic state in Xist preempts X inactivation choice without RNA stabilization. Mol Cell 21, 617–628.

Szabo, P., Tang, S. H., Rentsendorj, A., Pfeifer, G. P., and Mann, J. R. (2000). Maternal-specific footprints at putative CTCF sites in the H19 imprinting control region give evidence for insulator function. Curr Biol 10, 607–610.

Thorvaldsen, J. L., Fedoriw, A. M., Nguyen, S., and Bartolomei, M. S. (2006). Developmental profile of H19 differentially methylated domain (DMD) deletion alleles reveals multiple roles of the DMD in regulating allelic expression and DNA methylation at the imprinted H19/Igf2 locus. Mol Cell Biol 26, 1245–1258.

Turner, J. M., Mahadevaiah, S. K., Ellis, P. J., Mitchell, M. J., and Burgoyne, P. S. (2006). Pachytene asynapsis drives meiotic sex chromosome inactivation and leads to substantial postmeiotic repression in spermatids. Dev Cell *10*, 521–529.

Vigneau, S., Augui, S., Navarro, P., Avner, P., and Clerc, P. (2006). An essential role for the *DXPas34* tandem repeat and *Tsix* transcription in the counting process of X chromosome inactivation. Proc Natl Acad Sci USA *103*, 7390–7395.

White, W. M., Willard, H. F., Van Dyke, D. L., and Wolff, D. J. (1998). The spreading of X inactivation into autosomal material of an X;autosome translocation: evidence for a difference between autosomal and X-chromosomal DNA. Am J Hum Genet *63*, 20–28.

Wutz, A., and Jaenisch, R. (2000). A shift from reversible to irreversible X inactivation is triggered during ES cell differentiation. Mol Cell *5*, 695–705.

Wutz, A., Rasmussen, T. P., and Jaenisch, R. (2002). Chromosomal silencing and localization are mediated by different domains of *Xist* RNA. Nat Genet *30*, 167–174.

Xu, N., Donohoe, M. E., Silva, S. S., and Lee, J. T. (2007). Evidence that homologous X-chromosome pairing requires transcription and Ctcf protein. Nat Genet *39*, 1390–1396.

Xu, N., Tsai, C. L., and Lee, J. T. (2006). Transient homologous chromosome pairing marks the onset of X inactivation. Science *311*, 1149–1152.

Zhang, L. F., Huynh, K. D., and Lee, J. T. (2007). Perinucleolar targeting of the inactive X during S phase: evidence for a role in the maintenance of silencing. Cell *129*, 693–706.

Zuccotti, M., and Monk, M. (1995). Methylation of the mouse *Xist* gene in sperm and eggs correlates with imprinted *Xist* expression and paternal X-inactivation. Nat Genet *9*, 316–320.

Part III
Epigenetic Control of Developmental Processes

Polycomb Complexes and the Role of Epigenetic Memory in Development

Yuri B. Schwartz and Vincenzo Pirrotta

Abstract The availability of a many important developmental genes is determined by events that occurred at earlier developmental stages. In such genes, some kind of cellular memory encodes an epigenetic mark that is transmitted through many rounds of cell division and determines whether or how the gene will respond to the presence of activators. Polycomb mechanisms are perhaps the best known example of such epigenetic regulators. Polycomb complexes can bind to Polycomb Response Elements and establish a repressive chromatin state but they also leave an epigenetic mark on the affected genes such that the chromatin state will be recreated in the following cell cycle. Polycomb mechanisms and the nature and propagation of the epigenetic mark during development are reviewed with particular attention to the genetic and molecular evidence available from the fruit fly in which they were first discovered.

Keywords Polycomb mechanisms · Epigenetic mark · Histone modification · Chromatin replication · Homeotic genes

1 Introduction

Epigenetics is all about memory. Epigenetic information, like all other kinds, is only information if it can be retrieved at some time after it has been stored. Therefore, an epigenetic memory process must encode information that is stable enough to persist until it needs to be read out. Typically, this means the interval between DNA replication and the end of mitosis since, once the information is transmitted to the next cell cycle, the corresponding chromatin state will be recreated. In addition, for epigenetic information to be effectively deployed in developmental processes, the chromatin state associated with it must also be able to re-encode the epigenetic

---

V. Pirrotta (✉)
Department of Molecular Biology and Biochemsitry, Rutgers University.
604 Allison Road, Piscataway, NJ 08854, USA
e-mail: pirrotta@biology.rutgers.edu

information in the daughter cells produced by mitosis so that the memory is not diluted and lost during cell proliferation.

The most important epigenetic information associated with each gene concerns its availability for expression. Gene function can be turned on by supplying trans-acting transcriptional activators or repressors, therefore it does not strictly require epigenetic memory. However, whenever a transcription factor is produced, all genes that bind that factor will be necessarily targeted. In contrast, epigenetic information is specifically associated with each gene and modulates how that gene will respond to activators depending on its history. A gene that has been epigenetically switched off at some earlier stage in the history of a cell or its precursors will not respond even when its transcription factors are present in the nucleus. This in effect provides a way to make a gene available or unavailable, depending on its earlier history. The maintenance of the epigenetic state requires a mechanism to mark the chromatin of the target gene in such a way that after a round of cell division, the progeny cells can recreate the state that prevailed in the previous cell cycle. Thus, if the gene had been active, it is predisposed to be active again while if it had been repressed, the repressed state will be re-established.

The best example of the role of epigenetic memory during development is that mediated by Polycomb Group (PcG) complexes. PcG mechanisms control many hundreds of genes in the mammalian genome and are involved in most developmental decisions from differentiation and morphogenesis to X chromosome inactivation. They are also the best understood epigenetic mechanism due, to a large extent, to extensive study of their function in the fruit fly Drosophila melanogaster. In this article we will be concerned with the epigenetic memory of PcG repression and its interplay with the epigenetic marks associated with the transcriptionally active state. PcG mechanisms were first discovered in *Drosophila*, which still provides much of the evidence for their action. Much of the discussion will therefore focus on this model organism with comparison to what is known in mammals. For more details and for discussion of many issues not covered here, several recent reviews are available (Schwartz and Pirrotta, 2007; Ringrose and Paro, 2007; Schuettengruber et al. 2007; Schwartz and Pirrotta, 2008).

2 PcG Complexes

We will start with a brief review of PcG complexes and their activities. The genetics of PcG regulation indicated that more than a dozen different proteins were involved in the process and that they worked together (see for example Franke et al. 1992; Cheng et al. 1994). This was confirmed by molecular analysis of the PcG complexes, which showed that three different multiprotein Polycomb Repressive Complexes are involved: PRC1, PRC2 and PhoRC in *Drosophila* and very similar complexes in mammals (Saurin et al. 2001; Cao et al. 2002; Klymenko et al. 2006; Czermin et al. 2002; Müller et al. 2002; Kuzmichev et al. 2002; Levine et al. 2002).

PRC1 contains a core of four proteins, Polycomb (PC), Polyhomeotic (PH), Posterior sex combs (PSC) and dRING. PRC2 contains Enhancer of zeste [E(Z)], Extra sex combs (ESC) or its close homologue ESCL, Suppressor of zeste-12 [SU(Z)12], and the histone chaperone RpAp48. PhoRC contains Pleiohomeotic (PHO) and dSFMBT. PHO is the only PcG protein that is known to bind directly to a consensus motif on the DNA and the PhoRC complex is thought to contribute to the recruitment of the other two complexes. PRC1 and PRC2 have known histone modifying activities. PRC1, through the action of dRING and PSC, mono-ubiquitylates lysine 119 of histone H2A (Wang et al. 2004; de Napoles et al. 2004; Cao et al. 2005). The role of this modification is not clear but recent work has shown that it interferes with trancription initiation and/or elongation (Nakagawa et al. 2008; Zhou et al. 2008). This opens the possibility that ubiquitylated H2A (H2Aub) might be the actual effector of transcriptional repression. The PRC2 complex contains the methyltransferase E(Z) that can mono-, di- or trimethylate lysine 27 of histone H3 (Ebert et al. 2004). In the presence of an additional protein, Polycomblike (PCL), PRC2 predominantly trimethylates, producing H3 K27me3 (Nekrasov et al. 2007). Importantly, the chromodomain of the PC protein has affinity for methylated H3 K27 and binds preferentially to the trimethylated form (Fischle et al. 2003; Min et al. 2003). It is also important to note that PRC2 is also a global methyltransferase that mono- and dimethylates more than 60% of all genomic H3 K27 (Ebert et al. 2004). While the role of this widespread methylation is unknown, the trimethylated state of H3 K27 is found only at PcG target genes and serves therefore as a chromatin mark associated with the binding of PcG complexes at these genes.

3 Polycomb Response Elements: PREs

In *Drosophila*, genetic and molecular mapping has shown that genes responsive to PcG regulation contain regulatory regions called Polycomb Response Elements (Chan et al. 1994; Kassis, 1994; Fauvarque and Dura, 1993). These regions, usually several hundred bp in length are thought to contain binding motifs for several DNA binding proteins that recruit the PcG complexes. The precise nature of the recruitment process is not yet clear but it often involves PHO, GAGA factor (GAF) and DSP1, acting in concert since each by itself is found at many other genomic sites unrelated to PcG regulation (Fritsch et al. 1999; Horard et al. 2000; Déjardin et al. 2005). Additional and alternative recruiting proteins are probably important at different target genes and there is at present no DNA binding protein that has been found at all PcG binding sites.

In addition to PcG complexes, the PREs also recruit Trithorax (TRX) a methyltransferase that methylates lysine 4 of histone H3 (Orlando et al. 1998, Czermin et al. 2002; Nakamura et al. 2002; Kahn et al. 2006; Papp and Müller, 2006). TRX is a close relative of the yeast Set1 and the mammalian MLL methyltranferases and, like them, is normally a component of the COMPASS complex that is recruited at active promoters and is important for transcript elongation by RNA pol II (Miller et al. 2001). It is paradoxical therefore to find TRX also at PREs but it is consistent with genetic and functional data that show TRX to act as an antagonist of PcG repressive mechanisms. In some way not well understood, therefore, TRX binding at the PRE is implicated in the decision whether or not to recruit PcG complexes there. Loss of function of TRX causes ectopic repression by PcG mechanisms, whereby

PcG target genes are repressed even in tissues where they are normally active (Poux et al. 2002; Klymenko and Müller, 2004).

PREs are often found upstream of the gene(s) they regulate, frequently near the promoter. However, they can also be found downstream or even within an intron; they can act at considerable distances, several tens of kb from the promoter; they can control multiple genes.

4 PcG Regulation of Homeotic Genes

To understand how these components work together, we will survey their role in the epigenetic regulation of the best understood PcG target genes: the homeotic genes. In these genes, a simple paradigm explains much of their epigenetic regulation. In the early embryo, segmentation genes act as activators and repressors of different homeotic genes, producing in each case a specific domain of expression while expression is inhibited elsewhere (Fig. 1). These trans-acting regulatory proteins are short lived and disappear shortly after gastrulation but in their brief period of activity they set the domains of expression of each homeotic gene. It is around the same time that the function of PcG complexes first becomes apparent. When the early repressors disappear, the homeotic genes are kept in the repressed state by the PcG complexes. Therefore, in the cells in which a given homeotic gene was initially repressed, it will be maintained in the repressed state but wherever the gene was initially activated, it will be protected against PcG repression. Genetic analysis indicates that this protection is dependent on TRX (Poux et al. 2002; Klymenko and Müller, 2004). PcG and TRX proteins are also responsible for maintaining this antagonistic relationship and the resulting repressed or non-repressed state from one cell cycle to another through many rounds of cell division in the course of development.

In the *Drosophila* larva, imaginal disc expression is controlled by the PcG repression put in place in the early embryo (Pirrotta et al. 1995; Poux et al. 1996). Thus, although the enhancers that control imaginal disc expression have no intrinsic mechanism to confine activity to the appropriate segments, the segmental specificity established in the early embryo is carried over in the larva by the maintenance of PcG repression in the inappropriate segments. This implies the ability to retain a memory of the repressed state through at least a dozen mitotic cycles. A similar logic can be applied in principle to many other developmental decisions. Many genes that govern pattern formation and the development of structures in *Drosophila* are known to be regulated by early embryonic cues that activate the gene in some cells and repress it in other cells. In many cases such as those of *wingless, engrailed, Distalless* and many other pattern forming genes, expression at later stages is controlled by different signals and regulated by different enhancer elements but these elements only respond in cells that are descended from precursors in which the gene had been activated in the early embryo (see for example Ingham and Hidalgo, 1993; Moazed and O'Farrell, 1992; Cohen et al. 1993). From the preceding analysis of homeotic gene regulation, we recognize this as an early phase that establishes a

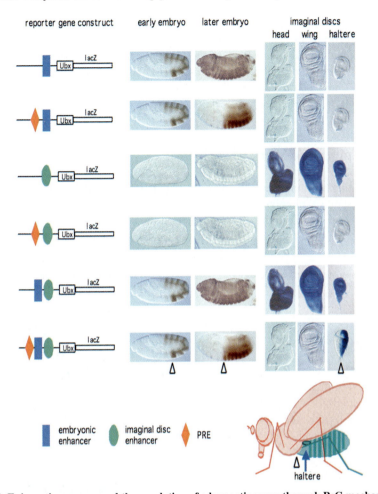

Fig. 1 Epigenetic memory and the regulation of a homeotic genes through PcG mechanisms. The interplay of enhancers and PRE in the expression of the *Ultrabithorax* (*Ubx*) gene is illustrated through a series of transgene constructs. A reporter gene expressing LacZ through the *Ubx* promoter is controlled by different combinations of a *Ubx* embryonic enhancer (blue rectangle), a larval imaginal disc enhancer (*green oval*) and PRE (*red lozenge*). For each combination the expression pattern is shown in the embryo (*brown stain*) or in the head, wing and haltere imaginal discs (*blue stain*). In the early embryo, the correct domain of expression of *Ubx* is set by the embryonic enhancer, which functions in each parasegment but is blocked by a repressor in the embryonic region anterior to the future parasegment 6 (indicated by *white arrowhead*). Shortly after however, the repressor disappears and the reporter gene is expressed in all segments. Addition of the PRE maintains repression in the anterior region. Imaginal disc enhancers activate expression at a later stage in head, wing and haltere discs. If combined with the PRE, they become repressed in the early embryo and remain silent in the imaginal discs. The correct expression pattern is created in the embryo and epigenetically maintained throughout development when all three elements are combined: the embryonic enhancer sets the pattern, the PRE maintains the repressed or non-repressed state and the imaginal disc enhancer now remains active only posterior to parasegment 6, not in the head or wings

domain of potential expression and a complementary domain in which the gene becomes silenced. In later developmental stages the ability to respond to cues is confined to the clonal descendants of these initial cells because silencing is maintained in the rest of the embryo. It is not surprising therefore that genomic analyses (see below) have shown that all these genes are PcG targets even if the details of PcG regulation have not been worked out in most cases.

5 The Epigenetic Mark

The preceding account shows that in some way the PcG complexes bound to a target gene establish an epigenetic mark that allows the gene to reassemble the PcG complexes and therefore the repressed state in the subsequent cell cycle. To constitute a functioning epigenetic memory, the mechanism must not only lay down a

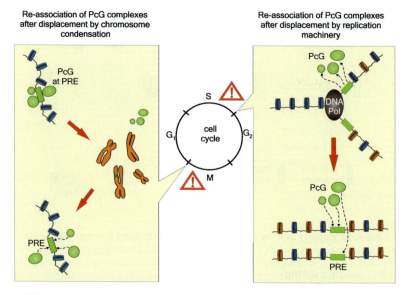

Fig. 2 Utilization of the epigenetic memory mark during cell cycle progression. Two moments in the cell cycle are likely to be critical for the faithful propagation of the epigenetic memory mark through multiple cell generations. As chromosomes replicate, the traversing DNA polymerase holoenzyme is likely to dislodge PcG complexes from the chromatin. After the passage of the replication fork, the PcG complex must reassemble on the PREs of both daughter chromosomes. The epigenetic mark is required to ensure that the assembly takes place only on the PREs of those genes that had been PcG-repressed before replication. Replication of chromatin also decreases the density of covalently marked nucleosomes (*blue discs*) approximately two-fold due to random distribution of old nucleosomes between daughter chromosomes and deposition of new unmarked nucleosomes (*orange disks*). The density of the mark must be restored before next replication cycle. At mitosis, chromosome condensation once again causes dissociation of PcG proteins from the chromatin. Upon completion of cell division PcG complexes must re-assemble at the PREs of the daughter cells but only at the genes that have been repressed before cell division

chromatin mark but it must also provide an apparatus to read the mark and to ensure that the mark is reconstituted from one cell cycle to the next. We have seen that PcG complexes lay down two kinds of chromatin marks, both in the form of histone modifications: histone H3 K27me3 and histone H2Aub. Can the modification of nucleosomal histones be inherited from one cell cycle to the next? In principle the replication of chromatin can account for the inheritance of histone marks (Fig. 2). An alternative view of the propagation of epigenetic states to the one proposed here has been argued by Henikoff (2008). In this view, an epigenetic state could be maintained through the active turnover of nucleosomes at regulatory elements such as PREs or promoters. Regardless of the specific details of the mechanism, it is known that when chromatin is replicated, the old nucleosomes partition randomly to each daughter DNA molecule (see discussion by (Annunziato, 2005). This is then followed by de novo deposition of new histones to reconstitute the full complement of nucleosomes. In this so-called "semi-conservative" replication of nucleosomes, the pre-existing methyl marks would be diluted in the daughter chromatin molecules to half their previous density, on the average, but could still serve as an epigenetic mark. To function as carrier of epigenetic memory, the mark must be "read" by the PcG mechanism and result in the reconstitution of the PcG complexes. We do not know what, if anything, "reads" the H2Aub mark. Quite possibly this mark functions more as the effector of PcG repression by inhibiting transcription initiation rather than as a carrier of epigenetic memory. In the case of the H3 K27me3 mark, however, a readout could be provided by the chromodomain of the PC protein.

The discovery that the PC chromodomain binds preferentially to H3 K27me3 (Fischle et al. 2003; Min et al. 2003) led to the early conclusion that this histone modification was the epigenetic mark that allowed the distinction between a gene that had previously been repressed from one that had not been repressed. In its simplest form, this conclusion was taken to mean that H3 K27me3 "recruited" PcG complexes to a target gene. There is very little evidence in *Drosophila* in favor of this direct recruitment of PRC1 by H3 K27me3 and, as we will show below, the evidence argues against this. The recruiters of PcG complexes are the PREs, specific DNA sequences, not histone modifications irrespective of sequence. Experiments with transgenic flies carrying reporter constructs have shown that excision of the PRE from the construct during development results in the loss of repression (Busturia et al. 1997). Therefore, the continued presence of the PRE is required for continued binding of PcG complexes and histone modifications are not sufficient for the maintenance of the repressed state. They are also not sufficient for self-propagation. Recruitment of PRC1 complexes alone would not suffice for the maintenance of the H3 K27me3 mark since that is generated by the PRC2 complex. Overall, therefore, we do not yet have a full account of the transmission of the epigenetic memory. In some way, the function of H3 K27me3 (and/or of H2Aub) as the epigenetic mark would be fulfilled if it could favor the re-establishment of the repressed state rather than the active or de-repressed state. The affinity of the PC chromodomain for the K27me3 mark could provide such a competitive edge to the PcG complexes recruited to the PRE by DNA-binding proteins. It could also provide a head start for the PRC2 complex to reconstitute the fully methylated complement after the dilution caused by a round of replication. To understand the nature of this mark, its relationship to the PcG complexes, and how it could provide for its self-renewal, we need to examine the distribution of each in the genome at the PcG target genes.

6 Genomic Distribution of PcG Complexes

The association of specific proteins or of histone modifications with specific sites in the genome can be determined by the very powerful technique of chromatin immunoprecipitation (ChIP) in which chromatin proteins are first crosslinked, typically with formaldehyde, then the chromatin is fragmented into pieces containing 200–800 bp and the pieces associated with the protein of interest are precipitated with a corresponding antibody. The DNA sequences associated with the protein of interest are then identified by hybridization to genomic tiling microarrays: the so-called "ChIP/chip" approach. The microarrays contain ordered arrays of oligonucleotides representing unique genomic sequences often spaced at intervals of 10–50 bp to give a high resolution representation of the entire non-repetitive part of the genome. The immunoprecipitated DNA fragments, labeled with a fluorescent tag are hybridized and the result is then read out and mapped on a genomic representation. This widely used technique and others that allow the retrieval of genomic DNA fragments that bind the protein of interest, now allow us to determine at high resolution the distribution of proteins or protein modifications for which a specific antibody is available.

The mapping of PcG proteins in the *Drosophila* genome (Schwartz et al. 2006; Négre et al. 2006; Tolhuis et al. 2006) showed that, as expected, different PRC1 or PRC2 proteins are found together at specific sites near target genes. The binding is usually highly localized in sharp peaks that correspond to PREs, whenever these had been previously identified by functional approaches. In the genome of *Drosophila* cultured cell lines, these PcG binding sites are found at several hundred genes in the genome, in most cases, genes that control developmental, differentiation or morphogenetic pathways (Schwartz et al. 2006). Histone H3 K27 trimethylation is almost always also found at genes that bind PcG proteins but, in contrast to the PcG proteins, the methylation mark is not sharply localized but spread over a large domain usually encompassing the entire target gene as well as its regulatory region. Such methylation domains are often many tens of kilobases long. To account for the difference in the localization of PcG proteins and the modification that they produce it has been proposed that the proteins, while remaining bound to the PRE, nevertheless loop to interact transiently with the nucleosomes over a large region, maintaining the methylated state (Kahn et al. 2006; Papp and Müller, 2006). This looping action would be greatly facilitated if some of the nucleosomes are already methylated at K27. In that case, the PC chromodomain would mediate the looping action by transiently binding to these methylated nucleosomes. As a result, the presence of the K27me3 mark after a round of replication would provide the necessary head start for the re-establishment of the full complement of methylation (Fig. 3). The difference in distributions makes it clear, however, that the H3

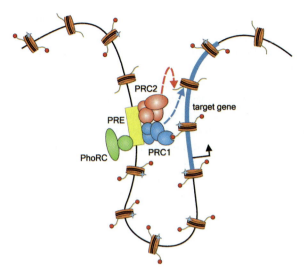

Fig. 3 Reconstitution of the epigenetic mark. As the chromatin replicates and nucleosomes are randomly partitioned between daughter chromosomes, the density of the epigenetic mark is diluted two-fold after each replication cycle. To ensure faithful inheritance of the epigenetic state, the mark must be restored in each cell cycle. In the model proposed here, the specific affinity of the PC chromodomain for tri-methylated H3 K27 promotes looping interactions between PcG complexes associated with the PRE (*yellow rectangle*) and a broad chromatin domain surrounding the target gene. Such looping would allow PRC2 (shown as a group of *red spheres*) and PRC1 (shown as blue spheres) to efficiently methylate H3K27 (*red ball*) and ubiquitylate H2AK119 (*blue star*) on the newly deposited nucleosomes

K27me3 by itself does not support the stable binding of PcG complexes. In fact, the equilibrium constant determined in vitro for the PC chromodomain interaction with H3 K27me3 is of the order of 10^{-6} M (Fischle et al. 2003), as compared to the equilibrium constants of the order of 10^{-11} M for the interaction of a typical DNA binding protein to its specific binding sequence. Another important feature of the K27 methylation domain is its very extent. The semiconservative replication of the nucleosomes guarantees only an average partitioning of the mark between the daughter chromatin molecules. If the methylation domain were limited to the regions immediately flanking the PRE, the probability of loss of the mark in one daughter molecule would be significant. The extent of the observed methylation domains guarantees that clusters of sufficiently high density of methylation would be transmitted to both daughter molecules.

Similar genome-wide analyses carried out in mammalian cells (Lee et al. 2006; Boyer et al. 2006; Bracken et al. 2006) have shown fundamental similarities between the *Drosophila* PcG complexes and the mammalian PcG complexes. In both types of organisms, the PcG targets are the regulators of all major developmental pathways. PcG binding is accompanied by broad domains of H3 K27me3. A major difference between mammals and *Drosophila* is that the PcG proteins do not display sharply localized binding that in *Drosophila* helps to identify putative PREs.

Instead, they form domains almost as broad as the K27 methylation domains. In fact, no mammalian PRE has yet been identified although in mammals also PcG recruitment must depend on specific DNA sequences. It is unlikely that mammalian PREs are as extensive as the observed binding domains. More likely, a functional PRE is buried within the binding domain and is responsible for the recruitment of the PcG complexes, which is then followed by a secondary spreading or expansion of the PcG binding domain. Whether this might be accounted for by a higher affinity of the mammalian PC chromodomain for the H3 K27me3 or by other mechanisms remains to be determined. Recent reports of a close molecular interaction between the PRC2 complex and both maintenance and de novo DNA methyltransferases (Viré et al. 2006; Villa et al. 2007) open the possibility that a synergy between histone methylation and DNA methylation might contribute to this spreading.

7 The Epigenetic Memory of the Active State

PcG regulation of genes is often thought of simply as the establishment of a repressed state that is inherited epigenetically. In fact, however, even in the case of homeotic gene regulation, the system involves an opposition between two states. If a homeotic gene is activated in the early embryo, it is not subject to repression by the PcG mechanism even though the PcG proteins are present in the nucleus and the gene contains a PRE. The gene is in some way rendered resistant to PcG repression. Furthermore, this early activity sets its own epigenetic mark such that the resistance to PcG repression, the anti-silenced state will be transmitted to progeny cells. As a result, in the domains where the homeotic gene was activated in the early embryo, PcG repression will not set in at later stages even if transcriptional activity switches on and off depending on specific enhancers and the availability of enhancer factors during development. In other words, the gene remains available for expression in the cellular progeny. This implies the existence of two cellular memories: the memory of the repressed state as well as the memory of the non-repressed state. Genetic evidence strongly suggests that the memory of the non-repressed state depends on TRX and on a second protein, ASH1, the product of the *absent or small homeotic discs-1 (ash1)* gene (Tripoulas et al. 1994; Byrd and Shearn,2003). Like TRX, ASH1 is a SET domain protein, a presumptive methyltransferase, but its target is not clear. Different reports have claimed that it methylates histone H3 K4, K9, K36 and histone H4 K20 (Beisel et al. 2002; Byrd and Shearn, 2003; Tanaka et al. 2007) but there has been no resolution of the conflicting claims. We have already seen that TRX binds to the PRE and in fact it is found there whether the associated gene is in the active or in the repressed state. Conflicting claims also have been made about the site of action of ASH1, arguing that it binds to an RNA-chromatin complex at the PRE to promote derepression or that it binds in the transcribed region when the gene is active (Sanchez-Elsner et al. 2006; Papp and Müller, 2006).

While the molecular aspects of TRX and ASH1 action in maintaining the non-repressed epigenetic state remain unresolved, the genetic results imply that when they are absent or insufficient, PcG target genes are unable to be expressed efficiently and tend to become repressed in domains where they should be active. These consequences are alleviated if PcG repression is also impaired, implying that the two systems are antagonistic.

8 Dynamic Range of PcG Repression

The functional antagonism between PcG repression on the one hand and TRX mechanisms on the other hand has far reaching implications. The all-or-none nature of PcG repression of homeotic genes is not a universal characteristic of PcG action. In *Drosophila*, the homeotic genes are appropriate targets for a mechanism that sets the epigenetic state once for all in early in development and maintains it ever after. However, many other PcG target genes revealed by the ChIP/chip analyses are less suited for a permanent shut down. For example, genes encoding morphogens such as *wingless* (*wg*) or *decapentaplegic* (*dpp*) are required at many stages. Genes like *engrailed* or *cyclin A* are known to be reactivated in certain cells at certain times (Lee et al. 2005; Martinez et al. 2006). More conclusively, some genes bind PcG complexes and contain extensive H3 K27 trimethylation but are nevertheless transcriptionally active (Schwartz et al. 2006). Clear examples of this situation are the *Psc* and *Su(z)2* genes, two closely related genes arranged back to back and divergently transcribed. Their products are components of PcG products and are required for PcG repression. They must therefore be expressed to enable PcG repression itself. This is a case of autoregulation that must be seen as a dynamic form of PcG repression where transcription can be up- or down-regulated by PcG mechanisms rather than silenced.

In the case of the strongest PREs, such as the *bxd* PRE of the *Ultrabithorax* gene, the result is more in keeping with the all-or-none behavior that increases the probability of derepression rather than modulating the level of repression. This gives rise to the characteristic variegated expression: one cell among many becomes derepressed and the derepressed state is maintained in the progeny of that cell (Fig. 4). However, in other cases, the overexpression of an activator or decrease in dosage of PcG, or of TRX results in a modulated change in the level of expression. In the *Drosophila* embryo, such a forced derepression induced by overexpression of the activator (in this case, GAL4) can result in a stably derepressed state that is maintained for the rest of development and can even be transmitted maternally to about one fourth of the progeny flies (Cavalli and Paro, 1998, 1999). Interestingly, the ability to induce a stable derepressed state decreases with developmental age: at later stages, overexpression of the activator produces transient derepression that returns to the repressed state after the activator fades away.

These observations indicate that there probably exists a considerable variation in the strength of a PRE or its ability to withstand derepressive influences but they certainly lead us to conclude that, in general, PcG repression exists in a dynamic continuum ranging from tight silencing to permissivity for transcriptional activity. The availability of PcG proteins, of TRX/ASH1 and of specific transactivators are among the factors that determine the degree of repression.

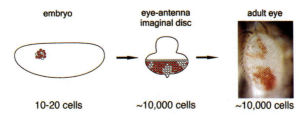

Fig. 4 Variegation illustrates the epigenetic memory of Polycomb repression. The epigenetic nature of PcG repression is most obvious from the effect of the PRE on the expression of *white* gene when the two are placed together in a reporter construct. The fly eye develops from a small primordial group of cells specified in the embryo (10–20 cells). At this stage, the *white* gene, responsible for the red pigmentation of the ommatidia in the eye of the adult fly, becomes stochastically repressed by PRE in some cells of the primordium (cells in which *white* is repressed are in white and cells in which it is not repressed are in red). As the cells proliferate and form the part of larval eye-antenna imaginal disc from which the adult eye will develop, the decision to keep the *white* gene repressed is propagated in the clonal descendants of the cells in which the gene was originally silenced. The stochastic repression in the primordium, followed by clonal expansion and maintenance of the repressed state results in the variegated pigmentation of the adult eye that is often observed in PRE-containing transgenes

Enzymatic activities that could effect the switch or mediate the relative predominance of repressive vs derepressive states have been characterized very recently. These are histone demethylases such as LID, which demethylates H3 K4 (Lee et al. 2007a; Eissenberg et al. 2007; Secombe et al. 2007), or UTX, which demethylates H3 K27 (Agger et al. 2007; Lan et al. 2007; Lee et al. 2007b), or specific proteases such as USP21, which deubiquitylates H2A (Nakagawa et al. 2008). In principle these activities could remove the epigenetic methylation mark and the repressive ubiquitylation mark. However, it may be too early to identify the precise role these activities play in normal transcriptional regulation. For example, a cycle of H2B ubiquitylation and deubiquitylation has been shown to be necessary for H3 K4 methylation and transcriptional elongation (Henry et al. 2003). The H3 K4 demethylation activity is associated with the COMPASS complex at active promoters and is likely to serve a similar cycling role in the promotion of transcriptional elongation. The H3 K27 demethylation activity of UTX may also be a normal function required to remove the pervasive global H3 K27 dimethylation prior to transcription initiation.

9 Mammalian PcG Target Genes, Pluripotency and Differentiation

In the course of differentiation, cells enter into pathways that lead to a restriction of the potential of gene expression to a specific subset of genes. Terminal differentiation ultimately results in exit from the cell cycle and effective silencing of the rest of the genome. Embryonic stem (ES) cells represent the opposite extreme: they are pluripotent, meaning that they have the potential to differentiate into any kind of tissue of the adult organism, and they can self-renew, that is they can proliferate while maintaining their pluripotent state. ES cells therefore present very interesting problems and enormous promise for biomedical applications. One intrinsic problem is that they can, in principle, express any gene and enter any differentiation pathway but at the same time they must not do so, at least not while they retain their pluripotency. Therefore the differentiation genes must be available but not expressed until the appropriate signals are presented. In ES cells, in fact, the differentiation genes are targets of PcG complexes and H3 K27 trimethylation (Lee et al. 2006; Boyer et al. 2006; Bracken et al. 2006; Squazzo et al. 2006). The epigenetic state of these genes in ES cells is not a completely repressed one and significant transcriptional activity has been detected. The chromatin signature associated with these genes is the presence of a smaller domain of H3 K4 trimethylation embedded within the K27me3 domain (Bernstein et al. 2006; Stock et al. 2007). The simultaneous presence of the marks associated with repression and with transcriptional activity has been taken to signify a "bivalent" epigenetic state: not fully repressed but poised for derepression. When ES cells are induced to differentiate, the bivalent state can be resolved. Some genes become completely repressed and lose the H3 K4 methylation. Others become fully active and lose the H3 K27 methylation as well as the PcG complexes (Mikkelsen et al. 2007). Some remain in the bivalent state (Stock et al. 2007). This pattern of events coincides very well with the view of PcG repression as a component of a dynamic relationship between PcG and TRX/ASH1 mechanisms where the extent of transcriptional activity depends on the relative availability of the two kinds of complexes, as well as on the presence of specific transcriptional activators.

10 Change Versus Stability

If epigenetic marks can be erased at will by the timely recruitment of a histone demethylase or deubiquityl protease, what is the point of an epigenetic memory? The answer to this question is, at least in part, that we have been misled into thinking that epigenetic memory has to be permanent or at least very long lived in order to be useful. The role it plays in the regulation of *Drosophila* homeotic genes is in fact unusually long lasting but it probably represents one extreme of a range of dynamic behavior. In a general sense, the epigenetic memory represents an additional dimension or a further layer of flexibility in a regulatory circuit, which allows earlier events to influence current outcomes to a greater or lesser degree. The memory can be abrogated under specific circumstances that require "reprogramming" of a gene. Or the degree of repression can be modulated by tilting the balance in favor of TRX/ASH1 activity or PcG protein activity. The role of PcG proteins in development strongly suggests that flexibly deployed epigenetic memory mechanisms have made possible the marvelously complex developmental programs of metazoans.

References

Agger, K., Cloos, P. A. C., Christensen, J., Pasini, D., Rose, S., Rappsilber, J., Issaeva, I., Canaani, E., Salcini, A. E., and Helin, K. (2007). UTX and JMJD3 are histone H3K27 demethylases involved in HOX gene regulation and development. Nature 449, 731–734.

Annunziato, A. T. (2005). Split Decision: What happens to nucleosomes during DNA replication? J Biol Chem 280, 12065–12068.

Beisel, C., Imhof, A., Greene, J., Kremmer, E., and Sauer, F. (2002). Histone methylation by the Drosophila epigenetic transcriptional regulator Ash1. Nature 419, 857–862.

Bernstein, B. E., Mikkelsen, T. S., Xie, X., Kamal, M., Huebert, D. J., Cuff, J., Fry, B., Meissner, A., Wernig, M., Plath, K., et al. (2006). A bivalent chromatin structure marks key developmental genes in embryonic stem cells. Cell 125, 315–326.

Boyer, L. A., Plath, K., Zeitlinger, J., Brambrink, T., Medeiros, L. A., Lee, T. I., Levine, S. S., Wernig, M., Tajonar, A., Ray, M. K., et al. (2006). Polycomb complexes repress developmental regulators in murine embryonic stem cells. Nature 441, 349–353.

Bracken, A. P., Dietrich, N., Pasini, D., Hansen, K. H., and Helin, K. (2006). Genome-wide mapping of Polycomb target genes unravels their roles in cell fate transitions. Genes Dev 20, 1123–1136.

Busturia, A., Wightman, C. D., and Sakonju, S. (1997). A silencer is required for maintenance of transcriptional repression throughout Drosophila development. Development 124, 4343–4350.

Byrd, K. N., and Shearn, A. (2003). ASH1, a Drosphila trithorax group protein, is required for methylation of lysine 4 residues on histone H3. Proc Natl Acad Sci USA 100, 11535–11540.

Cao, R., Tsukada, Y.-I., and Zhang, Y. (2005). Role of Bmi-1 and Ring1A in H2A ubiquitylation and Hox gene silencing. Mol Cell 20, 845–854.

Cao, R., Wang, L., Wang, H., Xin, L., Erdjument-Bromage, H., Tempst, P., Jones, R. S., and Zhang, Y. (2002). Role of histone H3 lysine 27 methylation in Polycomb-Group silencing. Science 298, 1039–1043.

Cavalli, G., and Paro, R. (1998). The Drosophila Fab-7 chromosomal element conveys epigenetic inheritance during mitosis and meiosis. Cell 93, 505–518.

Cavalli, G., and Paro, R. (1999). Epigenetic inheritance of active chromatin after removal of the main transactivator. Science 286, 955–958.

Chan, C.-S., Rastelli, L., and Pirrotta, V. (1994). A Polycomb response element in the Ubx gene that determines an epigenetically inherited state of repression. EMBO J 13, 2553–2564.

Cheng, N. N., Sinclair, D. A. R., Campbell, R. B., and Brock, H. W. (1994). Interactions of polyhomeotic with Polycomb group genes of Drosophila melanogaster. Genetics 138, 1151–1162.

Cohen, B., Simcox, A.A. and Cohen, S.M. (1993) Allocation of the thoracic imaginal primordia in the Drosophila embryo. Development 117, 597–608

Czermin, B., Melfi, R., McCabe, D., Seitz, H., Imhof, A., and Pirrotta, V. (2002). Drosophila Enhancer of Zeste/ESC complexes have a histone H3 methyltransferase activity that marks chromosomal Polycomb sites. Cell 111, 185–196.

de Napoles, M., Mermoud, J. E., Wakao, R., Tang, Y., A., Endoh, M., Appanah, R., Nesterova, T. B., Silva, J., Otte, A. P., Vidal, M., et al. (2004). Polycomb group proteins Ring1A/B link ubiquitylation of histone H2A to heritable gene silencing and X inactivation. Dev Cell 7, 663–676.

Déjardin, J., Rappailles, A., Cuvier, O., Grimaud, C., Decoville, M., Locker, D., and Cavalli, G. (2005). Recruitment of Drosophila Polycomb group proteins to chromatin by DSP1. Nature 434, 533–538.

Ebert, A., Schotta, G., Lein, S., Kubicek, S., Krauss, V., Jenuwein, T., and Reuter, G. (2004). Su(var) genes regulate the balance between euchromatin and heterochromatin in Drosophila. Genes Dev 18, 2973–2983.

Eissenberg, J. C., Lee, M. G., Schneider, J., Ilvarsonn, A., Shiekhattar, R., and Shilatifard, A. (2007). The trithorax-group gene in Drosophila little imaginal discs encodes a trimethylated histone H3 Lys4 demethylase. Nat Struct Mol Biol 14, 344–346.

Fauvarque, M.-O., and Dura, J.-M. (1993). polyhomeotic regulatory sequences induce developmental regulator-dependent variegation and targeted P-element insertions in *Drosophila*. Genes Dev *7*, 1508–1520.

Fischle, W., Wang, Y., Jacobs, S. A., Kim, Y., Allis, C. D., and Khorasanizadeh, S. (2003). Molecular basis for the discrimination of repressive methyl-lysine marks in histone H3 by Polycomb and HP1 chromodomains. Genes Dev *17*, 1870–1881.

Franke, A., DeCamillis, M., Zink, D., Cheng, N., Brock, H. W., and Paro, R. (1992). Polycomb and polyhomeotic are constituents of a multimeric protein complex in chromatin of *Drosophila melanogaster*. EMBO J*11*, 2941–2950.

Fritsch, C., Brown, J. L., Kassis, J. A., and Müller, J. (1999). The DNA-binding Polycomb group protein Pleiohomeotic mediates silencing of a *Drosophila* homeotic gene. Development *126*, 3905–3913.

Henikoff, S. (2008). Nucleosome destabilization in the epigenetic regulation of gene expression. Nat Rev Genet *9*, 15–26.

Henry, K. W., Wyce, A., Lo, W.-S., Duggan, L. J., Emre, N. C. T., Kao, C.-F., Pillus, L., Shilatifard, A., Osley, M. A., and Berger, S. L. (2003). Transcriptional activation via sequential histone H2B ubiquitylation and deubiquitylation, mediated by SAGA-associated Ubp8. Genes Dev *17*, 2648–2663.

Horard, B., Tatout, C., Poux, S., and Pirrotta, V. (2000). Structure of a Polycomb Response element and in vitro binding of Polycomb Group complexes containing GAGA factor. Mol Cell Biol *20*, 3187–3197.

Ingham, P.W. and Hidalgo, A. (1993) Regulation of *wingless* transcription in the *Drosophila* embryo. Development 117:283–291

Kahn, T. G., Schwartz, Y. B., Dellino, G. I., and Pirrotta, V. (2006). Polycomb complexes and the propagation of the methylation mark at the *Drosophila Ubx* gene. J Biol Chem *281*, 29064–29075.

Kassis, J. A. (1994). Unusual properties of regulatory DNA from the *Drosophila engrailed* gene: three "pairing-sensitive" sites within a 1.6 kb region. Genetics *136*, 1025–1038.

Klymenko, T., and Müller, J. (2004). The histone methyltransferases Trithorax and Ash1 prevent transcriptional silencing by Polycomb group proteins. EMBO Reports *5*, 373–377.

Klymenko, T., Papp, B., Fischle, W., Kocher, T., Schelder, M., Fritsch, C., Wild, B., Wilm, M., Muller, J. (2006). A Polycomb group protein complex with sequence-specific DNA-binding and selective methyl-lysine-binding activities. Genes Dev *20*, 1110–1122.

Kuzmichev, A., Nishioka, K., Erdjument-Bromage, H., Tempst, P., and Reinberg, D. (2002). Histone methyltransferase activity associated with a human multiprotein complex containing the Enhancer of Zeste protein. Genes Dev *22*, 2893–2905.

Lan, F., Bayliss, P. E., Rinn, J. L., Whetstine, J. R., Wang, J. K., Chen, S., Iwase, S., Alpatov, R., Issaeva, I., Canaani, E., et al. (2007). A histone H3 lysine 27 demethylase regulates animal posterior development. Nature *449*, 689–694.

Lee, M. G., Villa, R., Trojer, P., Norman, J., Yan, K.-P., Reinberg, D., Croce, L. D., and Shiekhattar, R. (2007b). Demethylation of H3K27 Regulates Polycomb Recruitment and H2A Ubiquitination. Science *318*, 447–450.

Lee, N., Maurange, C., Ringrose, L., and Paro, R. (2005). Suppression of Polycomb group proteins by JNK signalling induces transdetermination in *Drosophila* imaginal discs. Nature *438*, 234–237.

Lee, N., Zhang, J., Klose, R. J., Erdjument-Bromage, H., Tempst, P., Jones, R. S., and Zhang, Y. (2007a). The trithorax-group protein Lid is a histone H3 trimethyl-Lys4-demethylase. Nat Struct Mol Biol *14*, 341–343.

Lee, T. I., Jenner, R. G., Boyer, L. A., Guenther, M. G., Levine, S. S., Kumar, R. M., Chevalier, B., Johnstone, S. E., Cole, M. F., Isono, K. , et al. (2006). Control of developmental regulators by Polycomb in human embryonic stem cells. Cell *125*, 301–313.

Levine, S. S., Weiss, A., Erdjument-Bromage, H., Shao, Z., Tempst, P., and Kingston, R. E. (2002). The core of the Polycomb repressive complex is compositionally and functionally conserved in flies and humans. Mol Cell Biol *22*, 6070–6078.

Martinez, A.-M., Colomb, S., Dejardin, J., Bantignies, F., and Cavalli, G. (2006). Polycomb group-dependent Cyclin A repression in *Drosophila*. Genes Dev 20, 501–513.

Mikkelsen, T. S., Ku, M., Jaffe, D. B., Issac, B., Lieberman, E., Giannoukos, G., Alvarez, P., Brockman, W., Kim, T.-K., Koche, R. P., et al. (2007). Genome-wide maps of chromatin state in pluripotent and lineage-committed cells. Nature 448, 553–560.

Miller, T., Krogan, N. J., Dover, J., Erdjument-Bromage, H., Tempst, P., Johnston, M., Greenblatt, J. F., and Shilatifard, A. (2001). COMPASS: a complex of proteins associated with a trithorax-related SET domain protein. Proc Natl Acad Sci USA 98, 12902–12907.

Min, J., Zhang, Y., and Xu, R.-M. (2003). Structural basis for specific binding of Polycomb chromodomain to histone H3 methylated to Lys 27. Genes Dev 17, 1823–1828.

Moazed, D. and O'Farrell, P.H. (1992) Maintenance of the *engrailed* expression pattern by Polycomb group genes in *Drosophila*. Development 116:805–810

Müller, J., Hart, C. M., Francis, N. J., Vargas, M. L., Sengupta, A., Wild, B., Miller, E. L., O'Connor, M. B., Kingston, R. E., and Simon, J. A. (2002). Histone methyltransferase activity of a *Drosophila* Polycomb Group repressor complex. Cell 111, 197–208.

Nakagawa, T., Kajitani, T., Togo, S., Masuko, N., Ohdan, H., Hishikawa, Y., Koji, T., Matsuyama, T., Ikura, T., Muramatsu, M., and Ito, T. (2008). Deubiquitylation of histone H2A activates transcriptional initiation via trans-histone cross-talk with H3K4 di- and trimethylation. Genes Dev 22, 37–49.

Nakamura, T., Mori, T., Tada, S., Krajewski, S., Rozovskaia, T., Wassell, R., Dubois, G., Mazo, A., Croce, C. M., and Canaani, E. (2002). ALL-1 is a histone methyltransferase that assembles a supercomplex of proteins involved in transcriptional regulation. Mol Cell 10, 1119–1128.

Négre, N., Hennetin, J., Sun, L. V., Lavrov, S., Bellis, M., White, K. P., and Cavalli, G. (2006). Chromosomal distribution of PcG proteins during *Drosophila* development. PLoS Biology 4, e170.

Nekrasov, M., Klymenko, T., Fraterman, S., Papp, B., Oktaba, K., Köcher, T., Cohen, A., Stunnenberg, H. G., Wilm, M., and Müller, J. (2007). Pcl-PRC2 is needed to generate high levels of H3-K27 trimethylation at Polycomb target genes. EMBO J 26, 4078–4088.

Orlando, V., Jane, E. P., Chinwalla, V., Harte, P. J., and Paro, R. (1998). Binding of Trithorax and Polycomb proteins to the bithorax complex: dynamic changes during early *Drosophila* embryogenesis. EMBO J 17, 5141–5150.

Papp, B., and Müller, J. (2006). Histone trimethylation and the maintenance of transcriptional ON and OFF states by trxG and PcG proteins. Genes Dev 20, 2041–2054.

Pirrotta, V., Chan, C. S., McCabe, D., and Qian, S. (1995). Distinct Parasegmental and Imaginal Enhancers and the Establishment of the Expression Pattern of the *Ubx* Gene. Genetics 141, 1439–1450.

Poux, S., Horard, B., Sigrist, C. J. A., and Pirrotta, V. (2002). The *Drosophila* Trithorax protein is a coactivator required to prevent re-establishment of Polycomb silencing. Development 129, 2843–2893.

Poux, S., Kostic, C., and Pirrotta, V. (1996). *Hunchback*-independent silencing of late *Ubx* enhancers by a Polycomb Group Response Element. EMBO J 15, 4713–4722.

Ringrose, L., and Paro, R. (2007). Polycomb/Trithorax response elements and epigenetic memory of cell identity. Development 134, 223–232.

Sanchez-Elsner, T., Gou, D., Kremmer, E., and Sauer, F. (2006). Noncoding RNAs of Trithorax Response Elements Recruit *Drosophila* Ash1 to *Ultrabithorax*. Science 311, 1118–1123.

Saurin, A. J., Shao, Z., Erdjument-Bromage, H., Tempst, P., and Kingston, R. E. (2001). A *Drosophila* Polycomb group complex includes Zeste nd dTAFII proteins. Nature 412, 655–660.

Schuettengruber, B., Chourrout, D., Vervoort, M., Leblanc, B., and Cavalli, G. (2007). Genome regulation by Polycomb and Trithorax proteins. Cell 128, 735–745.

Schwartz, Y.B. and Pirrotta, V. (2008) Polycomb complexes and epigenetic states. Curr. Opin. Cell Biol., 20, 266–273.

Schwartz, Y. B., and Pirrotta, V. (2007). Polycomb silencing mechanisms and the management of genomic programmes. Nat Rev Genet 8, 9–22.

Schwartz, Y. B., Kahn, T. G., Nix, D. A., Li, X.-Y., Bourgon, R., Biggin, M., and Pirrotta, V. (2006). Genome-wide analysis of Polycomb targets in *Drosophila melanogaster*. Nat Genet *38*, 700–705.

Secombe, J., Li, L., Carlos, L., and Eisenman, R. N. (2007). The Trithorax group protein Lid is a trimethyl histone H3K4 demethylase required for dMyc-induced cell growth. Genes Dev *21*, 537–551.

Squazzo, S. L., O'Geen, H., Komashko, V. M., Krig, S. R., Jin, V. X., Jang, S.-w., Margueron, R., Reinberg, D., Green, R., and Farnham, P. J. (2006). Suz12 binds to silenced regions of the genome in a cell-type-specific manner. Genome Res *16*, 890–900.

Stock, J. K., Giadrossi, S., Casanova, M., Brookes, E., Vidal, M., Koseki, H., Brockdorff, N., Fisher, A. G., and Pombo, A. (2007). Ring1-mediated ubiquitination of H2A restrains poised RNA polymerase II at bivalent genes in mouse ES cells. Nat Cell Biol *9*, 1428–1435.

Tanaka, Y., Katagiri, Z., Kawahashi, K., IKioussis, D., and Kitajima, S. (2007). Trithorax-group protein ASH1 methylates histone H3 lysine 36. Gene *397*, 161–168.

Tolhuis, B., Muljrers, I., de Wit, E., Teunissen, H., Talhout, W., van Steensel, B., and van Lohuizen, M. (2006). Genome-wide profiling of PRC1 and PRC2 Polycomb chromatin binding in *Drosophila melanogaster*. Nat Genet *38*, 694–699.

Tripoulas, N. A., Hersperger, E., La Jeunesse, D., and Shearn, A. (1994). Molecular genetic analysis of the *Drosophila melanogaster gene absent or small homeotic discs 1 (ash1)*. Genetics *137*, 1027–1038.

Villa, R., Pasini, D., Gutierrez, A., Morey, L., Occhionorelli, M., Viré, E., Nomdedeu, J. F., Jenuwein, T., Pelicci, P. G., Minucci, S. , et al. (2007). Role of the Polycomb Repressive Complex 2 in Acute Promyelocytic Leukemia. Cancer Cell *11*, 513–525.

Viré, E., Brenner, C., Deplus, R., Blanchon, L., Fraga, M., Didelot, C., Morey, L., Van Eynde, A., Bernard, D., Vanderwinden, J.-M. , et al. (2006). The Polycomb group protein EZH2 directly controls DNA methylation. Nature *439*, 871–874.

Wang, H., Wang, L., Erdjument-Bromage, H., Vidal, M., Tempst, P., Jones, R. S., and Zhang, Y. (2004). Role of histone H2A ubiquitination in Polycomb silencing. Nature *431*, 873–878.

Zhou, W., Zhu, P., Wang, J. K., Pascual, G., Ohgi, K. A., Lozach, J., Glass, C. K., and Rosenfeld, M. G. (2008). Histone H2A monoubiquitination represses transcription by inhibiting RNA polymerase II transcriptional elongation. Mol Cell *29*, 69–80.

Genomic Imprinting – A Model for Roles of Histone Modifications in Epigenetic Control

Kirsten R. McEwen and Anne C. Ferguson-Smith

Abstract Genomic imprinting is a normal process found in plants and mammals. Imprinted genes are characterised by expression that is dependent on the parental-origin of the gene such that one of the two copies is expressed – either the maternally inherited copy or the paternally inherited copy. It is well-established that the regulation of activity and repression at imprinted domains is conferred by acquisition of DNA methylation at CG dinucleotides in eggs and sperm, which differentially marks the maternal and paternal chromosome homologues and influences gene expression after fertilisation. Differential histone modifications have also been identified at imprinted domains. Recently, the genome-wide distribution of several histone modifications has been described in mammalian cells. Here we extract this histone modification data specifically for imprinted domains and assess the extent to which regional modification might provide insight into the epigenetic control of gene activity and repression in mammals, and the functional relationship between histone modifications and DNA methylation at imprinted loci.

Keywords Genomic imprinting · DNA methylation · histone modifications · differentially methylated regions (DMRs) · imprinting control regions (ICRs)

1 Introduction

Genomic imprinting refers to the phenomenon whereby expression of a gene is restricted to only one of the parental chromosomes (Ferguson-Smith and Surani 2001). Either the gene copy inherited from the mother is expressed while the paternal copy is repressed, or *vice versa*. Approximately 95 mouse imprinted genes and 70 human imprinted genes have been identified to date (http://www.har.mrc.ac.uk/research/genomic_imprinting/, Morison et al. 2001, Schulz et al. 2008). In order to achieve this functional haploidy at selected genes,

A.C. Ferguson-Smith (✉)
Department of Physiology Development and Neuroscience, University of Cambridge, Downing Street, Cambridge CB2 3EG
e-mail: afsmith@mole.bio.cam.ac.uk

epigenetic mechanisms must be utilised to differentiate between the genetically identical sequences. Imprinted domains are therefore a useful model for the study of epigenetics as both the active and repressed state of a single gene can be compared at the same spatiotemporal point.

Distinguishable epigenetic marks are found on the maternal and paternal genomes in the respective gametes. These imprint marks are retained during differentiation and development to adulthood with the only exception being that of primordial germ cells, the cells destined to form egg and sperm (see Fig. 1). In these cells, all imprinting marks are erased and re-established according to parental origin, returning the embryo to a balanced state of maternally and paternally marked regions after fertilisation.

A number of key genomic features exist for the control of imprinted genes and DNA methylation has been shown to be an important factor. Primary marks originally established in the gametes show differential DNA methylation between the two parental chromosomes and are known as germline differentially methylated regions (gDMRs). The majority of these gDMRs have been shown to act as imprinting control regions (ICRs) by experimental deletion of the region leading to disruption of imprinting (for example, Lin et al. 2003, Williamson et al. 2006). Two classes of germline ICRs exist; those located at gene promoters and those at intergenic regions. Where an ICR is found at a promoter, the gene product transcribed from the unmethylated allele is in most cases a non-coding RNA. These non-coding RNAs can regulate imprinting of multiple genes in an imprinted domain with expression of the non-coding RNA correlating with repression of the protein-coding genes in cis (Mancini-Dinardo et al. 2006, Sleutels et al. 2002). This mechanism therefore occurs at regions of the genome where a number of imprinted genes are clustered together. Intergenic ICRs can also regulate clusters of imprinted genes, however the mechanisms of control are likely to differ between each cluster and are not in all cases well understood. Intriguingly, promoter ICRs are always methylated on the maternal chromosome, whereas intergenic ICRs are paternally methylated.

An additional method of control comprises regions that establish their differential methylation post-fertilisation rather than in the gametes. Importantly, these somatic DMRs (sDMRs) are dependent on differential methylation at the gDMR. These controlling elements can be found at imprinted genes within a cluster and those located at promoters may regulate allelic expression in a tissue- and temporal-dependent manner. For example, the imprinted gene *Tssc4* has a sDMR in tissues where the gene is imprinted that is absent in tissues where it is biallelically expressed (Lewis et al. 2004). Promoter sDMRs are methylated on the inactive allele of the imprinted gene.

Imprinted genes also exist outside of imprinting clusters. These singletons can be regulated by an ICR at the gene promoter, whereby differential methylation directly reflects gene activity (for example, Hikichi et al. 2003). Three types of singletons exist; tissue-specific, retrogenes and non-retrogenes.

Somatic promoter DNA methylation, although an important regulator of imprinted gene expression, does not act at all genes and for this reason further epigenetic mechanisms are thought to participate in the regulation of gene expression.

Genomic Imprinting

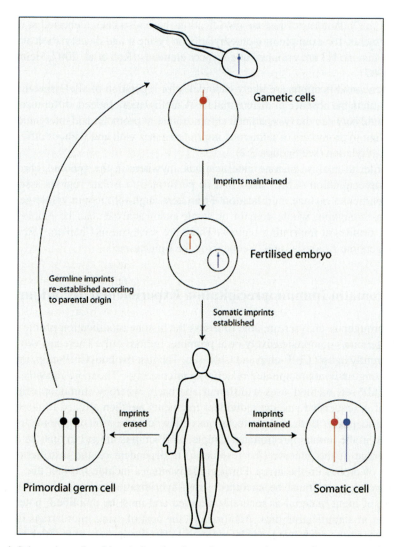

Fig. 1 Schematic cycle of imprinting that determines expression according to parental origin. Lines with overlapping circles represent the parental imprint marking of the genome within a cell; red represents maternal marking and blue represents paternal marking. Germline imprints initiated in the gametes are maintained during early development. In somatic cells additional secondary imprint marks become established dependent on the gametic imprints and these too are maintained in somatic cells. When new gametes develop, old imprints are erased allowing the establishment of new parental-origin specific marks

One such mechanism involves modification to the histone proteins that constitute the nucleosome within which DNA is wrapped and packaged. Addition of chemical groups to specific residues of the N-terminal tails of these histone proteins have been found to correlate with the expression status of a gene (see Chapter "Sequencing the

Epigenome"). Patterns of histone modifications have also been identified at regulatory elements, for example monomethylation at lysine 4 and diacetylation at lysine 9/14 of histone H3 are enriched at enhancer elements (Roh et al. 2007, Heintzman et al. 2007).

Histone modifications are likely candidates for regulation of allele-specific gene expression in the absence of differential DNA methylation. Indeed, differences have been found between the two parental chromosomes at promoter and intergenic ICRs in addition to promoters of numerous imprinted genes with and without differential DNA methylation (see Section 3.2).

In order to analyse histone modifications anywhere in the genome, chromatin immunoprecipitation (ChIP) must first be performed to isolate regions associated with a particular histone modification. From here, high-throughput whole-genome, medium-throughput whole-domain or single point analyses can be employed to identify profiles at imprinting regions. These are reviewed in Chapters "Strategies for Epigenome Analysis" and "Sequencing the Epigenome".

2 Chromatin Immunoprecipitation Experimental Techniques

High-throughput analyses are able to assess the histone modification profile across whole genomes comprehensively or at promoter regions only. There are two methods currently in use: ChIP-chip and ChIP-seq. The first method, ChIP-chip, involves hybridising immunoprecipitated material to microarrays. The more recently developed ChIP-seq method uses a different approach, whereby immunoprecipitated material is sequenced and the individual fragments are then aligned to the known genome sequence. Both of these techniques allow identification of genomic regions enriched in the immunoprecipitated sample. ChIP-chip is limited in that the degree of coverage of the genome (the resolution) is dependent on the distribution frequency of probes on the array. Further disadvantages include the fact that highly repetitive elements must be excluded, cross-hybridisation can occur and a large amount of input material is generally required and must be amplified, potentially resulting in amplification bias. Additionally, the cost of using microarrays is high. ChIP-seq, on the other hand, can be more cost-effective in spite of the high number of sequencing reads required (reviewed in Mellor et al. 2008). Genome coverage is high, however a small number of sequencing reads may not align to the known genome sequence (Mellor et al. 2008). A considerable advantage of ChIP-seq for the study of imprinted genes is the ability to recognise single nucleotide polymorphisms (SNPs), allowing parental alleles to be distinguished.

Medium- and low-throughput techniques assess the histone modification profile on a much smaller scale. Medium-throughput techniques involve applying ChIP samples to a tiling array, covering a small genomic region at high resolution, whereas low-throughput techniques assess the immunoprecipitated material at a single point using PCR (ChIP-PCR). The latter approach allows assessment of the two parental chromosomes using SNPs and if conducted properly, includes analysis of reciprocal hybrids so that the epigenetic state of each SNP can be attributed to parental origin rather than genetic background. It is also important to quantify the total amount of enrichment (i.e. on both chromosomes) of a particular histone modification at the site of interest as a five-fold difference in maternal to paternal enrichment may be insignificant if the total amount of the modification present is extremely low. The parental chromosomes can be distinguished after amplification of the ChIP material using either restriction site polymorphism, where a restriction site is lost due to the SNP, or single strand conformation polymorphism (SSCP). SSCP takes advantage of the different conformations formed by each of the two DNA strands as a direct result of the sequence and the products subsequently migrate to different positions on electrophoresis gels. The intensity of the two bands using either of these methods is then quantified to give the proportion of the particular histone modification on the respective chromosome. This must be normalised to the input chromatin (chromatin before immunoprecipitation) to account for potential differences in the proportion of maternal or paternal chromatin initially used (Gregory et al. 2001). The presence of SNPs within regions of interest does limit the locations able to be assessed on an allelic basis.

Parental origin-specific modifications can also be distinguished through ChIP analysis of chromatin isolated from uniparental disomy cells. Uniparental disomies contain two copies of a particular chromosome or chromosomal region from one parent with the corresponding deficiency from the other. The use of disomies therefore precludes the need for SNPs to distinguish parental origin (Grandjean et al. 2001). Similarly, a deletion of the region of interest on one of the parental chromosomes can allow the chromatin state of the remaining chromosome to be determined (Regha et al. 2007). These reduced-throughput methods assess a smaller region of the genome, but by their nature are amenable to more detailed analyses of the results.

A number of low-throughput studies assessing histone modifications at imprinted genes have been performed (see Table 2). However, the current pool of knowledge must be treated cautiously as only a limited number of cell types have been assessed. Additionally, many studies omit data from reciprocal cross experiments when SNP-containing hybrids are used. These experiments are essential as it has previously been observed that gene expression levels can vary depending on genetic background (Edwards et al. 2008). Any histone bias observed must be confirmed to be specific to the parental allele rather than the genetic background of the model system. It must also be verified that imprinted expression and DNA methylation patterns are normal in the system analysed as it has been determined that imprinting can be disrupted in some cell types, particularly high passage cultured cells. This is also true for any high-throughput studies assessing allelic marks.

3 Histone Modifications at Imprinted Loci

3.1 High-Throughput Analysis in Embryonic Stem Cells (ESCs) Without Reference to Allele-Specificity

By assessing the data from high-throughput whole genome or promoter-specific experiments, histone modification profiles at imprinted genes can be determined.

All human and mouse imprinted genes confirmed to date (http://www.har.mrc.ac.uk/research/genomic_imprinting/, Morison et al. 2001, Schulz et al. 2008) were searched in raw data files from such studies (Lee et al. 2006, Pan et al. 2007, Zhao et al. 2007, Guenther et al. 2007, Boyer et al. 2006, Mikkelsen et al. 2007). Where a particular known imprinted gene name was not found in the data files, alias gene names and accession numbers were utilised. A number of imprinted genes were absent in data files from all studies and are therefore not included in the analysis. This is most likely due to the unconfirmed status of these genes in current reference gene databases. Overall, histone modification profiles of 55 mouse imprinted genes and 42 human imprinted genes known to be imprinted in at least one tissue are here characterised. In ESCs, however, it is known that some of these genes are biallelically expressed.

3.1.1 The H3K4me3 and H3K27me3 Double Mark Is Overrepresented at Imprinted Gene Transcription Start Sites

Studies undertaken by a number of groups have assessed two histone modifications, trimethylation of histone H3 at lysine 4 (H3K4me3) and H3K27me3, in human and mouse embryonic stem cells (ESCs) (Pan et al. 2007, Zhao et al. 2007, Mikkelsen et al. 2007). Profiles at transcription start sites of imprinted genes are here characterised by averaging data from these three studies and the results are shown in Fig. 2. A higher proportion of imprinted genes carry both H3K4me3 and H3K27me3 marks compared to all known genes. This "bivalent" state has previously been characterised at non-imprinted genes that are expressed at low levels or not at all and is suggested to hold the gene in a poised state, where it can be readily turned on or off (Guenther et al. 2007, Mikkelsen et al. 2007, Azuara et al. 2006, Bernstein et al. 2006, Roh et al. 2006). In the case of imprinted genes, this double mark may represent an allelic difference with H3K4me3 on the active allele and H3K27me3 on the inactive allele. Importantly, the high-throughput studies assessed do not characterise the histone modifications in an allele-specific manner, therefore it is not known in which respect these marks act. A number of genes in these data sets display neither of these marks, reflecting the diverse nature of epigenetic states.

3.1.2 Histone Codes of Imprinted Genes

We assessed mouse ESC profiles of the four histone modifications H3K4me3, H3K27me3, H3K9me3 and H4K20me3 at transcription start sites of imprinted genes using the raw data of Mikkelsen and colleagues (Mikkelsen et al. 2007). The authors determined enriched genomic regions for H3K4me3 and H3K27me3 using a Window Interval method; for H3K9me3 and H4K20me3, a Hidden Markov Model methodology was employed (Mikkelsen et al. 2007). These two methods show different stringencies therefore H3K4me3 and H3K27me3 may be slightly overrepresented in the sample when compared to H3K9me3 and H4K20me3. Galaxy (http://g2.bx.psu.edu) was utilised to intersect genomic coordinates of enriched H3K9me3 and H4K20me3 regions with transcription start sites. H3K4me3

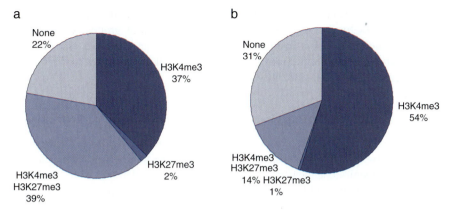

Fig. 2 H3K4me3 and H3K27me3 profiles at transcription start sites of (**a**) imprinted genes and (**b**) all genes in human and mouse ESCs. The percentage represents the proportion of genes exhibiting the histone modification profiles shown. Analysis performed on data obtained from Pan et al. 2007, Zhao et al. 2007, Mikkelsen et al. 2007. Percentages for each profile illustrated are an average of the results of these three studies

and H3K27me3 enriched transcription start sites were provided in raw data files (Mikkelsen et al. 2007). Of note, the antibody used against H3K9me3 cross-reacts to some degree with H3K27me3. Nevertheless, it can be seen by the results shown in Fig. 3 that three patterns emerge. These patterns consist of genes marked

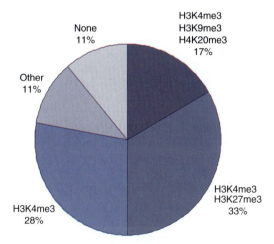

Fig. 3 Three patterns emerge at imprinted genes assessed for H3K4me3, H3K27me3, H3K9me3 and H4K20me3 in mouse ESCs ($n = 54$). The percentage represents the proportion of imprinted gene transcription start sites exhibiting the histone modification profiles illustrated. "Other" represents alternative combinations of these four modifications and "None" represents genes without any of these modifications. Analysis performed on data of enriched regions obtained from Mikkelsen et al. 2007

by H3K4me3 only, marked by both H3K4me3 and H3K27me3 or marked by H3K4me3, H3K9me3 and H4K20me3. This may represent groups of imprinted genes regulated in different manners or with other distinct properties (see below). By comparison, less than 0.1% of all known transcription start sites in the mouse genome carry H3K4me3, H3K9me3 and H4K20me3.

3.1.3 Distinguishing Developmental Repression from Imprinting Repression

Imprinted gene expression is often highly dynamic. The active alleles of imprinted genes are developmentally regulated and are therefore themselves repressed in a tissue- or temporal-dependent manner. An important consideration is the comparison between histone modifications correlating with heritable imprinted repression and those that might relate to the more canonical transcriptional repression at the active allele, the latter hereafter referred to as *developmental* repression. We have therefore characterised histone modifications associated with developmentally expressed and repressed imprinted genes and these results are depicted in Fig. 4 (raw data of gene expression and enriched histone modifications from Mikkelsen et al. 2007). The expression and histone modification status relates to the average of both alleles and does not differentiate between the two.

When developmental expression status is considered, it can be seen that expressed imprinted genes (i.e. mono-allelically expressed genes) display altered profiles of H3K4me3 and H3K27me3 at the transcription start site compared to repressed imprinted genes (i.e. biallelically repressed genes, see Fig. 4). The active mark H3K4me3 shows a higher prevalence at expressed compared to repressed genes whereas the repressive mark H3K27me3 is more frequent at repressed genes.

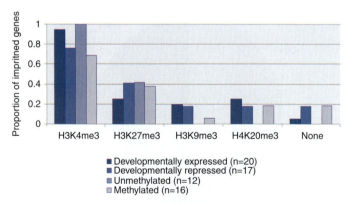

Fig. 4 Mouse ESC histone modification profiles at transcription start sites of imprinted genes according to *developmental* expression and promoter DNA methylation status. The proportion of genes with enrichment of a particular histone modification (*x axis*) is shown for each category of imprinted genes (*y axis*). Multiple histone modifications are in some cases present at a single gene. The number of genes assessed for each category is represented by the *n* value adjacent. Analysis was performed on raw data obtained from Mikkelsen et al. 2007 and Fouse et al. 2008 as described in Section 3.1.2. A gene was considered repressed if the signal intensity value was less than 25

Genomic Imprinting 243

From these results we interpret that these two modifications are associated with developmental regulation of expression though potentially in addition to a role in imprinting regulation. Data from a previous study of the *Igf2r/Air* locus supports a role for H3K27me3 in developmental repression of imprinted genes. Fibroblasts with a deletion of the locus on either the maternal or paternal chromosome were used to characterise allelic enrichment of particular histone modifications (Regha et al. 2007). At genes imprinted specifically in the placenta, but repressed in these fibroblasts (*Slc22a2* and *Slc22a3*), widespread H3K27me3 was found on both chromosomes. This profile was not observed at genes that display imprinted expression in these tissues.

A significant proportion of developmentally repressed genes are enriched for H3K4me3, consistent with a role in imprinting regulation (Fig. 4). Alternatively this may represent a bivalent chromatin state with H3K4me3 acting in a developmental manner to poise the gene for rapid activation, as discussed above. 25% of developmentally expressed genes are enriched for H3K27me3 at the transcription start site. This may also reflect a bivalent state, with H3K27me3 on the active allele. However, if H3K27me3 is enriched to a greater degree on the inactive allele compared to the active allele, a role in imprinting repression may be proposed. Studies assessing the allelic basis of these modifications will enable these two mechanisms of transcriptional regulation to be differentiated.

The modifications H3K9me3 and H4K20me3, which are generally regarded as repressive marks, are present at transcription start sites of both repressed and expressed imprinted genes (see Fig. 4). The presence of these modifications at developmentally expressed genes likely signifies an association of these marks with the inactive allele, although this is not confirmed. A slight increase in frequency of these marks is observed at developmentally expressed compared to repressed imprinted genes. This may be attributable to the fact that a greater proportion of developmentally expressed genes assessed in Fig. 4 possess a promoter DMR than do the developmentally repressed genes (discussed in Section 3.1.5). Nevertheless, the presence of H3K9me3 and H4K20me3 at expressed imprinted genes corresponds with a role for these modifications in imprinting regulation rather than developmental regulation of gene repression.

3.1.4 H3K9me3 and H4K20me3 Are more Frequent at Imprinted Genes with DNA Methylated Promoters than Without

DNA methylation plays an important role both in repression of inactive alleles of imprinted genes and in canonical (developmental) transcriptional repression. A recent study has assessed the DNA methylation status of promoters throughout the mouse genome (Fouse et al. 2008). We have assessed histone modification profiles from Mikkelsen and colleagues (Mikkelsen et al. 2007) in parallel with DNA methylation status from the raw data of Fouse and colleagues (Fouse et al. 2008) at imprinted genes and the results are shown in Fig. 4. Importantly, neither of these studies characterise allelic marks. A gene depicted as methylated in Fig. 4 may be methylated on one or both alleles and as mentioned above, histone modification enrichment is an average of both alleles. H3K9me3 and H4K20me3 are increased at transcription start sites of imprinted genes with DNA methylated promoters compared to biallelically unmethylated promoters. Previous studies have shown that DNA methylated regions such as heterochromatin are associated with H3K9me3 and H4K20me3 (Mikkelsen et al. 2007, Schotta et al. 2004, Barski et al. 2007, reviewed in Kouzarides 2007) and this association appears to also act at imprinted genes.

3.1.5 Clarifying Associations with Differentially Methylated Promoters

Differential DNA methylation between the promoters of each allele is found at some imprinted genes, whereby methylation is associated with the inactive allele. However, not all imprinted genes possess a promoter DMR and little is known of the epigenetic mechanisms of imprinting repression at genes that do not have this differential DNA methylation. We have compared the histone modifications enriched in mouse ESCs at imprinted genes with a promoter DMR and without, although allelic differences of enriched histone modifications are not characterised in the high-throughput studies assessed (see Fig. 5; raw data of enriched histone modifications from Mikkelsen et al. 2007). Germline and somatic promoter DMRs are not distinguished in these analyses.

It can be seen from the results shown in Fig. 5 that H3K9me3 and H4K20me3 are more prevalent at genes with a promoter DMR than without. Combined with the assessment above (Fig. 4) that these two modifications are more often associated with imprinted genes possessing DNA methylated promoters compared to unmethylated promoters *and* are found at developmentally expressed imprinted genes (hence are likely to be present on the inactive allele), it can be tentatively concluded that

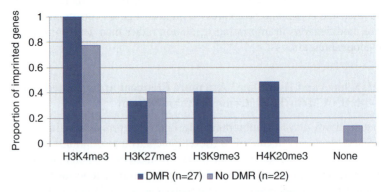

Fig. 5 Distinguishing histone modification profiles of imprinted genes by promoter DMR status. The proportion of genes with enrichment of a particular histone modification (*x axis*) is shown for each category of imprinted genes (*y axis*). Multiple histone modifications can be present at a single gene. The *n* value represents the number of genes assessed for each category. Analysis performed on raw data obtained from Mikkelsen et al. 2007

when present, H3K9me3 and H4K20me3 are usually located on the DNA methylated, inactive allele.

The two categories of promoter DMR status can be directly assessed with respect to developmental gene expression (raw expression data from Mikkelsen et al. 2007, results not shown). Of all imprinted genes assessed that are developmentally expressed and possess promoter DMRs, 45% display H4K20me3 enrichment and 36% display H3K9me3 enrichment ($n = 11$). Interestingly, of genes developmentally expressed *without* promoter DMRs, none display enrichment of these two histone marks ($n = 9$) suggesting that of the imprinted genes assessed, H3K9me3 and H4K20me3 are only present at developmentally expressed genes in the presence of promoter differential DNA methylation (presumably on the inactive allele). Of all developmentally *repressed* imprinted genes without DMRs that were assessed ($n = 13$), only one (*Gnas*) displays enrichment of H4K20me3 in ESCs and none are enriched for H3K9me3. These results further support the conclusion that H4K20me3 and H3K9me3 more commonly act to regulate imprinted repression than developmental repression.

A greater proportion of imprinted genes with promoter DMRs assessed in this analysis are developmentally expressed in ESCs relative to genes with no promoter DMR. The increase in H3K4me3 observed at transcription start sites in the presence of a promoter DMR may be a reflection of this (Fig. 5). When specifically considering imprinted genes that are developmentally expressed, almost all transcription start sites regardless of promoter DMR status are enriched with H3K4me3 (see Fig. 4). This implies that the role of H3K4me3 in transcriptional activation in either an imprinted or developmental manner is independent of promoter DMR status.

The analyses performed here on high-throughput data have provided useful insight into the association of histone modifications with different mechanisms of genomic repression. Provisionally, H3K27me3 appears to act more frequently at transcription start sites of imprinted genes to control developmental repression, whereas H3K9me3 and H4K20me3 correlate with repression of the inactive allele of imprinted genes possessing promoter DMRs, rather than with repression in a developmental manner. H3K4me3 is more likely to act in the control of both imprinted and developmental expression.

3.1.6 Analysis of Imprinting Control Regions

As mentioned above, the results described thus far refer to defined genes in the genome, yet a large proportion of imprinted genes are not confirmed in gene reference databases. Also of importance in relation to imprinting are intergenic regions such as paternally methylated ICRs. These are often overlooked in analyses of high-throughput studies. Furthermore, the results obtained from high-throughput studies do not provide information regarding the shape of a peak at a particular position, only the presence or absence of enrichment. It is for these reasons that viewing histone modification data from high-throughput experiments in a genome browser such as UCSC (http://genome.ucsc.edu/) or Ensembl (http://www.ensembl.org) can generate further insight into patterns of histone modifications. Computational analyses will hopefully be developed in the near future to incorporate these factors.

Imprinting control regions are key cis-acting elements harbouring a germline DNA methylation imprint and controlling the imprinting status of one or multiple imprinted genes. As noted above, most germline DMRs are methylated during oogenesis and are found at promoters of imprinted transcripts. Three are methylated during spermatogenesis and these are located at intergenic regions rather than at gene promoters. As a result of assessing peak shapes of four histone modifications, a very specific histone modification profile at all ICRs is found in mouse ESCs (analysis performed on raw data obtained from Mikkelsen et al. 2007). These ICRs are characterised by very high peaks of H3K4me3, H3K9me3 and H4K20me3 and this is the first analysis performed to recognise this specific profile (see Fig. 6 for a characteristic example). Intriguingly, this pattern is observed at both promoter and intergenic ICRs and is not a characteristic mark of somatic DMRs. H3K27me3 is observed at some, but not all ICRs again in a manner independent of the type of ICR (see Table 1). At the *Gnas* locus on mouse distal chromosome 2, two gDMRs

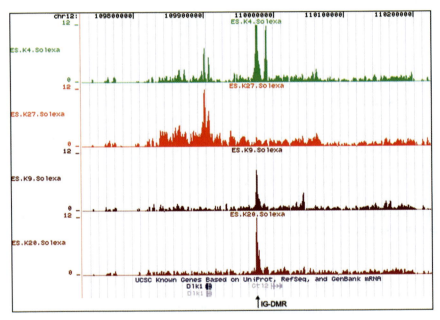

Fig. 6 Histone modification profile across the imprinted genes *Dlk1* and *Gtl2* in undifferentiated ESCs. An intergenic paternally methylated ICR (the IG-DMR, *black arrow*) is located between these two genes. The IG-DMR displays a histone modification profile characterised by high peaks of H3K4me3, H3K9me3 and H4K20me3, typical of all ICRs. Notably, a somatic DMR present at the *Gtl2* promoter does not display this profile. The *Gtl2* promoter does not exhibit any high H3K27me3 peaks, in contrast to the biallelically unmethylated *Dlk1* promoter which does show a significant H3K27me3 peak. Both *Gtl2* and *Dlk1* promoters have H3K4me3 peaks, likely reflecting the active maternal and paternal alleles respectively in ESCs. UCSC (Kent et al. 2002) image generated from data obtained from (Mikkelsen et al. 2007)

Genomic Imprinting

Table 1 Histone modification profiles of ICRs. Data tabulated from UCSC Kent et al. 2002) images of raw data tracks displaying ChIP-seq results from Mikkelsen et al. 2007 for the four histone marks H3K4me3, H3K27me3, H3K9me3 and H4K20me3

ICR profile	
H3K4me3, H3K9me3, H4K20me3	*H3K4me3, H3K9me3, H4K20me3, H3K27me3*
IG-DMR, Kcnq1ot1, Snrpn, H19 upstream, U2af1-rs1	Nespas, Air, Rasgrf upstream, Peg10, Grb10 brain-type promoter

exist, however only one of these has been shown to act as an ICR (the *Nespas* promoter DMR) (Williamson et al. 2006). Intriguingly, only the ICR gDMR exhibits this specific histone modification profile, implying that it is a true marker of an ICR. This may prove to be a useful tool for identifying ICRs for newly discovered imprinted genes. Limited analyses of parental chromosome-specific enrichment have been performed using SNP data, where it was found that some, but not all ICRs showed greater H3K4me3 enrichment on the unmethylated chromosome than the methylated chromosome (Mikkelsen et al. 2007). Although this specific ICR histone modification profile is always observed in ESCs, this is not the case for differentiated cells (Mikkelsen et al. 2007). This may reflect involvement of these marks in the establishment of imprinting early in development.

3.2 Medium- and Low-Throughput Analysis with Reference to Allele-Specificity

Studies focusing on smaller regions of the genome have provided information on the allelic nature of histone modifications at imprinted genes. Many of these studies do not assess overall levels of each histone modification analysed. The significance of allelic differences observed when overall modification levels are very low is questionable; however the detection of these modifications in high-throughput studies at some of these genes in the same cell types provides indirect evidence in support of their presence. As a result of assessing a number of studies of medium- and low-throughput techniques, H3K4 in the di- or trimethylated state and H3ac are found associated preferentially with the active allele while H3K9me2 and/or H3K9me3 is associated preferentially with the inactive allele ($n = 19$) at all imprinted genes studied to date in tissues where they are imprinted (data not shown) (Lewis et al. 2004, Gregory et al. 2001, Grandjean et al. 2001, Regha et al. 2007, Delaval et al. 2007, Fournier et al. 2002, Fulmer-Smentek and Francke 2001, Green et al. 2007, Han et al. 2008, Higashimoto et al. 2003, Hu et al. 2000, Lau et al. 2004, Lewis et al. 2006, Li et al. 2004, Pedone et al. 1999, Perk et al. 2002, Saitoh and Wada 2000, Umlauf et al. 2004, Verona et al. 2008, Vu et al. 2004, Wagschal et al. 2008, Wu et al. 2006, Xin et al. 2001, 2003, Yamasaki et al. 2005, Yamasaki-Ishizaki et al. 2007, Yang et al. 2003, Yoshioka et al. 2001). H3K27me3 is enriched to a greater degree on the inactive allele compared to the active allele in some cases and this may reflect a role in imprinted repression.

3.2.1 Allele-Specific Marks at Imprinting Control Regions (ICRs)

The profile at both maternally and paternally methylated ICRs is the same as for all imprinted genes for the modifications discussed above (see Table 2). The histone mark H4K20me3 is always found on the methylated chromosome of ICRs when assessed, however this mark has only been studied at one non-ICR region (the *Igf2r* promoter) and conflicting data was found within this single study comparing medium- and low-throughput techniques (Regha et al. 2007). H3K27me3 is found enriched on the methylated chromosome to a greater degree than the unmethylated chromosome for some, but not all ICRs. It is interesting to note that paternally methylated ICRs display allelic differences in histone modifications despite the fact that they are present at intergenic regions. The modifications H3K4me3, H3K9me3 and H4K20me3 consistently display parental allelic differences at ICRs and are also shown to be enriched at these regions through high-throughput techniques (compare Table 1 and Table 2). Together these results indicate that the peaks observed at ICRs in the high-throughput analyses are likely to be associated preferentially with one of the two parental chromosomes.

3.2.2 Distinguishing Between Imprinted Genes with and Without Promoter DMRs

Medium- and low-throughput histone modification studies of imprinted regions that have been performed to date (Carr et al. 2007, Lewis et al. 2004, Gregory et al. 2001, Grandjean et al. 2001, Regha et al. 2007, Delaval et al. 2007, Fournier et al. 2002, Fulmer-Smentek and Francke 2001, Green et al. 2007, Han et al. 2008, Higashimoto et al. 2003, Hu et al. 2000, Lau et al. 2004, Lewis et al. 2006, Li et al. 2004, Pedone et al. 1999, Perk et al. 2002, Saitoh and Wada 2000, Umlauf et al. 2004, Verona et al. 2008, Vu et al. 2004, Wagschal et al. 2008, Wu et al. 2006, Xin et al. 2001, 2003, Yamasaki et al. 2005, Yamasaki-Ishizaki et al. 2007, Yang et al. 2003, Yoshioka et al. 2001) can be assessed by promoter DMR status. A greater proportion of genes with a promoter DMR have H3K9me2 and/or H3K9me3 preferentially enriched on the inactive allele compared to genes without a promoter DMR (~75% compared to ~40% of those tested for H3K9me2/3, data not shown). This is consistent with the data assessment of high-throughput studies, where H3K9me3 was found to occur more often at transcription start sites of genes with promoter DMRs (see Section 3.1.5). Interestingly, all genes without a promoter DMR displaying an H3K9 methylation difference reside within an imprinting cluster containing numerous genes imprinted specifically in the placenta. This is discussed further in Section 3.2.4 below.

When comparing germline to somatic DMRs, H3K9me3 is always observed on the methylated chromosome at gDMRs yet only sometimes is a parental difference detected at sDMRs, providing evidence of an epigenetic difference between these two types of imprinting control regions in somatic cells. It will be interesting to determine whether H4K20me3 shows a distinct difference between sDMRs and gDMRs for allelic enrichment; this awaits additional experimental analysis.

Table 2 Allelic histone modification profiles at ICRs from medium- and low-throughput analyses. Bold type represents modifications tested in all cell types; * represents discrepancies found between studies

ICR	DNA methylated chromosome	Maternal chromosome histone marks	Paternal chromosome histone marks	No bias	Cell/tissue type studied	References
Air promoter	Maternal	H3K9me2 H3K9me3 H4K20me3	**H3ac H4ac** **H3K4me2** **H3K4me3** H3S10P		Brain, cultured brain cells, kidney, liver, fibroblasts	Regha et al. 2007, Fournier et al. 2002, Hu et al. 2000, Vu et al. 2004, Yamasaki et al. 2005 and Yang et al. 2003
Grb10 brain-type promoter	Maternal	**H3K9me3**	**H3ac H4ac** **H3K4me2**		Neurons	Yamasaki-Ishizaki et al. 2007
Kcnq1ot1 promoter	Maternal	H3K9me2 H3K9me3 H4K20me3 H3K27me3* H4R2me2s	**H3ac** H4ac **H3K4me2** H4K4me3		Liver, embryo, placenta, ESCs, TSCs, fibroblasts, A9 hybrids	Delaval et al. 2007, Higashimoto et al. 2003, Lewis et al. 2006, Umlauf et al. 2004, Wagschal et al. 2008, Yoshioka et al. 2001 and Reese et al. 2007
Nespas promoter	Maternal	**H3K9me3**	**H3ac H4ac** **H3K4me3**		Fibroblasts	Li et al. 2004

Table 2 (Continued)

ICR	DNA methylated chromosome	Maternal chromosome histone marks	Paternal chromosome histone marks	No bias	Cell/tissue type studied	References
Snrpn promoter / exon 1	Maternal	H3K9me2 H3K9me3 H4K20me3 H4R2me2s H3K27me3	H3ac H4ac H3K4me2 H3K4me3		Brain, liver, spleen, ESCs, fibroblasts, A9 hybrids, human lymphocytes	Gregory et al. 2001, Fournier et al. 2002, Fulmer-Smentek and Francke 2001, Lau et al. 2004, Perk et al. 2002, Saitoh and Wada 2000, Wu et al. 2006, Xin et al. 2003, Yoshioka et al. 2001 and Reese et al. 2007
U2af1-rs1 5′ UTR	Maternal	H3K9me2/3	**H3ac** H4ac* H3K4me H3K9me2		Brain, liver, fibroblasts, ESCs	Gregory et al. 2001 and Fournier et al. 2002
H19 upstream	Paternal	H3ac H4ac **H3K4me2** H3K4me3	**H3K9me3** H4K20me3	H4R3me2s **H3K27me3**	Liver, ESCs, fibroblasts	Delaval et al. 2007 Han et al. 2008, Yang et al. 2003, Reese et al. 2007 Singh and Srivastava 2008
IG-DMR	Paternal	H3ac **H3K4me2** H3K4me3	H3K9me3* H4K20me3 H4R3me2s	**H3K27me3**	Liver, ESCs, fibroblasts	Regha et al. 2007, Delaval et al. 2007 and Reese et al. 2007
Rasgrf upstream	Paternal	H3ac **H3K4me2 H3K27me3**	**H3K9me3 H4K20me3**		Liver, ESCs	Delaval et al. 2007

Genomic Imprinting

The H3K27me3 mark displays a difference in enrichment between parental alleles at some promoters without DMRs (where the modification is more enriched on the inactive allele), but not at promoters with DMRs of those assessed to date. Note there are two exceptions of promoter DMRs, *Snrpn* and *Tssc4*, which do display an H3K27me3 difference in some tissues and conflicting data exists for *Kcnq1ot1*, *H19* and *Cdkn1c* which also have promoter DMRs (Lewis et al. 2004, Gregory et al. 2001, Han et al. 2008, Lewis et al. 2006, Umlauf et al. 2004, Verona et al. 2008). The presence of an H3K27me3 allelic difference at non-DMR promoters (an example of this occurs at the *Igf2* promoter 2 (Grandjean et al. 2001, Han et al. 2008)) was not found to be a general rule, however in some cases it could play a role in repressing the inactive allele in the absence of differential DNA methylation.

Further insight can be gathered from low-throughput studies by assessing imprinted regions in greater detail. A number of imprinted genes are complex in that they can have many transcript variants and tissue-specific imprinting patterns in addition to developmental expression patterns. These features are discussed below in attempt to characterise associated epigenetic mechanisms.

3.2.3 Transcriptional Variants: Histone Modification Patterns Can Correlate with Imprinted Expression

Transcript variants of imprinted genes can show discrete imprinting patterns. Some transcripts may be imprinted while others are biallelically expressed and this can be achieved through the use of alternative promoters with different epigenetic characteristics. For example, at the imprinted locus on mouse distal chromosome 2, numerous alternative transcripts arise from the *Gnas* gene through the use of alternative promoters. *Nesp*, *Gnasxl* and *Exon1A* transcripts are ubiquitously imprinted, whereas the *Gnas* transcript itself is only imprinted in a small number of tissues (reviewed in Peters and Williamson 2007). The DNA methylation and histone modification profile reflects the expression state for these transcripts, with active marks enriched on the active allele and vice versa. In other words, when expression is imprinted, promoter DMRs are present and promoter histone modifications differ between the parental alleles whereas biallelic expression is accompanied by biallelic DNA hypomethylation and biallelic histone modifications at the promoter (Li et al. 2004, Sakamoto et al. 2004). An exception to this occurs in tissues where the *Gnas* transcript adopts imprinted expression. For the *Gnas* transcript, differential promoter DNA methylation is not observed alongside imprinted expression and instead the region remains biallelically hypomethylated as in tissues where the gene is not imprinted. Differential histone modifications are however acquired (Sakamoto et al. 2004). This emphasises the correlation of histone modification profiles with expression in the absence of any associated differential DNA methylation. This provides an example of how imprinted genes can be utilised as model systems for assessing epigenetic changes associated with gene regulation. Correlations between histone modifications and expression in an allelic manner have also been observed at a number of other imprinted genes, including *H19*, *Igf2r* and *NDN* (Lau et al. 2004, Verona et al. 2008, Vu et al. 2004).

Intriguingly, at promoter germline DMRs the histone modification profile does not always reflect expression patterns. An example of this occurs at the *Grb10* locus, which possesses two alternative promoters. *Grb10* is expressed from the maternal allele when expressed from the major-type promoter, yet in neurons this gene employs the brain-type promoter, resulting in paternal-specific expression (Yamasaki-Ishizaki et al. 2007). A gDMR exists at the brain-type promoter and is associated with differential H3K4me3 and H3K9me3 on the unmethylated and methylated alleles respectively in neurons (Yamasaki-Ishizaki et al. 2007). These differential histone modifications were also detected in cells that have no expression from this promoter on either allele (Yamasaki-Ishizaki et al. 2007), suggesting that differential histone modifications can exist at gDMRs in tissues where both alleles are inactive. The *Air* promoter on mouse chromosome 17 also harbours a gDMR and again differential histone modifications have been identified at this region in cells that have biallelic *Air* repression (Yamasaki et al. 2005). Many studies have shown that germline DMRs exist in differentiated tissues (for example, Ferguson-Smith et al. 1993, Liu et al. 2000). Somatic DMRs, however, show tissue-specificity (for example, Lewis et al. 2004, Lin et al. 2007); it will therefore be interesting to determine whether sDMRs also maintain differential DNA methylation and histone modifications in tissues where the gene is biallelically repressed. Furthermore, genes without any differential DNA methylation may or may not retain histone modification differences between the two parental alleles.

Some imprinted domains are interspersed with non-imprinted genes, for example the gene *Slc22a1* at the imprinted *Igf2r/Air* locus. Regha and colleagues have shown that this gene does not display a parental-specific difference in DNA methylation or a number of histone modifications in fibroblasts (Regha et al. 2007).

3.2.4 Tissue-Specific Imprinted Expression

Imprinted genes can also display tissue-dependent imprinting profiles where a gene is imprinted in only a subset of tissues, as described above for the *Gnas* transcript and *Grb10* variants. Another example occurs at the *Kcnq1* cluster on mouse distal chromosome 7. This cluster contains many genes biallelically expressed in the embryo and imprinted specifically in the trophoblast derivatives (extraembryonic tissues), where they are maternally expressed (Lewis et al. 2004). These genes (including *Ascl2*, *Cd81*, *Osbpl* and *Tssc4*) display an H3ac and H3K4me2 bias towards the maternal allele and an H3K9me2 bias towards the paternal allele in trophoblast lineages, with no bias observed in the embryo (Lewis et al. 2006, Umlauf et al. 2004, Wagschal et al. 2008). Allelic histone modification profiles at placental-specific imprinted genes of this domain therefore follow imprinting expression patterns, similar to imprinted versus non-imprinted transcript variants.

It has been shown that the maintenance of imprinting in extraembryonic tissue is less dependent on DNA methylation than in embryonic tissue, suggesting that epigenetic control is mediated differently in this lineage (Lewis et al. 2004, Umlauf et al. 2004, Lin et al. 2007, Sasaki et al. 1995). Alternative mechanisms to DNA methylation appear to maintain the imprinted status of placental-specific imprinted genes at the *Kcnq1* domain. Epigenetic modifications have been assessed at this region in the mouse when the maintenance DNA methylation enzyme, Dnmt1, has been deleted. Two forms of this enzyme exist: an oocyte specific variant and a somatic variant. When the somatic form (Dnmt1s) is deleted, methylation is acquired in the female germline at the *Kcnq1ot1* promoter ICR as per usual, but this methylation cannot be maintained after fertilisation (Lewis et al. 2004). Despite this, imprinting is only perturbed at genes ubiquitously imprinted and not at those normally imprinted specifically in the placenta, indicating maintenance of methylation does not regulate the placental imprinting of these genes. When the oocyte specific variant of Dnmt1 is deleted, imprints are affected at all imprinted genes of the domain, illustrating the requirement for germline methylation to establish imprinting of all genes in the cluster (Green et al. 2007). Together these findings allude to the possibility that differential methylation at the ICR is required only for the establishment of imprinting at these placental-specific imprinted genes and that the maintenance of imprinting may in fact be controlled by other epigenetic mechanisms such as differential histone modification (Green et al. 2007). H3K27me3 does not show a consistent allelic difference at placental-specific imprinted genes in the placenta, nor in the embryo or ESCs (Lewis et al. 2004, 2006, Umlauf et al. 2004, Wagschal et al. 2008). This is despite the fact that Ascl2, a placental-specific imprinted gene at the cluster, shows loss of imprinting when an H3K27 methylation enzyme, Eed, is knocked out in mice (Mager et al. 2003). This perhaps suggests that H3K27me3 acts to control imprinting of this gene indirectly.

An alternative repressive histone modification may act in the placenta to support imprinted repression of genes at the *Kcnq1* cluster. Of nine imprinted promoters without DMRs tested for allelic di- or tri-methylated H3K9 (see Section 3.2.2), the *Kcnq1* domain genes *Ascl2*, *Cd81*, *Kcnq1* and *Phlda2* are the only genes showing a difference in enrichment between the two parental alleles. This was detected in placental tissue and not in embryonic tissue or ESCs, despite the fact that two of these genes are imprinted in both the placenta and embryo (Lewis et al. 2004, 2006, Umlauf et al. 2004, Wagschal et al. 2008). Additionally, none of these genes show enrichment for H3K9me3 at the transcription start site in a high-throughput study of mouse ESCs (Mikkelsen et al. 2007), highlighting the importance of assessing different cell types. Further support for the role of H3K9 methylation in placental imprinting control is provided by analysis of mice lacking the H3K9 methylating enzyme G9a. Some loss of imprinting of placental-specific imprinted genes at the cluster occurs in placentas of this mutant (Wagschal et al. 2008). Together, these results suggest that H3K9 methylation may be an important factor in maintenance control of imprinting at a limited number of genes in place of DNA methylation.

Both differential histone modifications and sDMRs appear to play important roles in maintaining tissue-specific imprinting, yet it remains unclear as to how imprinting is initiated in one tissue or lineage but not another. Epigenetic profiles may be established before lineage specification and only utilised or read in the lineage or tissue where the gene is imprinted (as suggested for the *Kcnq1* domain). Imprinting of tissue-specific imprinted genes may initially be regulated directly by the ICR, with subsequent methylation at sDMRs and/or acquisition of differential histone modifications modulating tissue- and lineage-specific imprinting. Alternatively, sDMRs and differential histone modifications may be a consequence of transcriptional activity/repression conferred by a combination of the ICR and the presence of transcription factors. Absence of imprinting in particular tissues might also be caused by erasure of somatic epigenetic marks (for example, mouse imprinted X chromosome inactivation (Okamoto et al. 2004)). Alternatively, imprinting may be established at the gene or cluster exclusively in the tissue displaying imprinting expression at later developmental stages, although examples of this have not been found to date. It may be the case that different imprinting clusters employ alternative mechanisms for achieving lineage-specific imprinting.

4 Summary

Imprinted genes have transcriptional properties that must be controlled by epigenetic mechanisms. First and foremost, expression is dependent on parent of origin. Within this context, there exists transcript-specific and tissue-specific control of imprinting. Furthermore, like any other developmentally regulated gene, the normally active allele of an imprinted gene is also repressed or expressed in a tissue and temporally regulated manner. A working model for histone modification profiles at imprinted genes during developmental repression is illustrated in Fig. 7.

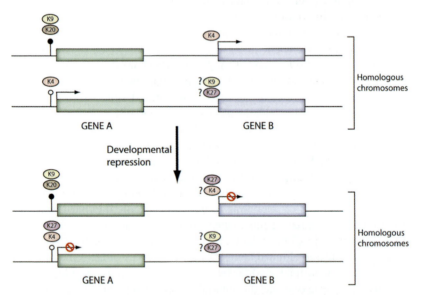

Fig. 7 Schematic of a working model for histone modification profiles at imprinted genes. All histone modifications illustrated represent the trimethylated state. Gene A has an ICR at the promoter whereas gene B has no differential DNA methylation and these two states confer distinct histone modification profiles. After developmental repression, both genes acquire H3K27me3 on the previously active allele. Transcriptional activators and repressors are key players in this process and may be a cause or consequence of the histone modification states shown

Imprinted genes have specific allelic profiles of histone modifications not currently known to occur in other regions of the genome. Modification patterns present at one of the two parental alleles can however in some cases represent patterns observed at non-imprinted genes with allelic equivalence. Interestingly, the presence of H3K9me3 and H4K20me3 on inactive alleles of imprinted genes is representative of the profile characterising heterochromatin and also pseudogenes within euchromatic regions (Regha et al. 2007, Mikkelsen et al. 2007, Barski et al. 2007). This suggests that the presence of these two marks combined may represent a more permanent mark of repression than other repressive histone modifications such as H3K27me3. The presence of H3K9me3 and H4K20me3 at imprinted regions may be linked to the expression of non-coding RNAs, a feature common to many imprinted domains.

Mechanisms other than histone tail modifications and DNA methylation are known to operate at imprinting clusters, including non-coding RNAs, histone protein variants and chromatin-looping. These provide additional layers of epigenetic complexity and further discussion of these mechanisms can be found in other chapters of this volume (see Chapters "Epigenetic Profiling of Histone Variants" and "MacroRNAs in the Epigenetic Control of X-Chromosome Inactivation").

Many questions remain regarding the epigenetic control of genomic imprinting that also apply in a more genome-wide context. Probably the most important question is whether the histone modification profile acts to establish and/or maintain patterns of imprinting or whether it is merely a consequence. Furthermore, how is lineage-specific imprinting regulated? Are non-imprinted genes within a cluster protected from imprinting or are imprinted genes in the domain specifically targeted? It remains to be fully ascertained how all the layers of complexity of imprinting regions are epigenetically regulated; nevertheless research within the field of genomic imprinting is constantly contributing to knowledge of epigenetic processes.

Key points

- ICRs have a unique histone modification profile: H3K4me3 on the unmethylated chromosome with H3K9me3 and H4K20me3 on the methylated chromosome
- H3K9me3 and H4K20me3 are associated with imprinted genes possessing differentially DNA methylated promoters
- H3K4me3 and H3K27me3 appear to mirror developmental regulation, whereas H3K9me3 and H4K20me3 may reflect imprinted repression
- Differential DNA methylation and histone modifications are consistent with expression patterns, potentially with the general exception of germline DMRs
- Differential histone modifications and somatic DMRs likely play roles in tissue-specific imprinting regulation

Acknowledgement We are grateful to the members of the Ferguson-Smith lab for helpful discussions and also to Marika Charalambous for comments on the manuscript. Work was supported by a New Zealand TEC studentship to KM, and grants from the Wellcome Trust and MRC.

References

Azuara, V., et al., *Chromatin signatures of pluripotent cell lines*. Nat Cell Biol, 2006. **8**(5): 532–8.
Barski, A., et al., *High-resolution profiling of histone methylations in the human genome*. Cell, 2007. **129**(4): 823–37.
Bernstein, B.E., et al., *A bivalent chromatin structure marks key developmental genes in embryonic stem cells*. Cell, 2006. **125**(2): 315–26.
Boyer, L.A., et al., *Polycomb complexes repress developmental regulators in murine embryonic stem cells*. Nature, 2006. **441**(7091): 349–53.
Carr, M.S., et al., *Allele-specific histone modifications regulate expression of the DLK1-GH2 imprinted domain*. Genomics, 2007. **89**(2): 280–90.
Delaval, K., et al., *Differential histone modifications mark mouse imprinting control regions during spermatogenesis*. EMBO J, 2007. **26**(3): 720–9.
Edwards, C.A., et al., *The Evolution of the DLK1-DIO3 Imprinted Domain in Mammals*. PLoS Biol, 2008. **6**(6): e135.
Ferguson-Smith, A.C. and M.A. Surani, *Imprinting and the epigenetic asymmetry between parental genomes*. Science, 2001. **293**(5532): 1086–9.
Ferguson-Smith, A.C., et al., *Parental-origin-specific epigenetic modification of the mouse H19 gene*. Nature, 1993. **362**(6422): 751–5.
Fournier, C., et al., *Allele-specific histone lysine methylation marks regulatory regions at imprinted mouse genes*. Embo J, 2002. **21**(23): 6560–70.
Fouse, S.D., et al., *Promoter CpG methylation contributes to ES cell gene regulation in parallel with Oct4/Nanog, PcG complex, and histone H3 K4/K27 trimethylation*. Cell Stem Cell, 2008. **2**(2): 160–9.
Fulmer-Smentek, S.B. and U. Francke, *Association of acetylated histones with paternally expressed genes in the Prader–Willi deletion region*. Hum Mol Genet, 2001. **10**(6): 645–52.
Grandjean, V., et al., *Relationship between DNA methylation, histone H4 acetylation and gene expression in the mouse imprinted Igf2-H19 domain*. FEBS Lett, 2001. **488**(3): 165–9.
Green, K., et al., *A developmental window of opportunity for imprinted gene silencing mediated by DNA methylation and the Kcnq1ot1 noncoding RNA*. Mamm Genome, 2007. **18**(1): 32–42.
Gregory, R.I., et al., *DNA methylation is linked to deacetylation of histone H3, but not H4, on the imprinted genes Snrpn and U2af1-rs1*. Mol Cell Biol, 2001. **21**(16): 5426–36.
Guenther, M.G., et al., *A chromatin landmark and transcription initiation at most promoters in human cells*. Cell, 2007. **130**(1): 77–88.
Han, L., D.H. Lee, and P.E. Szabo, *CTCF is the master organizer of domain-wide allele-specific chromatin at the H19/Igf2 imprinted region*. Mol Cell Biol, 2008. **28**(3): 1124–35.
Heintzman, N.D., et al., *Distinct and predictive chromatin signatures of transcriptional promoters and enhancers in the human genome*. Nat Genet, 2007. **39**(3): 311–8.
Higashimoto, K., et al., *Loss of CpG methylation is strongly correlated with loss of histone H3 lysine 9 methylation at DMR-LIT1 in patients with Beckwith-Wiedemann syndrome*. Am J Hum Genet, 2003. **73**(4): 948–56.
Hikichi, T., et al., *Imprinting regulation of the murine Meg1/Grb10 and human GRB10 genes; roles of brain-specific promoters and mouse-specific CTCF-binding sites*. Nucleic Acids Res, 2003. **31**(5): 1398–406.
Hu, J.F., et al., *Allele-specific histone acetylation accompanies genomic imprinting of the insulin-like growth factor II receptor gene*. Endocrinology, 2000. **141**(12): 4428–35.
Kent, W.J., et al., *The human genome browser at UCSC*. Genome Res, 2002. **12**(6): 996–1006.
Kouzarides, T., *Chromatin modifications and their function*. Cell, 2007. **128**(4): 693–705.

Lau, J.C., M.L. Hanel, and R. Wevrick, *Tissue-specific and imprinted epigenetic modifications of the human NDN gene.* Nucleic Acids Res, 2004. **32**(11): 3376–82.

Lee, T.I., et al., *Control of developmental regulators by Polycomb in human embryonic –stem cells.* Cell, 2006. **125**(2): 301–13.

Lewis, A., et al., *Imprinting on distal chromosome 7 in the placenta involves repressive histone methylation independent of DNA methylation.* Nat Genet, 2004. **36**(12): 1291–5.

Lewis, A., et al., *Epigenetic dynamics of the Kcnq1 imprinted domain in the early embryo.* Development, 2006. **133**(21): 4203–10.

Li, T., et al., *Activating and silencing histone modifications form independent allelic switch regions in the imprinted Gnas gene.* Hum Mol Genet, 2004. **13**(7): 741–50.

Lin, S.P., et al., *Asymmetric regulation of imprinting on the maternal and paternal chromosomes at the Dlk1-Gtl2 imprinted cluster on mouse chromosome 12.* Nat Genet, 2003. **35**(1): 97–102.

Lin, S.P., et al., *Differential regulation of imprinting in the murine embryo and placenta by the Dlk1-Dio3 imprinting control region.* Development, 2007. **134**(2): 417–26.

Liu, J., et al., *Identification of a methylation imprint mark within the mouse Gnas locus.* Mol Cell Biol, 2000. **20**(16): 5808–17.

Mager, J., et al., *Genome imprinting regulated by the mouse Polycomb group protein Eed.* Nat Genet, 2003. **33**(4): 502–7.

Mancini-Dinardo, D., et al., *Elongation of the Kcnq1ot1 transcript is required for genomic imprinting of neighboring genes.* Genes Dev, 2006. **20**(10): 1268–82.

Mellor, J., Dudek, and D. Clynes, *A glimpse into the epigenetic landscape of gene regulation.* Curr Opin Genet Dev, 2008. **18**(2): 116–22.

Mikkelsen, T.S., et al., *Genome-wide maps of chromatin state in pluripotent and lineage-committed cells.* Nature, 2007. **448**(7153): 553–60.

Morison, I.M., C.J. Paton, and S.D. Cleverley, *The imprinted gene and parent-of-origin effect database.* Nucleic Acids Res, 2001. **29**(1): 275–6.

Okamoto, I., et al., *Epigenetic dynamics of imprinted X inactivation during early mouse development.* Science, 2004. **303**(5658): 644–9.

Pan, G., et al., *Whole-genome analysis of histone H3 lysine 4 and lysine 27 methylation in human embryonic stem cells.* Cell Stem Cell, 2007. **1**(3): 299–312.

Pedone, P.V., et al., *Role of histone acetylation and DNA methylation in the maintenance of the imprinted expression of the H19 and Igf2 genes.* FEBS Lett, 1999. **458**(1): 45–50.

Perk, J., et al., *The imprinting mechanism of the Prader-Willi/Angelman regional control center.* EMBO J, 2002. **21**(21): 5807–14.

Peters, J. and C.M. Williamson, *Control of imprinting at the Gnas cluster.* Epigenetics, 2007. **2**(4): 207–13.

Reese, K.J., et al., *Maintenance of paternal methylation and repression of the imprinted H19 gene requires MBD3.* PLoS Genet, 2007. **3**(8): e137.

Regha, K., et al., *Active and repressive chromatin are interspersed without spreading in an imprinted gene cluster in the mammalian genome.* Mol Cell, 2007. **27**(3): 353–66.

Roh, T.Y., et al., *Genome-wide prediction of conserved and nonconserved enhancers by histone acetylation patterns.* Genome Res, 2007. **17**(1): 74–81.

Roh, T.Y., et al., *The genomic landscape of histone modifications in human T cells.* Proc Natl Acad Sci U S A, 2006. **103**(43): 15782–7.

Saitoh, S. and T. Wada, *Parent-of-origin specific histone acetylation and reactivation of a key imprinted gene locus in Prader-Willi syndrome.* Am J Hum Genet, 2000. **66**(6): 1958–62.

Sakamoto, A., et al., *Tissue-specific imprinting of the G protein Gsalpha is associated with tissue-specific differences in histone methylation.* Hum Mol Genet, 2004. **13**(8): 819–28.

Sasaki, H., et al., *Temporal and spatial regulation of H19 imprinting in normal and uniparental mouse embryos.* Development, 1995. **121**(12): 4195–202.

Schotta, G., et al., *A silencing pathway to induce H3-K9 and H4-K20 trimethylation at constitutive heterochromatin.* Genes Dev, 2004. **18**(11): 1251–62.

Schulz, R., et al., *WAMIDEX: A web atlas of murine genomic imprinting and differential expression.* Epigenetics, 2008. **3**(2): 89–96.

Singh, V. and M. Srivastava, *Enhancer blocking activity of insulator at H19-ICR is independent of chromatin barrier establishment.* Mol Cell Biol, 2008. **28**(11): 3767–75.

Sleutels, F., R. Zwart, and D.P. Barlow, *The non-coding Air RNA is required for silencing autosomal imprinted genes.* Nature, 2002. **415**(6873): 810–3.

Umlauf, D., et al., *Imprinting along the Kcnq1 domain on mouse chromosome 7 involves repressive histone methylation and recruitment of Polycomb group complexes.* Nat Genet, 2004. **36**(12): 1296–300.

Verona, R.I., et al., *The transcriptional status but not the imprinting control region determines allele-specific histone modifications at the imprinted H19 locus.* Mol Cell Biol, 2008. **28**(1): 71–82.

Vu, T.H., T. Li, and A.R. Hoffman, *Promoter-restricted histone code, not the differentially methylated DNA regions or antisense transcripts, marks the imprinting status of IGF2R in human and mouse.* Hum Mol Genet, 2004. **13**(19): 2233–45.

Wagschal, A., et al., *G9a histone methyltransferase contributes to imprinting in the mouse placenta.* Mol Cell Biol, 2008. **28**(3): 1104–13.

Williamson, C.M., et al., *Identification of an imprinting control region affecting the expression of all transcripts in the Gnas cluster.* Nat Genet, 2006. **38**(3): 350–5.

Wu, M.Y., T.F. Tsai, and A.L. Beaudet, *Deficiency of Rbbp1/Arid4a and Rbbp1l1/Arid4b alters epigenetic modifications and suppresses an imprinting defect in the PWS/AS domain.* Genes Dev, 2006. **20**(20): 2859–70.

Xin, Z., C.D. Allis, and J. Wagstaff, *Parent-specific complementary patterns of histone H3 lysine 9 and H3 lysine 4 methylation at the Prader-Willi syndrome imprinting center.* Am J Hum Genet, 2001. **69**(6): 1389–94.

Xin, Z., et al., *Role of histone methyltransferase G9a in CpG methylation of the Prader-Willi syndrome imprinting center.* J Biol Chem, 2003. **278**(17): 14996–5000.

Yamasaki, Y., et al., *Neuron-specific relaxation of Igf2r imprinting is associated with neuron-specific histone modifications and lack of its antisense transcript Air.* Hum Mol Genet, 2005. **14**(17): 2511–20.

Yamasaki-Ishizaki, Y., et al., *Role of DNA methylation and histone H3 lysine 27 methylation in tissue-specific imprinting of mouse Grb10.* Mol Cell Biol, 2007. **27**(2): 732–42.

Yang, Y., et al., *The histone code regulating expression of the imprinted mouse Igf2r gene.* Endocrinology, 2003. **144**(12): 5658–70.

Yoshioka, H., Y. Shirayoshi, and M. Oshimura, *A novel in vitro system for analyzing parental allele-specific histone acetylation in genomic imprinting.* J Hum Genet, 2001. **46**(11): 626–32.

Zhao, X.D., et al., *Whole-genome mapping of histone H3 Lys4 and 27 trimethylations reveals distinct genomic compartments in human embryonic stem cells.* Cell Stem Cell, 2007. **1**(3): 286–98.

The Epigenomic Landscape of Reprogramming in Mammals

Gabriella Ficz, Cassandra R. Farthing and Wolf Reik

Abstract Epigenetic reprogramming is commonly defined as the erasure or removal of an existing set of epigenetic marks, followed by establishment of a different set of marks. Epigenetic reprogramming can occur in specific genes or subsets of genes, for example during lineage-specific differentiation events. It can also take place on a more global level, for example when primordial germ cells undergo erasure of histone marks and DNA methylation in many genes and sequences in the genome, or in the early embryo after fertilisation, where gametic epigenetic programmes are replaced by those characteristic of totipotent and pluripotent embryonic cells and stem cells. Experimental epigenetic reprogramming on a large scale has been shown to be possible during animal cloning, and during the recent spectacular direct reprogramming of differentiated cells to ES like cells. However, these advances have also highlighted the fact that natural reprogramming needs to be understood mechanistically so that the experimental techniques can be improved and made fully efficient for potential applications in regenerative medicine. Mechanistic insights are now aided by the recent development of genome-wide epigenomic profiling techniques for histone modifications, transcription factors, and DNA methylation. The purpose of this chapter is to provide a brief summary of how these technical advances are illuminating a fascinating area of biology with immense promise for medicine.

Keywords Epigenetic programming · Pluripotency · DNA methylation · Histone modifications · Demethylation · Somatic cell nuclear transfer · iPS cells · ES cells · Germline reprogramming · Genomic imprints

---

W. Reik (✉)
Laboratory of Developmental Genetics and Imprinting, The Babraham Institute,
Cambridge CB22 3AT, U.K; Centre for Trophoblast Research, University of Cambridge, Cambridge CB2 3EG, UK

1 Naturally Occurring Epigenetic Reprogramming

Epigenetic reprogramming was first discovered in mouse embryos. While it had been appreciated that during development the patterns of DNA methylation of individual genes could change, investigations of methylation genome-wide showed that there was a remarkable loss of DNA methylation after fertilisation in preimplantation embryos up to the blastocyst stage (Dean et al. 2001; Howlett and Reik 1991; Mayer et al. 2000; Monk et al. 1987; Oswald et al. 2000; Santos et al. 2002), and later studies revealed that during development of primordial germ cells (PGCs) just after their arrival in the genital ridges, there was a similar genome-wide loss of DNA methylation (Hajkova et al. 2008; Hajkova et al. 2002; Lee et al. 2002; Seki et al. 2005 2007). More detailed analyses have shown that after fertilisation, the paternal genome is rapidly demethylated in the zygote before DNA replication, indicating an active removal of methylation. Sequences that are demethylated include Line1 repeats, several single copy genes including pluripotency genes (see below), but exclude Intracisternal A Particle elements (IAPs) and paternally methylated control regions (ICRs) in imprinted genes (Lane et al. 2003). The maternal genome may be protected from active demethylation by a mechanism which might be linked with chromatin organisation (see below) but may also involve the protein Dppa3 (Stella) whose presence in the zygote seems to protect some imprinted genes in the maternal genome from demethylation (Nakamura et al. 2007). Active demethylation of the paternal genome is largely conserved in mammals, including in humans, rodents, and ruminants, although the precise extent of demethylation may vary slightly (Dean et al. 2001; Young and Beaujean 2004).

The mechanisms of active demethylation are still unknown, but may involve deamination of 5-methylcytosine or its removal by glycosylases, that is the base excision repair pathway, in analogy to the pathway that has been identified in plants (Gehring et al. 2006; Kress et al. 2006; Morales-Ruiz et al. 2006; Morgan et al. 2004 2005). While the nucleotide excision repair pathway has also been implicated in demethylation (Barreto et al. 2007; Weiss et al. 1996), these claims have not been substantiated (Jin et al. 2008). Finally, while there is possible chemistry for the removal of the methyl group directly from the cytosine base by oxidative demethylation (Gerken et al. 2007), it is not clear at present whether enzymes exist that demethylate 5meC by this mechanism.

Genome-wide demethylation during preimplantation development is further completed by a passive mechanism, by which DNA is replicated largely in the absence of Dnmt1, the maintenance methyltransferase. This is apparently regulated by exclusion of the enzyme from the nucleus, resulting in replication dependent demethylation of Line1 retrotransposons and many other sequences (Carlson et al. 1992); however some Dnmt1 can enter the nucleus and is needed there to maintain methylation of imprinted genes and IAPs (Hirasawa et al. 2008). How the nucleo-cytoplasmic shuttling of the enzyme is regulated is a fascinating problem which is not understood.

In PGCs there may be two phases of reprogramming, one at around E8 where some DNA methylation is lost together with H3K9 dimethylation (Seki et al. 2005), and one that appears to coincide with the arrival of the PGCs in the gonads, in which large scale chromatin changes occur together with demethylation (Hajkova et al. 2008). The mechanistic links between the erasure of histone modifications and DNA methylation at this stage are not understood, however they have been interpreted as active demethylation followed by base excision repair which may trigger histone variant H2AZ exchange leading to the disappearance of histone marks (Hajkova et al. 2008). A major purpose of erasure of epigenetic marks in PGCs is the removal of parental imprints, but other sequences (eg Line1 elements) are also demethylated, and the inactive X chromosome is reactivated, revealing more widespread reprogramming in the germline. Nevertheless, some sequences such as IAPs are more resistant to demethylation, so the whole genome is not completely demethylated (Lane et al. 2003).

It is possible that there are other reprogramming cycles which have not been described as extensively so far. First, genome wide loss of methylation (based on meC antibody staining) has also been suggested to take place in mouse spermatocytes (Loukinov et al. 2002), and imprinted X chromosome inactivation is reprogrammed in mouse inner cell mass cells through downregulation of Xist and perhaps removal of histone marks associated with X inactivation in the preimplantation embryo (Mak et al. 2004; Okamoto et al. 2004). It is interesting to note that epigenetic reprogramming appears to be linked to the attainment of stem cell pluripotency in culture, since ES, EG, and mGS (multipotent germline stem) cells can be derived from celltypes which are undergoing epigenetic reprogramming (Surani and Reik 2007).

2 Experimental Epigenetic Reprogramming

There are three main methods by which somatic cells can be epigenetically reprogrammed to a more pluripotent state; fusion, cloning, and direct reprogramming to iPS cells. Reprogramming by fusion can be done with EC, ES, and EG cells, and results in tetraploid cells whose genome epigenetically largely resembles that of the pluripotent fusion partner, indicating extensive and dominant reprogramming (Cowan et al. 2005; Tada et al. 1997 2001). For example, fusion with ES cells induces reactivation of the X chromosome, and demethylation and activation of pluripotency genes, such as *Oct4* and *Nanog* (Tada et al. 2001). Fusion with EG cells also leads to demethylation of imprinted genes, indicating a reprogramming capacity which is similar to that of the PGCs from which the EG cells were derived (Tada et al. 1997). So far, the (dominant) factors that allow ES and EG cells to reprogramme somatic cells have remained unknown, although the ability of ES cells to induce reprogramming seems to depend on expression of *Nanog* (Silva et al. 2006). Permeabilised somatic cells have also been incubated in extracts from pluripotent cells and this has shown some temporary signs of reprogramming, but stable pluripotent cells have not been derived by this method (Collas and Taranger 2006).

Somatic cell nuclear transfer (SCNT) has been used in many animals in order to reprogramme somatic cells and derive cloned animals, or stem cells from cloned embryos (Yang et al. 2007). This method harnesses the natural reprogramming capacity of the oocyte or zygote into which the somatic nucleus is transferred. While SCNT clearly achieves reprogramming in the sense that live offspring are produced, this happens at a low frequency because the majority of the resulting embryos are epigenetically or otherwise abnormal and die in utero; even offspring that survive are often abnormal. No substantial improvements of the technique have been made in recent years, presumably because the mechanisms of reprogramming are poorly understood (Yang et al. 2007).

A spectacular advancement was made a couple of years ago, when Takahashi and Yamanaka showed that mouse fibroblasts could be directly reprogrammed to ES like cells (which they called induced pluripotent state, or iPS), with a combination of four factors (Oct4, Sox2, Klf4, c-myc), which were retrovirally transduced into the fibroblasts (Takahashi and Yamanaka 2006). More recently it has been shown that c-myc is not necessary for iPS induction (Nakagawa et al. 2008; Wernig et al. 2008), and that this direct reprogramming can be done from different somatic cells and also in human cells (discussed in more detail later within the chapter). While it is the case that apparently epigenetically normal iPS cells can be derived which give rise to germ cells in chimeras and hence germline transmission, the efficiency of deriving iPS cells remains low, and the mechanistic process of epigenetic reprogramming is not understood. Recent studies indicate that the erasure of DNA methylation may be one of the critical steps limiting the efficiency of cloning as well as direct reprogramming.

3 Genome Wide Approaches to the Understanding of Reprogramming

Most of the insights into reprogramming we have at this point have been obtained by either global or by gene specific analyses. Global analyses have been done by immunofluorescence of nuclei and chromosomes with antibodies to 5meC or specific histone modifications, by digestion patterns of total genomic DNA with methylation sensitive restriction enzymes, or by chemical analysis such as HPLC of the amounts of 5meC in genomic DNA (Barreto et al. 2007; Monk et al. 1987). Some of these methods have the advantage that they can be applied to small numbers of cells, which is particularly useful when analysing germ cells and early embryos. A disadvantage is that the analysis is very global and therefore resolution is low, and as far as immunofluorescence is concerned, proper quantitation is difficult. Gene specific analyses have been conducted for DNA methylation by southern blotting, methylation sensitive PCR, and bisulphite sequencing (and variants thereof). The first gene specific analyses of histone modification in early embryos have recently been published, and are based on developing a carrier ChIP (cChIP) method, by which a small number of mouse cells are mixed with a large number of Drosophila carrier cells, whose DNA is not amplified with the gene specific PCR primers (O'Neill et al. 2006). In all, sequence or gene specific analyses of reprogramming are still low in number. While there are some general conclusions that have emerged, much more detailed information needs to be gathered.

New technologies for Epigenomics are advancing rapidly, and are briefly reviewed here (see Chapters "Strategies for Epigenome Analysis" and "Sequencing the Epigenome" for more detail). ChIP on microarray (ChIP on chip) screens using specific antibodies to histones or histone modifications, or to meC (meDIP on chip), have been in use for a number of years, the state of the art technology being oligonucleotide tiling arrays. As far as methylation is concerned, there are some alternative techniques that involve arrays, including pull-downs with methyl-binding proteins, or hybridisation of bisulphite treated DNA to arrays (Farthing et al. 2008; Reinders et al. 2008; Weber et al. 2007). These techniques are being rapidly superseded by next generation sequencing (NGS). These new studies provide unprecedented insights into periodicity and sequence dependent patterns of methylation in the genome, and it will be fascinating to apply these techniques to reprogramming tissues (Cokus et al. 2008).

3.1 MeDIP Chip of Germ Cell, Pluripotent and Differentiated Tissues

A first study has recently been completed which uses meDIP chip to analyse methylation of all the promoters in the mouse genome, and which compares germline celltypes (EG cells, sperm), with early embryonic pluripotent (ES) and multipotent extraembryonic (TS), and with more differentiated cells, mouse embryonic fibroblasts (pMEF) (Fig. 1) (Farthing et al. 2008). EG cells are derived from PGCs (in this case E11.5 and 12.5 embryos), and are pluripotent just as ES cells but in addition are expected to have demethylated imprinted genes. Sperm is one of the (analysable) mature gametes reflecting the germ cell epigenotype just before fertilisation. ES and TS cells are derived from the ICM and the TE in the blastocyst, respectively, and therefore represent the first two cell lineages in the mammalian embryo. We were therefore able to analyse methylation in gene promoters genome wide in EG cells (e.g. after reprogramming occurs in PGCs), at the end of male gametogenesis, at the intersection between reprogramming in the preimplantation embryo and, potentially, programming of the first lineage specific methylation marks, and following the major de novo methylation programming phase in postimplantation embryos, represented by pMEFs. Because of the extensive de novo methylation of the genome during spermatogenesis, which includes imprinted and non-imprinted sequences, we expected the sperm genome to be substantially differently methylated from the EG and ES genomes. Extensive reprogramming after fertilisation would then convert the sperm epigenotype into an ES epigenotype. Comparing ES with TS cells might enable detection of genes differentially methylated between the two cardinal lineages, embryonic and extraembryonic, and thus reveal epigenetic principles of early cell lineage determination. Finally, a comparison between ES cells and pMEFs might be expected to reveal methylation of genes that are needed in pluripotent cell types, and which are stably repressed in differentiated somatic tissues.

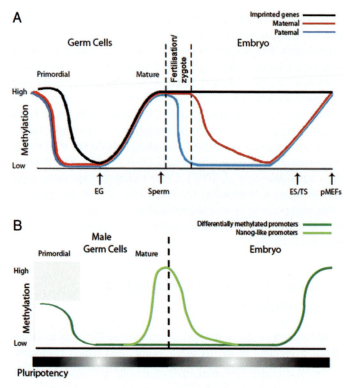

Fig. 1 The changing landscape of methylation during development. (**A**) Two waves of methylation reprogramming occur during development. During germ cell development a wave of demethylation followed by de novo methylation takes place before the germ cells are mature. At fertilisation paternally derived chromosomes undergo active demethylation and both maternal and paternal chromosomes are demethylated passively in a replication dependent manner. The methylation status of imprinted genes is conserved during this second wave of methylation reprogramming. As pluripotency is lost, methylation is gained during differentiation. (**B**) A model for the methylation reprogramming events at promoters differentially methylated during development. It is unclear from our studies whether promoter specific methylation is gained up to early PGC stages. Most promoters in the mouse genome, however, remain unmethylated during the germline-pluripotency life-cycle, EG and ES cells are hypomethylated, yet surprisingly we found that mature sperm was also hypomethylated to a similar extent at promoters. Some genes such as *Nanog* undergo cycles of de novo methylation during germ cell development and must be demethylated in the early embryo. Presumably this enables loss and re-establishment of pluripotency in a cyclical fashion (shaded bar). Demethylation of the promoters of these genes is thus critical for the pluripotent part of the germline cycle (*light region*), while re-methylation is crucial for the differentiation part of this cycle (*dark region*)

The output of meDIP chip is displayed on a genome browser interface (ChIP-Monk, Fig. 2a), which shows the hybridisation signal on each oligonucleotide tile across a promoter, in relation to the median of the cell type under study. Bars that point upwards from the median thus indicate more methylation, while bars pointing downwards indicate less methylation than the median. Selected patterns can then

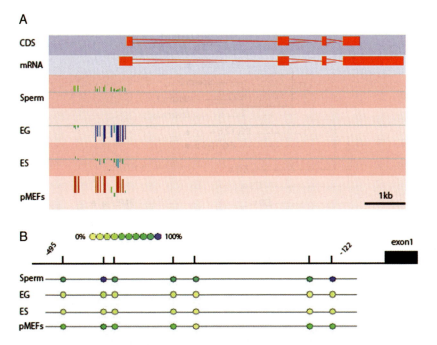

Fig. 2 Validation of meDIP candidate, *Nanog*, using Sequenom MassArray technology. (**A**) The genome-wide meDIP data were plotted into a ChIPMonk profile showing methylation at promoter regions. This example shows the promoter of *Nanog* in various cell types. The middle line represents the median signal intensity of the array. Each vertical bar represents the methylation signal at an individual oligonucleotide probe; above the median line indicates relative hypermethylation and below indicates relative hypomethylation. (**B**) A Sequenom profile of the *Nanog* promoter. Sequenom MassArray technology gives quantitative measurements of the methylation level and is comparable to the classical bisulphite sequencing analysis. Blue circles indicate complete methylation; yellow circles indicate no methylation at individual CpG units

be confirmed either by bisulphite sequencing or by Sequenom Massarray bisulphite analysis (Fig. 2b). It should be noted that peaks of methylation as measured by meDIP hybridisation to a particular oligonucleotide tile do not necessarily correspond in their location precisely to where the methylated CpGs are in the promoter area. This is because the fragments of DNA that are pulled down by the meC antibody have a certain size range (typically 300–800 bp), and will therefore hybridise to a number of tiles if they are close together. In order to compare methylation profiles between tissue types, and to identify groups of genes that show the biggest changes in methylation between tissues, we wrote evaluation algorithms that take patterns of hybridisation into account as well as absolute values. The best algorithm we have been able to develop so far results in validation of predicted methylation profiles (by Sequenom) of higher than 88%.

Global comparisons between different cell types show interesting, and some unexpected patterns (Fig. 3). What was expected was that ES and EG cells would resemble each other closely. What was unexpected was that sperm also

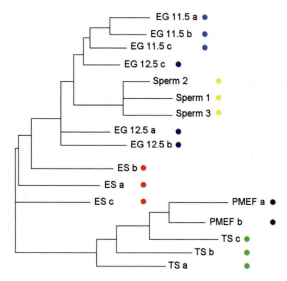

Fig. 3 Global comparisons of promoter methylation patterns between cell types. Pairwise correlation comparisons were made between all cell types to establish the similarity of promoter methylation and a correlation tree was plotted. Replicates of each cell type are indicated by colour. This clearly shows good correlation between the global promoter methylation patterns of ES cells, EG cells and sperm, but poor correlation of these with pMEFs and TS cells

resembles the two pluripotent cell types very closely. The most pronounced differences that occur in promoter methylation are between the pluripotent group (EG, ES, sperm) and pMEFs, and between ES cells and TS cells, respectively, and the great majority of these are in the form of hypomethylated promoters in pluripotent cells, and hypermethylated promoters in pMEFs and TS cells. Thus the general methylation signature of pluripotent or reprogrammed tissues appears to be hypomethylation. It was unexpected that sperm matches this pattern so well; however other recent studies have also found that promoters in human (Weber et al. 2007), and mouse sperm (Oakes et al. 2007) tend to be globally hypomethylated. This is interesting because it means that globally promoters do not have to be reprogrammed after fertilisation by demethylation in order to be expressible in the embryo. It does raise, however, the question of what sequences it is which are methylated in the sperm genome and then become reprogrammed after fertilisation (this is the pattern observed by immunofluorescence). Clearly Line1 repeats (of which there are about 100,000 copies in the genome) do become substantially demethylated in the zygote and cleavage stage embryo (Lane et al. 2003), and other repeat families and possibly also genes outside of the promoter regions may do the same. This needs to be investigated in more detail.

While most promoters therefore appear to be hypomethylated in sperm, we found a small group of genes where this was not the case. This group includes some interesting genes, such as *Nanog* and *Lefty1*, which are key regulators of pluripotency or early embryo patterning. *Oct4* and *Sox2* have also been found to be methylated, in cis-regulatory regions outside of their promoters, in sperm (Imamura et al. 2006). The reason for methylating this small group of pluripotency regulators might be that differentiation during spermatogenesis requires their tight silencing (akin to a group of pluripotency regulators becoming methylated in somatic cells such as pMEFs, see below). This raises the question whether methylation in these promoters becomes reprogrammed after fertilisation, as it ought to since the promoters are hypomethylated in ES cells. This was directly tested for the *Nanog* promoter which indeed showed complete demethylation towards the blastocyst stage by a combination of active and passive demethylation (Farthing et al. 2008). Because targeting the *Nanog* promoter with DNA methylation leads to it being silenced, it can therefore be concluded that methylation reprogramming in the preimplantation embryo is actually necessary for pluripotency and embryo development. It will be highly desirable to carry out a similar analysis for oocytes, which with developing miniaturisation of epigenomics techniques should be possible in the future (see Section 5.1).

3.2 Determination of Lineage Fate – Epigenetic Gatekeeper Genes

It is generally believed that lineage decisions in the mammalian embryo are brought about by differential expression of key determinants such as transcription factors (e.g. *Oct4, Nanog* and *Sox2* for the ICM derived embryonic lineage, *Tead4, Cdx2* and *Eomes* for the TE derived extraembryonic lineage). Expressions of such transcription factors or combinations of transcription factors then induce networks of gene expression and epigenetic modifications characteristic of the cell fate under study (Jaenisch and Young 2008). The epigenetic marks that are thus induced, which include histone modifications and DNA methylation, are thought to confer stability of the differentiated state, and to prevent transdifferentiation and dedifferentiation and hence keep development of complex organisms generally on track (Reik 2007). Many recent studies have confirmed that lineage determinants and epigenetic modifiers (such as polycomb genes) are important regulators of inner cell mass fate and ES cell pluripotency, for example, but the interplay between these different systems is not well understood (Jaenisch and Young 2008). What is also not understood is how differential patterns of transcription factor expression and differential epigenetic marks are first set up. For example, there are diverse theories about how in the mammalian preimplantation embryo the first body axis (the embryonic-abembryonic one) is established at the blastocyst stage, and with it the identity of inner cell mass and trophectoderm lineages. One school of thought suggests that earlier dividing cells in the morula are more likely to give rise to ICM cells, while later dividing cells have a greater tendency to contribute to TE (Rossant 2008). Another school suggests that there may be cytoplasmic determinants in the zygote whose asymmetric distribution amongst dividing blastomeres determines their fate; this model borrows from the well established deterministic systems in Drosophila or *C.elegans* which have relatively large egg cytoplasms (Zernicka-Goetz 2006). However mammalian eggs are relatively small, and this together with the fact that early blastomeres show remarkable developmental plasticity does not support a deterministic model. Nevertheless, it is possible that individual blastomeres from the 4 cell stage or so do have slight preferences for allocation to the ICM or TE, respectively, and this can apparently be associated with different levels of histone argine methylation (Torres-Padilla et al. 2007). It is interesting to note that at the late morula and early blastocyst stage the lineage determinants *Oct4, Nanog*, and *Cdx2* are mosaically expressed both in inside and outside cells, suggesting a stochastic element to lineage allocation at this stage (Dietrich and Hiiragi 2007).

As far as epigenetic modifications are concerned, apart from the reported differences in histone arginine methylation between blastomeres at the 4 cell stage (which might also be cell-cycle related), the earliest confirmed differences occur at the blastocyst stage, at which DNA methylation overall (as judged by immunofluorescence) increases in the inner cell mass but not so much in the TE (Dean et al. 2001; Santos et al. 2002). It is not known which sequences become methylated at this stage in the ICM, but based on the immunofluorescence patterns it can be speculated that centromeric heterochromatin might be one of the first targets, and that this might involve the de novo methyltransferase Dnmt3b (Branco et al. 2008). Based on this pattern, and the earlier observations that extraembryonic tissues in comparison to embryonic ones remain relatively undermethylated also later in development (Monk et al. 1987), we speculated that DNA methylation in the ICM might be associated with segregation between embryonic and extraembryonic lineages (Dean et al. 2001; Santos et al. 2002). Indeed recent work from the Hemberger and our lab confirms this hypothesis. Mouse ES cells cannot normally differentiate into the trophoblast lineage (while they can differentiate into many derivatives of the primary embryonic lineages). However, ES cells that are deficient in DNA methylation differentiate highly efficiently into trophoblast cells in vitro, apparently following the normal sequence of differentiation into trophoblast stem cells, intermediate trophoblast, and giant cells (Ng et al. 2008). In a genome-wide screen for promoter methylation between ES and TS cells, a very small number of genes with methylated promoters in ES and hypomethylated promoters in TS cells were identified. Amongst these, the extraembryonic transcription factor *Elf5* is of particular interest. It was found that *Elf5* is demethylated in methylation-deficient ES cells, and expressed during TS cell differentiation slightly downstream of *Cdx2* and *Eomes*. Elf5 deficiency abolished the maintenance of trophoblast stem cells. Elf5 was found by ChIP to bind to the *Cdx2* and *Eomes* promoters, and to activate *Cdx2* and *Eomes* transcription.

From these results it appears that Elf5 has a key role in trophoblast differentiation by being induced through Cdx2 and Eomes, but then establishing a positive feedback loop with these two factors in order to sustain TS cell expansion and maintenance (Ng et al. 2008). By contrast, in the epiblast lineage, in which early on *Cdx2* can be expressed in a stochastic fashion, *Elf5* cannot be induced because its promoter is methylated, and this does not allow a positive feedback loop to be established, thus aborting TS cell fate.

From these observations a new model of lineage 'canalisation' can be formulated, which involves the initial stochastic expression of lineage determinants such as *Cdx2* or *Oct4*, followed by positive reinforcement by an epigenetically regulated gatekeeper such as *Elf5*. This is attractive because of the established plasticity of mammalian blastomeres, which would later be canalised by epigenetically regulated gatekeepers. This model raises the question of when and how epiblast specific methylation of *Elf5* is established, since it is possible that this is a primary event in ICM allocation. It is also interesting to ask if reciprocal epigenetic gatekeepers exist that keep the TE lineage from transdifferentiating to embryonic cells, and if so what type of epigenetic marking system this might involve.

3.3 Epigenetic Inactivation of Pluripotency Genes in Somatic Cells

As outlined above, pluripotency regulators are expressed in ICM and epiblast, ES cells, and PGCs but are largely silenced in somatic lineages. A number of studies show that inactivation of these genes in somatic cells involves stable epigenetic silencing, including by DNA methylation. The genome wide profiling of DNA methylation in mouse promoters in pluripotent and other cell types has revealed a class of genes whose promoters are differentially methylated between ES cells and pMEFs, with the 70 most differentially methylated genes all being hypomethylated in ES cells and hypermethylated in pMEFs (Farthing et al. 2008). Many of these genes are also highly expressed in ES cells and silenced in pMEFs. This selection of genes is clearly enriched in pluripotency regulators; it contains *Nanog*, *Cripto*, *Rex1*, *Lefty1* amongst others. *Oct4* has also been shown to acquire promoter methylation during differentiation and silencing, and in this case the sequence of epigenetic silencing events has been characterised in more detail. It appears that the *Oct4* promoter first attracts H3K9 methylation which is mediated by the histone methyltransferase G9a, and this is followed by de novo DNA methylation of the promoter (Feldman et al. 2006). This silent state, as well as that of other pluripotency regulators, seems difficult to reverse since somatic nuclear transfer embryos (cloned embryos) often show defects in demethylating the DNA of the somatic nucleus including promoters of pluripotency genes, which fail to be appropriately activated as a consequence (Yang et al. 2007). Demethylation of pluripotency gene promoters may also be a limiting factor in the efficiency with which iPS cells can be generated (see below). However, in preimplantation embryos in vivo demethylation of the *Nanog* promoter from its completely methylated state in the sperm genome proceeds incredibly efficiently apparently by both active and passive demethylation (Farthing et al. 2008). The mechanistic understanding of this natural reprogramming and harnessing of the factors that are involved for the reprogramming of epigenetically inactivated pluripotency genes in somatic tissues therefore remains a critical goal in reprogramming research.

4 Epigenetic Reprogramming During Cloning and iPS Generation

Experimental reprogramming either through somatic cell nuclear transfer (SCNT), cell fusion or by direct reprogramming through the addition of a limited number of factors results in dramatic changes to the epigenome. It is extraordinary that this reprogramming can occur successfully at all in the absence of the normal reprogramming stages that occur during germline development and post fertilisation. Here we review the success of these experimental techniques from the point of view of epigenetic reprogramming.

SCNT has variable outcomes with cloned embryos dying throughout development as well as perinatally. Often those embryos analysed at later developmental stages had placental abnormalities (Inoue et al. 2002; Kang et al. 2002). The epigenetic profiles of cloned embryos from various species are just as varied, including abnormal inactivation of the X chromosome in females (Eggan et al. 2000; Xue et al. 2002), DNA methylation defects genome-wide and of specific gene and repetitive elements (Bourc'his et al. 2001; Dean et al. 2001; Humpherys et al. 2001; Kang et al. 2001), imprinting defects (Humpherys et al. 2001; Inoue et al. 2002; Mann et al. 2003; Yang et al. 2005) and inappropriate covalent histone modifications (Inoue et al. 2006; Kishigami et al. 2007; Santos et al. 2003). These epigenetic abnormalities are consistent with the observed gene expression defects which include failure to activate the key genes involved in establishing and maintaining pluripotency (Boiani et al. 2003; Boiani et al. 2002; Bortvin et al. 2003). Some or all of these defects in epigenetic reprograming likely underlie the premature deaths of successfully cloned animals as their offspring appear normal (Zhang et al. 2004).

Taking a comparative approach to the reprogramming that occurs post nuclear transfer, the active demethylation of the paternal pronucleus (Mayer et al. 2000; Oswald et al. 2000; Santos et al. 2002) is mirrored to some extent by some active demethylation within the early cloned embryo (Dean et al. 2001). However, there are defects observed in the passive, replication dependent, demethylation that should follow early active demethylation. This abnormal passive loss of DNA methylation has been suggested to occur because the somatic form of Dnmt1 remains in the donor nucleus and this may also be exasperated by abnormal translocation of the oocyte-specific form (Dnmt1o) into the nucleus (Chung et al. 2003) both perhaps preventing the normal reduction of methylation within non-imprinted genes. Imprinted genes are also affected, being found in one study to be abnormally expressed in dead but not surviving cloned calfs (Yang et al. 2005). The dynamics of methylation reprogramming during normal development appear to differ somewhat between species (Park et al. 2007; Young and Beaujean 2004) so it is likely that the extent to which any abnormalities in reprogramming the methylation profile of the donor epigenome affect the developmental outcome of the cloned embryo also vary between species and caution should be used in drawing conclusions across species.

The overall nuclear architecture of cells from cloned embryos has been observed to resemble that of the donor cell nucleus, particularly in the appearance of pericentric heterochromatin, (Beaujean et al. 2004; Dean et al. 2001; Martin et al. 2006) suggesting that often limited genome-wide reorganisation occurs post nuclear transfer. One of the major chromosome-wide reorganisations that must occur is the reactivation of the inactive X chromosome of the somatic donor nucleus. Normally the inactive X chromosome is reactivated in the germ line and then again in the cells of the inner cell mass after a period of imprinted Xi, whereas cells of the trophectoderm retain the paternally imprinted Xi (Mak et al. 2004; Sugimoto and Abe 2007). Several groups have analysed this process post nuclear transfer (Bao et al. 2005; Eggan et al. 2000; Senda et al. 2004) and whilst most agree that reactivation does occur, the extent of this and whether later inactivation occurs randomly as normal in the ICM is debated (Senda et al. 2004).

X chromosome inactivation involves both hypermethylation of the promoters of X-linked genes (Goto and Monk 1998; Weber et al. 2005) and the accumulation of repressive histone modifications and histone variants (Brinkman et al. 2006; Okamoto et al. 2004; Valley et al. 2006). Genome-wide abnormalities in histone modifications have also been observed post SCNT (Inoue et al. 2006; Santos et al. 2003; Wee et al. 2006). Post fertilisation asymmetry in histone acetylation normally occurs as the paternal epigenome gains acetylation more rapidly (Adenot et al. 1997; Sarmento et al. 2004), however, in cloned embryos by the 2 cell stage differences in both the level of acetylation and the residues modified are observed relative to control embryos (Inoue et al. 2006). The importance of correct reprogramming during cloning is highlighted by the finding that the success rate of SCNT greatly improved following treatment of cloned embryos with a histone deacetylase inhibitor and chromatin remodeller, trichostatin A (Kishigami et al. 2007).

In an attempt to identify particular genes or genomic regions affected by nuclear transfer (NT) Hikichi et al analysed changes in gene expression between parthenogenetic ES (pES) cells and NT-pES cells (Hikichi et al. 2008). Whilst only 7 genes were identified, these included the imprinted gene *U2af1-rs1* for which expression and bi-maternal methylation levels returned to normal post NT (hypermethylation was lost and "paternal" expression resumed). Moreover, loss of methylation was observed at this methylated promoter in NT-ES cell lines derived from several different somatic donor nuclei. However, other differentially methylated regions have retained the parthenogenetic methylation status in NT-pES cells (Hikichi et al. 2008; Hikichi et al. 2007), suggesting that reprogramming may be specific to this particular gene and that it, along with the other 6 genes identified, may be a candidate for determining developmental potential.

The molecular mechanisms that underlie the use of specified factors in direct reprogramming are not yet known, but the improvement of the technique to a stage where iPS cells are able to contribute to germline chimeras (Okita et al. 2007) clearly shows ability to reprogramme to a pluripotent state. Initial use of the four factors (Oct4, Sox2, Klf4 and c-myc) to reprogramme fibroblasts combined with selection based on the expression of *Fbx15* resulted in iPS cells that could differentiate to all three germ layers both in vitro and in vivo, however, they made no contribution to the germ line (Takahashi and Yamanaka 2006). Experimental reprogramming using cell fusion showed that hypermethylation at the promoters of pluripotency genes was lost (Cowan et al. 2005; Tada et al. 2001) and so true direct reprogramming should result in demethylation to the same extent. The starting tissue showed extensive methylation at the promoters of the key pluripotency regulators *Oct3/4* and *Nanog* consistent with silenced expression within these differentiated cells. However, the epigenetic profile of the Fbx15-iPS cells indicated that whilst loss of hypermethylation at the promoter of *Fbx15* had occurred, the promoters of *Oct3/4* and *Nanog* were only partially reprogrammed to the methylation status of ES cells. Moreover when chromatin marks at these specific promoters were analysed using ChIP, whilst histone H3 showed significantly increased acetylation and decreased dimethylation of lysine 9 relative to MEFs, levels were still abnormally low/high respectively in comparison to those in ES cells. Using *Nanog* expression to select for iPS cells was more successful in producing cells reprogrammed to a greater extent as indicated by the increased similarity of the methylation status of iPS cells at the promoters of *Nanog* and *Oct3/4* relative to ES cells and the germline competence of these cells (Okita et al. 2007). The methylation patterns of selected imprinted genes in these Nanog-iPS cells are similar to ES cells rather than EG cells indicating that direct reprogramming resembles more the reprogramming that occurs naturally post fertilisation and experimentally in SCNT rather than the reprogramming in the germline where imprints are erased.

Recently more careful consideration has been taken as to whether directly reprogrammed iPS cells regain ES cell-like chromatin states as well as being able to contribute to the germline. Mikkelsen et al have generated genome-wide maps of specific chromatin marks using ChIP-Seq, indicating great similarity between fully reprogrammed iPS cells and ES cells (Mikkelsen et al. 2008). Importantly this study also dissected the potentially intermediate states by analysing partially reprogrammed cells. These cells, whilst lacking expression of key pluripotency genes, had down-regulated structural and regulatory factors expressed in MEFs and upregulated several related to self-renewal and proliferation. Together with another study this indicates that reactivation of genes expressed in ES cells occurs in a sequential manner (Brambrink et al. 2008; Mikkelsen et al. 2008). Importantly Mikkelsen et al go on to suggest a correlation between the pattern of reactivation during direct reprogramming and the chromatin status in the starting tissue. Between the starting tissue and the intermediate stage, promoters categorised as having a certain CpG dinucleotide content and marked with H3K4me3 in MEFs were highly likely to get reactivated at the intermediate stage, whereas those marked with H3K27me3 or neither mark were not. When promoters with bivalent histone marks in ES cells, correlating with repressed developmental genes (Bernstein et al. 2006), were analysed the intermediate iPS cells had a higher proportion of bivalent marks at these promoters than the MEFs, but fewer than the completely reprogrammed iPS (Oct4-iPS) cells, consistent with partial dedifferentiation.

The differing timescales involved in the experimental reprogramming via nuclear transfer in comparison to production of iPS cells is hardly surprising given the paring down of factors involved. The final transition to pluripotency appears to involve reprogramming of chromatin marks back to a bivalent status and demethylation at key pluripotency-specific loci. Indeed Mikkelsen et al showed that treatment of partially reprogrammed cells with the DNA methyltransferase inhibitor 5-azacytidine increased the number of cells that make the transition to a fully reprogrammed iPS state (Mikkelsen et al. 2008). Further analysis of the partially reprogrammed cells and the mechanisms involved in making the final reprogramming step should produce candidates for understanding and increasing the efficiency of epigenetic reprogramming.

5 Outlook

5.1 Candidates and Screens for Reprogramming Factors

Embryonic stem cells are valuable undifferentiated cell types that have received much attention due to the wide range of potential they can offer for regenerative medicine (Murry and Keller 2008). They have the ability to develop into any type of adult cell and are able to maintain their pluripotency indefinitely, if provided with the right environment. The attractiveness of a method to easily and efficiently generate patient-specific pluripotent stem cells is clear (Jaenisch and Young 2008; Yamanaka 2007). Whilst differentiated cells (except some immune cells) and pluripotent cells contain the same genome, they differ in shape, function and differentiation potential. Since reverting the cellular identity of a differentiated cell to a pluripotent cell has been shown to be possible and since we know that major determinants in generating these differences are DNA methylation (at 5meC) and histone modifications, the identification of factors that are able to reprogramme these marks will be key to future therapeutic use.

To date, there have been several methods developed that can induce pluripotency in somatic cells: nuclear transfer into oocytes (Wakayama and Yanagimachi 2001), cellular fusions with embryonic stem cells (Cowan et al. 2005; Tada et al. 2001) or germ cells (Tada et al. 1997). In 2006, Takahashi et al reported the identification of four factors able to reprogram somatic cells to induced pluripotent cells (iPS cells) by means of retroviral transfection (Takahashi and Yamanaka 2006). The four genes (Oct4, Sox2, Klf4 and c-Myc) were the result of an exclusion screening strategy starting from 24 candidate genes for reprogramming of somatic cells. The authors based their candidate selection hypothesis on the fact that the genes must have an essential role in maintaining ES cell identity. The mechanisms these defined factors use to directly reprogramme the somatic cells are as yet undefined. As mentioned above, the identification of factors that are involved in demethylation of DNA may be particularly critical, but up to now no *bona fide* mammalian demethylase has been found. Demethylation of DNA can occur theoretically either by direct removal of the methyl group from the cytosine base, or by removal of the methyl group together with the cytosine (Morgan et al. 2005), and the most favoured are the indirect, repair-based removal of 5meC by DNA deaminases, glycosylases, or the theoretically possible direct removal by dioxygenases. Morgan et al showed that the cytidine deaminases AID and APOBEC1 can deaminate 5meC and are expressed in tissues in which reprogramming occurs (Morgan et al. 2004). Their role in demethylation in vivo needs to be assessed genetically. In 2006 two genes were identified in plants with 5meC DNA glycosylase activity, DME and ROS1 (Gehring et al. 2006; Gong et al. 2002; Morales-Ruiz et al. 2006). DME was identified in a screen for parent-of origin effects on seed viability (Choi et al. 2002) and ROS1 was found by screening for mutants that caused transcriptional gene silencing of an active transgene and endogenous gene with a homologous promoter (Gong et al. 2002). DME and ROS1 are closely related proteins with a glycosylase/lyase domain that are able to cleave the N-glycosydic bond and remove the 5meC base leaving a gap which is subsequently repaired through the base excision repair pathway (Gehring et al. 2006). This involves insertion of an unmethylated cystosine by a DNA polymerase and the nick is sealed by DNA ligase. There are no apparent othologues or homologues of these large bifunctional glycosylases in the mammalian genome.

Barreto et al describe a different type of screen where a Xenopus expression library was screened for factors that would reactivate luciferase expression from a promoter silenced by methylation (Barreto et al. 2007). In this screen, the stress-response gene Gadd45a was isolated in three independent active pools by sib selection. Gadd45a expression is induced by p53, is known to be implicated in the G2 cell cycle checkpoint and is involved in maintaining genomic stability. Gadd45 genes generally are stress inducible and play a role in many biological processes like cell cycle, senescence, and apoptosis. In the luciferase reporter assay used, the authors showed that Gadd45a was able to reactivate expression from a normally silenced methylated promoter by three fold. The expression of endogenous *Oct4* was also induced by Gadd45, similar to the effect of a combination of the methylation inhibitor 5-aza-2′deoxycytidine and the histone deacetylase inhibitor trichostatin A. In a subsequent report however the human GADD45a protein was not found to induce demethylation, and therefore the role of Gadd45 in demethylation, if any, remains unclear (Jin et al. 2008).

The elucidation of the mechanism of active DNA demethylation in mammals therefore remains a key objective for reprogramming. A number of approaches can be envisaged by which demethylases might be isolated. For example, assays can be constructed where demethylation is detected by activation of reporters normally repressed by DNA methylation (such as in the assay in which Gadd45a was isolated), or using in vitro methods where for example demethylation may enable specific amplification of a DNA fragment, revealing a factor that caused demethylation. Other selection schemes may be used such as those in bacterial cells where DNA demethylation may promote survival of the cells that express a DNA demethylase, allowing identification of the factor(s) involved.

5.2 Future Approaches to Epigenomic Profiling of Reprogramming

Current applications to analyse DNA methylation patterns of genomic regions include bisulphite sequencing and meDIP (methylated DNA immunoprecipitation) combined with hybridization to arrays (Weber et al. 2005; Zhang et al. 2006).

Recently, new DNA sequencing methodologies have been introduced, all in different stages of development (Bentley 2006), providing fast and cost-effective tools to analyse whole genomes. These methods also offer new opportunities for analysing methylated DNA. One of the new sequencing methods is the Solexa sequencing technology (Illumina GA) where single molecules are attached to a surface and amplified to form a cluster followed by sequencing in real time using fluorescently-labelled nucleotides. DNA after ChIP is sequenced at levels of 30 million reads per experiment, allowing deep coverage and precise positioning of histone modifications, transcription factor binding, and DNA methylation (ChIP-Seq and meDIP-Seq). Next generation sequencing has already been applied to whole genome bisulphite sequencing of Arabidopsis (BS-Seq) (Cokus et al. 2008), and is in principle applicable to single nucleotide mapping of methylation patterns in mammalian genomes too. Cokus et al. created sequence fragments that mapped successfully to the genome and covered 93% of all cytosines. This study generated a comprehensive view of the plant DNA methylation landscape determining the levels and the patterns of cytosine methylation in different contexts (CG, CHG and CHH – where H is A, C or T). There are several advantages of the BS-Seq compared to the microarray based methods, it is more sensitive: several previously undetected methylated regions have been described; it is more accurate: the microarray data rely on the antibody binding and DNA hybridization efficiency therefore detection is more noise-prone and variable; and BS-Seq is better for analysing repetitive sequences where microarrays suffer due to cross-hybridization; most importantly it is at a single base resolution. BS-Seq has proven to be a powerful methodology that can be applied to analyse methylated DNA in other organisms as well. The mouse and human epigenome is dynamic during development and within different cell types, therefore having such a fast and accurate sequencing technique available will enable us to have a more detailed understanding of how DNA methylation is linked to transcriptional control in developmental processes. A comparative approach between different cell types would be interesting in order to analyse the changing epigenomic landscape during development and in disease. A critical aspect that has to still be optimised is the amount of starting material (i.e. DNA) necessary for the bisulphite conversion, especially when dealing with the limited availability of cells such as germ cells and early embryos. Since the amount of DNA needed for the sequencing can be decreased significantly the limiting factor is the bisulphite conversion where much of the DNA is fragmented due to the harsh chemical treatment.

5.3 Applications to Medicine

Adult stem cells are capable of maintaining, generating and replacing terminally differentiated cells within their own tissues as a process of natural turnover and following tissue injury. Moreover, these cells have also been shown to be versatile, being able to differentiate across lineages, tissues, and germ layer boundaries (Hennessy et al. 2004). In addition, mesenchymal stem cells (MSC) may be a very promising alternative source of multipotent cells in tissue replacement therapies (Porada et al. 2006). Nevertheless, embryonic stem cells (ES cells) have many advantages over adult stem cells since they are easier to isolate, can be propagated indefinitely and are capable of generating terminally differentiated cells of all three embryonic germ layers. There are three main areas where ES cells can contribute to important developments in medicine: generation of new tissues and organs, cell replacement therapy and drug discovery (Keller 2005). Successful generation of pluripotent stem cells from somatic cells (SCNT, fusion and iPS cells) and advances in understanding the mechanisms underlying stem cell differentiation into various adult tissues have generated great hopes for personalised regenerative medicine where new tissues can be generated starting from the patient's own cells (Yamanaka 2007). Much is known about the developmental pathways from ES cells to differentiated cells and protocols have been developed to generate a large spectrum of cell types: hematopoietic cells, cardiomyocytes, oligodendrocytes, dopamine neurons and pancreatic β cells (Erceg et al. 2008; Kawasaki et al. 2000; Kroon et al. 2008; Laflamme et al. 2007; Murry and Keller 2008; Ott et al. 2008; van Laake et al. 2008). There are many challenges as well for clinical application of stem cells: tumourigenicity (natural tendency of undifferentiated ES cells to form teratomas), purity of the differentiated cells (this depends very much on the quality of the starting material), immune rejection, absolute control of the factors necessary to programme the cells down specific lineages (Murry and Keller 2008). The technique of direct reprogramming to form iPS cells must, in addition, address the consequences of the use of retroviral genes. Recently it has been shown that in the process of inducing pluripotency, the first 12 days are critical where the retrovirally transfected genes have to be active and later on the pluripotency will be self-sustained (Jaenisch and Young 2008). It remains to be shown whether delivering the proteins themselves during this critical time window will have the same potential to induce pluripotency. The use of small molecules in direct reprogramming is an additional appealing prospect for generating iPS cells, maintaining pluripotency and differentiating ES cells into adult cells (Xu et al. 2008).

References

Adenot, P.G., Mercier, Y., Renard, J.P., and Thompson, E.M. (1997). Differential H4 acetylation of paternal and maternal chromatin precedes DNA replication and differential transcriptional activity in pronuclei of 1-cell mouse embryos. Development (Cambridge, England) *124*, 4615–4625.

Bao, S., Miyoshi, N., Okamoto, I., Jenuwein, T., Heard, E., and Azim Surani, M. (2005). Initiation of epigenetic reprogramming of the X chromosome in somatic nuclei transplanted to a mouse oocyte. EMBO reports *6*, 748–754.

Barreto, G., Schafer, A., Marhold, J., Stach, D., Swaminathan, S.K., Handa, V., Doderlein, G., Maltry, N., Wu, W., Lyko, F., *et al.* (2007). Gadd45a promotes epigenetic gene activation by repair-mediated DNA demethylation. Nature *445*, 671–675.

Beaujean, N., Taylor, J., Gardner, J., Wilmut, I., Meehan, R., and Young, L. (2004). Effect of limited DNA methylation reprogramming in the normal sheep embryo on somatic cell nuclear transfer. Biology of Reproduction *71*, 185–193.

Bentley, D.R. (2006). Whole-genome re-sequencing. Current Opinion in Genetics & Development *16*, 545–552.
Bernstein, B.E., Mikkelsen, T.S., Xie, X., Kamal, M., Huebert, D.J., Cuff, J., Fry, B., Meissner, A., Wernig, M., Plath, K., et al. (2006). A bivalent chromatin structure marks key developmental genes in embryonic stem cells. Cell *125*, 315–326.
Boiani, M., Eckardt, S., Leu, N.A., Scholer, H.R., and McLaughlin, K.J. (2003). Pluripotency deficit in clones overcome by clone-clone aggregation: epigenetic complementation? EMBO Journal *22*, 5304–5312.
Boiani, M., Eckardt, S., Scholer, H.R., and McLaughlin, K.J. (2002). Oct4 distribution and level in mouse clones: consequences for pluripotency. Genes and Development *16*, 1209–1219.
Bortvin, A., Eggan, K., Skaletsky, H., Akutsu, H., Berry, D.L., Yanagimachi, R., Page, D.C., and Jaenisch, R. (2003). Incomplete reactivation of Oct4-related genes in mouse embryos cloned from somatic nuclei. Development (Cambridge, England) *130*, 1673–1680.
Bourc'his, D., Le Bourhis, D., Patin, D., Niveleau, A., Comizzoli, P., Renard, J.P., and Viegas-Pequignot, E. (2001). Delayed and incomplete reprogramming of chromosome methylation patterns in bovine cloned embryos. Current Biology *11*, 1542–1546.
Brambrink, T., Foreman, R., Welstead, G.G., Lengner, C.J., Wernig, M., Suh, H., and Jaenisch, R. (2008). Sequential expression of pluripotency markers during direct reprogramming of mouse somatic cells. Cell Stem Cell *2*, 151–159.
Branco, M., Oda, M., and Reik, W. (2008). Safeguarding parental identity: Dnmt1 maintains imprints during epigenetic reprogramming in early embryogenesis. Genes & Development *22(12)*, 1567–71.
Brinkman, A.B., Roelofsen, T., Pennings, S.W., Martens, J.H., Jenuwein, T., and Stunnenberg, H.G. (2006). Histone modification patterns associated with the human X chromosome. EMBO Reports *7*, 628–634.
Carlson, L.L., Page, A.W., and Bestor, T.H. (1992). Properties and localization of DNA methyltransferase in preimplantation mouse embryos: implications for genomic imprinting. Genes & Development *6*, 2536–2541.
Choi, Y., Gehring, M., Johnson, L., Hannon, M., Harada, J.J., Goldberg, R.B., Jacobsen, S.E., and Fischer, R.L. (2002). DEMETER, a DNA glycosylase domain protein, is required for endosperm gene imprinting and seed viability in arabidopsis. Cell *110*, 33–42.
Chung, Y.G., Ratnam, S., Chaillet, J.R., and Latham, K.E. (2003). Abnormal regulation of DNA methyltransferase expression in cloned mouse embryos. Biology of Reproduction *69*, 146–153.
Cokus, S.J., Feng, S., Zhang, X., Chen, Z., Merriman, B., Haudenschild, C.D., Pradhan, S., Nelson, S.F., Pellegrini, M., and Jacobsen, S.E. (2008). Shotgun bisulphite sequencing of the Arabidopsis genome reveals DNA methylation patterning. Nature *452*, 215–219.
Collas, P., and Taranger, C.K. (2006). Epigenetic reprogramming of nuclei using cell extracts. Stem Cell Reviews *2*, 309–317.
Cowan, C.A., Atienza, J., Melton, D.A., and Eggan, K. (2005). Nuclear Reprogramming of Somatic Cells After Fusion with Human Embryonic Stem Cells. Science (New York, NY *309*, 1369–1373.
Dean, W., Santos, F., Stojkovic, M., Zakhartchenko, V., Walter, J., Wolf, E., and Reik, W. (2001). Conservation of methylation reprogramming in mammalian development: aberrant reprogramming in cloned embryos. Proceedings of the National Academy of Sciences of the United States of America *98*, 13734–13738.
Dietrich, J.E., and Hiiragi, T. (2007). Stochastic patterning in the mouse pre-implantation embryo. Development (Cambridge, England) *134*, 4219–4231.
Eggan, K., Akutsu, H., Hochedlinger, K., Rideout, W., 3rd, Yanagimachi, R., and Jaenisch, R. (2000). X-Chromosome inactivation in cloned mouse embryos. Science (New York, NY *290*, 1578–1581.
Erceg, S., Lainez, S., Ronaghi, M., Stojkovic, P., Perez-Arago, M.A., Moreno-Manzano, V., Moreno-Palanques, R., Planells-Cases, R., and Stojkovic, M. (2008). Differentiation of human embryonic stem cells to regional specific neural precursors in chemically defined medium conditions. PLoS ONE *3*, e2122.

Farthing, C.R., Ficz, G., Ng, R.K., Chan, C.-F., Andrews, S., Dean, W., Hemberger, M., and Reik, W. (2008). Global mapping of DNA methylation in mouse promoters reveals epigenetic reprogramming of pluripotency genes PLoS Genetics 4(6), e1000116.

Feldman, N., Gerson, A., Fang, J., Li, E., Zhang, Y., Shinkai, Y., Cedar, H., and Bergman, Y. (2006). G9a-mediated irreversible epigenetic inactivation of Oct-3/4 during early embryogenesis. Nature Cell Biology 8, 188–194.

Gehring, M., Huh, J.H., Hsieh, T.F., Penterman, J., Choi, Y., Harada, J.J., Goldberg, R.B., and Fischer, R.L. (2006). DEMETER DNA glycosylase establishes MEDEA polycomb gene self-imprinting by allele-specific demethylation. Cell 124, 495–506.

Gerken, T., Girard, C.A., Tung, Y.C., Webby, C.J., Saudek, V., Hewitson, K.S., Yeo, G.S., McDonough, M.A., Cunliffe, S., McNeill, L.A., et al. (2007). The obesity-associated FTO gene encodes a 2-oxoglutarate-dependent nucleic acid demethylase. Science (New York, NY 318, 1469–1472.

Gong, Z., Morales-Ruiz, T., Ariza, R.R., Roldan-Arjona, T., David, L., and Zhu, J.K. (2002). ROS1, a repressor of transcriptional gene silencing in Arabidopsis, encodes a DNA glycosylase/lyase. Cell 111, 803–814.

Goto, T., and Monk, M. (1998). Regulation of X-chromosome inactivation in development in mice and humans. Microbiology and Molecular Biology Reviews 62, 362–378.

Hajkova, P., Ancelin, K., Waldmann, T., Lacoste, N., Lange, U.C., Cesari, F., Lee, C., Almouzni, G., Schneider, R., and Surani, M.A. (2008). Chromatin dynamics during epigenetic reprogramming in the mouse germ line. Nature 452, 877–881.

Hajkova, P., Erhardt, S., Lane, N., Haaf, T., El-Maarri, O., Reik, W., Walter, J., and Surani, M.A. (2002). Epigenetic reprogramming in mouse primordial germ cells. Mechanisms of Development 117, 15–23.

Hennessy, B., Korbling, M., and Estrov, Z. (2004). Circulating stem cells and tissue repair. Panminerva medica 46, 1–11.

Hikichi, T., Kohda, T., Wakayama, S., Ishino, F., and Wakayama, T. (2008). Nuclear transfer alters the DNA methylation status of specific genes in fertilized and parthenogenetically activated mouse embryonic stem cells. Stem Cells (Dayton, Ohio) 26, 783–788.

Hikichi, T., Wakayama, S., Mizutani, E., Takashima, Y., Kishigami, S., Van Thuan, N., Ohta, H., Thuy Bui, H., Nishikawa, S., and Wakayama, T. (2007). Differentiation potential of parthenogenetic embryonic stem cells is improved by nuclear transfer. Stem Cells (Dayton, Ohio) 25, 46–53.

Hirasawa, R., Chiba, H., Kaneda, M., Tajima, S., Li, E., Jaenisch, R., and Sasaki, H. (2008). Maternal and zygotic Dnmt1 are necessary and sufficient for the maintenance of DNA methylation imprints during preimplantation development. Genes & Development 22(12), 1607–16.

Howlett, S.K., and Reik, W. (1991). Methylation levels of maternal and paternal genomes during preimplantation development. Development (Cambridge, England) 113, 119–127.

Humpherys, D., Eggan, K., Akutsu, H., Hochedlinger, K., Rideout, W.M., 3rd, Biniszkiewicz, D., Yanagimachi, R., and Jaenisch, R. (2001). Epigenetic instability in ES cells and cloned mice. Science (New York, NY 293, 95–97.

Imamura, M., Miura, K., Iwabuchi, K., Ichisaka, T., Nakagawa, M., Lee, J., Kanatsu-Shinohara, M., Shinohara, T., and Yamanaka, S. (2006). Transcriptional repression and DNA hypermethylation of a small set of ES cell marker genes in male germline stem cells. BMC Developmental Biology 6, 34.

Inoue, K., Kohda, T., Lee, J., Ogonuki, N., Mochida, K., Noguchi, Y., Tanemura, K., Kaneko-Ishino, T., Ishino, F., and Ogura, A. (2002). Faithful expression of imprinted genes in cloned mice. Science (New York, NY 295, 297.

Inoue, K., Ogonuki, N., Miki, H., Hirose, M., Noda, S., Kim, J.M., Aoki, F., Miyoshi, H., and Ogura, A. (2006). Inefficient reprogramming of the hematopoietic stem cell genome following nuclear transfer. Journal of Cell Science 119, 1985–1991.

Jaenisch, R., and Young, R. (2008). Stem cells, the molecular circuitry of pluripotency and nuclear reprogramming. Cell 132, 567–582.

Jin, S.-G., Guo, C., and Pfeifer, G.P. (2008). GADD45A Does Not Promote DNA Demethylation. PLoS Genetics *4*, e1000013.

Kang, Y.K., Koo, D.B., Park, J.S., Choi, Y.H., Chung, A.S., Lee, K.K., and Han, Y.M. (2001). Aberrant methylation of donor genome in cloned bovine embryos. Nature genetics *28*, 173–177.

Kang, Y.K., Park, J.S., Koo, D.B., Choi, Y.H., Kim, S.U., Lee, K.K., and Han, Y.M. (2002). Limited demethylation leaves mosaic-type methylation states in cloned bovine pre-implantation embryos. The EMBO Journal *21*, 1092–1100.

Kawasaki, H., Mizuseki, K., Nishikawa, S., Kaneko, S., Kuwana, Y., Nakanishi, S., Nishikawa, S.I., and Sasai, Y. (2000). Induction of midbrain dopaminergic neurons from ES cells by stromal cell-derived inducing activity. Neuron *28*, 31–40.

Keller, G. (2005). Embryonic stem cell differentiation: emergence of a new era in biology and medicine. Genes & Development *19*, 1129–1155.

Kishigami, S., Bui, H.T., Wakayama, S., Tokunaga, K., Van Thuan, N., Hikichi, T., Mizutani, E., Ohta, H., Suetsugu, R., Sata, T., et al. (2007). Successful mouse cloning of an outbred strain by trichostatin A treatment after somatic nuclear transfer. Journal of Reproduction and Development *53*, 165–170.

Kress, C., Thomassin, H., and Grange, T. (2006). Active cytosine demethylation triggered by a nuclear receptor involves DNA strand breaks. Proceedings of the National Academy of Sciences of the United States of America *103*, 11112–11117.

Kroon, E., Martinson, L.A., Kadoya, K., Bang, A.G., Kelly, O.G., Eliazer, S., Young, H., Richardson, M., Smart, N.G., Cunningham, J., et al. (2008). Pancreatic endoderm derived from human embryonic stem cells generates glucose-responsive insulin-secreting cells in vivo. Nature Biotechnology *26*, 443–452.

Laflamme, M.A., Chen, K.Y., Naumova, A.V., Muskheli, V., Fugate, J.A., Dupras, S.K., Reinecke, H., Xu, C., Hassanipour, M., Police, S., et al. (2007). Cardiomyocytes derived from human embryonic stem cells in pro-survival factors enhance function of infarcted rat hearts. Nature Biotechnology *25*, 1015–1024.

Lane, N., Dean, W., Erhardt, S., Hajkova, P., Surani, M.A., Walter, J., and Reik, W. (2003). Resistance of IAPs to methylation reprogramming may provide a mechanism for epigenetic inheritance in the mouse. Genesis *35*, 88–93.

Lee, J., Inoue, K., Ono, R., Ogonuki, N., Kohda, T., Kaneko-Ishino, T., Ogura, A., and Ishino, F. (2002). Erasing genomic imprinting memory in mouse clone embryos produced from day 11.5 primordial germ cells. Development (Cambridge, England) *129*, 1807–1817.

Loukinov, D.I., Pugacheva, E., Vatolin, S., Pack, S.D., Moon, H., Chernukhin, I., Mannan, P., Larsson, E., Kanduri, C., Vostrov, A.A., et al. (2002). BORIS, a novel male germ-line-specific protein associated with epigenetic reprogramming events, shares the same 11-zinc-finger domain with CTCF, the insulator protein involved in reading imprinting marks in the soma. Proceedings of the National Academy of Sciences of the United States of America *99*, 6806–6811.

Mak, W., Nesterova, T.B., de Napoles, M., Appanah, R., Yamanaka, S., Otte, A.P., and Brockdorff, N. (2004). Reactivation of the paternal X chromosome in early mouse embryos. Science (New York, NY *303*, 666–669.

Mann, M.R., Chung, Y.G., Nolen, L.D., Verona, R.I., Latham, K.E., and Bartolomei, M.S. (2003). Disruption of imprinted gene methylation and expression in cloned preimplantation stage mouse embryos. Biology of Reproduction *69*, 902–914.

Martin, C., Beaujean, N., Brochard, V., Audouard, C., Zink, D., and Debey, P. (2006). Genome restructuring in mouse embryos during reprogramming and early development. Developmental Biology *292*, 317–332.

Mayer, W., Niveleau, A., Walter, J., Fundele, R., and Haaf, T. (2000). Embryogenesis: Demethylation of the zygotic paternal genome. Nature *403*, 501–502.

Mikkelsen, T.S., Hanna, J., Zhang, X., Ku, M., Wernig, M., Schorderet, P., Bernstein, B.E., Jaenisch, R., Lander, E.S., and Meissner, A. (2008). Dissecting direct reprogramming through integrative genomic analysis. Nature *454(7200)*, 49–55.

Monk, M., Boubelik, M., and Lehnert, S. (1987). Temporal and regional changes in DNA methylation in the embryonic, extraembryonic and germ cell lineages during mouse embryo development. Development (Cambridge, England) 99, 371–382.

Morales-Ruiz, T., Ortega-Galisteo, A.P., Ponferrada-Marin, M.I., Martinez-Macias, M.I., Ariza, R.R., and Roldan-Arjona, T. (2006). DEMETER and REPRESSOR OF SILENCING 1 encode 5-methylcytosine DNA glycosylases. Proceedings of the National Academy of Sciences of the United States of America 103, 6853–6858.

Morgan, H.D., Dean, W., Coker, H.A., Reik, W., and Petersen-Mahrt, S.K. (2004). Activation-induced cytidine deaminase deaminates 5-methylcytosine in DNA and is expressed in pluripotent tissues: implications for epigenetic reprogramming. The Journal of Biological Chemistry 279, 52353–52360.

Morgan, H.D., Santos, F., Green, K., Dean, W., and Reik, W. (2005). Epigenetic reprogramming in mammals. Human Molecular Genetics 14 Spec No 1, R47–58.

Murry, C.E., and Keller, G. (2008). Differentiation of embryonic stem cells to clinically relevant populations: lessons from embryonic development. Cell 132, 661–680.

Nakagawa, M., Koyanagi, M., Tanabe, K., Takahashi, K., Ichisaka, T., Aoi, T., Okita, K., Mochiduki, Y., Takizawa, N., and Yamanaka, S. (2008). Generation of induced pluripotent stem cells without Myc from mouse and human fibroblasts. Nat Biotech 26, 101–106.

Nakamura, T., Arai, Y., Umehara, H., Masuhara, M., Kimura, T., Taniguchi, H., Sekimoto, T., Ikawa, M., Yoneda, Y., Okabe, M., et al. (2007). PGC7/Stella protects against DNA demethylation in early embryogenesis. Nature Cell Biology 9, 64–71.

Ng, R.K., Dean, W., Dawson, C., Lucifero, D., Madeja, Z., Reik, W., and Hemberger, M. (2008). Epigenetic restriction of embryonic cell lineage fate by methylation of Elf5. Nature cell Biology 2008 Oct 5. PMID: 18836439.

O'Neill, L.P., VerMilyea, M.D., and Turner, B.M. (2006). Epigenetic characterization of the early embryo with a chromatin immunoprecipitation protocol applicable to small cell populations. Nature Genetics 38, 835–841.

Oakes, C.C., La Salle, S., Smiraglia, D.J., Robaire, B., and Trasler, J.M. (2007). Developmental acquisition of genome-wide DNA methylation occurs prior to meiosis in male germ cells. Developmental Biology 307, 368–379.

Okamoto, I., Otte, A.P., Allis, C.D., Reinberg, D., and Heard, E. (2004). Epigenetic dynamics of imprinted X inactivation during early mouse development. Science (New York, NY 303, 644–649.

Okita, K., Ichisaka, T., and Yamanaka, S. (2007). Generation of germline-competent induced pluripotent stem cells. Nature 448, 313–317.

Oswald, J., Engemann, S., Lane, N., Mayer, W., Olek, A., Fundele, R., Dean, W., Reik, W., and Walter, J. (2000). Active demethylation of the paternal genome in the mouse zygote. Current Biology 10, 475–478.

Ott, H.C., Matthiesen, T.S., Goh, S.K., Black, L.D., Kren, S.M., Netoff, T.I., and Taylor, D.A. (2008). Perfusion-decellularized matrix: using nature's platform to engineer a bioartificial heart. Nature Medicine 14, 213–221.

Park, J.S., Jeong, Y.S., Shin, S.T., Lee, K.K., and Kang, Y.K. (2007). Dynamic DNA methylation reprogramming: active demethylation and immediate remethylation in the male pronucleus of bovine zygotes. Developmental Dynamics 236, 2523–2533.

Porada, C.D., Zanjani, E.D., and Almeida-Porad, G. (2006). Adult mesenchymal stem cells: a pluripotent population with multiple applications. Current Stem Cell Research and Therapy 1, 365–369.

Reik, W. (2007). Stability and flexibility of epigenetic gene regulation in mammalian development. Nature 447, 425–432.

Reinders, J., Delucinge Vivier, C., Theiler, G., Chollet, D., Descombes, P., and Paszkowski, J. (2008). Genome-wide, high-resolution DNA methylation profiling using bisulfite-mediated cytosine conversion. Genome Research 18, 469–476.

Rossant, J. (2008). Stem cells and early lineage development. Cell 132, 527–531.

Santos, F., Hendrich, B., Reik, W., and Dean, W. (2002). Dynamic reprogramming of DNA methylation in the early mouse embryo. Developmental Biology *241*, 172–182.

Santos, F., Zakhartchenko, V., Stojkovic, M., Peters, A., Jenuwein, T., Wolf, E., Reik, W., and Dean, W. (2003). Epigenetic marking correlates with developmental potential in cloned bovine preimplantation embryos. Current Biology *13*, 1116–1121.

Sarmento, O.F., Digilio, L.C., Wang, Y., Perlin, J., Herr, J.C., Allis, C.D., and Coonrod, S.A. (2004). Dynamic alterations of specific histone modifications during early murine development. Journal of Cell Science *117*, 4449–4459.

Seki, Y., Hayashi, K., Itoh, K., Mizugaki, M., Saitou, M., and Matsui, Y. (2005). Extensive and orderly reprogramming of genome-wide chromatin modifications associated with specification and early development of germ cells in mice. Developmental Biology *278*, 440–458.

Seki, Y., Yamaji, M., Yabuta, Y., Sano, M., Shigeta, M., Matsui, Y., Saga, Y., Tachibana, M., Shinkai, Y., and Saitou, M. (2007). Cellular dynamics associated with the genome-wide epigenetic reprogramming in migrating primordial germ cells in mice. Development (Cambridge, England) *134*, 2627–2638.

Senda, S., Wakayama, T., Yamazaki, Y., Ohgane, J., Hattori, N., Tanaka, S., Yanagimachi, R., and Shiota, K. (2004). Skewed X-inactivation in cloned mice. Biochemical and Biophysical Research Communications *321*, 38–44.

Silva, J., Chambers, I., Pollard, S., and Smith, A. (2006). Nanog promotes transfer of pluripotency after cell fusion. Nature *441*, 997–1001.

Sugimoto, M., and Abe, K. (2007). X chromosome reactivation initiates in nascent primordial germ cells in mice. PLoS Genetics *3*, e116.

Surani, M., and Reik, W. (2007). Germ line and pluripotent stem cells. In Epigenetics (Cold Spring Harbor Press), pp. 315–327.

Tada, M., Tada, T., Lefebvre, L., Barton, S.C., and Surani, M.A. (1997). Embryonic germ cells induce epigenetic reprogramming of somatic nucleus in hybrid cells. The EMBO Journal *16*, 6510–6520.

Tada, M., Takahama, Y., Abe, K., Nakatsuji, N., and Tada, T. (2001). Nuclear reprogramming of somatic cells by in vitro hybridization with ES cells. Current Biology *11*, 1553–1558.

Takahashi, K., and Yamanaka, S. (2006). Induction of pluripotent stem cells from mouse embryonic and adult fibroblast cultures by defined factors. Cell *126*, 663–676.

Torres-Padilla, M.E., Parfitt, D.E., Kouzarides, T., and Zernicka-Goetz, M. (2007). Histone arginine methylation regulates pluripotency in the early mouse embryo. Nature *445*, 214–218.

Valley, C.M., Pertz, L.M., Balakumaran, B.S., and Willard, H.F. (2006). Chromosome-wide, allele-specific analysis of the histone code on the human X chromosome. Human Molecular Genetics *15*, 2335–2347.

van Laake, L.W., Passier, R., Doevendans, P.A., and Mummery, C.L. (2008). Human embryonic stem cell-derived cardiomyocytes and cardiac repair in rodents. Circulation Research *102*, 1008–1010.

Wakayama, T., and Yanagimachi, R. (2001). Mouse cloning with nucleus donor cells of different age and type. Molecular Reproduction and Development *58*, 376–383.

Weber, M., Davies, J.J., Wittig, D., Oakeley, E.J., Haase, M., Lam, W.L., and Schubeler, D. (2005). Chromosome-wide and promoter-specific analyses identify sites of differential DNA methylation in normal and transformed human cells. Nature Genetics *37*, 853–862.

Weber, M., Hellmann, I., Stadler, M.B., Ramos, L., Paabo, S., Rebhan, M., and Schubeler, D. (2007). Distribution, silencing potential and evolutionary impact of promoter DNA methylation in the human genome. Nature Genetics *39*, 457–466.

Wee, G., Koo, D.B., Song, B.S., Kim, J.S., Kang, M.J., Moon, S.J., Kang, Y.K., Lee, K.K., and Han, Y.M. (2006). Inheritable histone H4 acetylation of somatic chromatins in cloned embryos. Journal of Biological Chemistry *281*, 6048–6057.

Weiss, A., Keshet, I., Razin, A., and Cedar, H. (1996). DNA demethylation in vitro: involvement of RNA. Cell *86*, 709–718.

Wernig, M., Meissner A., Cassady, J.P., and Jaenisch, R. (2008). C-Myc is dispensable for direct reprogramming of mouse fibroblasts. Cell stem cell *2*, 10–12.

Xu, Y., Shi, Y., and Ding, S. (2008). A chemical approach to stem-cell biology and regenerative medicine. Nature *453*, 338–344.

Xue, F., Tian, X.C., Du, F., Kubota, C., Taneja, M., Dinnyes, A., Dai, Y., Levine, H., Pereira, L.V., and Yang, X. (2002). Aberrant patterns of X chromosome inactivation in bovine clones. Nature Genetics *31*, 216–220.

Yamanaka, S. (2007). Strategies and new developments in the generation of patient-specific pluripotent stem cells. Cell Stem Cell *1*, 39–49.

Yang, L., Chavatte-Palmer, P., Kubota, C., O'Neill, M., Hoagland, T., Renard, J.P., Taneja, M., Yang, X., and Tian, X.C. (2005). Expression of imprinted genes is aberrant in deceased newborn cloned calves and relatively normal in surviving adult clones. Molecular Reproduction and Development *71*, 431–438.

Yang, X., Smith, S.L., Tian, X.C., Lewin, H.A., Renard, J.-P., and Wakayama, T. (2007). Nuclear reprogramming of cloned embryos and its implications for therapeutic cloning. Nature Genetics *39*, 295–302.

Young, L.E., and Beaujean, N. (2004). DNA methylation in the preimplantation embryo: the differing stories of the mouse and sheep. Animal Reproduction Science *82– 83*, 61–78.

Zernicka-Goetz, M. (2006). The first cell-fate decisions in the mouse embryo: destiny is a matter of both chance and choice. Current Opinion in Genetics and Development *16*, 406–412.

Zhang, S., Kubota, C., Yang, L., Zhang, Y., Page, R., O'Neill, M., Yang, X., and Tian, X.C. (2004). Genomic imprinting of H19 in naturally reproduced and cloned cattle. Biology of Reproduction *71*, 1540–1544.

Zhang, X., Yazaki, J., Sundaresan, A., Cokus, S., Chan, S.W.L., Chen, H., Henderson, I.R., Shinn, P., Pellegrini, M., Jacobsen, S.E., *et al.* (2006). Genome-wide High-Resolution Mapping and Functional Analysis of DNA Methylation in Arabidopsis. Cell *126*, 1189–1201.

Epigenetic Gene Regulation—Lessons from Globin

Ann Dean and Steven Fiering

Abstract The globin loci, in particular the β globin locus, have been important models for identifying and understanding the mechanisms of transcriptional regulation in mammals. This is because they are multigenic, tissue specific, developmentally regulated and among the most highly transcribed genes in our genome. In general the chromatin structure of the mammalian β-globin locus reflects the transcriptional state of individual globin genes rather than having a uniform chromatin structure across the locus. A great deal of effort has been devoted to understanding how the β-globin locus control region (LCR) regulates transcription and influences chromatin structure. While studies of transgenes with and without the LCR suggest that the LCR primarily regulates transcription by influencing the overall locus chromatin structure, this does not appear to be the case in the endogenous mouse locus and the LCR appears to have multiple activities in various contexts. Recent studies have led to a new model of how the LCR influences transcriptional regulation and this model, if correct, will have a major influence on understanding transcriptional regulation in mammals. In this model, the LCR augments transcription by influencing the subnuclear localization of the locus in order to maintain the locus in concentrated regions of RNA pol II called transcription factories, in particular, in the transcription factories that contain active pol II with a hyperphosphorylated carboxy terminal domain (CTD). By keeping the locus in association with active transcription factories a large percentage of the time, the LCR appears to mediate the high levels of transcription associated with the β-like globin genes in erythroblasts.

Keywords Globin · epigenetics · chromatin · subnuclear localization · histone modification

The α and β-globin loci are among the first vertebrate loci to have served as models for understanding the connection between epigenetic alterations and developmentally regulated gene expression. By epigenetics, we wish to consider chromatin

S. Fiering (✉)
Depts. of Microbiology/Immunology and Genetics, Dartmouth Medical School, Rubin 622, DHMC, Lebanon, NH 03756
e-mail: fiering@dartmouth.edu

changes that are maintained or reestablished through metaphase and influence the transcription of a particular gene locus without altering the DNA sequence therein. We will discuss methylation of DNA cytosine residues and covalent modifications of histones including acetylation and methylation of the N-terminal tail residues of these proteins, although these represent only a sub-set of possible histone modifications. Recent work has established that these marks recruit proteins that have downstream effects on gene expression (for review see Berger, 2007). The epigenetic landscape and functional outcome in several developmentally regulated gene loci, such as the growth hormone locus and the T_H2 cell cytokine and MHC class II loci have been extensively studied [for review see (Dean, 2006)], but in a number of respects the β-globin locus has provided an exception to these findings and this locus shall be a focus of this review.

1 Characteristics of α and β Globin Regulation in Mammals

Hemoglobin, the respiratory protein in red cells, is a hetero-tetramer composed of two α-like and two β-like globin chains and four heme rings with a central iron atom in each that coordinately binds oxygen. In vertebrates, the α-like genes and the β-like genes typically are clustered together on two different chromosomes. As a group, the human hemoglobinopathies, α- or β-thalassemia and Sickle Cell Disease are the most common human genetic disorders. The transcriptional regulation of the multiple genes at each of the globin loci has been intensely investigated for many years because it is relevant to the hemoglobinopathies. This intense analysis in combination with the developmental complexity they exhibit has made these loci the source of considerable fundamental epigenetic insight.

There are discrete stages of erythropoiesis that involve expression of different globin genes and roughly correspond with the sites of erythropoiesis during development in mammals. For example, during embryonic erythropoiesis in the yolk sac of humans, the embryonic ζ-globin gene and, to a lesser extent, the α1 and α2 globin genes are expressed from the α-globin locus, while the predominant expressed β-like gene is ε-globin (Fig. 1). The large erythrocytes produced in the yolk sac are "primitive erythrocytes" and retain their nuclei. During the fetal stage of development, hematopoiesis produces "definitive" (enucleated) erythrocytes in the fetal liver. The α1 and α2 genes continue to be transcribed from the α locus, while the ζ gene is silenced. In the β locus the fetal Gγ and Aγ genes predominate, ε is silenced, and the adult β gene is expressed at low levels. The postnatal site of erythropoiesis is the bone marrow where definitive erythrocytes that are slightly smaller in size than those of the fetal liver are generated. While the α locus continues to express α1 and α2, the β gene is now the predominant gene expressed from the β locus with low levels of δ and very low levels of the γ genes. This developmental process in which the genes are sequentially expressed in the order of their 5′–3′ chromosomal arrangement is the "globin switch" which produces a series of different hemoglobin tetramers during development. A mechanistic understanding of the globin switch is

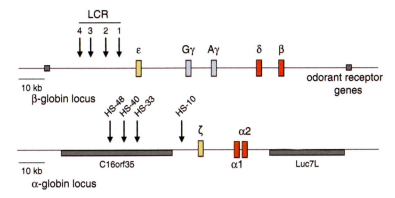

Fig. 1 The human β-globin locus and the human α-globin locus. Yellow genes are expressed only in the embryo (ε and ζ). Blue genes are fetal specific (γ). Red genes are adult specific (δ and β) or expressed at all three stages (α). Arrows denote erythroid specific DNase I hypersensitive sites. C16orf35 and Luc7L are constitutively expressed genes

far from complete, but what is known forms the center of epigenetic thinking about globin gene regulation.

Early investigations of the developmental control of globin genes focused on the expression of the human β-globin locus in transgenic mice. The mouse β-globin locus is organized similarly to the human locus but with only one globin "switch" from expression of the embryonic εy and βH1 genes to expression of the fetal/adult β-major and β-minor genes (see Fig. 2). The endogenous globin genes in differentiating red cells are expressed at remarkably high levels for genes with one or two copies per haploid genome. This is necessary to produce adequate globin protein for normal red cell development. The first transgenic mice carrying human globin genes showed quickly that the human genes and their proximal promoters carried sufficient information to drive tissue-specific expression in erythroid cells (Townes et al. 1985, Chada et al. 1985, Raich et al. 1990). In this milieu, the human locus behaves more like the mouse locus and undergoes only one switch with the embryonic and fetal genes expressed during embryonic development and the β gene expressed at the fetal and adult stage (Gaensler et al. 1993). However, the levels of the β globins were only a few percent of the endogenous mouse globins. Furthermore, a large proportion of the transgenes were highly susceptible to "position effects" associated with the integration sites and had no detectable globin expression (Townes et al. 1985, Chada et al. 1985).

Efforts were made to identify distal regulatory elements and a series of DNase hypersensitive (HS) sites were identified far upstream of the ε-globin the gene (Tuan et al. 1985; Forrester et al. 1986) (Figs. 1 and 2). Some of these HSs had enhancer activity when transfected into erythroid cells in tissue culture (Forrester et al. 1989). When linked to globin transgenes, HS1-4 conferred very high levels of expression to the genes, similar to the levels of endogenous mouse globins in erythroid cells (Grosveld et al. 1987). Eventually called the locus control region (LCR), this element was defined by its ability to confer "position independent" and "copy number

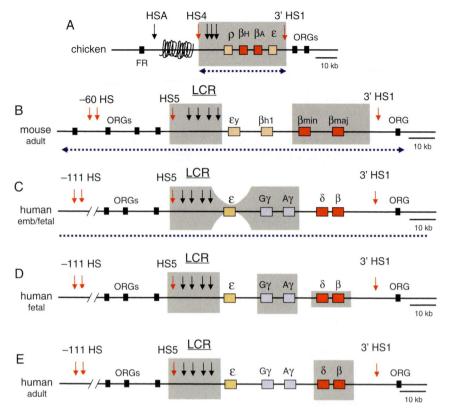

Fig. 2 **Chromatin modification patterns of the vertebrate loci reflect expression patterns**. The figure presents data obtained by chromatin immunoprecipitation across the chicken, mouse and human β-globin loci at various developmental stages. The grey shaded blocks are regions of positive histone modifications including acetylation of H3 and H4 and di-methylation of H3K4. The height of the blocks reflects the level of the modifications. The blue dotted line under the loci indicates the extent of general DNase sensitivity. Lines that terminate with arrowheads indicate the extent of the domain of sensitivity, while those without arrowheads indicate the extent of sensitivity without reaching a transition as far as was studied. Vertical arrows denote DNase I hypersensitive sites as in Fig. 2. (**A**) The chicken β-globin locus (data from Litt 2001a and b). (**B**) The mouse β-globin locus (data from (Bulger et al 2003). (**C**) The human β-globin locus in K562 cells (data from Kim et al 2007a), (**D**) The human β-globin locus in fetal and (**E**) adult erythroblasts (Mei Hsu and SF, unpublished)

dependent" expression to a transgene, characteristics that had not been seen with any transgene to that point. Thus, "LCR activity" appeared to be dominant over the influence of the integration site regardless of the state of chromatin at the site and this implied that a major functional activity of the LCR was in regulation of chromatin structure. Since that time many regulatory elements have been identified which have the critical attributes of an LCR with regard to controlling transgene expression (reviewed in Li et al. 2002).

Unlike the β-globin locus, which resides in a relatively gene poor chromosomal region with no "housekeeping" genes nearby, the α-globin locus is in a region that is densely populated with predominantly constitutively expressed genes (Fig. 1). Although their neighborhoods are very different, the transcription of the α-like and β-like genes must be coordinately regulated since imbalance of one type of protein over the other can cause thalassemia and make the red cells unstable. There is an enhancer (HS -40) for the human α genes that is 40 kb upstream of the genes (26 kb upstream in mice) that resembles a single one of the HSs associated with the β-globin LCR (Pondel, et al. 1992, Rombel et al. 1995). HS -40 does not have LCR activity in transgenes, suggesting that LCR activity is somehow not required for the α genes (Sharpe et al. 1993). There are other nearby erythroid specific HSs but the current consensus is that HS –40 is the most powerful regulatory element in this group of HSs (De Gobbi et al. 2007; Higgs et al. 2006).

2 β-Globin LCR Activity

While it is clear that the β-globin LCR is a potent enhancer of transcription, the original concept that it confers "copy number dependent and integration position independent" gene expression merits reconsideration and refinement. Large LCR-containing human β-globin locus transgenes consisting of 100+ kb of DNA in a YAC or BAC context can clearly strongly suppress position effects but not eliminate them (Porcu et al. 1997, Kaufman et al. 1999, Alami et al. 2000). The range of expression typically observed is 3 fold, so although there is a clear relationship between copy number and expression level (as compared to a transgene with no LCR in which there is no copy number/expression level relationship) the ability of the LCR to overcome the influence of local chromatin structure is not absolute. For example, in one report, a single copy BAC transgene with the entire intact locus did not express the globin genes at detectable levels (Kaufman et al. 1999).

Surprising epigenetic results were derived from two sets of studies done on a β-globin YAC that was engineered to invert the LCR relative to the genes under the influence of Cre (Tanimoto et al. 1999). This study showed clearly that the LCR is directional and when it is inverted the linked genes had much lower expression. A follow up study on these transgenic lines in which expression was assayed at the single cell level produced the surprising result that the LCR even in its normal orientation was not able to fully suppress position effect variegation (PEV) (Alami et al. 2000). While some of the transgenic lines expressed the human globin genes in every cell, most did not and showed clear PEV in which many cells had no apparent expression and others had a high level of expression. In the transgenic lines that variegated when the LCR was in its normal orientation, globin gene expression dropped 3 fold after inversion and variegation increased a similar 3 fold, sufficient to account for the reduction in expression. Variegation reflected a failure of the LCR to form HS in the non-expressing cells, highlighting the failure of the LCR to overcome local suppressive chromatin effects in a subset of cells.

These results leave us with the expectation that there are at least two levels of position effects, one level that is generally but not always suppressible by an LCR to achieve reasonable levels of expression from each transgene and another that more moderately affects expression levels and is less easily suppressed. Each of these types of position effects may be a reflection of epigenetic variability that can be moderated by the LCR. Recent transgenic studies which showed that even a small promoter element can confer the same sort of relative copy number dependence attributed to the LCR have brought into question whether the β-globin or other LCRs are really unique elements or are better considered to be powerful versions of classical transcriptional enhancers (Sabatino et al. 2000).

Central questions underlying studies of the β-globin locus have focused on how the LCR functions to regulate a transgene and what role the LCR plays in the endogenous β-globin locus. The expectation was that the LCR would be required to generate high level expression from the endogenous genes. This expectation had strong support from a β-thalassemia mutation in which very low levels of β globin were expressed from alleles that had an intact β gene but a deletion of the LCR (Forrester et al. 1990). A further experimental demonstration that the LCR is required for high level expression of the linked β globin genes was the deletion of the entire LCR from the mouse globin locus (Bender et al. 2000). The result was that the "switch" was intact with expression of the genes at the expected developmental stage. However, the levels of expression were only a few percent of normal. This definitive experiment proved that the LCR is required for high level expression but left open the mechanism underlying that function. It was further demonstrated that all cells expressed low levels of the genes; there were no cells with high levels. This observation ruled out the possibility that, at the endogenous locus, the LCR acts to increase the probability of expression in each cell but not the level of expression once expression is established. Unlike in a transgene, at the endogenous mouse locus, the LCR does not serve to suppress PEV.

3 β-Globin Chromatin Structure and Epigenetic Modification

Another key hypothesis that preceded experiments in which the LCR was deleted from the mouse β-globin locus was that the LCR was required to maintain an open chromatin structure in the locus. It had been observed early on that β-globin locus chromatin in erythroid cells (but not in nonerythroid cells) was sensitive to low levels of DNase I, referred to as "general" DNase sensitivity, consistent with a relatively "open" chromatin structure conducive to transcription (Forrester et al. 1986). Our clearest picture of the chromatin organization of the β-globin locus comes from studies of chicken erythroid cells. The chicken β-globin locus contains four developmentally regulated genes and an upstream LCR but instead of being arranged in the order in which they are expressed (as the mammalian globin genes are arranged), the ε and ρ embryonic genes flank the adult β genes (Fig. 2A). The locus is bordered by additional HS that bind the insulator factor CTCF (Farrell et al. 2002). The 5' site, cHS4, is a well characterized insulator (Chung et al. 1993) and separates the locus from a 16 Kb heterochromatic region while the 3' site, 3'HS1, borders a domain of odorant receptor genes not expressed in erythroid cells.

The chicken locus CTCF sites precisely circumscribe the extent of general DNase I sensitivity and of acetylated histones H3 and H4 and H3 lysine 4 methylation, positive epigenetic marks associated with active chromatin (Litt et al. 2001b; Litt et al. 2001a; Hebbes et al. 1994) (Fig. 2A). Within this region, the positive histone marks anti-correlate with H3 K9 methylation, a mark more characteristic of non-transcribed chromatin. This arrangement is consistent with the idea that the CTCF sites organize a domain that includes the β-globin genes and their LCR enhancer (Burgess-Beusse et al. 2002). Although predicted, there has not been an experimental demonstration that loss of CTCF binding affects the chromatin structure of the chicken locus. Both silent and active globin genes are located within this domain, indicating that the domain of modified histones *per se* is not determinative of gene activity in this system.

The chromatin picture of the mouse β-globin locus differs from and is more complex than the chicken locus chromatin. In the mouse β-globin locus orthologous 5' and 3' CTCF sites are found (HS5 and 3' HS1) but these sites form more fuzzy chromatin borders and the extents of DNase I general sensitivity and acetylated and K4 methylated histones do not correlate precisely with them (Forsberg et al. 2000; Bulger et al. 2003) (Fig. 2B). Furthermore, the positive histone marks form discontinuous domains, unlike the chicken locus noted above. For example, at the adult stage of erythroid differentiation, the histones in the LCR region and the active β-globin gene carry positive marks but histones in the intervening silent embryonic genes are not positively marked. However, in the silent embryonic region, DNase general sensitivity is retained, indicating that the positive histone modifications alone are not the cause of the altered chromatin structure.

The mouse β-globin locus is embedded within a cluster of odorant receptor genes. Interestingly, deletion or mutation of one or the other of the CTCF sites, or knock down of CTCF using RNA interference, did not perturb globin gene expression, indicating that these sites are not likely to act as insulators at their endogenous location (Bender et al. 1998; Farrell et al. 2000; Bender et al. 2006; Splinter et al. 2006). Chromatin structure in the human β-globin domain, which is also embedded in an odorant receptor cluster, resembles that at the mouse locus with indistinct borders that do not in general correspond to chromatin structural transitions (Kim, A et al. 2007a) (Fig. 2C-E). At the embryonic/fetal stage, as reflected in K562 cells, the LCR and actively transcribed γ-globin genes are modified by histone acetylation and H3 K4 methylation while the more weakly transcribed ε gene is modified at a lower level and the silent adult genes are not modified. Studies of the histone modification patterns of the human β-globin locus in primary human fetal liver and bone marrow erythroblasts paint a similar picture of positive histone modifications only at the LCR HS and around the actively transcribed genes (Mei Hsu and SF, unpublished).

Domains of positive histone modifications including H3 and H4 acetylation and H3 K4 methylation characterize other mammalian developmentally regulated loci such as the growth hormone, T_H2 cytokine and MHC class II loci. In the growth hormone locus, deletion of LCR HSI results in loss of the domain of histone modification, supporting the idea the LCR influences chromatin structure in an endogenous locus (Ho et al. 2002). However, the globin locus may function differently. When the LCR was deleted from the endogenous mouse globin locus, very little alteration in general DNase I sensitivity across the locus was detected (Bender et al. 2000). Thus, although globin transgenes without the LCR are often found to exist in "closed" chromatin (Milot et al. 1996), surprisingly, the LCR apparently does not serve to maintain open chromatin in the endogenous locus. Furthermore, histone acetylation was only modestly reduced in regions proximal to the LCR and not changed at the active β-globin gene promoter although transcription was only about 3% of normal (Schubeler et al. 2001). While it may be the case that histone modifications are maintained at a promoter with a low level of transcription, the lack of change in DNase sensitivity of the domain in the absence of the LCR argues, unexpectedly, that chromatin structure in the mouse β-globin locus is not dependent on the LCR.

4 β-Globin Regulatory Factors and Their Influence on Histone Modifications

GATA-1 and EKLF are erythroid specific transcription factors that are important regulators of β-like globin gene expression along with NF-E2 a heterodimer of which the large sub-unit, p45 is erythroid specific (reviewed in Stamatoyannopoulos, 2005; Mahajan et al. 2007). These proteins occupy LCR HSs and globin gene promoters. GATA-1 can homo-dimerize and hetero-dimerize with EKLF. All three proteins have been shown to interact with the histone and protein acetyltransferase CBP which is required for hematopoiesis and therefore assumed to play a role in histone and/or protein acetylation in the β-globin locus (Zhang and Bieker, 1998; Blobel et al. 1998; Cheng et al. 1997). The GATA-1 null erythroid cell line G1E (Weiss et al. 1997) and the NF-E2 null MEL cell line CB3 (Ben-David et al. 1992) have been profitably employed to define the roles of these proteins in epigenetic modification of the β-globin locus as they can be induced to differentiate by re-supplying the missing protein. Recruitment of CBP to the β-globin LCR HS is re-established under these circumstances (Letting et al. 2003; Kim et al. 2007c).

G1E cells do not express β-globin but expression can be induced by supplying GATA-1 from an estrogen receptor fusion construct by exposure to estrogen or tamoxifen. Before induction, the locus lacks histone acetylation and H3 K4 methylation marks. These marks are induced at the LCR HS and the β-globin genes along with transcription activation (Letting et al. 2003). Similarly, the marks are established within the β-globin locus when NF-E2 is re-expressed in CB3 cell clones stably expressing the protein (Johnson et al. 2001). Together these studies support an important role for GATA-1 and NF-E2 in establishing the pattern of histone modifications across the β-globin locus and suggest that their recruitment of histone modifying activities to the LCR is part of their mechanism of action. Studies in which the sites of interaction of these factors in LCR HS2 were ablated support a direct role for GATA-1 in recruitment of CBP to the LCR and indicate that NF-E2 but not GATA-1 helps recruit the MLL histone methyl transferase component Ash2L to the LCR [(Kim et al. 2007b) and AeRi Kim and AD, unpublished data].

Similar to the β-globin locus, in the MHC class II locus, the histone acetylation domain is lost after deletion of CIITA or RFX factors that bind to the LCR (Masternak et al. 2003). Since GATA-1 and NF-E2 recruit CBP to the LCR HSs, the results described above are difficult to reconcile with the results obtained after deletion of the LCR in which no substantive alteration of histone acetylation was observed. Possibly, these globin regulatory factors can bind to globin promoters independent of the LCR. This recently has been demonstrated for GATA-1 (Vakoc et al. 2005).

5 DNA Methylation, Does It Matter for β-Globin Regulation?

The β-globin locus was one of the first if not the first mammalian locus investigated for developmental changes in DNA methylation and their correlation with transcription (van der Ploeg and Flavell, 1980). These studies showed that CpGs in the promoters of the human β-like globin genes tended to be unmethylated in erythroblasts at the developmental stages at which they were expressed and methylated in erythroblasts that did not express them or in other cell types. A more recent study showed that there is a 20 kb area of DNA hypomethylation around the mouse embryonic genes in primitive erythrocytes. There is no data on functionality of this hypomethylated region but nothing similar has been reported for any other gene, so its very existence is intriguing (Hsu et al. 2007).

Most interest in DNA methylation is focused on CpG island genes and the β-globin locus has no CpG islands. However there have continued to be studies of methylation changes in the β-globin locus and continued interest in the possibility that DNA methylation affects β-globin regulation. The finding that the γ-globin genes could be transcriptionally activated to some extent postnatally, by exposure to 5-azacytidine the DNA methyltransferase inhibitor (Ley et al. 1983), stimulated interest in the role of DNA methylation in β-like globin regulation. DNA methylation is postulated to play a functional role in regulating the chicken globin switch (Singal et al. 1997). In the baboon, an animal with a β-globin switch similar to humans, treatment with 5-azacytidine strongly activates γ–globin expression postnatally (DeSimone et al. 1982). Recent studies of the human locus in a transgenic mouse suggest that methylation of the γ promoter plays a role in suppressing γ expression postnatally (Goren et al. 2006; Rupon et al. 2006). Although it is currently thought that DNA methylation is not the primary mechanism influencing globin switching in mammals, it is quite possibly one among multiple contributing mechanisms.

6 β-Globin LCR and Looping

The means by which an LCR or any other enhancer regulates transcription from a distant promoter has been intensely studied for years (Bulger and Groudine, 1999).

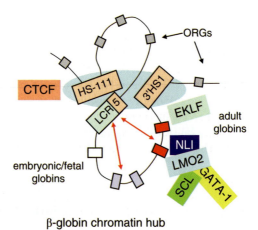

Fig. 3 Relationship between enhancer/promoter and insulator loops. Depicted is the close proximity among the flanking HSs of the β-globin locus that bind the insulator factor CTCF to form a chromatin hub (Tolhuis et al. 2002, Palstra et al. Nat. Gen. 2003). This association requires CTCF (Splinter et al. 2006). In more mature erythroid cells, the LCR and β-globin gene join in this close association in the "active" chromatin hub. The interaction of the LCR and β gene requires EKLF and a complex involving GATA-1/SCL/LMO2 and Ldb1/NLI (Drissen et al. 2004, Vakoc et al. 2005, Song et al. 2007)

It is clear that specific transcription factors bind to LCRs and recruit chromatin remodeling complexes of the SWI/SNF type and histone modifying complexes. Together, these factors and complexes are thought to alter the target promoters of the LCRs such that they become conducive to formation of an RNA pol II pre-initiation complex and to transcription initiation. From that understanding evolved questions about how the factors bound to distal LCRs, in the case of the β-globin gene up to 60 Kb distant, influence the promoter to increase transcription. The currently favored paradigm is that the region between the enhancer and promoter "loops" out to permit the factors bound to the LCRs to interact with other factors at the promoter. This model is supported by studies using 3C (chromosome conformation capture) and RNA-TRAP (tagging and recovery of associated proteins) that documented close proximity of the β-globin LCR and β-globin gene, presumed evidence of loop formation (Dekker et al. 2002; Carter et al. 2002; Tolhuis et al. 2002) (Fig. 3).

As previously mentioned, the α-globin genes and their upstream regulatory sequences are situated among housekeeping genes. The α-globin genes also form close interactions with their upstream regulatory elements and with the nearby housekeeping genes in erythroid cells, whereas, in non-erythroid cells the housekeepng genes retain their associations with each other but those with β-globin and the upstream regulatory sites are lost (Zhou et al. 2006) (Vernimmen et al. 2007). Numerous other examples now exist showing LCR/enhancer-gene proximity, for example, in the $T_H 2$ cytokine locus, the B cell Ig kappa locus and for odorant receptor genes and their enhancer on a separate chromosome (Spilianakis and Flavell, 2004; Liu and Garrard, 2005; Lomvardas et al. 2006).

In the β-globin locus, several factors required for transcription activation have been shown to be required for looping between the LCR and β-globin gene. These include GATA-1, FOG-1 and EKLF (Vakoc et al. 2005; Drissen et al. 2004). GATA-1 participates in a complex with erythroid specific factors SCL and LMO2 that interacts with both the β-globin LCR and gene and includes a non-DNA binding, ubiquitously expressed protein, Ldb1/NLI, which anchors the loop between the LCR and gene promoter (Song et al. 2007). Certain LCR or β-globin sequences appear to be dispensable, at least individually, for loop formation, however, looping (and gene activation) failed to occur if both LCR HS3 and the β-globin promoter were absent (Patrinos et al. 2004). The data favor the idea that the LCR-gene loop is required for high level transcription. This leaves open the question of how a low level of transcription is established in the absence of the LCR. Possibly, other long range associations are established that mediate some chromatin alterations at the β-globin promoter in the absence of the LCR: a high throughput 3C approach could reveal such interactions (Dostie et al. 2006). Alternatively basal transcription may occur in fully differentiated erythroid cells when activating factors bind the globin promoters independent of the LCR, as mentioned above (Vakoc et al. 2005).

7 β-Globin LCR and Sub-nuclear Localization

Studies on the subnuclear localization of the β-globin locus have opened a distinctly new perspective from which to understand the role of the LCR. The first relevant set of studies showed that as the locus becomes activated it assumes a new position within the nucleus by moving away from the heterochromatin that is generally found near the nuclear membrane (Francastel et al. 2001). One important set of studies concerns the localization of the locus in the concentrations of pol II known as transcription factories (TFs). It has generally been assumed that transcription occurred in a random distribution within the nucleus mediated by recruitment of soluble pol II to the promoter under the influence of transcription factors which organize, *de novo*, a transcription initiation complex. Other studies that more recently have received attention support a model in which pol II is concentrated in discrete sub-nuclear bodies with a very high density of pol II, the so called TFs (reviewed in Pombo et al. 2000). Once the viewpoint that a soluble pol II is recruited to the promoter is replaced by a model in which the transcribed locus has somehow been brought into an existing TF, the possible models for how transcription is regulated change considerably. An important new model is that *cis* regulatory elements like the LCR and the factors that bind such enhancers, influence the recruitment to and the retention of the locus in a TF (Osborne et al. 2004). They increase the time that a given locus is in association with a transcription factory and therefore increase the amount of transcription.

For this model to have validity the following requirements must be satisfied: 1) transcription should only occur when the locus co-localizes with a TF and when transcription is not occurring this localization should be lost. This supports the idea that the physical presence of a locus in a transcription factory is necessary, sufficient and rate-limiting for transcription. 2) the presence of a powerful enhancer/LCR like the β-globin LCR should mediate increased transcription in direct proportion to an increase in the amount of time the locus under its control spends in association with the TF and an increase in the amount of time the locus is being transcribed. This second condition would rule out models in which the LCR increases the amount of transcription that occurs during a given association with the TF rather than the fraction of time the locus associates with the TF at all.

A variety of recent studies support aspects of these requirements and the associated model of LCR functional activity. Studies that support condition 1 show that most genes are being transcribed a low percentage of the time and are in association with a TF only when being transcribed (Osborne et al. 2004). This implies that association with a TF is transient and a rate limiting step in the transcription process. However, the β and α globin loci in an erythroblast are both transcribed and associated with a TF as much as 95% of the time (Osborne et al. 2004). This unusual consistency of TF association and transcription is mediated by the LCR for the β globin locus, since when the LCR is deleted, the level of transcription is reduced 30–50 fold and the amount of time the locus is in association with a TF, is also greatly reduced (Ragoczy et al. 2006). However, this interesting study comes with a caveat; there appear to be two types of TFs, those with active pol II hyperphosphorylated at the C-terminal domain and those with inactive, hypophosphorylated polII. The LCR mediates association with TFs that have active pol II. Without the LCR, the locus is predominantly associated with TFs that do not appear to contain active pol II. These studies raise the important possibility that the LCR functions by somehow allowing the β-globin locus to spend an unusual amount of time in association with active pol II in a specific type of transcription factory.

The LCR appears to have multiple epigenetic functions in multiple contexts and integrating these functions into a unified model is a challenge. How does the β-globin LCR and the loop it forms with the β promoter relate to recruitment to a TF with active polII? The available data suggest that looping precedes transcription activation since transcription fails to occur when Ldb1/NLI which bridges the β-globin LCR-gene loop is ablated using shRNA (Song et al. 2007). This suggests that the order of events is looping, followed by movement in to a TF, followed by transcription which is consistent with detection of large amounts of pol II at the β-globin promoter after looping has occurred. Biochemical studies support certain aspects of this proposal (Kim et al. 2007c). If true, TFs would need to exist stably within nuclei in the absence of transcription. This has been shown to be the case after inhibition of transcription by DRB or by heat shock (Mitchell and Fraser, 2008). What happens to LCR/β-globin looping and to associations of β-globin genes with distal genes sharing the same factory? These authors found that associations with distal genes within a TF were retained after inhibition of transcription elongation by DRB, but they were lost, along with localization to the factory, after inhibition of initiation by heat shock. Under both conditions the LCR/β-globin loop remained stable, again supporting the idea that loop formation does not require transcription or TF localization and is an early step in the process by which the LCR mediates high level transcription of the β-like globin genes. Is looping required for movement to or maintenance in an active TF? If so, how does this chromatin conformation contribute to movement? These questions, along with the fundamental issue of what sort of motor allows directed movement of a locus to a TF will be important to address in future work.

Acknowledgment We thank Dr. Cecilia Trainor for comments on the manuscript. This work was funded by the Intramural Program of the NIDDK, NIH (A.D.) and NIH-NIDDK (RO1-DK54071) and NIH-NHLBI (RO1-HL73431) (S.F.)

References

Alami, R., Greally, J.M., Tanimoto, K., Hwang, S., Feng, Y.Q., Engel, J.D., Fiering, S., Bouhassira, E. (2000). ß-globin YAC transgenes exhibit uniform expression levels but position effect variegation in mice. Hum. Mol. Gen. 9, 631–636.

Ben-David, Y., Bani, M.R., Chabot, B., De, K.A., and Bernstein, A. (1992). Retroviral insertions downstream of the heterogeneous nuclear ribonucleoprotein A1 gene in erythroleukemia cells: evidence that A1 is not essential for cell growth. Mol. Cell Biol 12, 4449–4455.

Bender, M.A., Byron, R., Ragoczy, T., Telling, A., Bulger, M., and Groudine, M. (2006). Flanking HS-62.5 and 3′ HS1, and regions upstream of the LCR, are not required for beta-globin transcription. Blood 108, 1395–1401.

Bender, M.A., Reik, A., Close, J., Telling, A., Epner, E., Fiering, S., Hardison, R., and Groudine, M. (1998). Description and targeted deletion of 5′ hypersensitive site 5 and 6 of the mouse β-globin locus control region. Blood 92, 4394–4403.

Bender, M.A., Bulger, M., Close, J., Groudine, M. (2000) ß-globin gene switching and DNaseI sensitivity of the endogenous ß-globin locus in mice do not require the Locus Control Region. Mol. Cell 5, 387–393.

Berger, S.L. (2007). The complex language of chromatin regulation during transcription. Nature 447, 407–412.

Blobel, G.A., Nakajima, T., Eckner, R., Montminy, M., and Orkin, S.H. (1998). CREB-binding protein cooperates with transcription factor GATA-1 and is required for erythroid differentiation. Proc. Natl. Acad. Sci. U. S. A. 95, 2061–2066.

Bulger, M. and Groudine, M. (1999). Looping versus linking: toward a model for long-distance gene activation. Genes Dev. 13, 2465–2477.

Bulger, M., Schubeler, D., Bender, M.A., Hamilton, J., Farrell, C.M., Hardison, R.C., and Groudine, M. (2003). A complex chromatin landscape revealed by patterns of nuclease sensitivity and histone modification within the mouse β-globin locus. Mol. Cell. Biol. 23, 5234–5244.

Burgess-Beusse, B., Farrell, C., Gaszner, M., Litt, M., Mutskov, V., Recillas-Targa, F., Simpson, M., West, A., and Felsenfeld, G. (2002). The insulation of genes from external enhancers and silencing chromatin. Proc Natl Acad. Sci. U. S. A 99 Suppl 4, 16433–16437.

Carter, D., Chakalova, L., Osborne, C.S., Dai, Y., and Fraser, P. (2002). Long-range chromatin regulatory interactions in vivo. Nat. Genet. 32, 623–626.

Chada, K., Magram, J., Costantini, F. (1985). Developmental regulation of a cloned adult beta-gene in transgenic mice. Nature 315, 338–40.

Cheng, X., Reginato, M.J., Andrews, N.C., and Lazar, M.A. (1997). The transcriptional integrator CREB-binding protein mediates positive cross talk between nuclear hormone receptors and the hematopoietic bZip protein p45/NF-E2. Mol. Cell. Biol. 17, 1407–1416.

Chung, J.H., Whiteley, M., and Felsenfeld, G. (1993). A 5′ element of the chicken β-globin domain serves as an insulator in human erythroid cells and protects against position effect in Drosophila. Cell 74, 505–514.

Dean, A. (2006). On a chromosome far, far away: LCRs and gene regulation. Trends Genet. *22*, 38–45.

De Gobbi, M., Anguita, E., Hughes, J., Sloane-Stanley, J. A., Sharpe, J. A., Koch, C. M., Dunham, I., Gibbons, R. J., Wood, W. G., Higgs, D. R. (2007). Tissue-specific histone modification and transcription factor binding in alpha globin gene expression. Blood 110, 4503–10.

Dekker, J., Rippe, K., Dekker, M., and Kleckner, N. (2002). Capturing chromosome conformation. Science *295*, 1306–1311.

DeSimone, J., Heller, P., Hall, L., Zwiers, D. (1982) 5-Azacytidine stimulates fetal hemoglobin synthesis in anemic baboons. Proc. Natl. Acad. Sci. USA *79*, 4428–4431.

Dostie, J., Richmond, T.A., Arnaout, R.A., Selzer, R.R., Lee, W.L., Honan, T.A., Rubio, E.D., Krumm, A., Lamb, J., Nusbaum, C., Green, R.D., and Dekker, J. (2006). Chromosome Conformation Capture Carbon Copy (5C): a massively parallel solution for mapping interactions between genomic elements. Genome Res. *16*, 1299–1309.

Drissen, R., Palstra, R.J., Gillemans, N., Splinter, E., Grosveld, F., Philipsen, S., and de Laat, W. (2004). The active spatial organization of the β-globin locus requires the transcription factor EKLF. Genes Dev. *18*, 2485–2490.

Farrell, C.M., Grinberg, A., Huang, S.P., Chen, D., Pichel, J.G., Westphal, H., and Felsenfeld, G. (2000). A large upstream region is not necessary for gene expression or hypersensitive site formation at the mouse β-globin locus. Proc Natl. Acad. Sci. USA *97*, 14554–14559.

Farrell, C.M., West, A.G., and Felsenfeld, G. (2002). Conserved CTCF insulator elements flank the mouse and human β-globin loci. Mol Cell. Biol. *22*, 3820–3831.

Forrester, W.C., Novak, U., Gelinas, R., Groudine, M. (1989) Molecular analysis of the human beta-globin locus activation region. Proc. Natl. Acad. Sci. USA 86, 5439–5443.

Forrester, W.C., Epner, E., Driscoll, M.C., Enver, T., Brice, M., Papayannopoulou, T., and Groudine, M. (1990). A deletion of the human β-globin locus activation region causes a major alteration in chromatin structure and replication across the entire β-globin locus. Genes and Development *4*, 1637–1649.

Forrester, W.C., Thompson, C., Elder, J.T., and Groudine, M. (1986). A developmentally stable chromatin structure in the human β-globin gene cluster. Proc. Natl. Acad. Sci. USA *83*, 1359–1363.

Forsberg, E.C., Downs, K.M., Christensen, H.M., Im, H., Nuzzi, P.A., and Bresnick, E.H. (2000). Developmentally dynamic histone acetylation pattern of a tissue- specific chromatin domain. Proc. Natl. Acad. Sci. USA. *97*, 14494–14499.

Francastel, C., Magis, W., Groudine, M. (2001) Nuclear relocation of a transactivator subunit precedes target gene activation. Proc. Natl. Acad. Sci. USA *98*, 12120–12125.

Gaensler, K.M., Kitamura, M., Kan, Y.W. (1993). Germ-line transmission and developmental regulation of a 150-kb yeast artificial chromsome containing the human beta-globin locus in transgenic mice. Proc. Natl. Acad. Sci, USA 90, 11381–11385.

Goren, A., Simchen, G., Fibach, E., Szabo, P. E., Tanimoto, K., Chakalova, L., Pfeifer, G., Fraser, P. J., Engel, J. D., Cedar, H. (2006) Fine tuning of globin gene expression by DNA methylation. PLOS One *1*, e46.

Grosveld, F., van Assendelft, G.B., Greaves, D.R., and Kollias, G. (1987). Position-independent, high-level expression of the human β-globin gene in transgenic mice. Cell *51*, 975–985.

Hebbes, T.R., Clayton, A.L., Thorne, A.W., and Crane-Robinson, C. (1994). Core histone hyperacetylation co-maps with generalized DNase I sensitivity in the chicken β-globin chromosomal domain. EMBO J. *13*, 1823–1830.

Higgs, D. R., Vernimmen, D., De Gobbi, M., Anguita, E., Hughes, J., Buckle, V., Iborra, F., Garrick, D., Wood, W. G. (2006). How transcriptional and epigenetic programmes are played out on an individual mammalian gene cluster during lineage commitment and differentiation. Biochem. Soc. Symp. *73*, 11–22

Ho, Y., Elefant, F., Cooke, N., and Liebhaber, S. (2002). A defined locus control region determinant links chromatin domain acetylation with long-range gene activation. Mol. Cell *9*, 291–302.

Hsu, M., Mabaera, R., Lowrey, C. H., Martin, D. I., Fiering, S. (2007) CpG hypomethylation in a large domain encompassing the embryonic β-like globin genes in primitive erythrocytes. Mol. Cell. Biol. 27, 5047–5054.

Johnson, K.D., Christensen, H.M., Zhao, B., and Bresnick, E.H. (2001). Distinct mechanisms control RNA polymerase II recruitment to a tissue- specific locus control region and a downstream promoter. Mol. Cell *8*, 465–471.

Kim, A., Kiefer, C.M., and Dean, A. (2007a). Distinctive signatures of histone methylation in transcribed coding and noncoding human β-globin sequences. Mol. Cell. Biol. *27*, 1271–1279.

Kim, A., Song, S.H., Brand, M., and Dean, A. (2007b). Nucleosome and transcription activator antagonism at human beta-globin locus control region DNase I hypersensitive sites. Nucleic Acids Res. *35*, 5831–5838.

Kim, S.I., Bultman, S.J., Jing, H., Blobel, G.A., and Bresnick, E.H. (2007c). Dissecting Molecular Steps in Chromatin Domain Activation during Hematopoietic Differentiation. Mol. Cell Biol. *27*, 4551–4565.

Kaufman, R.M., Pham, C.T., Ley, T.J. (1999). Transgenic analysis of a 110-kb human ß-globin cluster-containing DNA fragment propagated as a bacterial artificial chromosome. Blood *94*, 3178–3184.

Ley, T.J., Anagnou, N.P., Noguchi, C.T. (1983) DNA methylation and globin gene expression patients treated with 5-azacytidine. Prog. Clin. Biol. Res. *134*, 457–474.

Letting, D.L., Rakowski, C., Weiss, M.J., and Blobel, G.A. (2003). Formation of a tissue-specific histone acetylation pattern by the hematopoietic transcription factor GATA-1. Mol. Cell. Biol. *23*, 1334–1340.

Li, Q., Peterson, K.R., Fang, X., and Stamatoyannopoulos, G. (2002). Locus control regions. Blood *100*, 3077–3086.

Litt, M.D., Simpson, M., Gaszner, M., Allis, C.D., and Felsenfeld, G. (2001a). Correlation between histone lysine methylation and developmental changes at the chicken beta-globin locus. Science *293*, 2453–2455.

Litt, M.D., Simpson, M., Recillas-Targa, F., Prioleau, M.N., and Felsenfeld, G. (2001b). Transitions in histone acetylation reveal boundaries of three separately regulated neighboring loci. EMBO J. *20*, 2224–2235.

Liu, Z. and Garrard, W.T. (2005). Long-range interactions between three transcriptional enhancers, active Vkappa gene promoters, and a 3′ boundary sequence spanning 46 kilobases. Mol. Cell. Biol. *25*, 3220–3231.

Lomvardas, S., Barnea, G., Pisapia, D.J., Mendelsohn, M., Kirkland, J., and Axel, R. (2006). Interchromosomal interactions and olfactory receptor choice. Cell *126*, 403–413.

Mahajan, M.C., Karmakar, S, Weissman, S.M. (2007) Control of beta globin genes. J. Cell. Biochem. 102, 801–810.

Masternak, K., Peyraud, N., Krawczyk, M., Barras, E., and Reith, W. (2003). Chromatin remodeling and extragenic transcription at the MHC class II locus control region. Nat. Immunol. *4*, 132–137.

Milot, E., Stroubolis, J., Trimborn, T., Wijgerde, M., de Boer, E., Langeveld, A., Tan-un, K., Vergeer, W., Yannoutsos, N., Grosveld, F., Fraser, P. (1996) Heterochromatin effects on the frequency and duration of LCR-mediated gene transcription. Cell *87*, 105–114.

Mitchell, J.A. and Fraser, P. (2008). Transcription factories are nuclear subcompartments that remain in the absence of transcription. Genes Dev. *22*, 20–25.

Osborne, C.S., Chakalova, L., Brown, K.E., Carter, D., Horton, A., Debrand, E., Goyenechea, B., Mitchell, J.A., Lopes, S., Reik, W., Fraser, P. (2004) Active genes dynamically colocalize to shared sites of ongoing transcription. Nature Gen. *36*, 1065–1071.

Palstra, R.J., Tolhuis, B., Splinter, E., Nijmeijer, R., Grosveld, F., de Laat, W. (2003) The β-globin nuclear compartment in development and erythroid differentiation. Nature Gen. *35*, 190–194.

Patrinos, G.P., de Krom, M., de Boer, E., Langeveld, A., Imam, A.M., Strouboulis, J., de Laat, W., and Grosveld, F.G. (2004). Multiple interactions between regulatory regions are required to stabilize an active chromatin hub. Genes Dev. *18*, 1495–1509.

Pombo, A., Jones, E., Iborra, F. J., Kimura, H., Sugaya, K., Cook, P. R., Jackson, D. A. (2000) Specialized transcription factories within mammalian nuclei. Crit. Rev. Eukaryot. Gene. Expr. *10*, 21–29.

Pondel, M.D., George, M., Proudfoot, N.J. (1992) The LCR-like alpha-globin positive regulatory element functions as an enhancer in transiently transfected cells during erythroid differentiation. Nucl. Acids Res. 20, 237–243.

Porcu, S., Kitamura, M., Witkowska, E., Zhang, Z., Mutero, A., Lin, C., Chang, J., Gaensler, K.M. (1997) The human beta-globin locus introduced by YAC transfer exhibits a specific and reproducible pattern of developmental regulation in transgenic mice. Blood 90, 4602–4609.

Ragoczy, T., Bender, M.A., Telling, A., Byron, R., Groudine, M. (2006) The locus control region is required for association of the murine beta-globin locus with engaged transcription factories during erythroid maturation. Genes Dev. 20 1447–1457.

Raich, N., Enver, T., Nakamoto, B., Josephson, B., Papayannopoulou, T., Stamatoyannopoulos, G. (1990) Autonomous developmental control of human embryonic globin gene switching in transgenic mice. Science, 250, 1147–1149.

Rombel, I., Hu, K.Y., Zhang, Q., Papayannopoulou, T., Stamatoyannopoulos, G., Shen, C.K. (1995) Transcriptional activation of human adult alpha-globin genes by hypersensitive site -40 enhancer: function of nuclear factor-binding motifs occupied in erythroid cells. Proc. Natl. Acad. Sci. USA 92, 6454–6458.

Rupon, J. W., Wang, S. Z., Gaensler, K., Lloyd, J., Ginder, G. D. (2006) Methyl binding domain protein 2 mediates gamma-globin gene silencing in adult human betaYAC transgenic mice. Proc. Natl. Acad. Sci. USA *103*, 6617–6622.

Sabatino, D. E., Wong, C., Cline, A. P., Pyle, L., Garrett, L. J., Gallagher, P. G., Bodine, D. M. (2000) A minimal ankyrin promoter linked to a human gamma-globin gene demonstrates erythroid specific copy number dependent expression with minimal position or enhancer dependence in transgenic mice. J. Biol. Chem. 275, 28549–28554.

Schubeler, D., Groudine, M., Bender, M.A. (2001) The murine ß-globin locus control region regulates the rate of trancription but not the hyperacetylation of histones at the active genes. Proc. Natl. Acad. Sci. USA 98, 11432–11437.

Sharpe, J.A., Wells. D.J., Whitelaw, E., Vyas, P., Higgs, D.R., Wood, W.G. (1993) Analysis of the human alpha-globin gene cluster in transgenic mice. Proc. Natl. Acad. Sci. USA 90, 11262–11266.

Singal, R., Ferris, R., Little, J.A., Wang, S.Z., Ginder, GD. (1997) Methylation of the minimal promoter of an embryonic globin gene sliences transcription in primary erythroid cells. Proc. Natl. Acad. Sci. USA *94*, 13724–13729.

Song, S.-H., Hou, C., and Dean, A. A positive role for NLI/Ldb1 in long-range β-globin locus control region function. Mol.Cell 28, 810–822. 12-14-2007.

Spilianakis, C.G. and Flavell, R.A. (2004). Long-range intrachromosomal interactions in the T helper type 2 cytokine locus. Nat. Immunol. *5*, 1017–1027.

Splinter, E., Heath, H., Kooren, J., Palstra, R.J., Klous, P., Grosveld, F., Galjart, N., and de Laat, W. (2006). CTCF mediates long-range chromatin looping and local histone modification in the beta-globin locus. Genes Dev. *20*, 2349–2354.

Stamatoyannopoulos, G. (2005). Control of globin gene expression during development and erythroid differentiation. Exp. Hematol. *33*, 259–271.

Tanimoto, K., Liu, Q., Bungert, J., Engel, J.D. (1999) Effects of altered gene order or orientation of the locus control region on human ß-globin gene expression in mice. Nature *398*, 344–347.

Tolhuis, B., Palstra, R.J., Splinter, E., Grosveld, F., and de Laat, W. (2002). Looping and interaction between hypersensitive sites in the active -globin locus. Mol. Cell *10*, 1453–1465.

Townes, T.M., Lingrel, J.B., Chen, H.Y., Brinster, R.L., Palmiter, R.D. (1985) Eythroid-specific expression of human beta-globin genes in transgenic mice. EMBO J. 4: 1715–1723

Tuan, D., Solomon, W., Li, Q., and London, I.M. (1985). The "beta-like-globin" gene domain in human erythroid cells. Proc. Natl. Acad. Sci. U. S. A. *82*, 6384–6388.

Vakoc, C.R., Letting, D.L., Gheldof, N., Sawado, T., Bender, M.A., Groudine, M., Weiss, M.J., Dekker, J., and Blobel, G.A. (2005). Proximity among distant regulatory elements at the -globin locus requires GATA-1 and FOG-1. Mol. Cell *17*, 453–462.

van der Ploeg, L. H., Flavell, R.A. (1980) DNA methylation in the human gamma delta beta-globin locus in erythroid and nonerythroid tissues. Cell *19*,847–858.

Vernimmen, D., De Gobbi, M., Sloane-Stanley, J.A., Wood, W.G., and Higgs, D.R. (2007). Long-range chromosomal interactions regulate the timing of the transition between poised and active gene expression. EMBO J. *26*, 2041–2051.

Weiss, M.J., Yu, C., and Orkin, S.H. (1997). Erythroid-cell-specific properties of transcription factor GATA-1 revealed by phenotypic rescue of a gene-targeted cell line. Mol. Cell Biol. *17*, 1642–1651.

Zhang, W. and Bieker, J.J. (1998). Acetylation and modulation of erythroid Kruppel-like factor (EKLF) activity by interaction with histone acetyltransferases. Proc. Natl. Acad. Sci. U. S. A. *95*, 9855–9860.

Zhou, G.L., Xin, L., Song, W., Di, L.J., Liu, G., Wu, X.S., Liu, D.P., and Liang, C.C. (2006). Active chromatin hub of the mouse alpha-globin locus forms in a transcription factory of clustered housekeeping genes. Mol. Cell Biol *26*, 5096–5105.

Meiotic Silencing, Infertility and X Chromosome Evolution

James M.A. Turner

1 Introduction

Pairing or synapsis of homologous chromosomes during meiosis is essential for normal chromosome segregation and the generation of genetically balanced offspring. For this reason, meiotic synapsis is subject to close surveillance and cells in which homologues fail to associate are rapidly removed from the germ cell pool. According to the classical model, meiotic cells with synaptic errors are identified and eliminated by a 'pachytene checkpoint', which shares mechanistic similarities with the mitotic DNA damage checkpoint. However, in mammals, the existence of a pachytene checkpoint has recently been called into question. The sex chromosomes – X and Y chromosomes – are largely asynapsed during normal male meiosis, but this clearly does not trigger pachytene arrest. A more parsimonious explanation for how chromosome pairing failure causes germ cell loss has now been provided by the discovery of meiotic silencing. In this review, I will discuss what is known about meiotic silencing in different organisms. Furthermore, I will discuss how meiotic silencing in mammals has shaped the gene content of the X chromosome and how it may have been co-opted as a means of dosage compensation.

2 Meiosis and the Threat of Unpaired Chromosomes

In sexually reproducing organisms, meiosis represents a pivotal point in germ cell differentiation. It is characterised by two fundamental steps. First, maternal and paternal homologous chromosomes are drawn together into close physical proximity within the nucleus by a protein scaffold known as the synaptonemal complex (SC). Then, the resulting 'synapsed' chromosome pair engages in recombination, in which resected DNA double strand breaks (DSBs) situated at multiple sites along the chromosome length invade the homologous chromosome.

J.M.A. Turner (✉)
Division of Stem Cell Research and Developmental Genetics, MRC National Institute for Medical Research, London NW7 1AA, UK

In mammals, meiotic recombination is initiated at 200–400 sites throughout the genome, yet around 90% of recombination intermediates are resolved as so-called gene conversion events – non-crossovers (NCOs) – where genetic material is not exchanged (Baudat and de Massy, 2007). The remaining 10% become crossovers (COs), physical connections that tether maternal and paternal homologues. Although few in number, COs constitute the *raison d'etre* of meiosis – in most organisms they are absolutely required for the generation of haploid gametes, because they ensure that homologous chromosomes segregate properly during the meiotic divisions. When CO formation is disturbed, the resulting gametes have the wrong chromosome number, and this in turn leads to aneuploid offspring, as seen in Down syndrome (Trisomy 21; Hassold et al. 2007).

Because normal recombination and synapsis are essential for CO formation, their progression is carefully monitored, and cells exhibiting errors in either of these processes are eliminated before reaching the meiotic divisions. In mice, mutations in genes required for meiotic recombination (such as *Dmc1* or *Msh5*) or (synapsis such as *Sycp1-3* or *Syce2*) cause complete pachytene arrest and infertility (Yoshida et al. 1998; Pittman et al. 1998; De Vries et al. 1999, 2005; Edelmann et al. 1999; Yuan et al. 2000; Yang et al. 2006; Bolcun-Filas et al. 2007). A similar phenotype is seen in *Saccharomyces cerevisiae* synapsis and recombination mutants. In this organism the arrest can be relieved by mutations in *Rad17*, *Rad24* and *Mec1* (Lydall et al. 1996; Roeder and Bailis, 2000). These genes also function in the mitotic G2/M checkpoint, where they delay cell division in the face of persistent DNA damage. In both yeast and mice, the initiation of recombination – the formation of DNA DSBs – precedes synapsis, and therefore when synapsis is disturbed, the resulting unsynapsed chromosomes are replete with unresolved DNA DSBs (Mahadevaiah et al. 2001; Padmore et al. 1991). It is currently believed that errors in synapsis or recombination cause arrest through a checkpoint pathway that is triggered by unresolved DNA DSBs, reminiscent of the situation in mitotic cells (Odorisio et al. 1998).

While it is certainly convenient to suppose that defective synapsis and recombination trigger meiotic arrest in mammals through a 'pachytene checkpoint', there is a fly in the ointment – the X and Y chromosomes of male meiotic cells. Although regarded as 'homologues' these chromosomes have diverged from one over the last 240–320 million years following recombination suppression (Lahn, and Page, 1999). As such, they are unsynapsed along much of their length during normal male meiosis. Immunocytological analysis shows that the X chromosome (but not the Y chromosome) acquires meiotic DNA DSBs and that these persist throughout pachytene – during and after the point at which the pachytene checkpoint is thought to operate (Ashley, 1995; Moens et al. 1997). This presents a conundrum: why does the constitutively unsynapsed and DNA DSB-enriched X chromosome not trigger pachytene arrest in all male meiotic cells? This has led researchers to reconsider whether a pachytene checkpoint analogous to that described in yeast really does control germ cell losses associated with asynapsis in mammals. An alternative explanation is that unsynapsed chromosomes trigger meiotic arrest through another process; meiotic silencing.

3 Meiotic Silencing of Unsynapsed Chromosomes – from Fungi to Mice

Aside from being unsynapsed, the mammalian X and Y chromosomes display another distinctive feature during meiosis – they are transcriptionally silent. This silencing, known as Meiotic Sex Chromosome Inactivation (MSCI), occurs as soon as synapsis of the autosomal homologues is complete, at the zygotene to pachytene transition, and results in the formation of the sex body (Solari, 1974; McKee, and Handel, 1993; Turner, 2007). MSCI has been described in a vast array of organisms in which the sex chromosomes are poorly paired, including *Caenorhabditis elegans* (Goldstein, 1982), mammals (Solari, 1974) and recently, flies (Hense et al. 2007). Although this degree of conservation suggests that MSCI is important, we remained ignorant of its function until a landmark paper appeared from the Metzenberg lab describing a similar silencing process in the fungus *Neurospora crassa*, named Meiotic Silencing by Unpaired DNA (Shiu et al. 2001).

In *Neurospora*, meiosis place takes within the zygote, following fusion of haploid nuclei from parents of opposite mating type. The resulting four haploid products then undergo a round of mitosis, generating eight ascospores that are arranged in a linear array within the spindle-shaped ascus (Raju, 1992). Ascospore development requires the *Ascospore maturation-1* (*Asm-1*) gene (Aramayo and Metzenberg, 1996). Heterozygous loss-of-function mutations in *Asm-1* are ascospore-autonomous; those ascospores inheriting the mutant allele are inviable, while those inheriting the wild-type allele develop normally. Curiously however, complete deletion of one of the two copies of *Asm-1* causes inviability of all ascospores, including those with the wild type allele. The phenotype cannot be corrected by expression of a wild type copy of *Asm1* inserted at an ectopic location (Aramayo and Metzenberg, 1996). This and other observations led (Shiu et al. 2001) to conclude that close physical apposition, or meiotic pairing, of the *Asm1* genes is required for their correct expression during meiosis. In the absence of pairing – as seen in the *Asm1* deletion mutant – a signal results in silencing of all additional copies of *Asm1*. This process is known as Meiotic Silencing by Unpaired DNA (MSUD; Shiu et al. 2001). MSUD may act as a means of defense by preventing the expression of invading transposable elements. When these elements integrate into the host genome, they will be hemizygous and therefore sensed us unpaired, and as a consequence they will be silenced by MSUD (Shiu et al. 2001).

When we apply these observations on chromosome pairing in *Neurospora* to mammalian sex chromosomes, the existence of MSCI begins to make sense. The X chromosome has no synaptic partner during male meiosis, and therefore MSCI could be viewed as the cumulative effect of MSUD operating at each unpaired X-gene locus. In support of this idea, data from both *C. elegans* and mammals show unequivocally that asynapsis drives MSCI (Bean et al. 2004; Turner et al. 2006). In *C. elegans* males have an XO and hermaphrodites an XX genotype. The single unsynapsed X chromosome of male early pachytene cells becomes enriched in repressive histone marks, most notably histone H3 dimethylated on lysine 9 (H3K9me2; Bean et al. 2004). In contrast, when there is complete X chromosome synapsis, as in XX hermaphrodites and in XX sex-reversed (*tra-2*) males, there is no enrichment for H3K9me2, suggesting that the appearance of this mark on the X chromosome in the XO male is related to its asynapsed state (Bean et al. 2004). Furthermore, males carrying a mutation that prevents autosomal synapsis (*him-8*) display enrichment of H3K9me2 on unsynapsed autosomes as well as on the unsynapsed X chromosome (Bean et al. 2004). Thus, any meiotic chromosome can acquire this repressive histone mark if unsynapsed.

Experiments in mice paint a similar picture. Both the X and Y chromosome are silenced at the onset of pachytene in normal (XY) males, but not when an additional Y chromosome is provided. In XYY males the two Y chromosomes often synapse completely and the resulting YY bivalents escape MSCI (Turner et al. 2006). Conversely, in male mice with chromosome rearrangements that disrupt autosomal synapsis, the resulting unsynapsed autosomal segments are transcriptionally silenced (Turner et al. 2005; Baarends et al. 2005; Homolka et al. 2007). An example of this is seen in the T(X;16)16H male mouse, which carries a reciprocal translocation between the X chromosome and one of the two chromosome 16 homologues (Ford, and Evans, 1964). This translocation disrupts normal chromosome 16 :chromosome 16 synapsis, and the unsynapsed chromosome 16 segments are transcriptionally silenced and become spatially sequestered with the X and Y chromosomes in the sex body (Turner et al. 2005). Rather surprisingly meiotic silencing is not restricted to males either in mice or *C. elegans*; in both XO female mice and XO *C. elegans*, the absence of the normal X chromosome pairing partner triggers silencing of the remaining unsynapsed X chromosome (Bean et al. 2004; Baarends et al. 2005; Turner et al. 2005).

4 MSUD and MSUC – Vanishing Similarities, Emerging Differences?

Although the abbreviation 'MSUD' was originally extended to describe silencing of unsynapsed chromosomes in organisms other than *Neurospora*, it is now clear – at least in mammals – that this term is no longer appropriate. Meiotic silencing in *Neurospora* and mammals differs in a number of key respects and this may suggest that they are fundamentally different biological processes.

First of all, while MSUD is strictly homology-driven, meiotic silencing in mammals is not. Experiments in *Neurospora* show that two sequences with as little as 6% nucleotide divergence can trigger silencing (Pratt et al. 2004). In contrast, synapsis between entirely non-homologous sequences can overcome silencing in mice. For example, in up to 30% of oocytes in XO females the single X chromosome is able to self synapse to form a hairpin structure, which allows escape from silencing and thus continued expression of X genes (Turner et al. 2005). Secondly, the term MSUD – Meiotic Silencing *by* Unpaired DNA – refers to the observation that unpaired genes can trigger silencing of closely related sequences located at distant sites in the genome – in *trans* (Shiu et al. 2001). In mice, MSCI certainly does not trigger *trans*-silencing. Evidence for this comes from studies of mice carrying an X-sequence containing YAC transgene integrated at an autosomal site (Okamoto et al. 2005). In contrast to the silent endogenous X-locus, the autosomal transgene is robustly expressed during pachytene due to its location on a synapsed homologous bivalent. Thus, in mammals, meiotic silencing does not involve cross-talk between identical DNA sequences located in different pairing environments. As these distinct properties have emerged, we have been forced to create another abbreviation to describe meiotic silencing in mammals – Meiotic Silencing of Unsynapsed Chromatin (MSUC; Schimenti, 2005).

Mechanistically, MSUD and MSUC share few common properties. MSUD silences genes at the post-transcriptional level, and accordingly involves several members of the RNA-interference (RNAi) pathway, most notably *Sad-1*, a putative RNA-dependent RNA polymerase (RdRP; Shiu et al. 2001), *Sms-2*, an Argonaute-like protein (Lee et al. 2003) and *Sms-3*, a Dicer-like protein (Kelly et al. 2007). A model for MSUD has been proposed in which regions of unpaired DNA generate aberrant transcripts that are converted into dsRNA by Sad1, and these dsRNAs then trigger the RNAi pathway (Kelly and Aramayo 2007). In contrast, RNA FISH, immunostaining and microarray approaches have shown that MSUC in mammals operates at the level of transcription (Baarends et al. 2005; Turner et al. 2005; Homolka et al. 2007). MSUC in mice requires a histone H2A variant, H2AX, which is phosphorylated at serine-139 by the kinase ATR (Fernandez-Capetillo et al. 2003). Targeting of ATR to the XY bivalent, in turn, requires the tumour suppressor BRCA1 (Turner et al. 2004; Fig. 1a). A notable feature of these three proteins is that they are also required for DNA DSB repair. This has led to the suggestion that the unresolved recombination intermediates present on unsynapsed chromosomes act as docking sites for BRCA1, which then recruits downstream silencing proteins (Bellani et al. 2005). If this were the case, then we would expect MSUC / MSCI to be dependent upon the presence of meiotic DNA DSBs. However, in *Spo11* null male pachytene cells – which have no DSBs and extensive asynapsis – an MSUC response is preserved (Mahadevaiah et al. 2008). BRCA1 appears on asynapsed axes with normal kinetics, and this is followed by accumulation of ATR, phosphorylation of H2AX and silencing. Nevertheless, the extent of this silencing response is limited. In contrast to other asynaptic mutants, in *Spo11*-null pachytene cells BRCA1 targets only a subpopulation of the unsynapsed chromosomes and so most unsynapsed chromosome remain transcriptionally active (Bellani et al. 2005; Mahadevaiah et al. 2008). Although these data show that MSUC is DNA DSB-independent, they do support the conclusion that DNA DSBs enhance targeting of the silencing response to unsynapsed chromosomes.

In mice, shortly after H2AX phosphorylation, a number of other chromatin modifications affect unsynapsed chromosomes. These include H2A ubiquitylation (Baarends et al. 1999) and widespread replacement of the canonical S-phase histones H3.1 and H3.2 for the histone variant H3.3 (van der Heijden et al. 2007). These transitions may be important in the maintenance of silencing to later stages of spermatogenesis. Like *C. elegans*, mammalian unsynapsed chromosomes are also enriched in H3K9me2 (Khalil et al. 2004; see Turner, 2007, for a more detailed description of components of the MSUC pathway in mice).

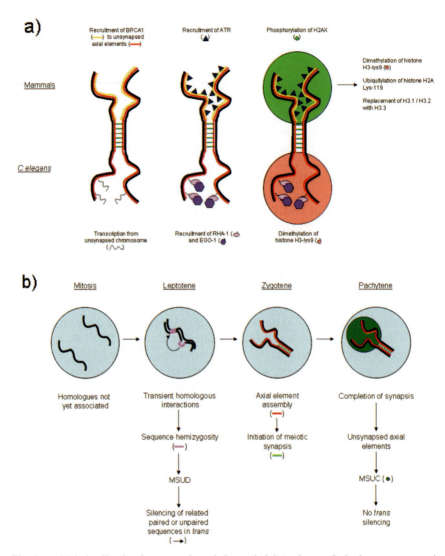

Fig. 1 (**a**) Meiotic silencing in mammals and *Caenorhabditis elegans*. In both cases, asynapsis at pachytene triggers the silencing response. In the case of mammals, unsynapsed axial elements recruit BRCA1, and BRCA1 then directly or indirectly recruits the kinase ATR. ATR subsequently phosphorylates histone H2AX. Downstream chromatin changes are numerous – the most significant are listed. In *Caenorhabditis elegans*, transcription from unsynapsed chromosomes results in recruitment of the RNA helicase RHA-1 and the RdRP EGO-1. These proteins co-operate to either directly recruit histone modifying enzymes or initiate RNAi-dependent heterochromatin assembly to result in dimethylation of histone H3 at lysine-9. (**b**) a potential model by which MSUD and MSUC can co-exist. Prior to meiosis, homologues are not associated. During leptotene, unstable homologous interactions permit trans-sensing – any sequence that is hemizygous initiates an RNAi-dependent silencing response – MSUD – which not only silences the hemizygous sequence but also any related sequence, whether paired or not. Later, during zygotene, meiotic synapsis initiates via the synaptonemal complex. Any chromosome unsynapsed at the zygotene – pachytene transition is detected by the second meiotic silencing process – MSUC – this results in transcriptional silencing but, unlike MSUD, related sequences in *trans* are not affected.

In *C. elegans* the distinction between MSUD and MSUC is less clear. *In-situ* hybridization data suggest that meiotic silencing occurs at the level of transcription, like mammalian MSUC (Bean et al. 2004). However, like *Neurospora* MSUD, silencing requires members of the RNAi machinery, most notably EGO-1, a putative RdRP (Maine et al. 2005). Studies in *S. pombe* have identified crosstalk between the post-transcriptional and transcriptional silencing pathways; the core RNAi components Dicer, Argonaute and RdRP are also required for heterochromatin formation and transcriptional silencing at centromeres and the mating-type locus, and this silencing involves H3K9me2 (Martienssen et al. 2005; Fig. 1a). It is therefore conceivable that in *C. elegans*, as in *Neurospora*, aberrant transcripts originating from unsynapsed chromosomes are the initiating event in the silencing response, but these transcripts could then direct transcriptional rather than post-transcriptional silencing via recruitment of chromatin-modifying enzymes that generate H3K9Me2 (Maine et al. 2005). With this in mind, the fact that MSUC in mice occurs at the transcriptional (RNA) level does not itself preclude the possibility that RNAi is somehow involved. One recent study has found that mouse MAEL, a protein whose *Drosophila* orthologue is implicated in RNAi (Findley et al. 2003) localizes both to sex body during pachytene and to the spermatid chromatoid body, where it interacts with *Argonaute*-like proteins MILI and MIWI, suggesting a possible link between RNAi and MSUC (Costa et al. 2006). However, any potential involvement of RNAi in mammalian MSUC will require much deeper investigation.

The perceived lack of similarity between *Neurospora* MSUD and mammalian MSUC may reflect an incorrect assumption – namely that 'pairing', as defined in MSUD, and 'synapsis', as defined in MSUC, are the same thing. It is clear that MSUC in mice occurs as a response to the presence of unsynapsed chromosomes during pachytene. However, although MSUD must involve some form of *trans*-sensing between homologous sequences, there is no evidence in *Neurospora* that this is related to meiotic synapsis. In many organisms, synapsis is preceded by a poorly-understood homologous pairing process that initiates during early leptotene and is functionally distinct from meiotic recombination and synapsis (Zickler, and Kleckner, 1998). This could represent an ideal opportunity for the *trans*-sensing required for MSUD to take place. Homologous pairing prior to meiotic synapsis has not been observed in mammals, but a phenomenon reminiscent of MSUD has been described, in which hemizygous transgenes can induce a heritable epigenetically repressed state on the homologous allele. This was subsequently shown to be due to paramutation, another RNA-mediated process (Rassoulzadegan et al. 2002). Therefore a mechanism analogous to *Neurospora* MSUD may be operating in mammals, but this could be occurring at a different time-point and in a mechanistically distinct way to MSUC (Fig. 1b).

5 The MSUC Model of Meiotic Arrest

Having established that unsynapsed chromosomes are silenced during meiosis, we can now begin to rethink how chromosome pairing failure might lead to pachytene arrest in mammals. The XO female and T(X;16)16H male mouse models already described above both have significant germ cell losses in pachytene. In XO females this causes a markedly shortened reproductive lifespan (Burgoyne and Baker, 1985), while in T(X;16)16H males it results in complete sterility (Odorisio et al. 1998).

When MSUC initiates, all genes within an unsynapsed chromosome segment will be silenced, with the effect that the meiotic cell will then be null with respect to all those genes. If there is even one gene within the unsynapsed chromosome segment that is required for progression through pachytene, then one would predict that meiosis will arrest. In the case of the XO female, silencing of the whole unsynapsed X chromosome would obviously not be compatible with cell survival during meiosis and it is therefore no surprise that there is such a precipitous loss of germ cells in the XO ovary. One would predict that the minority of XO oocytes that evade elimination – and permit limited fertility – would be those in which the X chromosome achieves full self-synapsis, allowing escape from MSUC. This is exactly what has been found. Studies in both XO mice and humans have shown that oocytes with hairpin X chromosomes progress to later stages of pachytene than those without (Speed, 1986).

Under the MSUC model, assuming that meiosis-critical genes are uniformly distributed among autosomes, the likelihood of an unsynapsed autosomal segment containing a meiosis-critical gene decreases in direct proportion to the length of that segment. Thus, mouse mutants with relatively short lengths of unsynapsed autosomal DNA would display less marked pachytene arrest. This prediction is borne out when comparing the phenotype of the T(X;16)16H male to other chromosomally aberrant models. The T(1;13)70H/T(1;13)1Wa double translocation hetereozygote male contains an autosome-autosome translocation that results in the formation of an unsynapsed loop during pachytene (Peters et al. 1997). This loop is relatively small compared to length of unsynapsed autosomal DNA in the T(X;16)16H male, and accordingly, T70H males are often fertile (Peters et al. 1997), in contrast to the complete spermatogenic arrest seen in T(X;16)16H males.

If silencing of unsynapsed chromosomes is detrimental to germ cell survival, an obvious question is how normal (XY) male meiotic cells tolerate the silencing of the X chromosome by MSCI. After all, silencing of the single unsynapsed X chromosome is detrimental to XO female meiosis, so why is it not equally harmful to normal male meiosis? In reality, despite the complete silencing of the X chromosome by MSCI, XY pachytene cells are not nullizygous for X gene products. The mouse genome is replete with duplicated, autosomally-located copies of essential X-linked genes (Wang, 2004). These copies have arisen during evolution by retroposition of X-derived transcripts and they are expressed exclusively in the testis during MSCI. Thus, silencing of the X chromosome by MSCI is tolerated by activation of this X-retrogene system. The transcription factors required for expression of these retrogenes are testis-specific (Yoshioka et al. 2007) and thus these genes are not activated in XO oocytes, explaining why the XO oocyte is unable to tolerate inactivation of the single X chromosome through MSUC.

6 Limits to the MSUC Model of Pachytene Arrest

MSUC provides a simple and compelling explanation for how chromosomal asynapsis causes pachytene arrest and it is certainly a more attractive than the pachytene checkpoint explanation. However, new studies now show that MSUC alone cannot explain germ cell losses in all meiotic mutants. A good case in point is the XYY male mouse. XYY mice have significant pachytene germ cell losses and they are usually sterile (Rodriguez, and Burgoyne, 2000). However, in contrast to the T(X;16)16H male, they do not have autosomal asynapsis and so there is no inappropriate silencing of autosomal genes by MSUC. Why then, are germ cells lost?

It turns out that escape from MSCI is as lethal to male germ cells as MSUC. During early pachytene in XYY meiosis, most meiotic cells have three unsynapsed sex chromosomes. In this case the X chromosome and the two Y chromosomes are silenced by MSUC / MSCI (Turner et al. 2006). As already discussed, the remaining early pachytene cells – around 22% – show complete YY synapsis, and the resulting YY bivalents escape silencing (Turner et al. 2006). Interestingly, the same analysis at late pachytene gives a different picture – *all* germ cells have three unsynapsed sex chromosomes, and cells with YY bivalents are rare or absent. This suggests that those early pachytene cells with YY bivalents are eliminated at some stage prior to late pachytene (Turner et al. 2006). But why should cells with YY bivalents be at a disadvantage compared to those without? One obvious consequence of Y chromosome synapsis is that the resulting YY bivalents will express Y genes that should normally be silenced by MSUC / MSCI, and so inappropriate expression of one or more Y genes could be toxic to mid-pachytene cells.

Other experimental models support the notion that MSCI is essential for male meiosis. In T(X;16)16H males, the X chromosome occasionally undergoes non-homologous synapsis with chromosome 16 and in doing so escapes MSCI (Turner et al. 2006). Like XYY cells with YY bivalents, these pachytene cells are eliminated at mid pachytene. Also, an autosome-autosome translocation model has been described in which the unsynapsed autosomal segments 'interfere' with normal MSCI and, once again, this is associated with significant pachytene losses (Homolka et al. 2007). Finally, mutations in the MSCI proteins BRCA1 and H2AX cause complete pachytene arrest (Xu et al. 2003; Fernandez-Capetillo et al. 2003), but in contrast to most targeted mutations, this only affects males, suggesting that the pachytene failure is due to defective MSCI.

7 The Influence of MSCI on X Chromosome Evolution

Despite their independent origins, the X chromosomes of flies, mammals and worms share a common feature – they are deficient in spermatogenesis genes, i.e. genes expressed exclusively or predominantly in the testis (Parisi et al. 2003; Reinke et al. 2004; Khil et al. 2004). Before we knew about the influence of MSCI on

X-linked gene expression this finding was surprising, because the evolutionary model of 'sexually antagonistic genes' predicted that spermatogenesis genes should be enriched on the X chromosome (Rice, 1984). The rationale for this enrichment is as follows: imagine that an X-linked gene acquires a mutation that confers an advantage to male germ cell development and a disadvantage to female germ cell development – i.e. it is sexually 'antagonistic'. If this mutation is recessive, its phenotypic effect will be immediately manifested in males because the gene is present in only one copy (males are XY), while in females it will be masked by the presence of the second X chromosome (females are XX). Because the mutation results in enhanced male reproductive capability, it will spread rapidly through the population and eventually females will arise that are homozygous for the mutation. Homozygosity will diminish female reproductive fitness, and so there will then be strong selective pressure for new mutations that limit the expression of that gene to the male germ line, i.e. to make the gene spermatogenesis-specific (Rice, 1984). This chain of events should result in the accumulation of spermatogenesis genes on the X chromosome. Why then is the X chromosome depleted of spermatogenesis genes?

The answer is one of timing. In a recent study, Khil et al. (2004) found that testis-expressed genes were under-represented on the mouse X chromosome, but when the data were re-analysed according to the testis cell type in which the genes were expressed, the picture looked very different. Spermatogenesis comprises three broad stages – in the first stage, spermatogonial stem cells undergo a series of mitotic division to generate differentiated spermatogonia. These spermatogonia then commit themselves to meiosis, which converts diploid precursor cells into haploid daughter cells. The resulting daughter cells undergo spermatid differentiation – spermiogenesis – during which their DNA undergoes increasing compaction, resulting in the formation of mature sperm. Khil et al. (2004) found that genes expressed in spermatogonia were actually *over*-represented on the X chromosome, consistent with the sexual antagonism model outlined above. However, genes expressed in meiosis or during spermiogenesis were under-represented on the X chromosome. Because meiotic cells and spermatids outnumber spermatogonia, when all these data were combined the overall picture was that the X chromosome was depleted for spermatogenesis genes (Khil et al. 2004).

The fact that the X chromosome has few meiotic genes makes sense – MSCI would obviously provide a strong evolutionary barrier against the accumulation of spermatogenesis genes on this chromosome. However, the finding that post-meiotic genes are under-represented on the X chromosome was surprising. Available data at that time told us that MSCI was transient and that the X and Y chromosomes were reactivated as cells exit meiosis (Hendriksen et al. 1995; Khalil et al. 2004; Fig. 2a). Therefore, there should be no evolutionary pressure to evict spermiogenesis genes from the X chromosome. However, subsequent experiments showed that the X chromosome actually retains a transcriptionally repressed state throughout spermiogenesis.

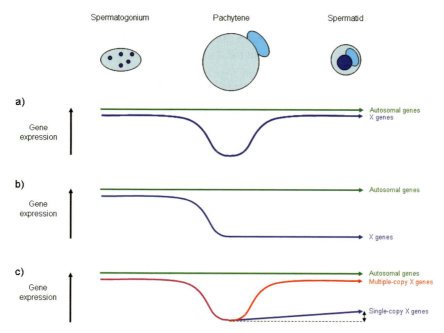

Fig. 2 An evolving model for the expression of spermatogenesis genes on the X chromosome. (**a**) the original model proposed that MSCI was transient, with X chromosome reactivation following exit from meiosis. (**b**) this model was superseded by a model in which the X chromosome retains a largely transcriptionally repressed state through to the end of spermatogenesis. (**c**) in the most recent model, repression of single-copy X-linked genes is retained, albeit in an imperfect fashion. However, multiple-copy genes show robust expression during spermiogenesis

8 X Chromosome Repression During Spermiogenesis

Aside from explaining the data of Khil et al. (2004), there was another reason for re-examining the transcriptional status of the X chromosome in spermatids. This related to female somatic X chromosome inactivation (XCI), the process in which one of the two X chromosomes of female somatic cells is inactivated in order to ensure equal dosage of X-linked genes between males and females. In mice, XCI takes two forms – in the extraembryonic lineages XCI is paternally silenced, a phenomenon resembling genomic imprinting while in the epiblast it is random, affecting either the maternal or paternal X chromosome with equal probability. Early studies had implied that XCI begins in the female mouse embryo at the blastocyst stage, and therefore that there was no X chromosome dosage compensation prior to that point (reviewed in Ferguson-Smith, 2004). However, two subsequent studies presented data to the contrary – both showed that paternal XCI initiated much earlier, with one finding XCI from the 4 cell stage (Okamoto et al. 2004) and the other even earlier, at the 2 cell stage (Huynh, and Lee, 2003). In their study, Okamoto et al. (2004) found a good correlation between the timing of X gene silencing and the expression of *Xist*, the RNA that mediates XCI, from the future inactive X chromosome (reviewed in Heard and Disteche, 2006). This led them to conclude that XCI initiates *de-novo* in the embryo from the 4 cell stage onwards. In contrast, Huynh and Lee (Huynh, and Lee, 2003) proposed something quite different – because they found evidence for XCI at the 2 cell stage, they questioned whether the paternal X chromosome could be inherited in an already inactive – or 'pre-inactivated' state. This 'pre-inactivation' would be initiated by MSCI in the paternal germ line, rather than by *Xist* in the female embryo. If this 'pre-inactivation' hypothesis were true then MSCI clearly could not be transient as we had previously suspected, but would instead have to be maintained from meiosis right through spermiogenesis.

Subsequent studies showed this to be the case – the X chromosome is heterochromatic and enriched in repressive histone marks, like H3K9me2 and H2AZ in spermatids (Khalil et al. 2004; Greaves et al. 2006), and microarray and real-time PCR analysis estimated that around 87% of X-linked genes retain a repressed state in the post-meiotic period (Namekawa et al. 2006; Fig. 2b). This later form of silencing was shown to be a direct result of earlier pachytene asynapsis, because unsynapsed autosomes also retained a repressed state in the post-meiotic period (Turner et al. 2006). X chromosome repression in the post-meiotic period requires the ubiquitin-conjugating enzyme HR6B – mice deficient in this enzyme display increased H3 lysine-4 dimethylation and H2A threonine-120 phosphorylation on the X chromosome in spermatids and a concomitant increase in expression of X-linked transcripts (Baarends et al. 2007).

The pre-inactivation idea was attractive for two reasons. Firstly, experiments in *C. elegans* provided a wonderful precedent for a link between MSCI and imprinted XCI. As in the mouse, the paternal X chromosome of XX *C. elegans* is in an epigenetically inactive state early in embryogenesis – this is manifested as a lack of enrichment of activating histone modifications on the X chromosome in the male pronucleus (Bean et al. 2004). This inactive 'imprint' is gradually diluted with subsequent cell divisions, with the paternal X chromosome resembling the autosomes in its histone signature by the 20 cell stage. Interestingly, the stability of this imprint is reduced when embryos are sired by XX (*tra-2*) rather than XO fathers – the paternal X chromosome becomes enriched in activating histone marks much earlier than the 20 cell stage (Bean et al. 2004). Because XX fathers do not have MSCI, this suggests that MSCI and imprinted repression of the paternal X chromosome in the early embryo are linked (Bean et al. 2004). Secondly, not all mammals that use XCI as a means of dosage compensation have an *Xist* gene. A notable class is the marsupials (metatherians), which diverged from the placental mammals (eutherians) some 180 million years ago (Duret et al. 2006; Hore et al. 2007; Davidow et al. 2007; Shevchenko et al. 2007). In these organisms, XCI is exclusively paternally inactivated – there is no random XCI, and they exhibit MSCI, which is maintained into spermatids (reviewed in Vandeberg, 1983). This has led to the proposition that MSCI is the evolutionarily ancient mechanism underlying XCI (Cooper, 1971; Huynh, and Lee, 2003; McCarrey, 2001).

In reality however, further studies in both embryos and male germ cells show that the situation in mice is far more complicated. A transgene containing *Xist* and flanking genes that has been integrated onto an autosome – and therefore does not undergo MSCI – still exhibits paternally inactivated XCI in early embryos, and this inactivation occurs concomitantly with expression of *Xist* from the transgene at the 4–8 cell stage (Okamoto et al. 2005). This shows that MSCI is not required for inactivated XCI and that *Xist* is sufficient for inactivation to take place. One could still argue that inactivation of other X-linked genes requires, or is potentiated by MSCI, but this possibility is further hampered by a recent re-analysis of X gene expression in spermatids (Mueller et al. 2008). RNA FISH shows that silencing of X chromosome genes during pachytene is robust – essentially all genes studied so far are silenced in all pachytene cells. However, silencing in spermatids is incomplete – most X-genes show reactivation in a small proportion of spermatids (Mueller et al. 2008). Although this finding does not contradict the conclusion that the X chromosome is largely repressed post-meiosis, it does show that the few X-linked genes are truly 'pre-inactivated'. Nevertheless, the imperfect nature of post-meiotic X chromosome repression has led to another important discovery that has forced us to re-examine, yet again, our conclusions about the distribution of spermatogenesis genes on the X chromosome.

9 Leaky X-Inactivation in Spermatids and the Evolution of Multiple Copy Genes

As already outlined, the prevailing view is that X chromosomes are enriched in spermatogenesis genes expressed before meiosis and depleted of spermatogenesis genes expressed after meiosis (Khil et al. 2004). The depletion of meiotic and post-meiotic genes on the mouse X chromosome is thought to be an evolutionary consequence of MSCI and its maintenance into spermatid differentiation. Interestingly, there are a handful of examples in the literature of X-linked genes that do not fit this model – they are testis-specific but they are expressed exclusively in spermatids (Clotman et al. 2000; Toure et al. 2004; Reynard et al. 2007). A common property of these genes is that they are present as multiple copies on the X chromosome. The conclusion that the mouse X chromosome is deficient in post-meiotic genes was based primarily on analysis of single-copy genes and so multiple-copy genes were not studied – could multiple-copy genes behave in a way that contravenes current models of X gene content?

This question has now been addressed in a systematic study characterizing the genomic organization and expression of X-linked multiple-copy genes in the mouse (Mueller et al. 2008). The big surprise was that multiple-copy genes are highly abundant on the X chromosome; there are at least 33 gene families, representing around 273 genes, or 18% of the total number of protein-coding genes. Strikingly, most of these genes are expressed predominantly or exclusively in spermatids, like the previously described multiple-copy X-linked genes. Therefore, contrary to the view that the X chromosome is depleted of post-meiotic spermatogenesis genes (Khil et al. 2004), a large number of previously overlooked X-linked genes show exclusive post-meiotic expression.

But why is there a relationship between multiple-copy genes and expression in spermatids? The important clue here was the fact that post-meiotic repression of the X chromosome is incomplete. RNA FISH analysis showed that single-copy genes were reactivated in a minority of X-containing spermatids – however in contrast, multiple copy genes were expressed in a larger proportion of spermatids, and the percentage of expressing spermatids increased with gene copy number (Mueller et al. 2008). In addition, the expression levels of multiple-copy genes were found to be similar to those of single-copy autosomal genes by microarray analysis. These findings suggest that gene amplification is necessary in order for them to counteract the repressive chromatin environment on the spermatid X chromosome and generate sufficient expression levels to carry out important late spermatogenic functions. Therefore, the model of spermatogenic gene distribution on the X chromosome has had to be refined once more – the mouse X chromosome is enriched in genes expressed both before *and* after meiosis, but those X-linked genes expressed before tend to be single copy, while those expressed after tend to be multiple-copy (Mueller et al. 2008; Fig. 2c).

10 Concluding Remarks

Meiotic silencing presents a new model for how chromosome pairing failure leads to germ cell arrest but this needs to be investigated further. An informative experiment would be to ablate silencing genetically in order to see whether this permits fertility in models with chromosome asynapsis. Although the role of meiotic silencing in dosage compensation in eutherian mammals remains highly controversial, there is general agreement that it could represent the evolutionarily ancient mechanism of dosage compensation in metatherians, and it would therefore be useful to compare the extent of X chromosome silencing in the marsupial male germ-line with that in early embryos. But how could the epigenetically inactive state created by meiotic silencing be transmitted to the embryo? Histone modifications or variants present one possible means of transmitting epigenetic information across generations. Although it is often assumed that histones are completely shed prior to protamine deposition during spermiogenesis, this is not the case. In human sperm for instance, approximately 15% of nuclear basic proteins are histones (Tanphaichitr et al. 1978), and histone variants have been found in the mature sperm of flies and *C. elegans*, e.g. histone H3.3 (Ooi et al. 2006; Chu et al. 2006) and mammals, e.g. histones H2AL1 and H2AL2 (Govin et al. 2007).

Another interesting avenue for research is how rapidly multiple-copy genes on the X chromosome are evolving – are these genes conserved among different mammals? Furthermore, what functions do they serve in spermatogenesis, and could variations in their copy numbers be associated with X-linked sterility in men? In conclusion, although initiating as a chance discovery in *Neurospora*, meiotic silencing now has profound implications for our understanding of X chromosome evolution, dosage compensation and human infertility.

References

Aramayo, R. and Metzenberg, R. L. (1996). Meiotic transvection in fungi. *Cell* **86**, 103–113.

Ashley, T. (1995). Dynamic changes in Rad51 distribution during meiosis in male and female vertebrates. *Chromosome* **104**, 19–28.

Baarends, W.M., Hoogerbrugge, J.W., Roest, H.P., Ooms, M., Vreeburg, J., Hoeijmakers, J.H. and Grootegoed, J.A. (1999). Histone ubiquitination and chromatin remodeling in mouse spermatogenesis. *Dev Biol.* **207**, 322–333.

Baarends, W.M., Wassenaar, E., van der Laan, R., Hoogerbrugge, J., Sleddens-Linkels, E., Hoeijmakers, J.H., de Boer, P. and Grootegoed, J.A. (2005). Silencing of unpaired chromatin and histone H2A ubiquitination in mammalian meiosis. *Mol Cell Biol.* **25**, 1041–1053.

Baarends W.M., Wassenaar E, Hoogerbrugge J.W., Schoenmakers S, Sun Z.W. and Grootegoed J.A. (2007). Increased phosphorylation and dimethylation of XY body histones in the Hr6b-knockout mouse is associated with derepression of the X chromosome. *J Cell Sci.* **120**, 1841–1851.

Baudat F and de Massy B. (2007). Regulating double-stranded DNA break repair towards crossover or non-crossover during mammalian meiosis. *Chromosome Res.* **15**, 565–577.

Bean, C.J., Schaner, C.E. and Kelly, W.G. (2004). Meiotic pairing and imprinted X chromatin assembly in Caenorhabditis elegans. *Nat Genet.* **36**, 100–105.

Bellani, M.A., Romanienko, P.J., Cairatti, D.A. and Camerini-Otero, R.D. (2005). SPO11 is required for sex-body formation, and Spo11 heterozygosity rescues the prophase arrest of Atm-/- spermatocytes. *J Cell Sci.* **118**, 3233–3245.

Bolcun-Filas E, Costa Y, Speed R, Taggart M, Benavente R, De Rooij D.G, Cooke H.J. (2007). SYCE2 is required for synaptonemal complex assembly, double strand break repair, and homologous recombination. *J Cell Biol.* **176**, 741–747.

Burgoyne P. and Baker T. G. (1985). Perinatal oocyte loss in XO mice and its implications for the aetiology of gonadal dysgenesis in XO women. *J Reprod Fertil.* **75**, 633–645.

Chu D.S., Liu H., Nix P., Wu T.F., Ralston E.J., Yates J.R 3rd. and Meyer B.J. (2006). Sperm chromatin proteomics identifies evolutionarily conserved fertility factors. *Nature.* **443**, 101–105.

Clotman F., De Backer O., De Plaen E., Boon T. and Picard J. (2000). Cell- and stage-specific expression of mage genes during mouse spermatogenesis. *Mamm Genome.* **11**, 696-699.

Cooper D.W. (1971). Directed genetic change model for X chromosome inactivation in eutherian mammals. *Nature.* **230**, 292–294.

Costa Y., Speed R.M, Gautier P, Semple C.A., Maratou K., Turner J.M. and Cooke H.J. (2006). Mouse MAELSTROM: the link between meiotic silencing of unsynapsed chromatin and microRNA pathway? *Hum Mol Genet.* **15**, 2324–34.

Davidow L.S., Breen M., Duke S.E., Samollow P.B., McCarrey J.R. and Lee J.T. (2007). The search for a marsupial XIC reveals a break with vertebrate synteny. *Chromosome Res.* **15**, 137–146.

de Vries S.S., Baart E.B., Dekker M., Siezen A., de Rooij D.G., de Boer P., te Riele H. (1999). Mouse MutS-like protein Msh5 is required for proper chromosome synapsis in male and female meiosis. *Genes Dev.* **13**, 523–531.

De Vries, F.A., de Boer, E., van den Bosch, M., Baarends, W.M., Ooms, M., Yuan, L., Liu, J.G., van Zeeland, A.A., Heyting, C. and Pastink, A. (2005). Mouse Sycp1 functions in synaptonemal complex assembly, meiotic recombination, and XY body formation.*Genes Dev.* **19**, 1376–1389.

Duret L., Chureau C., Samain S., Weissenbach J. and Avner P. (2006). The Xist RNA gene evolved in eutherians by pseudogenization of a protein-coding gene. *Science.* **312**, 1653–1655.

Edelmann W., Cohen P.E., Kneitz B., Winand N., Lia M., Heyer J., Kolodner R., Pollard J.W. and Kucherlapati R. (1999). Mammalian MutS homologue 5 is required for chromosome pairing in meiosis. *Nat Genet.* **21**, 123–127.

Ferguson-Smith A.C. (2004). X Inactivation: Pre- or Post-Fertilisation Turn-off? *Current Biol.* **14**, R323–R325.

Fernandez-Capetillo, O., Mahadevaiah, S.K., Celeste, A., Romanienko, P.J., Camerini-Otero R,D., Bonner, W.M., Manova, K., Burgoyne, P. and Nussenzweig A. (2003). H2AX is required for chromatin remodeling and inactivation of sex chromosomes in male mouse meiosis. *Dev Cell* **4**, 497–508.

Findley S.D., Tamanaha M., Clegg N.J. and Ruohola-Baker H. (2003). Maelstrom, a Drosophila spindle-class gene, encodes a protein that colocalizes with Vasa and RDE1/AGO1 homolog, Aubergine, in nuage. *Development.* **130**, 859–871.

Ford, C.E. and Evans E.P. (1964). A reciprocal translocation in the mouse between the X chromosome and a short autosome. *Cytogenetics* **3**, 295–305.

Goldstein, P. (1982) The synaptonemal complexes of *Caenorhabditis elegans*: pachytene karyotype analysis of male and hermaphrodite wild-type and him mutants. *Chromosoma* **86**, 577–593.

Govin, J., Escoffier, E., Rousseaux, S., Kuhn, L., Ferro, M., Thevenon, J., Catena, R., Davidson, I., Garin, J., Khochbin, S. and Caron, C. (2007). Pericentric heterochromatin reprogramming by new histone variants during mouse spermiogenesis.*J Cell Biol*, **176**, 283–294.

Greaves, I.K., Rangasamy, D., Devoy, M., Marshall Graves, J.A. and Tremethick, D.J. (2006). The X and Y chromosomes assemble into H2A.Z, containing facultative heterochromatin, following meiosis. *Mol Cell Biol.* **26**, 5394–5405.

Hassold T., Hall H. and Hunt P. (2007). The origin of human aneuploidy: where we have been, where we are going. *Hum Mol Genet.* **16**, R203–R208.

Heard E. and Disteche C.M. (2006). Dosage compensation in mammals: fine-tuning the expression of the X chromosome. *Genes Dev.* **20**, 1848–1867.

Hendriksen, P.J., Hoogerbrugge, J.W., Themmen, A.P., Koken, M.H., Hoeijmakers, J.H., Oostra, B.A., van der Lende, T. and Grootegoed, J.A. (1995). Postmeiotic transcription of X and Y chromosomal genes during spermatogenesis in the mouse. *Dev Biol.* **170**, 730–733.

Homolka D., Ivanek R., Capkova J., Jansa P. and Forejt J. (2007). Chromosomal rearrangement interferes with meiotic X chromosome inactivation. *Genome Res.* **17**, 1431–1437.

Hore T.A., Koina E., Wakefield M.J. and Marshall Graves J.A. (2007). The region homologous to the X-chromosome inactivation centre has been disrupted in marsupial and monotreme mammals. *Chromosome Res.* **15**, 147–161.

Huynh, K.D. and Lee, J.T. (2003). Inheritance of a pre-inactivated paternal X chromosome in early mouse embryos. Nature *426*, 857–862.

Kelly, W.G. and Aramayo, R. (2007). Meiotic silencing and the epigenetics of sex. *Chromosome Res.* **15**(5), 633–51.

Khalil, A.M., Boyar, F.Z. and Driscoll, D.J. (2004) Dynamic histone modifications mark sex chromosome inactivation and reactivation during mammalian spermatogenesis. *Proc. Natl. Acad.Sci.* **101**, 16583–16587

Khil, P.P., Smirnova, N.A., Romanienko, P.J. and Camerini-Otero, R.D. (2004). The mouse X chromosome is enriched for sex-biased genes not subject to selection by meiotic sex chromosome inactivation. *Nat Genet.* **36**, 642–664.

Lahn B.T., Page D.C. (1999). Four evolutionary strata on the human X chromosome. *Science.* **286**, 964–967.

Lee, D.W., Pratt, R.J., McLaughlin, M. and Aramayo, R. (2003). An argonaute-like protein is required for meiotic silencing. *Genetics* **164**, 821–828

Lydall D., Nikolsky Y., Bishop D.K. and Weinert T. (1996). A meiotic recombination checkpoint controlled by mitotic checkpoint genes. *Nature.* **383**, 840–843.

Mahadevaiah, S.K., Bourc'his, D., de Rooj, D.G., Bestor, T.H., Turner, J.M.A. and Burgoyne, P.S. (2008). Extensive meiotic asynapsis in mice antagonises meiotic silencing of unsynapsed chromatin and consequently disrupts meiotic sex chromosome inactivation. *J Cell Biol.* **182**(2), 263–76.

Mahadevaiah, S.K., Turner, J.M., Baudat, F., Rogakou, E.P., de Boer, P., Blanco-Rodriguez, J., Jasin, M., Keeney, S., Bonner, W.M. and Burgoyne, P.S. (2001). Recombinational DNA double-strand breaks in mice precede synapsis. *Nat Genet.* **27**, 271–276.

Maine, E. M., J. Hauth, T. Ratliff, V. E. Vought, X. She et al., (2005). EGO-1, a putative RNA-dependent RNA polymerase, is required for heterochromatin assembly on unpaired dna during *C. elegans* meiosis. *Curr Bio.* **15**, 1972–1978.

Martienssen, R. A., Zaratiegui, M. and Goto, D. B. (2005), RNA interference and heterochromatin in the fission yeast *Schizosaccharomyces pombe*. *Trends Genet* **21**: 450–456.

McCarrey JR. (2001). X-chromosome inactivation during spermatogenesis: The original dosage compensation mechanism in mammals? In: Xue G, Xue Y, Xu Z, Holmes R, Hammond GL, Lim HA, editors. Gene families: Studies of DNA, RNA, enzymes and proteins. New Jersey: World Scientific. pp. 59–72.

McKee, B.D. and Handel, M.A. (1993). Sex chromosomes, recombination, and chromatin conformation. *Chromosoma* **102**, 71–80.

Moens, P.B., Chen, D.J., Shen, Z., Kolas, N., Tarsounas, M., Heng, H.H.Q. and Spyropoulos, B. (1997). Rad51 immunocytology in rat and mouse spermatocytes and oocytes. *Chromosome.* **106**(4), 207–15.

Mueller J., Mahadevaiah L., Park S.K., Klarburton P.J., Page D.C. and Turner, J.M. (2008). The mouse X Chromosome is enriched for multicopy tested genes showing post-meiotic expression. *Nat Genet.* **40**(6), 794–799.

Namekawa, S.H., Park, P.J., Zhang, L.F., Shima, J.E., McCarrey, J.R., Griswold, M.D. and Lee, J.T. (2006). Postmeiotic sex chromatin in the male germline of mice. *Curr Biol.* **16**, 660–667.

Odorisio T., Rodriguez T.A., Evans E.P., Clarke A.R. and Burgoyne P.S. (1998). The meiotic checkpoint monitoring synapsis eliminates spermatocytes via p53-independent apoptosis. *Nat Genet.* **18**, 257–261.

Okamoto, I., Otte, A.P., Allis, C.D., Reinberg, D. and Heard, E. (2004). Epigenetic dynamics of imprinted X inactivation during early mouse development. Science **303**, 644–649.

Okamoto I., Arnaud D., Le Baccon P., Otte A.P., Disteche C.M., Avner P. and Heard E. (2005). Evidence for de novo imprinted X-chromosome inactivation independent of meiotic inactivation in mice. *Nature.* **438**, 369–373.

Ooi S.L., Priess J.R. and Henikoff S. (2006). Histone H3.3 variant dynamics in the germline of Caenorhabditis elegans. *PLoS Genet.* **2**, e97.

Padmore R., Cao L. and Kleckner N. (1991). Temporal comparison of recombination and synaptonemal complex formation during meiosis in S. cerevisiae. *Cell.* **66**, 1239–1256.

Parisi M, Nuttall R, Naiman D, Bouffard G, Malley J, et al. (2003) Paucity of genes on the *Drosophila* X chromosome showing male-biased expression. *Science.* **299**, 697–700.

Peters A.H., Plug A.W. and de Boer P. (1997). Meiosis in carriers of heteromorphic bivalents: sex differences and implications for male fertility. *Chromosome Res.* **5**, 313–324.

Pittman D.L., Cobb J., Schimenti K.J., Wilson L.A., Cooper D.M., Brignull E., Handel M.A., Schimenti J.C. (1998). Meiotic prophase arrest with failure of chromosome synapsis in mice deficient for Dmc1, a germline-specific RecA homolog. *Mol Cell.* **1**, 697–705.

Pratt, R.J., Lee D.W. and Aramayo, R. (2004). DNA Methylation Affects Meiotic trans-sensing, Not Meiotic Silencing, in Neurospora. *Genetics.* **168**, 1925–1935.

Raju, N. B., (1992) Genetic control of the sexual cycle in Neurospora. *Mycological Research* **96**, 241–262.

Rassoulzadegan, M., Magliano, M. and Cuzin, F. (2002). Transvection effects involving DNA methylation during meiosis in the mouse. *EMBO J.* **21**, 440–450

Reinke V., Gil I.S., Ward S. and Kazmer K. (2004). Genome-wide germline-enriched and sex-biased expression profiles in Caenorhabditis elegans. *Development.* **131**, 311–323.

Reynard L.N., Turner J.M., Cocquet J., Mahadevaiah S.K., Touré A., Höög C. and Burgoyne P.S. (2007). Expression analysis of the mouse multi-copy X-linked gene Xlr-related, meiosis-regulated (Xmr), reveals that Xmr encodes a spermatid-expressed cytoplasmic protein, SLX/XMR. *Biol Reprod.* **77**, 329–335.

Rice, W.R. (1984). Sex-chromosomes and the evolution of sexual dimorphism. *Evolution* **38**, 735–742.

Rodriguez T.A. and Burgoyne P.S. (2000). Evidence that sex chromosome asynapsis, rather than excess Y gene dosage, is responsible for the meiotic impairment of XYY mice. *Cytogenet Cell Genet.* **89**, 38–43.

Roeder G.S and Bailis J.M. (2000). The pachytene checkpoint. *Trends Genet.* **16**, 395–403.

Schimenti, J. (2005). Synapsis or silence. *Nat Genet.* **37**, 11–13.

Shevchenko, A., Zakharova, I., Elisaphenko, E., Kolesnikov, N., Whitehead, S., Bird, C., Ross, M., Weidman, J., Jirtle, R., Karamysheva, T., Rubtsov, N., VandeBerg, J., Mazurok, N., Nesterova, T., Brockdorff, N. and Zakian, S. (2007). Genes flanking Xist in mouse and human are separated on the X chromosome in American marsupials. *Chromosome Res.* **15**(2), 127–86.

Shiu PK, Raju NB, Zickler D, and Metzenberg RL. (2001). Meiotic silencing by unpaired DNA. *Cell* **107**, 905–916.

Solari, A. J. (1974). The behavior of the XY pair in mammals. *Rev. Cytol.* **38**, 273–317.

Speed, R.M. (1986). Oocyte development in XO foetuses of man and mouse: the possible role of heterologous X-chromosome pairing in germ cell survival. *Chromosoma* **94**, 115–124.

Tanphaichitr N., Sobhon P., Taluppeth N. and Chalermisarachai P. (1978). Basic nuclear proteins in testicular cells and ejaculated spermatozoa in man. *Exp Cell Res.* **117**, 347–356.

Toure, A., Szot, M., Mahadevaiah, S.K., Rattigan, A., Ojarikre, O.A. and Burgoyne, P.S. (2004). A new deletion of the mouse Y chromosome long arm associated with the loss of Ssty expression, abnormal sperm development and sterility.*Genetics* **166**, 901–912.

Turner, J.M., Aprelikova, O., Xu, X., Wang, R., Kim, S., Chandramouli, G.V., Barrett, J.C., Burgoyne, P.S. and Deng, C.X. (2004). BRCA1, histone H2AX phosphorylation, and male meiotic sex chromosome inactivation. *Curr Biol.* **14**, 2135–2142.

Turner, J.M., Mahadevaiah, S.K., Fernandez-Capetillo, O., Nussenzweig, A., Xu, X., Deng, C.X. and Burgoyne, P.S. (2005). Silencing of unsynapsed meiotic chromosomes in the mouse. *Nat Genet.* **37**, 41–47.

Turner, J.M., Mahadevaiah, S.K., Ellis, P.J., Mitchell, M.J. and Burgoyne PS. (2006). Pachytene asynapsis drives meiotic sex chromosome inactivation and leads to substantial postmeiotic repression in spermatids. *Dev Cell.* **10**, 521–529.

Turner, J.M. (2007). Meiotic sex chromosome inactivation. *Development.* **134**, 1823–1831.

VandeBerg J.L. (1983). Developmental aspects of X chromosome inactivation in eutherian and metatherian mammals. *J Exp Zool.* **228**(2), 271–86.

van der Heijden G.W., Derijck A.A., Pósfai E., Giele M., Pelczar P., Ramos L., Wansink D.G., van der Vlag J., Peters A.H. and de Boer P. (2007). Chromosome-wide nucleosome replacement and H3.3 incorporation during mammalian meiotic sex chromosome inactivation. *Nat Genet.* **39**, 251–258.

Wang, P.J. (2004). X chromosomes, retrogenes and their role in male reproduction. *Trends Endocrinol Metab.* **15**, 79–83.

Xu, X., Aprelikova, O., Moens, P., Deng, C.X. and Furth, P.A.(2003). Impaired meiotic DNA-damage repair and lack of crossing-over during spermatogenesis in BRCA1 full-length isoform deficient mice. *Development* **130**, 2001–2012.

Yang F., De La Fuente R., Leu N.A., Baumann C., McLaughlin K.J. and Wang P.J. (2006). Mouse SYCP2 is required for synaptonemal complex assembly and chromosomal synapsis during male meiosis. *J Cell Biol.* **173**, 497–507.

Yoshida K., Kondoh G., Matsuda Y., Habu T., Nishimune Y. and Morita T. (1998). The mouse RecA-like gene Dmc1 is required for homologous chromosome synapsis during meiosis. *Mol Cell.* **1**, 707–718.

Yoshioka H., Geyer C.B., Hornecker J.L., Patel K.T. and McCarrey J.R. (2007). In Vivo Analysis of Developmentally and Evolutionarily Dynamic Protein-DNA Interactions Regulating Transcription of the Pgk2 Gene during Mammalian Spermatogenesis. *Mol Cell Biol.* **27**, 7871–7885.

Yuan L., Liu J.G., Zhao J., Brundell E., Daneholt B. and Höög C. (2000). The murine SCP3 gene is required for synaptonemal complex assembly, chromosome synapsis, and male fertility. *Mol Cell.* **5**, 73–83.

Zickler D, and Kleckner N. (1998). The leptotene-zygotene transition of meiosis. *Annu Rev Genet.* **32**, 619–697.

Part IV
The Epigenome in Health and Disease

Genome Defense: The Neurospora Paradigm

Michael R. Rountree and Eric U. Selker

Abstract Eukaryotes deploy an array of defensive mechanisms to limit the destructive effects of "selfish" DNA. These protective mechanisms include both transcriptional gene silencing (TGS) and RNA-based post-transcriptional gene silencing (PTGS) mechanisms. The filamentous fungus *Neurospora crassa* defends its genome with incredible tenacity utilizing two TGS mechanisms, *r*epeat-*i*nduced point mutation (RIP) and DNA methylation and two PTGS mechanisms, quelling and meiotic *si*lencing of unpaired DNA (MSUD).

Keywords DNA methylation · Genome defense · MSUD · Quelling · RIP

1 Introduction

The genomes of organisms are subject to attack by selfish DNA elements, including transposons, retrotransposons and viruses. If left unchallenged, such elements can pose significant risk to an organism resulting in genome rearrangements, insertional mutagenesis, and alterations in expression of genes in their vicinity. To insulate their genomes from the destructive effects of these intrusive elements, organisms have evolved an array of protective mechanisms that act like genome immune systems. These genome defense systems may exist in all organisms, as selfish DNA appears ubiquitous. In eukaryotes, these genome defense systems have evolved to include both transcriptional gene silencing (TGS) and post-transcriptional gene silencing (PTGS) mechanisms. In this chapter, we discuss the genome defense systems of the model organism, *Neurospora crassa*. Studies of Neurospora's genome defense systems have resulted in great strides in our understanding of the control of DNA methylation and RNA silencing-related phenomena.

E.U. Selker (✉)
Institute of Molecular Biology, University of Oregon, Eugene, OR 97403
e-mail: selker@molbio.uoregon.edu

2 Neurospora: The Ultimate Genome Defender

The Neurospora genome consists of ~40 megabases of DNA, including ~10,000 genes on seven chromosomes (Galagan et al. 2003). While slim in comparison to the genomes of higher eukaryotes, Neurospora's svelte genome may in fact be due to success fending off invasive DNA. Of all eukaryotes studied to date, Neurospora may be the most veracious defender of its genome from selfish DNA. This possibility is underscored by the fact that the genome sequence of the commonly used laboratory strain of Neurospora shows no evidence of active transposons or retrotransposons (Galagan et al. 2003). Neurospora has evolved four distinct but somewhat interrelated genome defense systems: repeat-induced point mutation (RIP), DNA methylation, quelling, and meiotic silencing of unpaired DNA (MSUD). Two of these mechanisms, RIP and DNA methylation, are intricately linked and the discussion of these will be interlaced. Quelling and MSUD are RNAi-like defense systems and their similarities and differences to RNAi systems of other eukaryotes will be discussed.

3 RIP: A Formidable Barrier

RIP is a curious genome defense system that first senses duplicated sequences in the haploid genomes within the special dikaryotic tissue that exists after fertilization and prior to karyogamy (Fig. 1) (Selker 1991, 1999). RIP then subjects both sequences to numerous polarized transition mutations (G:C to A:T) (Cambareri et al. 1989). In a single passage through the sexual cycle, up to ~30% of the G:C pairs in a duplicated sequence can be mutated (Cambareri et al. 1991). Sequences that are substantially (~20-30%) diverged are no longer susceptible to RIP. The size and linkage of the duplicated sequence also play roles in how readily the duplication is detected by the RIP machinery. Tandem duplications of at least 400 bp are readily detected and subjected to RIP at frequencies of >99%, while unlinked duplications of at least 1 kb are targets of RIP ~50% of the time (Watters et al. 1999). There does not appear to be an upper size limit to RIP, as large chromosomal duplications are sensitive to RIP (Perkins et al. 1997, Bhat and Kasbekar 2001), although there is evidence that the RIP machinery can be "titrated out" by large duplications (Bhat and Kasbekar 2001). Cs preceding As (dinucleotide CpA) are most susceptible to RIP. This sequence preference produces a recognizable signature (i.e. the resulting TpA dinucleotides) that makes computational identification of RIP'd sequences straightforward (Margolin et al. 1998). Another hallmark of RIP is that sequences mutated by RIP are typically methylated at their remaining cytosines, at least in vegetative cells (Selker et al. 1993). The function and control of the DNA methylation associated with RIP is discussed below.

Of thousands of Neurospora strains collected in the wild, only one, named Adiopodoumé, is known to harbor an active transposon, a LINE-like retrotransposon called *Tad* (Kinsey 1989). The remaining wild-collected strains assayed to date showed no sign of active transposons. In contrast, RIP-inactivated copies of *Tad*

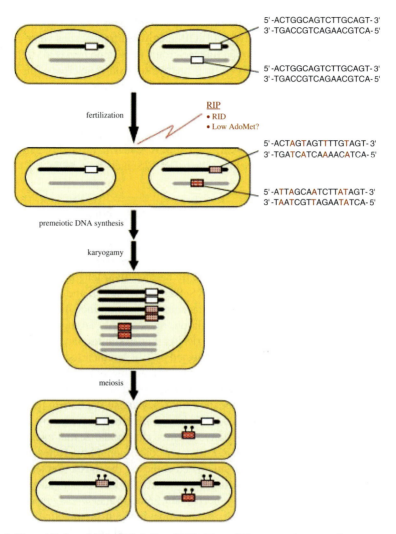

Fig. 1 Repeat-Induced Point Mutation (RIP). Two of Neurospora's seven chromosomes are represented in nuclei of opposite mating types. The open boxes represent any homologous gene or chromosomal segment. In the nucleus on the right, this sequence was duplicated during vegetative growth. During the sexual cycle after fertilization but prior to karyogamy, the RIP process (represented by the red lightening bolt) detects the duplicated sequence(s) and riddles both copies with numerous C:G to T:A transition mutations (represented by the patterned boxes). A short hypothetical portion of the duplicated sequence is shown to the right with RIP mutations (C:G to T:A) indicated in red. The exact mechanism of RIP is not known, but the DMT homologue, RID, is essential for the process. It has been proposed that the transition mutations result from deamination of cytosine or 5-methyl cytosine residues, perhaps catalyzed by RID in conditions of low AdoMet. Heterogenous DNA methylation (represented by *black lollipops*) is typically found at the remaining cytosines within sequences altered by RIP and can lead to transcriptional silencing

elements and the DNA-type transposon, *Punt*, were obvious (Margolin et al. 1998, Kinsey et al. 1994). Additional types of RIP-inactivated transposons were discovered around the centromeric region of linkage group VII (Cambareri et al. 1998) and in sequences isolated on the basis of their methylation status (Selker et al. 2003). The extent of RIP's proficiency to inactivate mobile elements was revealed by the genome sequence of the wild-type strain of *N. crassa*. While additional types of transposons were identified, no recognizable transposon has escaped RIP (Galagan et al. 2003). Analysis of the distribution of inactivated transposons in the genomes of numerous laboratory and wild-collected strains revealed variability suggesting Neurospora is still actively combating selfish-DNA (Selker et al. 2003).

3.1 RIP: Awesome Protector, but Evolutionary Hurdle

Neurospora does harbor a few repeated genes that are known to persist despite the effectiveness of RIP. The 5S rRNA and tRNA genes are dispersed throughout the genome and their evasion of RIP is apparently because their length (<150 bp) falls below that required for RIP (Grayburn and Selker 1989). Indeed, the first recognized relic of RIP, "ζ-η", consists of a 0.8 kb tandem duplication including a 5S rRNA gene (Grayburn and Selker 1989). In addition, the tandemly arranged 9 kb rDNA repeats, encoding the 17S, 5.8S and 25S rRNAs, persists in the face of RIP. These repeats are certainly large enough to be detected by RIP, but their location within the nucleolus organizer region (NOR) may provide protection from RIP (Selker 1990). Indeed, when copies of the rDNA repeats are introduced or found naturally outside the repeat cluster (presumably outside the NOR) they are susceptible to RIP (Selker et al. 2003, Selker 1990, Davis 2000). The insulating effect provided by the NOR may relate to its copy number plasticity observed during the sexual cycle (Butler and Metzenberg 1989, 1990, 1993). RIP-mutated copies could be detected and eliminated followed by amplification of unmutated copies of the rDNA (Selker 1990).

Following its discovery in Neurospora, evidence of RIP or similar processes appeared in other fungi. A silencing mechanism found in *Ascobolus immerses* and also reported for *Coprinus cinereus*, methylation induced premeiotically (MIP), does not cause transition mutations characteristic of RIP, but relies on methylation to silence duplicated sequences (Rossignol and Faugeron 1994, Freedman and Pukkila 1993). Other fungi perform RIP, but the preferred sequence context for mutations appears to vary, with closely related fungi sharing similar contexts (Ikeda et al. 2002). Although there is substantial variation in the frequency of RIP amongst wild-collected *N. crassa* strains (Bhat and Kasbekar 2001), RIP appears to be more efficient and severe in *N. crassa* than in other fungi tested. For example, in *M. grisea*, *P. anserine*, and *L. maculans*, RIP detects duplicated sequences less efficiently and produces fewer mutations (Ikeda et al. 2002, Graia et al. 2001, Nakayashiki et al. 1999). The relative inefficiency of RIP in these fungi is underscored by the presence of intact or nearly identical mobile elements and the presence of active transposons in *M. grisea* (Kachroo et al. 1994, Kito et al. 2003) and *F. oxysporum* (Chalvet et al. 2003, Davière and Daboussi 2001).

Organisms utilize gene duplications to evolve new gene functions (Lynch and Conery 2000, Walsh 1995). While a mighty weapon against invasive elements, does the more "severe form" of RIP in *N. crassa* present too great an evolutionary hurdle to the evolution of new gene function through gene duplication? Neurospora's genome sequence reveals that ~20% of its genes are in multigene families, but nearly all of the paralogs are 30% or more divergent and/or too short to be detected by RIP (Galagan et al. 2003) suggesting that all paralogs in *N. crassa* arose before the evolution of the "severe form" of RIP. Thus, the "severe form" of RIP is probably an evolutionary hurdle preventing substantial gene evolution via gene duplication in Neurospora (Galagan and Selker 2004).

3.2 Mechanism of RIP

The mechanism of RIP has not been elucidated because classic genetic and biochemical approaches are complicated by the specialized microscopic, dikaryotic ascogenous tissue in which the process occurs. However, the transition mutations and the cytosine methylation that is typically associated with sequences altered by RIP are suggestive of a mechanism involving deamination of cytosines or 5-methylcytosines to produce uracil or thymine, followed by a round of DNA replication to lock in the change (Selker 1990, Mautino and Rosa 1998). In fact, the addition of a methyl group to the 5-position on the cytosine ring by DNA methyltransferases (DMT) involves a reaction intermediate prone to spontaneous deamination (Selker 1990). Studies with bacterial DMTs demonstrated that these enzymes can carry out the initial steps of methyl group transfer but proceed from the intermediate to direct deamination, especially when AdoMet, the methyl donor, is limiting (Yebra and Bhagwat 1995, Zingg et al. 1996). Consistent with this idea, when the in vivo level of AdoMet is decreased by mutation of genes in the AdoMet pathway or increased by overexpression of AdoMet synthetase, the severity of RIP appeared inversely correlated to the cellular level of AdoMet (Rosa and Mautino 2004). Interestingly, a mutation in *P. anserine* (a close relative of Neurospora) that slowed development during the sexual cycle when RIP occurs led to an increase in RIP (Bouhouche et al. 2004), suggesting that extended time in the specialized ascogenous tissue may be conducive to the RIP process. A DMT homologue, Masc1, is responsible for the cytosine methylation that is observed after MIP, the homology-based defense system of *A. immersus* that is closely related to RIP (Malagnac et al. 1997). Moreover, the Neurospora homologue of Masc1, RID (*RIP Defective*) (Table 1a), is essential for RIP (Freitag et al. 2002).

The *rid* gene was identified in the genome sequence as one of two predicted proteins with a series of conserved motifs found in all known DMTs (Goll 2005). The other DMT homologue, *defective in methylation 2* (*DIM-2*), was originally uncovered in a mutant screen to identify genes involved in DNA methylation (see below). DIM-2 is essential for all DNA methylation in vegetative tissues, but is not involved in RIP (Kouzminova and Selker 2001). Conversely, *rid* mutants do not show defects in DNA methylation in vegetative tissue, fertility, growth or development (Freitag

Table 1 Neurospora's genome defense systems

Gene	Protein group	Function (known or proposed)
(a) Repeat Induced Point Mutation (RIP)		
Rid	DMT	Methylation of cytosines and/or deamination of cytosines/5-methylcytosines
(b) DNA Methylation		
dim-2	DMT	Methylation of cytosines (CpN)
dim-5	HMT	Trimethylation of histone H3K9
hpo	HP1	Recognition of trimethylated histone H3K9 and interaction with DIM-2
(c) Quelling		
qde-1	RdRP	Generation of dsRNA from aberrant RNA
qde-2	Argonaute	Degradation of mRNA as part of RISC
qde-3	RecQ-like DNA helicase	?
dcl-1/dcl-2	Dicer	Generation of siRNA from dsRNA
Qip	3'-5' exonuclease	Conversion of siRNA into single strands
rpa-1	RPA	Interaction with QDE-1
(d) Meiotic Silencing by Unpaired DNA (MSUD)		
sad-1	RdRP	Generation of dsRNA from aberrant RNA
sad-2	?	Localization of SAD-1 to perinuclear region
sms-2	Argonaute	Degradation of mRNA as part of RISC
dcl-1	Dicer	Generation of siRNA from dsRNA

et al. 2002). It is not currently known whether RID has DNA methyltransferase and/ or deaminase activity. The discovery of methylated sequences lightly altered by RIP that do not serve as de novo methylation signals suggests the DNA methylation was likely established, perhaps by RID, during the sexual phase and maintained through vegetative growth by DIM-2 (Singer et al. 1995). The mechanism of RIP clearly requires further study; no information is available on the presumptive machinery involved in sensing duplications. It is noteworthy; however, that inactivation is a pair-wise process and is nucleus-limited. When strains with duplication are crossed, either both copies or neither copy is affected, never just one copy (Selker and Garrett 1988). Similarly, triplicate sequences are inactivated in pairs (Fincham et al. 1989).

4 DNA Methylation in Neurospora

DNA methylation is perhaps the best known process that counters selfish DNA. Indeed, it has been proposed that its primary function in vertebrates is to suppress the abundant and potentially invasive transposable elements in the genome (Yoder et al. 1997). Unlike the DNA methylation found in vertebrates, DNA methylation in Neurospora is not restricted to symmetrical sequences (e.g. CpG or CpNpG) with ~1.5% of total cytosines methylated (Foss et al. 1993, Selker and Stevens 1985). In fact, it appears that any cytosine residue in a methylated region can be methylated. The level of methylation at a particular cytosine residue is typically heavy but heterogeneous within a population of nuclei (Selker et al. 1993). To date, DNA methylation has not been found in any of the protein-coding genes, but a low level is found associated with the ~170 copies of the ~9 kb rDNA unit (Selker et al. 2003, Perkins et al. 1986). The vast majority of DNA methylation is found at sequences altered by RIP (Galagan et al. 2003, Selker et al. 2003). The majority of these methylated sequences are relics of transposons subjected to RIP, consistent with the idea that DNA methylation plays a role in genome defense.

4.1 Function of DNA Methylation: Squelching the Noise?

Why does Neurospora methylate sequences altered by RIP? This methylation does not simply reflect vestiges of methylation established during the RIP process. Although there are some examples of such, as indicated by the observation that some methylation depends on preexisting methylation (i.e. it represents "maintenance methylation"), Neurospora possesses a robust system that detects most sequences altered by RIP and methylates them de novo (Singer et al. 1995). Over the last few decades, it has become clear that DNA methylation is involved in TGS in a number of organisms, including Neurospora (Rountree and Selker 1997, Zhou et al. 2001). Interestingly, while DNA methylation of the promoter region of genes in higher eukaryotes leads to an inhibition in transcription initiation, it appears to exert its effect downstream of transcription initiation in Neurospora (Rountree and Selker 1997). There is no evidence that DNA methylation plays a role in the development of Neurospora. Thus, the likely function of DNA methylation in Neurospora is to suppress the expression of sequences altered by RIP. The RIP process typically leads to numerous transition mutations, often creating aberrant stop codons in genes. Although methylation is dispensable in Neurospora, a situation could arise where expression of RIP-altered sequences could lead to the production of dominant negative proteins, or even RNA, with deleterious effects. We surmise that it is in the best interest of the organism to suppress such expression.

DNA methylation has also been shown to inhibit the expression and transposition of a native (i.e. not subjected to RIP) *Tad* retrotransposon experimentally introduced into Neurospora during vegetative growth (Zhou et al. 2001). The *Tad* element was methylated regardless of copy number within the genome. Thus, DNA methylation not only silences invasive elements inactivated by RIP, but can also suppress the activity of such elements that may invade the Neurospora genome during the vegetative phase of growth. Interestingly, the RNAi machinery of Neurospora, also appears to play a role in repression of *Tad* (see below) (Nolan et al. 2005).

4.2 Control of DNA Methylation: Cis-Acting Factors

When methylation is stripped from sequences mutated by RIP, either by drug treatment or molecular cloning followed by transformation back into Neurospora, the sequences typically trigger de novo methylation in vegetative cells (Singer et al. 1995, Selker et al. 1987). The DNA methylation does not depend on the sequence duplication that originally triggered RIP and is relatively independent of chromosomal position. How do mutations created by RIP trigger DNA methylation? Studies of the cis-acting signals of RIP-altered sequences that trigger de novo methylation concluded that RIP sequences contain multiple, additive, positive signals that promote DNA methylation (Miao et al. 2000). The mutations triggered by RIP result in an increase in A:T richness and higher densities of the TpA dinucleotide. These attributes alone are not essential features of the DNA methylation signal but they do promote methylation (Tamaru and Selker 2003). A sensitive in vivo targeting system, developed to test the ability of sequences to trigger de novo methylation in Neurospora, demonstrated the following: (1) A and T residues were required on both strands to induce de novo methylation. (2) Multiples of the sequence $(TAAA)_n$ or $(TTAA)_n$ were the most potent methylation signals. (3) Weak signals could by strengthened by extending their length. (4) Methylation was inhibited by the presence of G:C base pairs with Cs 5′ of ApT dinucleotides being the most inhibitory (Tamaru and Selker 2003).

4.3 Control of DNA Methylation: Trans-acting Factors

There is a long standing observation that DNA methylation is typically associated with heterochromatin and the link has been drawn tighter over the past few years. The first experiments to connect chromatin and DNA methylation in Neurospora made use of the histone deacetylase (HDAC) inhibitor Trichostatin-A (TSA). Addition of TSA to the growth medium caused a reduction of DNA methylation in some chromosomal regions (Selker 1998). Consistent with this result, at least one HDAC is involved in DNA methylation (K. Smith, J. Dobosy, and EUS, unpublished results).

What factor(s) recognizes the RIP-altered sequence and mediates DNA methylation? Presumably, such a factor would have to show relatively indiscriminate binding to A:T-rich sequences. Proteins containing an A:T-hook motif (e.g. high mobility group proteins) are known to bind in the minor groove of A:T-rich sequences (Reeves 2001). Treatment with Distamycin A, an analog of the A:T-hook motif, interferes with methylation in Neurospora consistent with the idea that an A:T hook protein is crucial in this process (Tamaru and Selker 2003). The existence of a protein(s) that preferentially binds to DNA with RIP mutations has been detected in gel mobility shift experiments. Interestingly, this activity, called methyl/RIP binding protein 1 (MRBP-1), has the strongest affinity for methylated DNA with RIP mutations (Selker et al. 2002).

Hunts for mutants d*efective* in *DNA* m*ethylation* (*dim*) have uncovered important members of the DNA methylation machinery (Foss et al. 1993). Two resulting mutants, *dim-2* and *dim-5*, completely abolish DNA methylation in vegetative tissue (Table 1b). To date, mutations that result in a complete loss of DNA methylation have not been described in other eukaryotes. This is most likely due to partial redundancy of the methylation machinery in higher eukaryotes. For example, at least three DMTs are used in both plants and mammals to establish methylation patterns (Goll 2005). In addition, unlike the case with Neurospora, DNA methylation is essential in many higher eukaryotes (Goll 2005).

As mentioned earlier, DIM-2 encodes the DMT responsible for all DNA methylation in vegetative tissue of Neurospora (Kouzminova and Selker 2001). Characterization of the *dim-5* mutant unequivocally linked chromatin to the control of DNA methylation. DIM-5 is a SET domain protein with histone H3 methyltransferase (HMT) activity, that specifically trimethylates histone H3 lysine 9 (hH3K9me) (Tamaru and Selker 2001, Tamaru et al. 2003). Consistent with this finding, chromatin immunoprecipitation assays showed that hH3K9me was highly enriched at chromosomal regions harboring DNA methylation and that this methylation is absent in *dim-5* strains. In addition, amino acid substitution of the hH3K9 residue, with either Leu or Arg, led to a loss of DNA methylation. Thus, the critical and perhaps sole target of DIM-5 is the hH3K9 residue (Tamaru et al. 2003) (Fig. 2). These results imply that all vegetative DNA methylation is dependent on trimethylation of hH3K9 by DIM-5. Methylation of hH3K9 has also been shown to be important for at least some DNA methylation in plants and animals (Jackson et al. 2002, Malagnac et al. 2002, Lehnertz et al. 2003).

These findings raised the question of how the trimethylation "mark" established by DIM-5 is "read" to target DNA methylation. Studies in *Drosophila melanogaster*, *S. pombe*, and mammals demonstrated that HP1, via its chromodomain, binds to hH3K9me and is important for silencing in heterochromatin (Bannister et al. 2001, Eissenberg and Elgin 2000, Jacobs et al. 2001, Lachner et al. 2001). The HP1 homolog in Neurospora, encoded by the *hpo* gene (Table 1b), is essential for DNA methylation and requires the catalytic activity of DIM-5 for localization to heterochromatic foci (Freitag et al. 2004a). These results indicate that HP1 reads the hH3K9me mark established by DIM-5. Recent work provided evidence that HP1 directly links hH3K9me and DNA methylation. Yeast two-hybrid assays identified an N-terminal domain of DIM-2 that interacts with the Chromo Shadow Domain (CSD) of HP1 (S. Honda and E.U.S., in preparation). Notably, HP1 homologs have also been shown to interact and/or colocalize with DMTs and methyl-binding proteins in mammals (Bachman et al. 2001, Reese et al. 2003, Fujita et al. 2003, Fuks et al. 2003). In contrast, the *Arabidopsis* HP1 homolog, TFL2/LHP1, is dispensable for DNA methylation (Malagnac et al. 2002). A working model for the control of DNA methylation of sequences altered by RIP based on these results is depicted in Fig. 2.

5 Quelling: Post-transcriptional Gene Silencing

Quelling is a post-transcriptional gene silencing (PTGS) phenomenon that occurs in the vegetative phase of the Neurospora life cycle. The discovery of quelling followed the establishment of DNA-mediated transformation for Neurospora. A number of Neurospora researchers noted peculiar behavior of transformants but the Macino lab first reported a systematic characterization of the vegetative phase

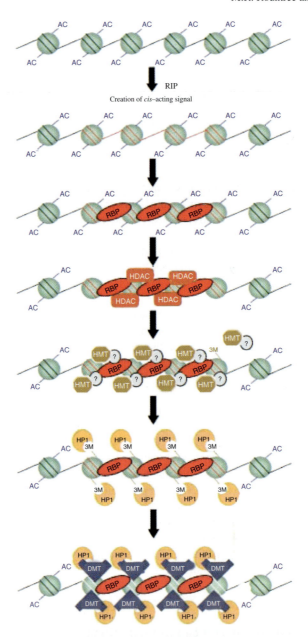

Fig. 2 Model for the Control of DNA Methylation of RIP'd Sequences. RIP mutations typically create a signal for de novo methylation (represented by the red DNA). This signal could then be recognized by an as yet unclassified protein, here symbolized RBP (*R*IP *B*inding *P*rotein). RBP in turn could directly or indirectly recruit HDAC(s) to deacetylate histones in the RIP'd region. Removal of the acetyl group (AC) from particular histone residues would allow a complex containing the histone methyltransferase (HMT), DIM-5, and one or more unidentified proteins (represented by the "?"), access to trimethylate hH3K9. The chromo-domain protein, HP1, then binds to the trimethylated hH3K9 (3M). The DMT, DIM-2, directly interacts with HP1 and methylates cytosine residues within the associated DNA

silencing and named the phenomenon quelling. Briefly, they demonstrated that a significant percentage of transformants show sequence-specific silencing of the transformed DNA along with homologous native sequences (Romano and Macino 1992). Genes vary in their sensitivity to quelling and tranformants carrying multiple copies of transforming DNA, often in tandem arrays, trigger quelling more readily for those genes that are sensitive. In heterokaryons, where genetically distinct nuclei share a common cytoplasm, quelling was found to be dominant (i.e. a transformed "quelled" nucleus could induce silencing of homologous sequences in non-transformed nuclei) (Cogoni et al. 1996). This result implicated a diffusible cytoplasmic factor as the silencing agent, such as an RNA element. The identification of genes required for quelling provided valuable insight into the mechanism of this process and ultimately revealed that it is closely related to RNAi silencing systems in other eukaryotes (Table 1c).

5.1 Mechanism of Quelling

The working model (Fig. 3) for quelling, similar to the model proposed for RNAi systems, is that transforming DNA generates an "aberrant" transcript that elicits action by the RNAi machinery, ultimately resulting in degradation of homologous mRNA. Specifically, QDE-1, an RNA-dependent RNA polymerase (RdRP), QDE-3, a RecQ-like presumptive DNA helicase, and replication protein A (RPA), are thought to be involved in the generation of double stranded RNA (dsRNA) from

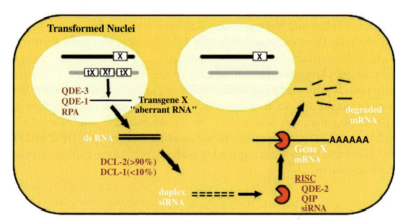

Fig. 3 Model for the Mechanism of Quelling. A heterokaryon is represented with two nuclei, one that has been transformed with multiple copies of a transgene (tX). The action of the RecQ-like DNA helicase (QDE-3), replication protein A (RPA) and the RdRP, QDE-1, results in the conversion of a putative aberrant RNA, produced by the multicopy integration of tX, into dsRNA. The dsRNA is then cleaved into siRNAs primarily through the action of the Dicer, DCL-2. Formation of an active RISC, involves removal of the passenger strand of the siRNA through the action of QIP. The siRNAs then guide the RISC, composed of the Argonaute protein, QDE-2, to degrade homologous mRNA produced by the tX and endogenous gene X

a postulated aberrant RNA produced from the multicopy insertion of a transgene (Cogoni and Macino 1999a, 1999b, Nolan et al. 2008). Two partially redundant Dicer proteins, DCL-1 and DCL-2, cleave the dsRNA to create the 21–25 nucleotide small inhibitory RNA (siRNA), with the majority (>90%) of this activity being conducted by DCL-2 (Catalanotto et al. 2004). The siRNA then guides the RNA-induced silencing complex (RISC) to degrade homologous mRNA. The core of RISC is QDE-2, an Argonaute protein thought to be involved with nicking the passenger strand of the siRNA and then degrading homologous mRNA (Catalanotto et al. 2002). The *Q*DE-2-*i*nteracting *p*rotein, QIP, is also critical to RISC function, apparently serving as an exonuclease to facilitate removal of the nicked passenger strand of the siRNA (Table 1c and Fig. 3) (Maiti et al. 2007).

5.2 Role of Quelling in Genome Defense

PTGS mechanisms (RNAi, quelling, cosuppression) appear common in eukaryotes and their proposed role is to combat the expansion of transposable elements (Waterhouse et al. 2001). Evidence supporting such a role came from identification of transposon-specific siRNAs in both Arabidopsis and Drosophila (Llave et al. 2002, Aravin et al. 2003). In addition, genes essential for RNAi were found to be essential for transposon control in Chlamydomonas and *C. elegans* (Wu-Scharf et al. 2000, Ketting et al. 1999, Tabara et al. 1999). In Neurospora, two studies demonstrated that components of the quelling machinery play a role in genome protection by helping to silence transposons inactivated by RIP and repressing the active *Tad* retrotransposon (Nolan et al. 2005, Chicas et al. 2004). In the first, siRNAs were detected for transposon relics and their presence was shown to be dependent on QDE-1, QDE-3, and both Dicer enzymes, DCL1/DCL2 (Chicas et al. 2004). Furthermore, this study indicated that despite DNA methylation, relics of RIP are transcribed and the transcript levels increase in mutants of the RNAi pathway. This observation is consistent with studies of alleles of the *am* and *mtr* gene generated by RIP that demonstrated a low level of transcripts from these alleles despite their dense methylation (Rountree and Selker 1997). In the second study, Nolan *et al.* (2005) demonstrated that some components of the quelling machinery, QDE-2 and Dicer, but not QDE-1 and QDE-3, are required to partially repress the expansion of active *Tad* retrotransposons.

5.3 No Relationship Between PTGS and TGS in Neurospora

In some eukaryotes, direct links have been drawn between PTGS and TGS. In fission yeast, plants and Drosophila, components of the RNAi machinery are involved in transcriptional silencing through the establishment of heterochromatin by promoting histone H3 lys9 methylation and, in the case of Drosophila, the localization of HP1 (Pal-Bhadra et al. 2004, Volpe et al. 2002, Hall et al. 2002, Zilberman et al. 2003, Liu et al. 2004). In addition, de novo methylation is impaired in RNAi mutants of Arabidopsis (Chan et al. 2004). A link between PTGS and TGS is not evident in Neurospora, however. siRNAs produced from a silent transgene, containing hH3K9 methylation, were unable to direct hH3K9 methylation of the endogenous gene in trans (Chicas et al. 2005). Moreover, analysis of mutants defective in components of Neurospora's RNAi machinery showed no effect on the establishment or maintenance of DNA methylation at sequences altered by RIP, methylation of hH3K9, nor HP1 localization (Chicas et al. 2004, Freitag et al. 2004b). Likewise, although DNA methylation is often found associated with the transformed sequences silenced by quelling, the silencing was not affected when DNA methylation was absent in a *dim-2* (DMT) or *dim-5* (HMT) mutant background (Cogoni et al. 1996, Chicas et al. 2005).

6 MSUD: Meiotic Silencing of Unpaired DNA

MSUD operates exclusively during meiosis to silence any gene that fails to pair with an identical or nearly identical sequence on the homologous chromosome (Fig. 4a and b) (Shiu et al. 2001 Aramayo and Metzenberg 1996). Described simply, MSUD is a two-step mechanism that involves sensing of unpaired DNA and subsequent silencing of any transcripts that correspond to the unpaired sequence. For a discussion on meiotic silencing in mammals see Chapter "Meiotic Silencing, Infertility and X Chromosome Evolution" by James Turner.

This phenomenon was first uncovered by Metzeberg and colleagues while investigating a puzzling ascus dominant phenotype produced by an as*cospore* m*aturation-1* (*asm-1*) deletion allele (Aramayo and Metzenberg 1996). Specifically, crosses of an *asm-1* deletion with a wild type strain produced inviable ascospores at a frequency of >99%. Since the *asm-1* allele was a deletion, it seemed unlikely that a dominant negative protein was being produced. As summarized in Fig. 4, careful analysis demonstrated: (1) A functional copy of the *asm-1* gene at an ectopic location failed to rescue the ascus dominant phenotype, suggesting that inadequate gene dosage was not responsible for the defect (Fig. 4c). (2) Consistent with this result, only one functional copy was required in meiosis as long as the functional allele had a pairing partner (i.e. the gene serving as the pairing partner could harbor mutations preventing its expression) (Fig. 4d). (3) Presence of pairable ectopic alleles (at the same chromosomal location) could complement the mutations, i.e. MSUD did not occur (Fig. 4e). (4) One ectopic copy can elicit MSUD and silence paired alleles at their native locus. Thus, MSUD results from the presence of unpaired alleles rather than the absence of paired alleles (Fig. 4f). Additional studies with meiotically expressed genes, including a GFP reporter, have demonstrated the generality of this phenomenon (Raju et al. 2007).

Aramayo and colleagues have shown that certain RIP'd and methylated alleles were able to elicit MSUD (Fig. 4g). Interestingly, some fail to do so in a *dim-2* background (Fig. 4h), suggesting that DNA methylation can inhibit pairing (Pratt et al. 2004). However, alleles with a high number of mutations by RIP, resulting in significant sequence divergence, were found to elicit MSUD regardless of

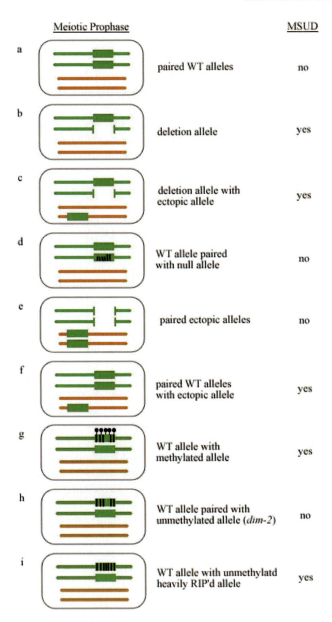

Fig. 4 Experiments that elucidated MSUD; see text for descriptions of each. Nuclei with two of Neurospora's seven chromosome pairs are represented during meiotic prophase. The green box represents a gene that is active during meiosis. Deletions are represented by gaps in the chromosomes. RIP mutations are represented by vertical lines in the gene. The black "lollipops" represent DNA methylation

their methylation status (Fig. 4i). Presumably, sequence divergence beyond some threshold prevents efficient pairing (Shiu et al. 2001, Pratt et al. 2004, Shiu and Metzenberg 2002). In addition to the methylation status, the size and content of an unpaired region influence initiation of MSUD. Larger unpaired regions trigger silencing more effectively than smaller unpaired regions. Importantly, the unpaired region must include ~700 bp of sequence corresponding to a gene transcript (Lee et al. 2004). This result is consistent with a RNA-mediated PTGS mechanism rather than a TGS mechanism.

6.1 Mechanism of MSUD

The first mutant hunt for genes involved in MSUD uncovered a gene, *Suppressor of ascus dominance 1* (*Sad-1*), which encodes an RdRP homologue, suggesting MSUD, like quelling, involves an RNAi-like mechanism (Table 1d) (Shiu et al. 2001). The second gene found to be involved in MSUD, *Sad-2*, encodes a protein not previously identified as a component in RNAi silencing systems (Shiu et al. 2006). SAD-2 colocalizes with SAD-1 and is required for targeting it to the perinuclear region (Shiu et al. 2006, Bardiya et al. 2008), where siRNAs are found concentrated in mammalian cells (Grünweller et al. 2003, Chiu et al. 2004). A reverse-genetics approach identified a second Argonaute-like protein-encoding gene in Neurospora, *Suppressor of meiotic silencing-2* (*Sms-2*), and showed that it too is required for MSUD (Table 1d) (Lee et al. 2003). Tests on strains defective for Neurospora's two Dicer-like ribonucleases, DCL-1 and DCL-2, demonstrated that DCL-1, but not DCL-2, is required for MSUD and that it colocalizes with SAD-1, SAD-2, and SMS-2 in the perinuclear region (Table 1d) (Alexander et al. 2008). MSUD is proposed to be induced by the generation of an aberrant RNA from the unpaired DNA (Lee et al. 2003). MSUD is then thought to involve steps analogous to those in quelling and other RNAi silencing systems (Nakayashiki 2005, Kelly and Aramayo 2007). In addition, two Spore killer strains, *Sk-2* and *Sk-3*, were shown to suppress MSUD (Raju et al. 2007). The authors propose that the ~30 cM-long haplotype region found in these Spore killer strains contains a suppressor of MSUD.

Notably, many of the components of the MSUD machinery are required for progression through meiosis. While heterozygous crosses of *Sad-1, Sad-2,* and *Sms-2* strains produced viable ascospores, homozygous crosses for any of these mutations produced barren perithecia (Shiu et al. 2001, Shiu et al. 2006, Lee et al. 2003). One intriguing possibility is that the unpaired mating type region may require regulation by the MSUD machinery. Alternatively, these MSUD pathway components may be required to produce small RNAs that regulate sexual development.

7 Conclusion: Running Neurospora's Genome Defense Gauntlet

The possibility of an invasive element, such as a transposon, invading and multiplying throughout Neurospora's genome was rendered unlikely by the evolution of the severe form of RIP. This is evident from the observation that most strains lack active transposons (Galagan et al. 2003, Selker et al. 2003). While RIP is highly effective at protecting Neurospora's genome, because it only occurs in premeiotic dikaryotic cells it leaves the genome susceptible to invasion by and/or expansion of transposons during the remainder of the life cycle. Neurospora's three other genome defense systems should guard against such incursions. In haploid vegetative cells, Neurospora deploys two mutually but potentially overlapping defense systems, a PTGS mechanism, quelling, and a TGS mechanism, DNA methylation, to silence active elements that may invade. Both also appear to play a role in silencing sequences that have been altered by RIP (Selker et al. 2003, Chicas et al. 2004). Although not directly tested to date, the mechanism of MSUD should silence any transposed sequence in meiotic cells, regardless of whether these sequences are altered by RIP or present in single copy (Shiu et al. 2001). Neurospora's four genome defense mechanisms present a gauntlet of defenses for an invasive DNA element to navigate.

Acknowledegment We thank Zachary Lewis for comments on the manuscript. Work in the laboratory of E.U.S. was supported by U.S. Public Health Service Grant GM-35690 from the National Institutes of Health.

References

Alexander WG, Raju NB, Xiao H, Hammond TM, Perdue TD, Metzenberg RL, Pukkila PJ, Shiu PK: DCL-1 colocalizes with other components of the MSUD machinery and is required for silencing. *Fungal Genet Biol* 2008 **45**(5):719–727 (Epub 2007).

Aramayo R, Metzenberg RL: Meiotic transvection in fungi. *Cell* 1996, **86**(1):103–113.

Aravin A, Lagos-Quintana M, Yalcin A, Zavolan M, Marks D, Snyder B, Gaasterland T, Meyer J, Tuschl T: The small RNA profile during Drosophila melanogaster development. *Dev Cell* 2003, **5**(2):337–350.

Bachman KE, Rountree MR, Baylin SB: Dnmt3a and Dnmt3b are transcriptional repressors that exhibit unique localization properties to heterochromatin. *J Biol Chem* 2001, **276**(34):32282–32287.

Bannister AJ, Zegerman P, Partridge JF, Miska EA, Thomas JO, Allshire RC, Kouzarides T: Selective recognition of methylated lysine 9 on histone H3 by the HP1 chromo domain. *Nature* 2001, **410**(6824):120–124.

Bardiya N, Alexander WG, Perdue TD, Barry EG, Metzenberg RL, Pukkila PJ, Shiu PK: Characterization of interactions between and among components of the meiotic silencing by unpaired DNA machinery in Neurospora crassa using bimolecular fluorescence complementation. *Genetics* 2008, **178**(1):593–596.

Bhat A, Kasbekar DP: Escape from repeat-induced point mutation of a gene-sized duplication in neurospora crassa crosses that are heterozygous for a larger chromosome segment duplication. *Genetics* 2001, **157**(4):1581–1590.

Bouhouche K ZD, Debuchy R, Arnaise S.: Altering a gene involved in nuclear distribution increases the repeat-induced point mutation process in the fungus Podospora anserina. *Genetics* 2004, **167**(1):151–159.

Butler DK, Metzenberg RL: Premeiotic change of nucleolus organizer size in Neurospora. *Genetics* 1989, **122**:783–791.

Butler DK, Metzenberg RL: Expansion and contraction of the nucleolus organizer region of Neurospora: changes originate in both proximal and distal segments. *Genetics* 1990, **126**(2):325–333.

Butler DK, Metzenberg RL: Amplification of the nucleolus organizer region during the sexual phase of Neurospora crassa. *Chromosoma* 1993, **102**(8):519–525.

Cambareri EB, Aisner R, Carbon J: Structure of the chromosome VII centromere region in *Neurospora crassa*: degenerate transposons and simple repeats. *Mol Cell Biol* 1998, **18**(9):5465–5477.

Cambareri EB, Jensen BC, Schabtach E, Selker EU: Repeat-induced G-C to A-T mutations in *Neurospora*. *Science* 1989, **244**(4912):1571–1575.

Cambareri EB, Singer MJ, Selker EU: Recurrence of repeat-induced point mutation (RIP) in *Neurospora crassa*. *Genetics* 1991, **127**(4):699–710.

Catalanotto C, Azzalin G, Macino G, Cogoni C: Involvement of small RNAs and role of the qde genes in the gene silencing pathway in Neurospora. *Genes Dev* 2002, **16**(7):790–795.

Catalanotto C, Pallotta M, ReFalo P, Sachs MS, Vayssie L, Macino G, Cogoni C: Redundancy of the two dicer genes in transgene-induced posttranscriptional gene silencing in Neurospora crassa. *Mol Cell Biol* 2004, **24**(6):2536–2545.

Chalvet F GC, Kaper F, Langin T, Daboussi MJ.: Hop, an active Mutator-like element in the genome of the fungus Fusarium oxysporum. *Mol Biol Evol* 2003, **20**(8):1362–1375.

Chan SW, Zilberman D, Xie Z, Johansen LK, Carrington JC, Jacobsen SE: RNA silencing genes control de novo DNA methylation. *Science* 2004, **303**(5662):1336.

Chicas A, Cogoni C, Macino G: RNAi-dependent and RNAi-independent mechanisms contribute to the silencing of RIPed sequences in Neurospora crassa. *Nucleic Acids Res* 2004, **32**(14):4237–4243.

Chicas A, Forrest EC, Sepich S, Cogoni C, Macino G: Small interfering RNAs that trigger posttranscriptional gene silencing are not required for the histone H3 Lys9 methylation necessary for transgenic tandem repeat stabilization in Neurospora crassa. *Mol Cell Biol* 2005, **25**(9):3793–3801.

Chiu YL, Ali A, Chu CY, Cao H, Rana TM: Visualizing a correlation between siRNA localization, cellular uptake, and RNAi in living cells. *Chem Biol* 2004, **11**(8):1165–1175.

Cogoni C, Irelan JT, Schumacher M, Schmidhauser TJ, Selker EU, Macino G: Transgene silencing of the *al-1* gene in vegetative cells of Neurospora is mediated by a cytoplasmic effector and does not depend on DNA-DNA interactions or DNA methylation. *EMBO J* 1996, **15**(12):3153–3163.

Cogoni C, Macino G: Gene silencing in Neurospora crassa requires a protein homologous to RNA-dependent RNA polymerase. *Nature* 1999a, **399**(6732):166–169.

Cogoni C, Macino G: Posttranscriptional gene silencing in Neurospora by a RecQ DNA helicase. *Science* 1999b, **286**(5448):2342–2344.

Davière JM LT, Daboussi MJ.: Potential role of transposable elements in the rapid reorganization of the Fusarium oxysporum genome. *Fungal Genet Biol* 2001, **34**(3):177–192.

Davis RH: Neurospora: Contributions of a Model Organism: Oxford University Press, Oxford; 2000.

Eissenberg JC, Elgin SC: The HP1 protein family: getting a grip on chromatin. *Current Opin Genet Dev* 2000, **10**(2):204–210.

Fincham JRS, Connerton IF, Notarianni E, Harrington K: Premeiotic disruption of duplicated and triplicated copies of the *Neurospora crassa am* (glutamate dehydrogenase) gene. *Curr Genet* 1989, **15**(5):327–334.

Foss HM, Roberts CJ, Claeys KM, Selker EU: Abnormal chromosome behavior in Neurospora mutants defective in DNA methylation. *Science* 1993, **262**:1737–1741.

Freedman T, Pukkila PJ: *De novo* methylation of repeated sequences in *Coprinus cinereus*. *Genetics* 1993, **135**:357–366.

Freitag M, Hickey PC, Khlafallah TK, Read ND, Selker EU: HP1 is essential for DNA methylation in Neurospora. *Mol Cell* 2004a, **13**(3):427–434.

Freitag M, Lee DW, Kothe GO, Pratt RJ, Aramayo R, Selker EU: DNA methylation is independent of RNA interference in Neurospora. *Science* 2004b, **304**(5679):1939.

Freitag M, Williams RL, Kothe GO, Selker EU: A cytosine methyltransferase homologue is essential for repeat-induced point mutation in *Neurospora crassa*. *Proc Natl Acad Sci U S A* 2002, **99**(13):8802–8807.

Fujita N, Watanabe S, Ichimura T, Tsuruzoe S, Shinkai Y, Tachibana M, Chiba T, Nakao M: Methyl-CpG binding domain 1 (MBD1) interacts with the Suv39h1-HP1 heterochromatic complex for DNA methylation-based transcriptional repression. *J Biol Chem* 2003, **278**(26):24132–24138.

Fuks F, Hurd PJ, Deplus R, Kouzarides T: The DNA methyltransferases associate with HP1 and the SUV39H1 histone methyltransferase. *Nucleic Acids Res* 2003, **31**(9):2305–2312.

Galagan JE, Calvo SE, Borkovich KA, Selker EU, Read ND, Jaffe D, FitzHugh W, Ma LJ, Smirnov S, Purcell S*et al*: The genome sequence of the filamentous fungus Neurospora crassa. *Nature* 2003, **422**(6934):859–868.

Galagan JE, Selker EU: RIP: the evolutionary cost of genome defense. *Trends Genet* 2004, **20**(9):417–423.

Goll MG BT: Eukaryotic cytosine methyltransferases. *Annu Rev Biochem* 2005, **74**:481–514.

Graia F, Lespinet O, Rimbault B, Dequard-Chablat M, Coppin E, Picard M: Genome Quality Control: RIP (repeat-induced point mutation) comes to Podospora. *Mol Microbiol* 2001, **39**:1–11.

Grayburn WS, Selker EU: A natural case of RIP: Degeneration of DNA sequence in an ancestral tandem duplication. *Mol Cell Biol* 1989, **9**(10):4416–4421.

Grünweller A, Gillen C, Erdmann VA, Kurreck J: Cellular uptake and localization of a Cy3-labeled siRNA specific for the serine/threonine kinase Pim-1. *Oligonucleotides* 2003, **13**(5):345–352.

Hall IM, Shankaranarayana GD, Noma KI, Ayoub N, Cohen A, Grewal SI: Establishment and Maintenance of a Heterochromatin Domain. *Science* 2002, **297**:2232–2237.

Ikeda K, Nakayashiki H, Kataoka T, Tamba H, Hashimoto Y, Tosa Y, Mayama S: Repeat-induced point mutation (RIP) in Magnaporthe grisea: implications for its sexual cycle in the natural field context. *Mol Microbiol* 2002, **45**(5):1355–1364.

Jackson JP, Lindroth AM, Cao X, Jacobsen SE: Control of CpNpG DNA methylation by the KRYPTONITE histone H3 methyltransferase. *Nature* 2002, **416**(6880):556–560.

Jacobs SA, Taverna SD, Zhang Y, Briggs SD, Li J, Eissenberg JC, Allis CD, Khorasanizadeh S: Specificity of the HP1 chromo domain for the methylated N-terminus of histone H3. *EMBO J* 2001, **20**(18):5232–5241.

Kachroo P, Leong SA, Chattoo BB: *Pot2*, an inverted repeat transposon from the rice blast fungus *Magnaporthe grisea*. *Mol Gen Genet* 1994, **245**(3):339–348.

Kelly WG, Aramayo R: Meiotic silencing and the epigenetics of sex. *Chromosome Res* 2007, **15**(5):633–651.

Ketting RF, Haverkamp TH, van Luenen HG, Plasterk RH: Mut-7 of C. elegans, required for transposon silencing and RNA interference, is a homolog of Werner syndrome helicase and RNaseD. *Cell* 1999, **99**(2):133–141.

Kinsey JA: Restricted distribution of the Tad transposon in strains of *Neurospora*. *Curr Genet* 1989, **15**:271–275.

Kinsey JA, Garrett-Engele PW, Cambareri EB, Selker EU: The Neurospora transposon Tad is sensitive to repeat-induced point Mutation (RIP). *Genetics* 1994, **138**:657–664.

Kito H TY, Sato J, Fukiya S, Sone T, Tomita F.: Occan, a novel transposon in the Fot1 family, is ubiquitously found in several Magnaporthe grisea isolates. *Curr Genet* 2003, **42**(6):322–331.

Kouzminova EA, Selker EU: *Dim-2* encodes a DNA-methyltransferase responsible for all known cytosine methylation in Neurospora. *EMBO J* 2001, **20**(15):4309–4323.

Lachner M, O'Carroll D, Rea S, Mechtler K, Jenuwein T: Methylation of histone H3 lysine 9 creates a binding site for HP1 proteins. *Nature* 2001, **410**(6824):116–120.

Lee DW, Pratt RJ, McLaughlin M, Aramayo R: An argonaute-like protein is required for meiotic silencing. *Genetics* 2003, **164**(2):821–828.

Lee DW, Seong KY, Pratt RJ, Baker K, Aramayo R: Properties of unpaired DNA required for efficient silencing in Neurospora crassa. *Genetics* 2004, **167**(1):131–150.

Lehnertz B, Ueda Y, Derijck AA, Braunschweig U, Perez-Burgos L, Kubicek S, Chen T, Li E, Jenuwein T, Peters AH: Suv39h-mediated histone h3 lysine 9 methylation directs DNA methylation to major satellite repeats at pericentric heterochromatin. *Curr Biol* 2003, **13**(14):1192–1200.

Liu J, Carmell MA, Rivas FV, Marsden CG, Thomson JM, Song JJ, Hammond SM, Joshua-Tor L, Hannon GJ: Argonaute2 is the catalytic engine of mammalian RNAi. *Science* 2004, **305**(5689):1437–1441.

Llave C, Kasschau KD, Rector MA, Carrington JC: Endogenous and Silencing-Associated Small RNAs in Plants. *Plant Cell* 2002, **14**(7):1605–1619.

Lynch M, Conery JS: The evolutionary fate and consequences of duplicate genes. *Science* 2000, **290**(5494):1151–1155.

Maiti M, Lee HC, Liu Y: QIP, a putative exonuclease, interacts with the Neurospora Argonaute protein and facilitates conversion of duplex siRNA into single strands. *Genes Dev* 2007, **21**(5):590–600.

Malagnac F, Bartee L, Bender J: An Arabidopsis SET domain protein required for maintenance but not establishment of DNA methylation. *EMBO J* 2002, **21**(24):6842–6852.

Malagnac F, Wendel B, Goyon C, Faugeron G, Zickler D, Rossignol JL, Noyer-Weidner M, Vollmayr P, Trautner TA, Walter J: A gene essential for de novo methylation and development in Ascobolus reveals a novel type of eukaryotic DNA methyltransferase structure. *Cell* 1997, **91**(2):281–290.

Margolin BS, Garrett-Engele PW, Stevens JN, Yen-Fritz D, Garrett-Engele C, Metzenberg RL, Selker EU: A methylated Neurospora 5S rRNA pseudogene contains a transposable element inactivated by RIP. *Genetics* 1998, **149**:1787–1797.

Mautino MR, Rosa AL: Analysis of models involving enzymatic activities for the occurrence of C–>T transition mutations during repeat-induced point mutation (RIP) in Neurospora crassa. *J Theor Biol* 1998, **192**(1):61–71.

Miao VP, Freitag M, Selker EU: Short TpA-rich segments of the zeta-eta region induce DNA methylation in *Neurospora crassa*. *J Mol Biol* 2000, **300**(2):249–273.

Nakayashiki H: RNA silencing in fungi: mechanisms and applications. *FEBS Lett* 2005, **579**(26):5950–5970.

Nakayashiki H, Nishimoto N, Ikeda K, Tosa Y, Mayama S: Degenerate MAGGY elements in a subgroup of Pyricularia grisea: a possible example of successful capture of a genetic invader by a fungal genome. *Mol Gen Genet* 1999, **261**(6):958–966.

Nolan T, Braccini L, Azzalin G, De Toni A, Macino G, Cogoni C: The post-transcriptional gene silencing machinery functions independently of DNA methylation to repress a LINE1-like retrotransposon in Neurospora crassa. *Nucleic Acids Res* 2005, **33**(5):1564–1573.

Nolan T, Cecere G, Mancone C, Alonzi T, Tripodi M, Catalanotto C, Cogoni C: The RNA-dependent RNA polymerase essential for post-transcriptional gene silencing in Neurospora crassa interacts with replication protein A. *Nucleic Acids Res* 2008, **36**(2):532–538.

Pal-Bhadra M, Leibovitch BA, Gandhi SG, Rao M, Bhadra U, Birchler JA, Elgin SC: Heterochromatic silencing and HP1 localization in Drosophila are dependent on the RNAi machinery. *Science* 2004, **303**(5658):669–672.

Perkins DD, Margolin BS, Selker EU, Haedo SD: Occurrence of repeat induced point mutation in long segmental duplications of Neurospora. *Genetics* 1997, **147**(1):125–136.

Perkins DD, Metzenberg RL, Raju NB, Selker EU, Barry EG: Reversal of a *Neurospora* translocation by crossing over involving displaced rDNA, and methylation of the rDNA segments that result from recombination. *Genetics* 1986, **114**:791–817.

Pratt RJ, Lee DW, Aramayo R: DNA methylation affects meiotic trans-sensing, not meiotic silencing, in Neurospora. *Genetics* 2004, **168**(4):1925–1935.

Raju NB, Metzenberg RL, Shiu PK: Neurospora spore killers Sk-2 and Sk-3 suppress meiotic silencing by unpaired DNA. *Genetics* 2007, **176**(1):43–52.

Reese BE BK, Baylin SB, Rountree MR.: The methyl-CpG binding protein MBD1 interacts with the p150 subunit of chromatin assembly factor 1. *Mol Cell Biol* 2003, **23**(9):3226–3236.

Reeves R: Molecular biology of HMGA proteins: hubs of nuclear function. *Gene* 2001, **277**(1–2):63–81.

Romano N, Macino G: Quelling: transient inactivation of gene expression in *Neurospora crassa* by transformation with homologous sequences. *Mol Microbiol* 1992, **6**(22):3343–3353.

Rosa AL FH, Mautino MR.: In vivo levels of S-adenosylmethionine modulate C:G to T:A mutations associated with repeat-induced point mutation in Neurospora crassa. *Mutat Res* 2004, **548**(1–2):85–95.

Rossignol J-L, Faugeron G: Gene inactivation triggered by recognition between DNA repeats. *Experientia* 1994, **50**:307–317.

Rountree MR, Selker EU: DNA methylation inhibits elongation but not initiation of transcription in *Neurospora crassa*. *Genes Dev* 1997, **11**:2383–2395.

Selker EU: Premeiotic instability of repeated sequences in *Neurospora crassa*. *Annu Rev Genet* 1990, **24**:579–613.

Selker EU: Repeat-induced point mutation (RIP) and DNA methylation. In: *More gene manipulations in fungi*. Edited by Bennet JW, Lasure L. New York: Academic Press, Inc.; 1991: 258–265.

Selker EU: Trichostatin A causes selective loss of DNA methylation in Neurospora. *Proc Natl Acad Sci U S A* 1998, **95**(16):9430–9435.

Selker EU: Gene silencing: repeats that count. *Cell* 1999, **97**(2):157–160.

Selker EU, Freitag M, Kothe GO, Margolin BS, Rountree MR, Allis CD, Tamaru H: Induction and maintenance of nonsymmetrical DNA methylation in Neurospora. *Proc Natl Acad Sci U S A* 2002, **99 Suppl 4**:16485–16490.

Selker EU, Fritz DY, Singer MJ: Dense non-symmetrical DNA methylation resulting from repeat-induced point mutation (RIP) in Neurospora. *Science* 1993, **262**:1724–1728.

Selker EU, Garrett PW: DNA sequence duplications trigger gene inactivation in *Neurospora crassa*. *Proc Natl Acad Sci USA* 1988, **85**(18):6870–6874.

Selker EU, Jensen BC, Richardson GA: A portable signal causing faithful DNA methylation *de novo* in*Neurospora crassa*. *Science* 1987, **238**:48–53.

Selker EU, Stevens JN: DNA methylation at asymmetric sites is associated with numerous transition mutations. *Proc Natl Acad Sci USA* 1985, **82**:8114–8118.

Selker EU, Tountas NA, Cross SH, Margolin BS, Murphy JG, Bird AP, Freitag M: The methylated component of the Neurospora crassa genome. *Nature* 2003, **422**(6934):893–897.

Shiu PK, Metzenberg RL: Meiotic silencing by unpaired DNA: properties, regulation and suppression. *Genetics* 2002, **161**(4):1483–1495.

Shiu PK, Raju NB, Zickler D, Metzenberg RL: Meiotic silencing by unpaired DNA. *Cell* 2001, **107**(7):905–916.

Shiu PK, Zickler D, Raju NB, Ruprich-Robert G, Metzenberg RL: SAD-2 is required for meiotic silencing by unpaired DNA and perinuclear localization of SAD-1 RNA-directed RNA polymerase. *Proc Natl Acad Sci U S A* 2006, **103**(7):2243–2248.

Singer MJ, Marcotte BA, Selker EU: DNA methylation associated with repeat-induced point mutation in *Neurospora crassa*. *Mol Cell Biol* 1995, **15**(10):5586–5597.

Tabara H, Sarkissian M, Kelly WG, Fleenor J, Grishok A, Timmons L, Fire A, Mello CC: The rde-1 gene, RNA interference, and transposon silencing in C. elegans. *Cell* 1999, **99**(2):123–132.

Tamaru H, Selker EU: A histone H3 methyltransferase controls DNA methylation in Neurospora crassa. *Nature* 2001, **414**(6861):277–283.

Tamaru H, Selker EU: Synthesis of Signals for De Novo DNA Methylation in *Neurospora crassa*. *Mol Cell Biol* 2003, **23**(7):2379–2394.

Tamaru H, Zhang X, McMillen D, Singh PB, Nakayama J, Grewal SI, Allis CD, Cheng X, Selker EU: Trimethylated lysine 9 of histone H3 is a mark for DNA methylation in Neurospora crassa. *Nat Genet* 2003, **34**(1):75–79.

Volpe TA, Kidner C, Hall IM, Teng G, Grewal SI, Martienssen RA: Regulation of Heterochromatic Silencing and Histone H3 Lysine-9 Methylation by RNAi. *Science* 2002, **297**(5588):1833–1837.

Walsh J: How often do duplicated genes evolve new functions? *Genetics* 1995, **139**(1):421–428.

Waterhouse P, Wang M, Lough T: Gene silencing as an adaptive defence against viruses. *Nature* 2001, **411**(6839):834–842.

Watters MK, Randall TA, Margolin BS, Selker EU, Stadler DR: Action of repeat-induced point mutation on both strands of a duplex and on tandem duplications of various sizes in Neurospora. *Genetics* 1999, **153**(2):705–714.

Wu-Scharf D, Jeong B, Zhang C, Cerutti H: Transgene and transposon silencing in Chlamydomonas reinhardtii by a DEAH-box RNA helicase. *Science* 2000, **290**(5494):1159–1162.

Yebra MJ, Bhagwat AS: A cytosine methyltransferase converts 5-methylcytosine in DNA to thymine. *Biochemistry* 1995, **34**(45):14752–14757.

Yoder JA, Walsh CP, Bestor TH: Cytosine methylation and the ecology of intragenomic parasites. *Trends Genet* 1997, **13**(8):335–340.

Zhou Y, Cambareri EB, Kinsey JA: DNA methylation inhibits expression and transposition of the Neurospora Tad retrotransposon. *Mol Gen Genet* 2001, **265**:748–754.

Zilberman D, Cao X, Jacobsen SE: ARGONAUTE4 control of locus-specific siRNA accumulation and DNA and histone methylation. *Science* 2003, **299**(5607):716–719.

Zingg JM, Shen JC, Yang AS, Rapoport H, Jones PA: Methylation inhibitors can increase the rate of cytosine deamination by (cytosine-5)-DNA methyltransferase. *Nucleic Acids Res* 1996, **24**(16):3267–3275.

Integrating the Genome and Epigenome in Human Disease

Claes Wadelius

Abstract Transcription factors (TFs) and the core components of the epigenome, DNA methylation and histone modifications interact in the epigenetic machinery. Expression of three-four key selected transcription factors can dedifferentiate differentiated cells into induced pluripotent stem cells with a totally distinct epigenome. Out of the around 2,000 nuclear proteins, around 350 are known to cause disease when mutated. The conditions range from rare syndromes to common diseases. Mutations are found in all components of the epigenetic machinery, e.g. proteins mediating DNA methylation and those binding to methylated cytosine, histone proteins and enzymes adding or removing modifications to histone tails, those binding to the modifications as well as proteins in the basal transcription machinery. Sequence specific transcription factors are the most abundant nuclear proteins and mutations in them cause a wide range of diseases affecting different organs in the developing or mature organism. Even if a mutated protein is present in most or all cell-types, a specific disease is often found only in one or a few types. The reason for this is unclear and an interesting topic for future research. One hypothesis is that the disease is caused by the mutated protein interacting with other tissue restricted proteins. Technical breakthroughs like chromatin immunoprecipitation and analysis on next generation sequencers (ChIP-seq) mean that these processes can be systematically studied.

Keywords Transcription factors · Histone modifying enzymes · Methyl binding proteins · Mutation · Genome association · Human disease

1 Introduction

There are different opinions on which are the biological phenomena that should be included in the subject epigenetics. It is widely accepted that DNA methylation

C. Wadelius (✉)
Department of Genetics and Pathology, Rudbeck Laboratory, Uppsala University, SE-75185 Uppsala, Sweden
e-mail: Claes.Wadelius@genpat.uu.se

and histone modifications are part of epigenetics since they are stably transmitted to daughter cells after cell division. Recent dramatic developments in stem cell research make it relevant to consider broadening the view of epigenetics. It has been shown that differentiated cells e.g. skin fibroblasts can be reprogrammed to a dedifferentiated state called induced pluripotent stem (iPS) cells (Takahashi et al. 2007, Park et al. 2008) (See Chapter "The Epigenomic Landscape of Reprogramming in Mammals"). This is achieved by ectopic expression of three-four transcription factors. These iPS cells show all signs of being stem cells as determined by gene expression, cell morphology and promoter methylation pattern. By subjecting them to defined stimuli, they can be differentiated into cells from all three germ cell layers. The conclusion is that a few transcription factors are able to totally reprogramme the epigenetic profile of these cells. In consequence, the action of transcription factors can be regarded as an integral part of the epigenetic machinery. A recent definition by Adrian Bird (Bird 2007) suggests that epigenetics is "the structural adaptation of chromosomal regions so as to register, signal and perpetuate altered activity states" which could include the action of transcription factors.

The opinion that transcription factors are part of epigenetics is further supported by the various layers of interplay between transcription factors and either DNA methylation or histone modification. The binding of the TF FOXA1 is strongly correlated to the appropriate histone modification at the binding sites (Lupien et al. 2008). Other factors have decreased affinity for a binding site when the CpG dinucleotide of its motif is methylated, For example USF1 binds differentially to a methylated and unmethylated CACGTG (Griswold and Kim 2001) (Fig. 1 a). A mutation or SNP in the motif can also affect the binding (Fig. 1b). Furthermore, mutations in genes encoding transcription factors often severely affect the function and epigenetic profile of a cell type. This is illustrated e.g. by mutations in p53 and MYC that are mutated in several cancers. In fact, if you look at how frequently different proteins are mutated in cancer, transcription factors are the most overrepresented (Futreal et al. 2004, Mitelman et al. 2004). There are around 2,000 genes encoding transcription factors and other nuclear proteins in the human genome. A recent survey has shown that at least 350 ($\sim$17.5%) of them are mutated in human disease (see reference Wadelius and Peltonen). These diseases have characteristic phenotypes and epigenotypes in one or several cell types. In summary, there are definite interactions between transcription factors and proteins of the epigenetic machinery. In this chapter I will describe the action of proteins controlling DNA methylation, histone modifications and transcription factors, and mutations causing malfunction.

The knowledge of genetic causes of disease is increasing rapidly. The loci for most Mendelian conditions have been genetically mapped using DNA samples from families segregating monogenic diseases and polymorphic DNA markers. Most monogenic diseases were mapped using highly informative microsatellite markers involving a fairly labor intensive process. The causative mutations have subsequently been identified for a majority of them and most of them are located in exons causing changes to the protein code (Fig. 2). A number of these genes encode proteins controlling epigenetic processes and some conceptually important ones will be discussed in this chapter.

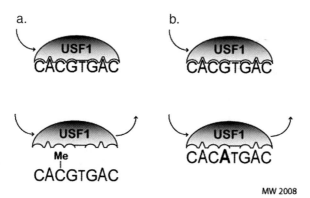

Fig. 1 Effect of methylation of DNA on transcription factor binding. (**a**) Methylation of CpG interferes with the binding of USF1. (**b**) Allelic variant of the E-box CACGTGAC has much lower affinity for USF1

	Regulatory element	Exon
Mendelian disease	x	xxxx
Common disease	xxxx	x
Cancer	xx	xx

Fig. 2 Mutations in monogenic diseases are mostly in coding regions, in complex diseases outside exons and sometimes affecting gene regulatory elements. In cancer, mutations are likely to occur both in exons and in regulatory modules

Despite large efforts it has been difficult to map genetic variants predisposing to common diseases using linkage analysis. The main reason is that alleles mediating risk for the common diseases act in a fundamentally different way. In most instances multiple loci contribute to a common disease, each with a small effect. This means that each locus has a marginal effect on disease risk and large families with the same causative allele are therefore not found (Risch and Merikangas 1996). In recent years, the strategy has changed to performing association studies in cases and controls, which dramatically increases the statistical power. Most common single nucleotide polymorphisms (SNPs) in the human genome have been identified and their frequencies determined in the major human ethnic groups (Frazer et al. 2007). In parallel, genotyping technologies have gone through a technical revolution. Currently 500,000 – 1,000,000 variable positions can be genotyped at a reasonable cost even in large cohorts. The HapMap project has shown that the genome is organized in haplotype blocks consisting of discrete regions of variable size, with a set of neighboring polymorphic markers, which are transmitted unchanged from one generation to the next. By typing SNPs that tag haplotypes (tagSNPs) new technologies permit you to capture the majority of the relevant polymorphic information in the genome. A flow of whole genome association studies with information of alleles predisposing to common disease are now published, and collected at NIH.[1]

---

[1] dbGaP. The DataBase of Genotype and Phenotype.www.ncbi.nlm.nih.gov/sites/entrez?Db=gap.

Genetic variants predisposing to common phenotypes are in general not located in exons and do not change the protein code (Fig. 2). They are rather located in non-coding regions and could affect transcription rate, stability of the transcript, alternative splicing, RNA transport and structure or target of noncoding RNAs. It has been suggested and sometimes shown that disease-related SNPs are associated with differential gene expression (Law et al. 2006). In other words, they affect the regulatory code. The mechanism mediating differences in gene expression is not known, but it is reasonable to assume that some of the differences are caused by variable affinity between a transcription factor and the two alleles (Fig. 1b). Differential binding of gene regulatory proteins to alleles of SNPs can be studied experimentally (Maynard et al. 2008), and pilot projects have shown that a transcription factor preferentially interacts with the allele most closely resembling the consensus sequence (Ameur et al. submitted). If this was studied systematically for all TFs in the most important cell types, it would provide information about mechanisms for common diseases and phenotypes. There are also inherited differences in gene expression between individuals and populations (Stranger et al. 2007) that could be explained by studying their epigenetic profile. To get an integrated view of these phenomena the status of chromatin modifications needs to be determined. The currently ongoing ENCODE and the new AHEAD projects (Birney et al. 2007, Pennisi 2008) could provide a framework for such an effort.

What is the magnitude of the work that needs to be done to characterize the gene regulatory code? First, each cell type is unique and needs to be studied individually. Second, we do not know the absolute number of regulatory regions. Evolutionary constraint acts on ~5% of the genome as a clear signal of functional importance (Birney et al. 2007). Around 1.5% is found in exons, leaving 3.5% to explain. Different studies have shown that at least some regions participate in gene regulation e.g. as enhancers directing embryonal development (Visel et al. 2008). Other studies have shown that many gene regulatory sequences are not constrained (Birney et al. 2007, Odom et al. 2007, Borneman et al. 2007), i.e. solid data show that gene regulatory proteins often bind to bases that are not under evolutionary conservation. This means that gene regulation evolves more quickly than the protein sequence. From evolutionary studies we can not tell what portion of the genome that regulates gene activity, but current data suggest that it is well above 3.5%. These numbers are supported by studies of regulatory regions. Recent data from studies of DNaseI hypersensitive sites suggest that an average cell type has ~100 000 regulatory regions (Boyle et al. 2008). When summarized over all cell types, we can assume that there are at least >500,000 regions in the genome with a regulatory function. Previous knowledge of promoters and enhancers indicate that they are 500-1,000 bp each, suggesting a total size of the regulatory DNA of 250,000,000 – 500,000,000 bp i.e. 8-16% of the human genome (Levine and Tjian 2003).

The human genome encodes around 2,000 transcription factors and other nuclear proteins out of which roughly 1,000 are expressed at detectable levels in an average cell. Detailed studies have shown that in the order of 10-20 proteins bind to promoters and enhancers (Levine and Tjian 2003). Each of the proteins are chosen from the 1,000 available, meaning that for a regulatory element with 10 proteins there are $1,000^{10}$ i.e. 10^{30} possible combinations and with 20 proteins there are $1,000^{20}$ i.e. 10^{60} combinations. These numbers exceed the number of regulatory elements by many orders of magnitudes, meaning that only a small fraction of all possible combinations are actually used. However, this shows that the cell has the potential to make an extreme number of combinations of regulatory factors and, thus, regulate each gene in a unique way. Each protein also can undergo post-translational modifications which allows for further dynamics and a way to react to environmental stimuli. As always, science depends on efficient methods to study a biological phenomenon and as described we have good assays to study the genome. Recently, technical breakthroughs have enabled large scale studies of the epigenome. Histone modifications and TF binding sites can be mapped genome wide with high precision (Barski et al. 2007, Johnson et al. 2007) and large scale assays for DNA methylation have also been developed (Jacinto et al. 2008). We can now get an unbiased view of key epigenetic features across the genome and correlate them to different diseases. The coming years will therefore be a harvest time for epigenomics research.

An important task for the future is to study genetic variation in gene regulatory regions and in genes controlling the epigenetic machinery. When this has been done we have a framework for an integrated view of genetics and epigenetics and their contribution to human disease. Most of the work thus lies ahead of us, but from pilot studies we can draw conclusions of some general principles and a number of them will be described in the rest of the chapter.

2 Primary Defects in DNA Methylation and Their Diseases

Only three proteins are known to have a DNA-methylating activity and consequently primary defects in the respective genes give rise to few diseases. On the other hand abnormal DNA-methylation is found in many genes in cancer and other conditions but those issues are only briefly discussed in this chapter. The proteins that are known to methylate DNA are DNMT1, DNMT3A and DNMT3B. Five proteins interact with methylated C (me-C) namely MBD1, MBD2, MBD3, MBD4 and MeCP2 (Fig. 3). These processes are fundamental for the function of the cell, and it is surprising that mutations in these proteins show manifestations in only selected cell types.

Mutations in both alleles of the gene DNMT3B lead to a recognizable syndrome of severe, often lethal immunodeficiency, centromeric instability and facial anomalies (ICF) syndrome (see reference OMIM) (OMIM #242860) i.e. it is inherited as an autosomal recessive trait (Xu et al. 1999). Cytogenetic analysis show severe disturbances of the pericentromeric regions of chromosomes 1, 9 and 16, known to contain satellite DNA. Most patients with this phenotype have been shown to harbour mutations in the DNA methyltransferase sequence motifs of DNMT3B and a recognisable lack of de novo methylation of the pericentric heterochromatic repeats. Some patients with ICF have no recognisable mutations in this gene, and may have a slightly different methylation phenotype (Jiang et al. 2005).

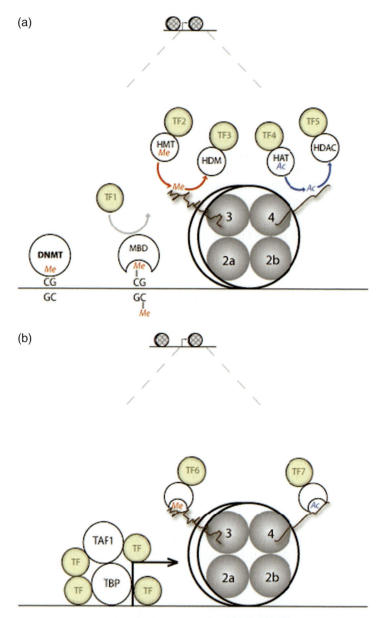

Fig. 3 (**a**) In inactive genes DNA Methyl Transferases (DNMT) methylate CpG which are then bound by Methyl Binding Domain (MBD) containing proteins. Both meC and MBD can prevent binding of transcription factors (TF). Histone modifying enzymes interact with TFs to target modifications to histone tails of appropriate genes. Histone Methyl Transferases (HMT) add methyl groups which are removed by Histone DeMethylases (HD). Acetyl groups are added by Histone Acetyl Transferases (HAT) and removed by Histone DeAcetylases (HDAC). (**b**) At active genes the nucleosome upstream of the transcription start site is replaced by the preinitiation complex including TATA-box binding protein (TBP), the general transcription factor TAF1 and several transcription factors. Specific proteins bind to modified histone tails and interact with various transcription factors

Among me-C binding proteins, only MeCP2 is known to contain mutations that cause a human disease, namely the Rett syndrome (OMIM #312750) which almost exclusively occurs in females (OMIM, Amir et al. 1999). The gene for MeCP2 is located on the X chromosome, in Xq28. It is an X-linked dominant disease caused by sporadic mutations, with male lethality and if males are affected, they have 2 X chromosomes or are somatic mosaics for mutations in the gene. The patients develop normally during the first year and then get progressive neurological symptoms. MeCP2 binds to methylated DNA and represses transcription in vitro from methylated, but not unmethylated promoters (Nan et al. 1997). Developmental studies have shown that the protein is expressed in most neurons and becomes abundant as the cells mature (Shahbazian et al. 2002) which is compatible with the cell type restricted behavior of the disease.

3 Defects in Histones, Histone Modifying Enzymes and General Transcription Factors and Their Diseases

A number of histones and histone modifying enzymes cause recognizable diseases when they are affected by mutations (Fig. 3). As with DNA methylation it is remarkable that defects in these basal processes affect only a very limited repertoire of cells (Table 1). What is less surprising is that mutations in these proteins most often result in malignant transformation including both solid tumors and leukemia. Another common result is a syndrome, i.e. a mixture of clinical symptoms from different cells and tissues, which is logical since basic machineries are perturbed. It also happens that mutations in one gene cause both a tumor and a syndrome, as with EHMT1 and EP300.

Mutations in genes encoding two histones have been significantly associated with cancer: HIST1H1B with colorectal cancer (Sjoblom et al. 2006) and HIST1H4I with non-Hodgkin's Lymphoma (NHL).[2] The mechanism leading to malignant transformation of specific cell types due to mutations in structural chromatin proteins remains unclear. Future work will show if these findings are false positives in large scale screening programs or represent real associations.

As described in other chapters there are several covalent modifications to histones that are associated to different cellular processes. Methylation and acetylation of various residues of H3 and H4 are found in distinct regions of the genome, and there are specific enzymes that add or remove these marks (Fig. 3). Mutations are found in genes performing all these processes and the most common outcome is cancer. SMYD3 is a H3K4 methyltransferase and the same activity is suggested for MLL. Both SMYD3 and MLL are associated to cancer. For SMYD3 a high activity allele of the promoter is associated with different solid tumors (Tsuge et al. 2005) and translocations involving MLL are found in many aggressive leukemias (Futreal et al. 2004). A ChIP-study using promoter arrays showed that MLL localizes with

---

[2] SCGC. Sanger Cancer Gene Census: www.sanger.ac.uk/genetics/CGP/Census.

Table 1 Mutated histones, histone modifying enzymes and general transcription factors

Group	Gene name	Symbol	OMIM ID	Disease	References
3	bromodomain containing 4	BRD4	608749	lethal midline carcinoma of young people	(SCGS)
3	bromodomain and WD repeat domain containing 3	BRWD3	300553	X-linked mental retardation	(Field et al. 2007)
2a	euchromatic histone-lysine N-methyltransferase 1	EHMT1	114480 610253	Breast cancer CaMP score 1.3; 9q34 subtelomeric deletion sdr	(Sjoblom et al. 2006, Kleefstra et al. 2006)
2b	E1A binding protein p300	EP300	114500 114480 260350 601626 180849	Colorectal;breast and pancreatic cancer; AML; Rubenstein-Taybi syndrome	(Futreal et al. 2004, Zimmermann et al. 2007)
5	general transcription factor IIH, polypeptide 5	GTF2H5	608780	Trichothiodystrophy	(Giglia-Mari et al. 2004)
5	GTF2I repeat domain containing 1	GTF2IRD1	194050	Williams-Beuren syndrome	(Tassabehji et al. 2005)
2b	histone deacetylase 4	HDAC4	114480	Breast cancer CaMP score 1.6	(Sjoblom et al. 2006)
1	histone 1, H1b	HIST1H1B	114500	Colorektal cancer CaMP score 2.5	(Sjoblom et al. 2006)
1	histone cluster 1, H4i	HIST1H4I	605027	NHL	(SCGC)
2a	myeloid/lymphoid or mixed-lineage leukemia	MLL	601626	AML; ALL	(Futreal et al. 2004)
2b	MYST histone acetyltransferase (monocytic leukemia) 3	MYST3 (RUNXBP2)	601626	AML	(Futreal et al. 2004)
2b	MYST histone acetyltransferase (monocytic leukemia) 4	MYST4	601626	AML	(Futreal et al. 2004)
2a	nuclear receptor binding SET domain protein 1	NSD1	601626	AML	(SCGC)
4	SWI/SNF related, matrix associated, actin dependent regulator of chromatin, subfamily a-like 1	SMARCAL1	242900	Schimke immuno-osseus dysplasia	(Boerkoel et al. 2002)

Table 1 (continued)

Group	Gene name	Symbol	OMIM ID	Disease	References
4	SWI/SNF related, matrix associated, actin dependent regulator of chromatin, subfamily b, member 1	SMARCB1	609322	Rhabdoid predisposition syndrome; malignant rhabdoid tumors	(SCGC)
2a	Smcy homolog, X-linked	SMCX	300534	syndromic X-linked mental retardation	(Jensen et al. 2005)
2a	SET and MYND domain containing 3	SMYD3	114500 114550 114800	colorectal, hepatocellular carcinomas, breast cancer	(Tsuge et al. 2005)
3	suppressor of zeste 12 homolog (Drosophila)	SUZ12	606245	endometrial stromal tumours	(SCGC)
5	TAF1 RNA polymerase II, TATA box binding protein (TBP)-associated factor, 250kDa	TAF1	314250	X-linked dystonia-parkinsonism (XDP)	(Makino et al. 2007)
5	TAF15 RNA polymerase II, TATA box binding protein (TBP)-associated factor, 68kDa	TAF15	601574	extraskeletal myxoid chondrosarcomas, ALL	(SCGC)
5	TATA box binding protein	TBP	607136	spinocerebellar ataxia 17, Parkinson disease included	(Stevanin et al. 2003)
5	transcription elongation factor A (SII), 1	TCEA1	181030	salivary adenoma	(SCGC)
2a	Wolf-Hirschhorn syndrome candidate 1(MMSET)	WHSC1	254500	MM	(SCGC)
2a	Wolf-Hirschhorn syndrome candidate 1-like 1	WHSC1L1	601626	AML	(SCGC)

1. Histones, 2. Histone modifying enzymes, 2a. Histone methylation, 2b. Histone acetylation, 3. Proteins binding histone modifications, 4. Chromatin modifying complex, 5. General transcription factors and elongation factors.

RNA polymerase II and in regions with H3K4me3 (Guenther et al. 2005). Interactions with transcription factors and other proteins may confer some specificity and direct these proteins to a subset of genes. Future ChIP-sequencing studies on normal and malignant cells may identify genes that are specific to the malignant process. Inherited mutations in the H3K4me3 demethylase SMCX does not result in cancer, but rather syndromic X-linked mental retardation (Jensen et al. 2005). Mutations in the methyltransferases NSD1 and EHMT1, mediating H3K36, H4K20 and H3K9 methylation, which are associated with transcription elongation, DNA-repair and silencing of heterochromatin, are found in AML (see footnote 2)[3] breast cancer (Sjoblom et al. 2006) and the 9q34 subtelomeric deletion syndrome (Kleefstra et al. 2006). Acetylation of H3 and H4 is associated with actively transcribed genes and a mutation in genes adding the modification, like EP300 and MYST4, are found in solid tumors (Futreal et al. 2004) and leukemia (Futreal et al. 2004). At the same time mutations in HDAC4, one of the enzymes removing the mark, has been found in breast cancer (Sjoblom et al. 2006). So a conclusion is that mutations in enzymes mediating epigenetic signals of both activation and inactivation of genes are associated with specific malignancies and rare congenital syndromes.

Designated proteins bind to specific histone modifications and mediate various nuclear processes (Fig. 3). The bromodomain-containing proteins, BRD4 and BRDW3, bind to acetylated histones and mutations in these proteins have been found in cancer (see footnote 2) and mental retardation (Field et al. 2007). SUZ12 participates in the polycomb complex to repress genes by establishing the H3K27me3 mark. Mutations in SUZ12 have been detected in endometrial tumors and this may thus impair inactivation of some genes (see footnote 2).

During gene activation chromatin modifying enzymes cooperate with chromatin remodeling complexes and SMARCAL1 and SMARCB1 take part in the processes. Mutations in these proteins have been found in Schimke immuno-osseus dysplasia (Boerkoel et al. 2002) and muscle (rhabdoid) tumors (see footnote 2).

Mutations in general transcription factors can cause specific diseases (Fig. 3). Most remarkable is that mutations in TAF1 and TBP are found in the neurological diseases X-linked dystonia-parkinsonism (Makino et al. 2007) and spinocerebellar ataxia 17 (Stevanin et al. 2003), with similarities to Parkinsons disease. Why defects in these proteins, most likely found in all cells and at all active promoters, only give symptoms in selected neurons remains to be understood. Mutations in the TBP-associated factor TAF15 and the transcription elongation factor TCEA1 are found in cases with solid tumors (see footnote 2) and leukemia (see footnote 2).

4 Constitutional Mutations of Transcription Factors and Disease

There are around 2,000 genes for proteins involved in the gene regulatory machinery. As mentioned, there are few proteins involved in DNA methylation, and a

---

[3] See footnote 2.

slightly higher number involved in the maintenance of core chromatin proteins, making sequence specific TFs by far the largest group (Fig. 3). The high number of genes makes them a large target for mutations and their diverse functions result in a wide range of clinical manifestations. It is well known from model organisms and human studies that TFs are essential for a normal embryonal development and consequently mutations in many TFs cause congenital syndromes. Today mutations in >133 genes encoding TFs are known to cause syndromes, autosomal dominant, autosomal recessive and X-linked recessive diseases, that each are relatively rare. However, taken together they are not infrequent findings in a pediatric clinic, where most cases are identified (Wadelius and Peltonen submitted). It is worth noting that mutations in this category can result in two or more diseases with manifestations in different cell types, even if the mutation takes place in a single gene. As mentioned, mutations in a gene can lead both to cancer and a non-malignant disease. In this chapter examples of autosomal dominant, autosomal recessive, X-linked recessive diseases and congenital syndromes will be presented (Table 2). To categorize a disease as rare or common is a matter of definition, but diseases affecting many people are important from a population perspective and some will be described.

An interesting example is a gene which is present in close to half the human population, and which has a substantial effect on the phenotype. The inheritance is Y-linked dominant and the gene encodes SRY, sex determining region Y, which is the TF that induces the embryo to develop into a male. The gene is located in the Y-specific portion of the short arm of the Y chromosome, very close to the pseudoautosomal region which is present on both the X and Y chromosome short arms. There are rare cases of XX males in which the SRY gene is present on one of the X chromosomes, as well as XY females that lack the SRY on the Y chromosome (Jager et al. 1990). SRY is thus a master regulator that induces a developmental program involving many downstream genes, some of them also transcription factors. Another factor in this developmental pathway is SOX9. Mutations in this gene cause a severe congenital disease characterized by bowing of the long bones and other malformations. In addition, around two thirds of children with both X and Y chromosomes have genital malformations and may develop into females. Mutations in this autosomal gene are only found in one of the alleles meaning that they have an autosomal dominant mode of action (Foster et al. 1994). The defects inactivate the proteins, making this a haploinsufficiency or gene dosage effect, i.e. that the amount of protein transcribed from the normal allele is not enough for normal development.

The consequence of having three gene doses is illustrated e.g. in Down syndrome, or trisomy 21, with multiple symptoms from most organs. A critical region on chromosome 21 has been suggested to give key features, and based on animal studies it has been proposed that SIM2 contributes to this (Chen et al. 1995). This can now be tested experimentally. Patients with DiGeorge syndrome have malformations of the thymus, the parathyroid and the heart, which are caused by a deletion of 1.5-3 Mb of chromosome 22q11 in a majority of the cases. Most symptoms can be ascribed to the TBX1 gene where rare patients have point mutations (Yagi

Table 2 Mutated transcription factors in rare diseases (selected)

Gene name	Symbol	OMIM ID	Disease	References
autoimmune regulator	AIRE	240300	Autoimmune polyendocrinopathy syndrome, type I (also called APECED)	(Nagamine et al. 1997, The Finnish-German APECED Consortium 1997)
Androgen receptor	AR	300068 313200 312300 146450 176807	Androgen insensitivity syndrome; Kennedy spinal and bulbar muscular atrophy; Breast cancer, male, with Reifenstein syndrome; Perineal hypospadias; Prostate cancer	(Wooster et al. 1992, Brown et al. 1998, La Spada et al. 1991, Batch et al. 1993, Visakorpi et al. 1995, Taplin et al. 1995)
cone-rod homeobox	CRX	120970 602225	Cone-rod retinal dystrophy-2; Leber congenital amaurosis, type 7; retinitis pigmentosa	(Freund et al. 1997, Freund et al. 1998, Sohocki et al. 1998)
FOXP2	FOXP2	602081	Speech-language disorder-1, developmental verbal dyspraxia	(Lai et al. 2001)
FOXP3	FOXP3	304790	Immunodysregulation, polyendocriopathy and enteropathy, X-linked, IPEX	(Wildin et al. 2001)
LIM homeobox transcription factor 1, beta	LMX1B	161200 137750	Nail-patella syndrome; Nail-patella syndrome with open-angle glaucoma	(Dreyer et al. 1998)
paired-like homeobox 2b	PHOX2B	209880 142623 256700	Congenital Central Hypoventilation Syndrome; Neuroblastoma (NB), Hirschsprung disease (HSCR)	(Futreal et al. 2004, Amiel et al. 2003, Trochet et al. 2004)

Table 2 (continued)

Gene name	Symbol	OMIM ID	Disease	References
peroxisome proliferative activated receptor, gamma	PPARG	125853 604367	Obesity, Modifier of type 2 diabetes; Familial partial lipodystrophy; Follicular thyroid carcinoma	(Futreal et al. 2004, Barroso et al. 1999, Altshuler et al. 2000)
short stature homeobox	SHOX	127300 249700	Leri-Weill dyschondrosteosis; Langer mesomelic dysplasia	(Shears et al. 1998, Belin et al. 1998)
single-minded homolog 2	SIM2	600892	some of the complex Down Syndrome phenotypes	(Chen et al. 1995)
SRY (sex determining region Y)-box 9	SOX9	114290	Campomelic dysplasia with autosomal sex reversal	(Foster et al. 1994)
sex determining region Y	SRY	306100	Gonadal dysgenesis, XY type (Bird 2007); Sex reversal	(Jager et al. 1990)
T-box transcription factor	TBX1	188400 207095 192430	DiGeorge syndrome; conotruncal anomaly face syndrome; velocardiofacial syndrome	(Yagi et al. 2003)

et al. 2003). It has been suggested that both deletion, i.e. an inactivation, and activating point mutations can result in the same disease. As we learn more about which regions in the genome that are subject to copy number variation, and consequently variation in protein dose we can expect that additional transcription factors and other genes will be associated with disease.

The nail-patella syndrome is a considerably milder autosomal dominant disease characterized by slow growing nails with ridges and absent or small patella, as well as kidney problems and glaucoma. This is a historic genetic disease since it was linked to the ABO blood group already in 1955. However, it took over 40 years before Dryer et al. (Dreyer et al. 1998) found that it is caused by mutations in the LMX1B gene that disrupted DNA binding or caused premature stop codons. Language clearly is an extremely complex phenotype and disturbances, if genetic, are caused by many genes. An intriguing finding is that rare families have a speech and language disorder due to mutations in FOXP2, inherited as an autosomal dominant phenotype. Those mutations have been found in regions interacting with DNA or causing stop codons (Lai et al. 2001). Specific brain regions in the cortex and basal ganglia have functional and structural defects in affected persons, showing that the identified factors are required for normal maturation of language (Vargha-Khadem et al. 1998).

Several TFs control the function of the immune system and cause distinct diseases when mutated. APECED is an autosomal recessive disease with multiple autoimmune features from endocrine and nonendocrine organs. Mutations are found in AIRE which normally has an important role in negative selection of T cells and elimination of autoreactive T cells in the thymus (Nagamine et al. 1997, The Finnish-German APECED Consortium 1997). IPEX is a severe X-linked recessive disease affecting several organs and includes insulin dependent (type 1) diabetes mellitus. It is caused by mutations in the FOXP3 gene and the manifestations can mainly be ascribed to the effect in regulatory T cells (Wildin et al. 2001). It may serve as a model to understand more about the processes leading to type 1 diabetes. Initial ChIP-chip experiments to explore the development of autoimmunity (Zheng et al. 2007) suggest that FOXP3 may mediate both up- and downregulation of protein coding genes and control genes for microRNAs. More knowledge in this field can be expected from future studies.

PPARG belongs to the nuclear hormone receptor subfamily of TFs and is well suited to illustrate the fact that the same TF can be involved in rare diseases, common diseases and cancer. Some rare sequence variants resulting in amino acid substitutions give rise to the autosomal dominant familial partial lipodystrophy. Patients have abnormal distribution of body fat, insulin resistance, type 2 diabetes and additional endocrine features (Barroso et al. 1999). Large scale studies have shown that the proline-12 to alanine substitution is a significant risk factor for type 2 diabetes (Zeggini et al. 2005, Scott et al. 2007) which is a common disease of increasing prevalence in the population. Somatic mutations, i.e. mutations that develop in individual organs or cells, are found in follicular thyroid carcinoma and colon cancer (Futreal et al. 2004). How different mutations in

PPARG affect the various outcomes in gene regulation and disease remains to be determined.

5 The Genome and Epigenome in Common Diseases

Both the genome and epigenome are important for the risk of developing common diseases. There is now a flood of results from whole genome association studies which pinpoints the common genetic variants, mostly SNPs, that confer risk to develop a common diseases (see footnote 1). As previously mentioned, most of the variants are located in non-coding sequences and the mode of action needs to be determined (Fig. 2). However, it is assumed that many of them modulate the expression of a nearby gene which will be reflected in the epigenetic profile of the relevant cell. Much more research is needed to investigate these phenomena.

A number of genes for transcription factors have been associated with common diseases and phenotypes and they are summarized in Table 3. The list includes several types of maturity onset diabetes of the young (MODY) that in them selves are not common but they are models for type 2 diabetes. Some mutations in IPF1 cause the rare MODY4 (Stoffers et al. 1997) whereas others occur in type 2 diabetes (Macfarlane et al. 1999). The same picture is found for KLF11 which causes MODY7 and predisposes to type 2 diabetes (Neve et al. 2005). As described above PPARG predisposes to type 2 diabetes (Scott et al. 2007) and causes both rare diseases (Barroso et al. 1999) and some forms of cancer (Futreal et al. 2004).

A striking conclusion form Table 3 is that most TFs currently associated with disease are involved in type 2 diabetes and regulation of blood lipid levels. This could be due to a selection bias because research has focused on these important risk factors for coronary artery disease. Even so, many TFs have been associated with type 2 diabetes, whereas TFs are rarely found to be involved in other common diseases. TCF7L2 (Grant et al. 2006) and other TFs have a known activity in beta cells but others, like USF1 and CHREBP, are associated with related phenotypes manifested in liver, fat and muscle tissue (Pajukanta et al. 2004, Kooner et al. 2008). There is an overlap between type 2 diabetes and the metabolic syndrome which, as the name suggests, is a combination of several features and all of them do not need to be present in all patients. Each TF regulates many genes and since several TFs contribute to these diseases, all downstream genes need to be considered. The symptoms also develop in different organs, and in this case beta cells, liver, fat, skeletal muscle, inflammatory and vascular endothelial cells are important and relevant to study epigenetically.

It is worth noting that several genes are involved both in diabetes and cancer, PPARG in type 2 diabetes (Scott et al. 2007) and follicular thyroid carcinoma (Futreal et al. 2004), TCF1 in MODY3 (Yamagata et al. 1996a) and hepatocellular carcinoma (Futreal et al. 2004) and breast cancer (Sjoblom et al. 2006) and TCF7L2 in type 2 diabetes (Grant et al. 2006) and colorectal cancer (Sjoblom et al. 2006). Furthermore, obesity is associated with increased cancer incidence

Table 3 Mutated transcription factors in common diseases (selected)

Gene name	Symbol	OMIM ID	Disease	References
GATA binding protein 2	**GATA2**	125850	Early onset coronary artery disease	(Connelly et al. 2006)
hepatocyte nuclear factor 4, alpha	**HNF4A**		Maturity-onset diabetes of the young, MODY, type 1	(Yamagata et al. 1996b)
insulin promoter factor 1	**IPF1**	260370 125853	Pancreatic agenesis; MODY 4; Type 2 diabetes	(Stoffers et al. 1997, Macfarlane et al. 1990)
Interferon regulatory factor 5	**IRF5**	152700	Systemic lupus erythematosus	(Sigurdsson et al. 2005)
Kruppel-like factor 11	**KLF11**	610508 125853	MODY7; Type 2 diabetes	(Neve et al. 2005)
MADS box transcription enhancer factor 2, polypeptide A (myocyte enhancer factor 2A)	**MEF2A**	608320	Coronary artery disease, myocardial infarction	(Wang et al. 2003)
MLX- interacting protein-like	**MLXIPL**	605678	Plasma triglycerides	(Kooner et al. 2008)
neurogenic differentiation 1	**NEUROD1**	606394	Maturity-onset diabetes of the young, MODY, type 6	(Malecki et al. 1999)
peroxisome proliferative activated receptor, alpha	**PPARA**	170998	Val162 associated with significantly increased serum concentrations of total and LDL cholesterol, apoB, and apoC3	(Tai et al. 2002)
peroxisome proliferative activated receptor, gamma	**PPARG**	12583 604367	Obesity, Modifier of type 2 diabetes; Familial partial lipodystrophy; Follicular thyroid carcinoma	(Futreal et al. 2004, Barroso et al. 1999, Altshuler et al. 2000)

Table 3 (continued)

Gene name	Symbol	OMIM ID	Disease	References
sterol regulatory element binding transcription factor 1, SREBP1	**SREBF1**	125853	Diabetes mellitus, type 2, and levels of total and LDL cholesterol	(Laudes et al. 2004, Vernia et al. 2006)
transcription factor 1, hepatic (HNF1)	**TCF1**	600496 114550 114480	Maturity-onset diabetes of the young, MODY, type 3; liver adenoma, hepatocellular carcinomas; Breast cancer CaMP score 1.6	(Futreal et al. 2004, Sjoblom et al. 2006, Yamagata et al. 1996b)
transcription factor 2, hepatic	**TCF2**	137920	Maturity-onset diabetes of the young, MODY, type 5; hypoplastic glomerulocystic kidney disease	(Horikawa et al. 1997)
transcription factor 7 (T-cell specific, HMG-box)	**TCF7**	125853	type 1 diabetes	(Noble et al. 2003)
transcription factor 7-like 2 (T-cell specific, HMG-box)	**TCF7L2**	125853 114500	Type 2 diabetes; Colorektal cancer CaMP score 2.8	(Sjoblom et al. 2006 Grant et al. 2006)
transcription factor CP2	**TFCP2**	104300	Alzheimer disease, protection against	(Lambert et al. 2000)
Upstream transcription factor 1	**USF1**	602491	Familial combined hyperlipidemia	(Pajukanta et al. 2004)

(Pischon et al. 2008) which indicates that the same basic biological processes are involved in metabolic and malignant diseases.

6 Mutations in Transcription Factors and Cancer

These are still early days in finding point mutations in genes associated with cancer. New high throughput methods like array-based exon selection and next generation sequencing are likely to provide a wealth of data in the years to come. The newly formed International Cancer Genome Consortium (ICGC) has planned to sequence exons and perhaps the whole genome in 500 tumors, each from the 50 most common cancers. This very ambitious project will continue for several years, and with time we will have a more comprehensive view of the genetic defects that cause cancer. Already, some large scale pilot studies have been published (Futreal et al. 2004, Sjoblom et al. 2006) (see footnote 2). A general pattern is that mutations are present in many different genes but only a small set of genes are frequently affected. In other systematic studies chromosomal rearrangements have been found and in complementary molecular investigations the genes identified (Mitelman et al. 2004). Much work has been performed on selected candidate genes that have been sequenced in tumor collections. In all, a large number of mutated genes have been found. A recurring pattern is that TFs is the class of proteins that most frequently is disrupted. Out of the close to 2,000 nuclear proteins, more than 200 have been found to harbor molecular defects in tumors (see reference Wadelius and Peltonen). It is clearly beyond the scope of this presentation to summarize everything that is known about TF mutations and cancer, but some illustrative examples are presented in Table 4 and in the preceding tables.

Testosterone binds to the androgen receptor, which is a TF that regulates the expression of downstream genes in the prostate and other organs. It is not unexpected that mutations in the gene occur in prostate cancer and in male breast cancer associated with Reifenstein syndrome (Wooster et al. 1992). Similarly, the estrogen receptor, which binds estrogen, is frequently subject to gene amplification in female breast cancer (Holst et al. 2007). Another member of the nuclear receptor family, the retinoic receptor alpha, RARA, is a classic model in tumor biology. In acute promyelocytic leukemia, translocations are found between this gene and the gene for PML, which appears to result in haploinsufficiency detrimental to the development of promyelocytes to myelocytes (Futreal et al. 2004). The translocation is present on one allele, whereas the other allele of RARA and PML are wild type. Patients are treated with higher than normal doses of retinoic acid which drives the remaining normal allele to induce a maturation of the cell (Huang et al. 1988). This could be regarded as a fine example of personalized medicine since the genotype with the PML-RARA translocation can be specifically treated.

PPARG has been mentioned before and is associated with several diseases including follicular thyroid carcinoma (Futreal et al. 2004). This is a cancer of the tissue producing the hormone T4, which sets the general metabolism in the organism. In this cancer, mutations have also been found in the PAX8 gene (Futreal

Table 4 Mutated transcription factors in cancer (selected)

Gene name	Symbol	OMIM ID	Disease	References
Androgen receptor	AR	300068 313200 312300 146450 176807	Androgen insensitivity syndrome; Kennedy spinal and bulbar muscular atrophy; Breast cancer, male, with Reifenstein syndrome; Perineal hypospadias; Prostate cancer	(Wooster et al. 1992, Brown et al. 1988, La Spada et al. 1991, Batch et al. 1993, Visakorpi et al. 1995, Taplin et al. 1995)
estrogen receptor 1	ESR1	133430 114480	Estrogen resistance; Breast cancer (gene amplification)	(Holst et al. 2007, Smith et al. 1994)
homeo box A11	HOXA11	142958 605432	CML; radioulnar synostosis and amegakaryocytic thrombocytopenia	(Futreal et al. 2004, Thompson and Nguyen 2000)
homeo box A13	HOXA13	601626 140000	AML; Hand-foot-uterus syndrome;	(Futreal et al. 2004, Mortlock and Innis 1997)
homeobox A3	HOXA3	114480	Breast cancer CaMP score1.6	(Sjoblom et al. 2006)
homeo box A9	HOXA9	601626	AML	(Futreal et al. 2004.)
homeo box C11	HOXC11	601626	AML	(Futreal et al. 2004.)
homeo box C13	HOXC13	601626	AML	(Futreal et al. 2004.)
homeo box D11	HOXD11	601626	AML	(Futreal et al. 2004.)
homeo box D13	HOXD13	601626 186000	AML; Synpolydactyly	(Futreal et al. 2004, Akarsu et al. 1996)

Table 4 (continued)

Gene name	Symbol	OMIM ID	Disease	References
myeloid/lymphoid or mixed-lineage leukemia	MLL	601626	AML; ALL	(Futreal et al. 2004,)
paired box gene 8	PAX8	218700 188550	Hypothyroidism, congenital, due to thyroid dysgenesis or hypoplasia; follicular thyroid carcinoma	(Futreal et al. 2004, Macchia et al. 1998)
peroxisome proliferative activated receptor, gamma	PPARG	125853 604367	Obesity, Modifier of type 2 diabetes; Familial partial lipodystrophy; Follicular thyroid carcinoma	(Futreal et al. 2004, Barroso et al. 1999, Altshuler et al. 2000)
retinoic acid receptor, alpha	RARA	180240	Acute promyelocytic leukemia	(Futreal et al. 2004,)
SMAD, mothers against DPP homolog 2	SMAD2	114500	Colorektal cancer CaMP score 3.1	(Sjoblom et al. 2006)
SMAD, mothers against DPP homolog 3	SMAD3	114500	Colorektal cancer CaMP score 1.9	(Sjoblom et al. 2006)
SMAD, mothers against DPP homolog 4	SMAD4	260350 114500	Pancreatic cancer; Colorektal cancer CaMP score 4.6	(Futreal et al. 2004, Sjoblom et al. 2006)
tumor protein p53	TP53	151623 114480 114500 191170 137800	Li-Fraumeni syndrome; Breast cancer CaMP score >10; Colorectal cancer CaMP score >10, 114500 lung, sarcoma, adrenocortical, glioma, multiple other tumour types	(Futreal et al. 2004, Sjoblom et al. 2006, Malkin et al. 1990)

et al. 2004) which is more intuitive, since PAX8 is central for development of the thyroid and congenital mutations in the gene result in hypothyroidism and thyroid hypoplasia (Macchia et al. 1998).

Cancer-associated mutations often affect central pathways. This is illustrated by the HOX gene cluster. These genes are essential for normal development and in addition mutations in eight HOX genes have been found various cancers, mostly AML (Table 4) (Futreal et al. 2004). Another example is the TGFβ pathway, which is of central interest in cancer biology. TGFβ binds to cell surface receptors and activate signaling molecules called SMADs, which are TFs that migrate to the nucleus and regulate transcription of many genes (Heldin et al. 1997). In addition, mutations in the same SMADs, SMAD2, SMAD3 and SMAD4 are found in colorectal and pancreatic cancer (Futreal et al. 2004, Sjoblom et al. 2006), indicating that normal TGFb signaling is required for proper differentiation of the colon and pancreas epithelium. TP53 is the classical cancer protein, which has multiple functions in the cell, one of them acting as a TF. Mutations in this gene is frequently found in cancer and many studies have been performed on the transcriptional consequences (Riley et al. 2008).

Furthermore, it is well established that there are epigenetic defects in cancer. They include global hypomethylation of DNA in human tumors, hypermethylation of DNA at tumor suppressor genes and genes for microRNAs, accompanied by abnormal histone modification patterns. This has been the basis for the development of therapies aimed at correcting these defects. This area has been the subject of many publications and reviews (Esteller 2008).

7 Perspectives for the Future

Mutations in gene regulatory proteins cause many different diseases originating from a range of cell types. Until recently, it has not been possible to find the downstream genes to obtain knowledge of the disease mechanisms in an efficient way. With the advent of genome wide ChIP-chip and especially the high resolution ChIP-seq technology (Barski et al. 2007) it is possible to determine these gene regulatory networks. The requirement is that suitable cells are available in the numbers needed for the experiments. For cancer and many of the common diseases that is likely to be the case. For congenital syndromes and developmental disorders it may be hard or impossible to access relevant human cells, and these experiments may need to be performed in model organisms. This limitation should not cloud the perspective that at this point we can start to understand a new dimension of biology. Indeed, the first genome wide ChIP studies have been conducted and provided a wealth of information. Given the large number of potential projects described in this chapter and Wadelius & Peltonen (see reference Wadelius and Peltonen) there is room for a new generation of experimental and computational biologists that can explore this fascinating field.

An even greater challenge is to understand the action of SNPs associated with common diseases. It is suspected that inherited differences in gene expression are part of the answer and allelic differences in DNA-protein interaction may prove to be a key mechanism. This issue can be addressed by characterizing global gene regulatory networks in cells from a panel of tissue donors of diverse allelic heterogeneity. To characterize the total gene regulatory network in a specified cell is a massive effort and to do it multiple times is a daunting task. Technical improvements are needed to make it possible as well as ways to handle and interpret the data. Never the less, it is something which is likely to happen in the not to distant future.

References

Akarsu AN, Stoilov I, Yilmaz E, Sayli BS, Sarfarazi M. Genomic structure of HOXD13 gene: a nine polyalanine duplication causes synpolydactyly in two unrelated families. Hum Mol Genet. 1996 Jul;5(7):945–52.

Altshuler D, Hirschhorn JN, Klannemark M, Lindgren CM, Vohl MC, Nemesh J, et al. The common PPARgamma Pro12Ala polymorphism is associated with decreased risk of type 2 diabetes. Nat Genet. 2000 Sep;26(1):76–80.

Ameur A, Rada-Iglesias A, Komorowski J, Wadelius C. Novel algorithm and ChIP-analysis identifies candidate functional SNPs (submitted).

Amiel J, Laudier B, Attie-Bitach T, Trang H, de Pontual L, Gener B, et al. Polyalanine expansion and frameshift mutations of the paired-like homeobox gene PHOX2B in congenital central hypoventilation syndrome. Nat Genet. 2003 Apr;33(4):459–61.

Amir RE, Van den Veyver IB, Wan M, Tran CQ, Francke U, Zoghbi HY. Rett syndrome is caused by mutations in X-linked MECP2, encoding methyl-CpG-binding protein 2. Nat Genet. 1999 Oct;23(2):185–8.

Barroso I, Gurnell M, Crowley VE, Agostini M, Schwabe JW, Soos MA, et al. Dominant negative mutations in human PPARgamma associated with severe insulin resistance, diabetes mellitus and hypertension. Nature. 1999 Dec 23–30;402(6764):880–3.

Barski A, Cuddapah S, Cui K, Roh TY, Schones DE, Wang Z, et al. High-resolution profiling of histone methylations in the human genome. Cell. 2007 May 18;129(4):823–37.

Batch JA, Evans BA, Hughes IA, Patterson MN. Mutations of the androgen receptor gene identified in perineal hypospadias. J Med Genet. 1993 Mar;30(3):198–201.

Belin V, Cusin V, Viot G, Girlich D, Toutain A, Moncla A, et al. SHOX mutations in dyschondrosteosis (Leri-Weill syndrome). Nat Genet. 1998 May;19(1):67–9.

Bird A. Perceptions of epigenetics. Nature. 2007 24 May 2007;447:396–8.

Birney E, Stamatoyannopoulos JA, Dutta A, Guigo R, Gingeras TR, Margulies EH, et al. Identification and analysis of functional elements in 1% of the human genome by the ENCODE pilot project. Nature. 2007 Jun 14;447(7146):799–816.

Boerkoel CF, Takashima H, John J, Yan J, Stankiewicz P, Rosenbarker L, et al. Mutant chromatin remodeling protein SMARCAL1 causes Schimke immuno-osseous dysplasia. Nat Genet. 2002 Feb;30(2):215–20.

Borneman AR, Gianoulis TA, Zhang ZD, Yu H, Rozowsky J, Seringhaus MR, et al. Divergence of transcription factor binding sites across related yeast species. Science. 2007 Aug 10;317(5839):815–9.

Boyle AP, Davis S, Shulha HP, Meltzer P, Margulies EH, Weng Z, et al. High-resolution mapping and characterization of open chromatin across the genome. Cell. 2008 Jan 25;132(2):311–22.

Brown TR, Lubahn DB, Wilson EM, Joseph DR, French FS, Migeon CJ. Deletion of the steroid-binding domain of the human androgen receptor gene in one family with complete androgen insensitivity syndrome: evidence for further genetic heterogeneity in this syndrome. Proc Natl Acad Sci U S A. 1988 Nov;85(21):8151–5.

Chen H, Chrast R, Rossier C, Gos A, Antonarakis SE, Kudoh J, et al. Single-minded and Down syndrome? Nat Genet. 1995 May;10(1):9–10.

Connelly JJ, Wang T, Cox JE, Haynes C, Wang L, Shah SH, et al. GATA2 is associated with familial early-onset coronary artery disease. PLoS Genet. 2006 Aug 25;2(8):e139.

Dreyer SD, Zhou G, Baldini A, Winterpacht A, Zabel B, Cole W, et al. Mutations in LMX1B cause abnormal skeletal patterning and renal dysplasia in nail patella syndrome. Nat Genet. 1998 May;19(1):47–50.

Esteller M. Epigenetics in cancer. N Engl J Med. 2008 Mar 13;358(11):1148–59.

Field M, Tarpey PS, Smith R, Edkins S, O'Meara S, Stevens C, et al. Mutations in the BRWD3 gene cause X-linked mental retardation associated with macrocephaly. Am J Hum Genet. 2007 Aug;81(2):367–74.

Foster JW, Dominguez-Steglich MA, Guioli S, Kowk G, Weller PA, Stevanovic M, et al. Campomelic dysplasia and autosomal sex reversal caused by mutations in an SRY-related gene. Nature. 1994 Dec 8;372(6506):525–30.

Frazer KA, Ballinger DG, Cox DR, Hinds DA, Stuve LL, Gibbs RA, et al. A second generation human haplotype map of over 3.1 million SNPs. Nature. 2007 Oct 18;449(7164):851–61.

Freund CL, Gregory-Evans CY, Furukawa T, Papaioannou M, Looser J, Ploder L, et al. Cone-rod dystrophy due to mutations in a novel photoreceptor-specific homeobox gene (CRX) essential for maintenance of the photoreceptor. Cell. 1997 Nov 14;91(4):543–53.

Freund CL, Wang QL, Chen S, Muskat BL, Wiles CD, Sheffield VC, et al. De novo mutations in the CRX homeobox gene associated with Leber congenital amaurosis. Nat Genet. 1998 Apr;18(4):311–2.

Futreal PA, Coin L, Marshall M, Down T, Hubbard T, Wooster R, et al. A census of human cancer genes. Nat Rev Cancer. 2004 Mar;4(3):177–83.

Giglia-Mari G, Coin F, Ranish JA, Hoogstraten D, Theil A, Wijgers N, et al. A new, tenth subunit of TFIIH is responsible for the DNA repair syndrome trichothiodystrophy group A. Nat Genet. 2004 Jul;36(7):714–9.

Grant SF, Thorleifsson G, Reynisdottir I, Benediktsson R, Manolescu A, Sainz J, et al. Variant of transcription factor 7-like 2 (TCF7L2) gene confers risk of type 2 diabetes. Nat Genet. 2006 Mar;38(3):320–3.

Griswold MD, Kim JS. Site-specific methylation of the promoter alters deoxyribonucleic acid-protein interactions and prevents follicle-stimulating hormone receptor gene transcription. Biol Reprod. 2001 Feb;64(2):602–10.

Guenther MG, Jenner RG, Chevalier B, Nakamura T, Croce CM, Canaani E, et al. Global and Hox-specific roles for the MLL1 methyltransferase. Proc Natl Acad Sci U S A. 2005 Jun 14;102(24):8603–8.

Heldin CH, Miyazono K, ten Dijke P. TGF-beta signalling from cell membrane to nucleus through SMAD proteins. Nature. 1997 Dec 4;390(6659):465–71.

Holst F, Stahl PR, Ruiz C, Hellwinkel O, Jehan Z, Wendland M, et al. Estrogen receptor alpha (ESR1) gene amplification is frequent in breast cancer. Nat Genet. 2007 May;39(5):655–60.

Horikawa Y, Iwasaki N, Hara M, Furuta H, Hinokio Y, Cockburn BN, et al. Mutation in hepatocyte nuclear factor-1 beta gene (TCF2) associated with MODY. Nat Genet. 1997 Dec;17(4):384–5.

Huang ME, Ye YC, Chen SR, Chai JR, Lu JX, Zhoa L, et al. Use of all-trans retinoic acid in the treatment of acute promyelocytic leukemia. Blood. 1988 Aug;72(2):567–72.

ICGC. International Cancer Genome Consortium.

Jacinto FV, Ballestar E, Esteller M. Methyl-DNA immunoprecipitation (MeDIP): hunting down the DNA methylome. Biotechniques. 2008 Jan;44(1):35, 7, 9 passim.

Jager RJ, Anvret M, Hall K, Scherer G. A human XY female with a frame shift mutation in the candidate testis-determining gene SRY. Nature. 1990 Nov 29;348(6300):452–4.

Jensen LR, Amende M, Gurok U, Moser B, Gimmel V, Tzschach A, et al. Mutations in the JARID1C gene, which is involved in transcriptional regulation and chromatin remodeling, cause X-linked mental retardation. Am J Hum Genet. 2005 Feb;76(2):227–36.

Jiang YL, Rigolet M, Bourc'his D, Nigon F, Bokesoy I, Fryns JP, et al. DNMT3B mutations and DNA methylation defect define two types of ICF syndrome. Hum Mutat. 2005 Jan;25(1):56–63.

Johnson DS, Mortazavi A, Myers RM, Wold B. Genome-wide mapping of in vivo protein-DNA interactions. Science. 2007 Jun 8;316(5830):1497–502.

Kleefstra T, Brunner HG, Amiel J, Oudakker AR, Nillesen WM, Magee A, et al. Loss-of-function mutations in euchromatin histone methyl transferase 1 (EHMT1) cause the 9q34 subtelomeric deletion syndrome. Am J Hum Genet. 2006 Aug;79(2):370–7.

Kooner JS, Chambers JC, Aguilar-Salinas CA, Hinds DA, Hyde CL, Warnes GR, et al. Genome-wide scan identifies variation in MLXIPL associated with plasma triglycerides. Nat Genet. 2008 Feb;40(2):149–51.

La Spada AR, Wilson EM, Lubahn DB, Harding AE, Fischbeck KH. Androgen receptor gene mutations in X-linked spinal and bulbar muscular atrophy. Nature. 1991 Jul 4;352(6330):77–9.

Lai CS, Fisher SE, Hurst JA, Vargha-Khadem F, Monaco AP. A forkhead-domain gene is mutated in a severe speech and language disorder. Nature. 2001 Oct 4;413(6855):519–23.

Lambert JC, Goumidi L, Vrieze FW, Frigard B, Harris JM, Cummings A, et al. The transcriptional factor LBP-1c/CP2/LSF gene on chromosome 12 is a genetic determinant of Alzheimer's disease. Hum Mol Genet. 2000 Sep 22;9(15):2275–80.

Laudes M, Barroso I, Luan J, Soos MA, Yeo G, Meirhaeghe A, et al. Genetic variants in human sterol regulatory element binding protein-1c in syndromes of severe insulin resistance and type 2 diabetes. Diabetes. 2004 Mar;53(3):842–6.

Law AJ, Lipska BK, Weickert CS, Hyde TM, Straub RE, Hashimoto R, et al. Neuregulin 1 transcripts are differentially expressed in schizophrenia and regulated by 5' SNPs associated with the disease. Proc Natl Acad Sci U S A. 2006 Apr 25;103(17):6747–52.

Levine M, Tjian R. Transcription regulation and animal diversity. Nature. 2003 Jul 10;424(6945):147–51.

Lupien M, Eeckhoute J, Meyer CA, Wang Q, Zhang Y, Li W, et al. FoxA1 translates epigenetic signatures into enhancer-driven lineage-specific transcription. Cell. 2008 Mar 21;132(6):958–70.

Macchia PE, Lapi P, Krude H, Pirro MT, Missero C, Chiovato L, et al. PAX8 mutations associated with congenital hypothyroidism caused by thyroid dysgenesis. Nat Genet. 1998 May;19(1):83–6.

Macfarlane WM, Frayling TM, Ellard S, Evans JC, Allen LI, Bulman MP, et al. Missense mutations in the insulin promoter factor-1 gene predispose to type 2 diabetes. J Clin Invest. 1999 Nov;104(9):R33–9.

Makino S, Kaji R, Ando S, Tomizawa M, Yasuno K, Goto S, et al. Reduced Neuron-Specific Expression of the TAF1 Gene Is Associated with X-Linked Dystonia-Parkinsonism. Am J Hum Genet. 2007 Mar;80(3):393–406.

Malecki MT, Jhala US, Antonellis A, Fields L, Doria A, Orban T, et al. Mutations in NEUROD1 are associated with the development of type 2 diabetes mellitus. Nat Genet. 1999 Nov;23(3):323–8.

Malkin D, Li FP, Strong LC, Fraumeni JF, Jr., Nelson CE, Kim DH, et al. Germ line p53 mutations in a familial syndrome of breast cancer, sarcomas, and other neoplasms. Science. 1990 Nov 30;250(4985):1233–8.

Maynard ND, Chen J, Stuart RK, Fan JB, Ren B. Genome-wide mapping of allele-specific protein-DNA interactions in human cells. Nat Methods. 2008 Apr;5(4):307–9.

Mitelman F, Johansson B, Mertens F. Fusion genes and rearranged genes as a linear function of chromosome aberrations in cancer. Nat Genet. 2004 Apr;36(4):331–4.

Mortlock DP, Innis JW. Mutation of HOXA13 in hand-foot-genital syndrome. Nat Genet. 1997 Feb;15(2):179–80.

Nagamine K, Peterson P, Scott HS, Kudoh J, Minoshima S, Heino M, et al. Positional cloning of the APECED gene. Nat Genet. 1997 Dec;17(4):393–8.

Nan X, Campoy FJ, Bird A. MeCP2 is a transcriptional repressor with abundant binding sites in genomic chromatin. Cell. 1997 Feb 21;88(4):471–81.

Neve B, Fernandez-Zapico ME, Ashkenazi-Katalan V, Dina C, Hamid YH, Joly E, et al. Role of transcription factor KLF11 and its diabetes-associated gene variants in pancreatic beta cell function. Proc Natl Acad Sci U S A. 2005 Mar 29;102(13):4807–12.

Noble JA, White AM, Lazzeroni LC, Valdes AM, Mirel DB, Reynolds R, et al. A polymorphism in the TCF7 gene, C883A, is associated with type 1 diabetes. Diabetes. 2003 Jun;52(6):1579–82.

Odom DT, Dowell RD, Jacobsen ES, Gordon W, Danford TW, MacIsaac KD, et al. Tissue-specific transcriptional regulation has diverged significantly between human and mouse. Nat Genet. 2007 Jun;39(6):730–2.

OMIM. Online Mendelian Inheritance in Man: www.ncbi.nlm.nih.gov/sites/entrez?db=OMIM.

Pajukanta P, Lilja HE, Sinsheimer JS, Cantor RM, Lusis AJ, Gentile M, et al. Familial combined hyperlipidemia is associated with upstream transcription factor 1 (USF1). Nat Genet. 2004 Apr;36(4):371–6.

Park IH, Zhao R, West JA, Yabuuchi A, Huo H, Ince TA, et al. Reprogramming of human somatic cells to pluripotency with defined factors. Nature. 2008 Jan 10;451(7175):141–6.

Pennisi E. Research funding. Are epigeneticists ready for big science? Science. 2008 Feb 29;319(5867):1177.

Pischon T, Nothlings U, Boeing H. Obesity and cancer. Proc Nutr Soc. 2008 May;67(2):128–45.

Riley T, Sontag E, Chen P, Levine A. Transcriptional control of human p53-regulated genes. Nat Rev Mol Cell Biol. 2008 May;9(5):402–12.

Risch N, Merikangas K. The future of genetic studies of complex human diseases. Science. 1996 Sep 13;273(5281):1516–7.

SCGC. Sanger Cancer Gene Census: www.sanger.ac.uk/genetics/CGP/Census/.

Scott LJ, Mohlke KL, Bonnycastle LL, Willer CJ, Li Y, Duren WL, et al. A genome-wide association study of type 2 diabetes in Finns detects multiple susceptibility variants. Science. 2007 Jun 1;316(5829):1341–5.

Shahbazian MD, Antalffy B, Armstrong DL, Zoghbi HY. Insight into Rett syndrome: MeCP2 levels display tissue- and cell-specific differences and correlate with neuronal maturation. Hum Mol Genet. 2002 Jan 15;11(2):115–24.

Shears DJ, Vassal HJ, Goodman FR, Palmer RW, Reardon W, Superti-Furga A, et al. Mutation and deletion of the pseudoautosomal gene SHOX cause Leri-Weill dyschondrosteosis. Nat Genet. 1998 May;19(1):70–3.

Sigurdsson S, Nordmark G, Goring HH, Lindroos K, Wiman AC, Sturfelt G, et al. Polymorphisms in the tyrosine kinase 2 and interferon regulatory factor 5 genes are associated with systemic lupus erythematosus. Am J Hum Genet. 2005 Mar;76(3):528–37.

Sjoblom T, Jones S, Wood LD, Parsons DW, Lin J, Barber TD, et al. The consensus coding sequences of human breast and colorectal cancers. Science. 2006 Oct 13;314(5797):268–74.

Smith EP, Boyd J, Frank GR, Takahashi H, Cohen RM, Specker B, et al. Estrogen resistance caused by a mutation in the estrogen-receptor gene in a man. N Engl J Med. 1994 Oct 20;331(16):1056–61.

Sohocki MM, Sullivan LS, Mintz-Hittner HA, Birch D, Heckenlively JR, Freund CL, et al. A range of clinical phenotypes associated with mutations in CRX, a photoreceptor transcription-factor gene. Am J Hum Genet. 1998 Nov;63(5):1307–15.

Stevanin G, Fujigasaki H, Lebre AS, Camuzat A, Jeannequin C, Dode C, et al. Huntington's disease-like phenotype due to trinucleotide repeat expansions in the TBP and JPH3 genes. Brain. 2003 Jul;126(Pt 7):1599–603.

Stoffers DA, Zinkin NT, Stanojevic V, Clarke WL, Habener JF. Pancreatic agenesis attributable to a single nucleotide deletion in the human IPF1 gene coding sequence. Nat Genet. 1997 Jan;15(1):106–10.

Stranger BE, Nica AC, Forrest MS, Dimas A, Bird CP, Beazley C, et al. Population genomics of human gene expression. Nat Genet. 2007 Oct;39(10):1217–24.

Tai ES, Demissie S, Cupples LA, Corella D, Wilson PW, Schaefer EJ, et al. Association between the PPARA L162V polymorphism and plasma lipid levels: the Framingham Offspring Study. Arterioscler Thromb Vasc Biol. 2002 May 1;22(5):805–10.

Takahashi K, Tanabe K, Ohnuki M, Narita M, Ichisaka T, Tomoda K, et al. Induction of pluripotent stem cells from adult human fibroblasts by defined factors. Cell. 2007 Nov 30;131(5):861–72.

Taplin ME, Bubley GJ, Shuster TD, Frantz ME, Spooner AE, Ogata GK, et al. Mutation of the androgen-receptor gene in metastatic androgen-independent prostate cancer. N Engl J Med. 1995 May 25;332(21):1393–8.

Tassabehji M, Hammond P, Karmiloff-Smith A, Thompson P, Thorgeirsson SS, Durkin ME, et al. GTF2IRD1 in craniofacial development of humans and mice. Science. 2005 Nov 18;310(5751):1184–7.

The Finnish-German APECED Consortium. An autoimmune disease, APECED, caused by mutations in a novel gene featuring two PHD-type zinc-finger domains. (Autoimmune Polyendocrinopathy-Candidiasis-Ectodermal Dystrophy). Nat Genet. 1997 Dec;17(4):399–403.

Thompson AA, Nguyen LT. Amegakaryocytic thrombocytopenia and radio-ulnar synostosis are associated with HOXA11 mutation. Nat Genet. 2000 Dec;26(4):397–8.

Trochet D, Bourdeaut F, Janoueix-Lerosey I, Deville A, de Pontual L, Schleiermacher G, et al. Germline mutations of the paired-like homeobox 2B (PHOX2B) gene in neuroblastoma. Am J Hum Genet. 2004 Apr;74(4):761–4.

Tsuge M, Hamamoto R, Silva FP, Ohnishi Y, Chayama K, Kamatani N, et al. A variable number of tandem repeats polymorphism in an E2F-1 binding element in the 5' flanking region of SMYD3 is a risk factor for human cancers. Nat Genet. 2005 Oct;37(10):1104–7.

Vargha-Khadem F, Watkins KE, Price CJ, Ashburner J, Alcock KJ, Connelly A, et al. Neural basis of an inherited speech and language disorder. Proc Natl Acad Sci U S A. 1998 Oct 13;95(21):12695–700.

Vernia S, Eberle D, Hernandez Mijares A, Foufelle F, Casado M. A rare missense mutation in a type 2 diabetes patient decreases the transcriptional activity of human sterol regulatory element binding protein-1. Hum Mutat. 2006 Feb;27(2):212.

Visakorpi T, Hyytinen E, Koivisto P, Tanner M, Keinanen R, Palmberg C, et al. In vivo amplification of the androgen receptor gene and progression of human prostate cancer. Nat Genet. 1995 Apr;9(4):401–6.

Visel A, Prabhakar S, Akiyama JA, Shoukry M, Lewis KD, Holt A, et al. Ultraconservation identifies a small subset of extremely constrained developmental enhancers. Nat Genet. 2008 Feb;40(2):158–60.

Wadelius C, Peltonen L. Mutated transcription factors and human disease (submitted).

Wang L, Fan C, Topol SE, Topol EJ, Wang Q. Mutation of MEF2A in an inherited disorder with features of coronary artery disease. Science. 2003 Nov 28;302(5650):1578–81.

Wildin RS, Ramsdell F, Peake J, Faravelli F, Casanova JL, Buist N, et al. X-linked neonatal diabetes mellitus, enteropathy and endocrinopathy syndrome is the human equivalent of mouse scurfy. Nat Genet. 2001 Jan;27(1):18–20.

Wooster R, Mangion J, Eeles R, Smith S, Dowsett M, Averill D, et al. A germline mutation in the androgen receptor gene in two brothers with breast cancer and Reifenstein syndrome. Nat Genet. 1992 Oct;2(2):132–4.

Xu GL, Bestor TH, Bourc'his D, Hsieh CL, Tommerup N, Bugge M, et al. Chromosome instability and immunodeficiency syndrome caused by mutations in a DNA methyltransferase gene. Nature. 1999 Nov 11;402(6758):187–91.

Yagi H, Furutani Y, Hamada H, Sasaki T, Asakawa S, Minoshima S, et al. Role of TBX1 in human del22q11.2 syndrome. Lancet. 2003 Oct 25;362(9393):1366–73.

Yamagata K, Furuta H, Oda N, Kaisaki PJ, Menzel S, Cox NJ, et al. Mutations in the hepatocyte nuclear factor-4alpha gene in maturity-onset diabetes of the young (MODY1). Nature. 1996a Dec 5;384(6608):458–60.

Yamagata K, Oda N, Kaisaki PJ, Menzel S, Furuta H, Vaxillaire M, et al. Mutations in the hepatocyte nuclear factor-1alpha gene in maturity-onset diabetes of the young (MODY3). Nature. 1996b Dec 5;384(6608):455–8.

Zeggini E, Parkinson JR, Halford S, Owen KR, Walker M, Hitman GA, et al. Examining the relationships between the Pro12Ala variant in PPARG and Type 2 diabetes-related traits in UK samples. Diabet Med. 2005 Dec;22(12):1696–700.

Zheng Y, Josefowicz SZ, Kas A, Chu TT, Gavin MA, Rudensky AY. Genome-wide analysis of Foxp3 target genes in developing and mature regulatory T cells. Nature. 2007 Feb 22;445(7130):936–40.

Zimmermann N, Acosta AM, Kohlhase J, Bartsch O. Confirmation of EP300 gene mutations as a rare cause of Rubinstein-Taybi syndrome. Eur J Hum Genet. 2007 Aug;15(8):837–42.

A Changing Epigenome in Health and Disease

Esteban Ballestar and Manel Esteller

Abstract In mammals, epigenetic modifications play an essential role both in establishing transcription profiles and in organizing DNA architecture within the cell nucleus. Specifically, the role of epigenetic modifications in regulating X-chromosome inactivation, genomic imprinting and tissue-specific expression is widely recognized. In addition, the implied role of epigenetic modifications in cell differentiation and development has recently been highlighted by the recognition of the roles of epigenetic regulators or processes in a number of human diseases, including genetic disorders such as Alpha-thalassemia/mental retardation, X-linked (ATRX), Facioscapulohumeral muscular dystrophy (FSHD), Immunodeficiency-Centromere Instability-Facial anomalies (ICF) and Rett syndrome. Particular attention has been focused on the study of epigenetic alterations in cancer, which is the subject of intense multidisciplinary efforts and has an impact not only in understanding the mechanisms of epigenetic regulation but also in guiding the development of novel and promising therapies for cancer treatment. Initial data about epigenetic changes in cardiovascular, neurological and autoimmune disorders are also starting to emerge. The examples discussed herein not only summarize the widespread association of epigenetic alterations with disease, but also bring to central stage the importance of accomplishing different epigenome projects to understand this fundamental human biological process.

Keywords Hypermethylation · Hypomethylation · Genome-wide · Methylation arrays · Cancer epigenetics

---

E. Ballestar (✉)
Chromatin and Disease Group, Cancer Epigenetics and Biology Programme (PEBC), Catalan Institute of Oncology (ICO-IDIBELL), 08907 L'Hospitalet de Llobregat, Barcelona, Spain
e-mail: eballestar@iconcologia.net

1 The Importance of Epigenetic Plasticity in Defining Cell Identity and Function

Epigenetic marks provide cells with a dynamic signaling system of the genome to regulate gene expression profiles and nuclear organization in a manner adapted to particular physiological situations. These epigenetic marks are established and maintained by different groups of enzymes which are specifically targeted to their correct genomic locations through different nuclear factors, some of which directly respond to environmental signals or constitute the final step of a cell signaling cascade. Two major groups of enzymes are responsible for the establishment and maintenance of epigenetic marks: DNA methyltransferases (DNMTs) and histone modification enzymes, like histone acetyltransferases (HATs), histone deacetylases (HDACs) or histone methyltransferases (HMTs).

DNA methylation is a major epigenetic modification with direct implications for the establishment of expression patterns in multicellular organisms (Jaenisch and Bird, 2003). In general, DNA methylation is considered to be a stable epigenetic mark, although mechanisms of active DNA demethylation have been proposed to occur in specific physiological contexts, including development and cell differentiation (Reik et al. 2001; Wilson and Merkenschlager, 2006). Very little is known about the enzymatic activities involved in active demethylation. The ability to demethylate DNA actively has been attributed to various factors, including MBD2 (Bhattacharya et al. 1999) and Gadd45a (growth arrest and DNA-damage-inducible protein 45a) (Barreto et al. 2007), a nuclear protein involved in maintaining genomic stability, DNA repair, and suppression of cell growth. In the first case, MBD2 was reported to catalyze the hydrolysis of 5-methylcytosine to yield cytosine and water (Bhattacharya et al. 1999). However, the chemistry necessary to directly demethylate 5-methylcytosine is challenging, requiring the disruption of a C–C bond and there have been unsuccesful attempts to reproduce the ability to demethylate by MBD2 (Wolffe et al. 1999). It is most likely that DNA repair-mediated mechanisms involve a DNA repair endonuclease, and Barreto et al. (2007) have proposed that Gadd45a plays a role in targeting the DNA repair endonuclease XPG to sites that become demethylated in *Xenopus laevis* oocytes. However, there is also some controversy on the direct implication of Gadd45a in this process (Jin et al. 2008).

In contrast with the lack of robust evidences on the enzymatic activities involved in active demethylation, several DNMTs have been identified (for an extensive review, please see Bestor, 2000), one of which appears to be devoted to the mechanisms of maintenance of methylation patterns across DNA replication cycles (DNMT1) whereas two of them have been proposed to be implicated in de novo methylation (DNMT3A and DNMT3B). In mammals, DNA methylation is restricted to the genomic context of CpG dinucleotides, whose abundance in the genome is much lower than expected based on GC content and exhibit a non uniform distribution. Typically, regions several hundreds of base pairs long that contain a high density of CpG sites are referred to as CpG islands (Gardiner-Garden and

Frommer, 1987) and generally associate with promoters. In mammalian genomes, CpG islands are in and near approximately 40% of promoters of genes (about 70% in human promoters) (Saxonov et al. 2006). It has been proposed that cytosine methylation occurring at repetitive and parasitic sequences plays a role in their stabilization (Robertson, 2000). Also, methylation of repetitive elements appears to contribute in the maintenance of nuclear architecture and organization of heterochromatic domains (Espada et al. 2004). On the other hand, most promoter CpG islands remain unmethylated under physiological conditions (Siegfried and Cedar, 1997). Methylation and subsequent transcriptional repression are confined to a relatively small set of genes, including those in the inactive X-chromosome of females (Wolf and Migeon, 1982), imprinted genes (Reik et al. 1987) and tissue-specific genes (Futscher et al. 2002; Song et al. 2005). Interestingly, very few genes have been consistently reported to be methylated in a tissue specific-manner, however it is likely that the use of genome-wide methods to map DNA methylation patterns will lead to the generation of complete maps of tissue-specific promoter methylation (Esteller, 2007).

The mechanisms by which promoter CpG island methylation leads to gene silencing involve changes in the modification of profile of histones. This process takes place through the direct recruitment of histone-modification enzymes by DNMTs (Burgers et al. 2002) and other nuclear factors such as methyl-CpG binding domain (MBD) proteins (Hendrich and Bird, 1998; Ballestar et al. 2005). Additional mechanistic connections between elements of the histone modification and DNA methylation machineries exist. For instance, Polycomb group (PcG) protein EZH2, which catalyzes methylation of K27 of histone H3, interacts with DNMTs to target DNA methylation (Vire et al. 2006).

In fact, histone modifications constitute a fundamental source of epigenetic information. Core histones are the protein component of the octameric complex around which the DNA is wrapped. Combinations or sequential addition of these modifications to histone-tail amino acid residues have different functional consequences for gene activity and chromatin organization (Wang et al. 2004). For instance, reversible acetylation of histone lysines at their N-terminal tails is generally associated with transcriptional activation (Chahal et al. 1980), although there are some particularities on the functional consequences that depend on the specific lysine that it is acetylated (see for example Rundlett et al. 1998; Shogren-Knaak et al. 2006). On the other hand, methylation of histones can occur in lysine and arginine residues; the functional consequences depend on the type of residue and specific site that is modified (Rao et al. 2005; Lachner et al. 2001; Schotta et al. 2004). For instance, methylation of H3 at K4 (Santos-Rosa et al. 2002) and R17 (Bauer et al. 2002) is closely linked to transcriptional competence, whereas methylation of H3 at K9, or H4 at K20, is associated with transcriptional repression (Lachner et al. 2001; Schotta et al. 2004).

Although DNA methylation is mechanistically linked with the modification status of histones, not every post-translational modification at the core histone tails depends on the methylation status of the DNA. Therefore, histone modification patterns can be established through DNA methylation-associated mechanisms or, alternatively, in a DNA methylation-independent fashion. In the latter case, recruitment of histone modification enzymes at specific genomic loci depends on the availability of particular transcription factors or through the ligand-dependent response of nuclear receptors which in turn recruit histone modification enzymes.

In multicellular organisms, cells usually respond to environmental or intracellular signals in a manner that depends on the participation of transcription factors which often recruit epigenetic enzymes (Feil, 2006). Within any particular organism, different cell lineages share a common genome although available sets of transcription factors and epigenetic marks are cell type specific and functionally interconnected. The balance between epigenetic modifications, transcription factors and their ability to respond to environmental stimuli is delicate and guarantees proper cell function. Epigenetic modifications and the required sets of transcription factors are also transmitted through successive rounds of DNA replication and cell division. However, disruption of a variety of pathways results in different types of epigenetic alterations.

In this review, we discuss different epigenetic alterations associated with disease, particularly in cancer, and the need for studying upstream mechanisms contributing to their occurrence in order to better understand cell behavior and address the design of specific compounds able to reverse them.

2 Epigenetic Changes in Cancer

Over the last few years, we have witnessed major progress in understanding the mechanisms involved in epigenetic alterations associated with aberrant behavior in disease. This is particularly important in the field of cancer research, where epigenetic alterations were recognized early. Cells from most cancer types suffer dramatic changes in their DNA methylation content and distribution. Tumor cells suffer a decrease in the global content of 5-methylcytosine, which can be mainly attributed to loss of methylation at repetitive sequences (Feinberg and Vogelstein, 1983; Ehrlich, 2002; Estécio et al. 2007). However, the promoter CpG islands of many tumor suppressor genes undergo hypermethylation (Fig. 1), and this process represents an important mechanism by which these genes are inactivated (Jones and Baylin, 2002). Systematic analysis of the profile of promoter CpG islands hypermethylation has encouraged the view that the profiles of promoter methylation are tumor-type specific (Costello et al. 2000; Esteller et al. 2001a–c).

There are several lines of evidence that imply an active role of hypermethylation of tumor-suppressor genes in the development of cancer. In the first place, hypermethylation is an early event in cancer. This is the case of p16INK4a, p14ARF and MGMT (Esteller et al. 2000a, b) in colorectal adenomas and hMLH1 in endometrial hyperplasias (Esteller et al. 1999a) and gastric adenomas (Fleisher et al. 1999). Another clue that highlights the functional relevance of promoter CpG island hypermethylation in tumorigenesis is its occurrence in the absence of genetic mutations. Both events (genetic and epigenetic) abolish normal gene function and their coincidence in the same allele would be redundant from an evolutionary point of view.

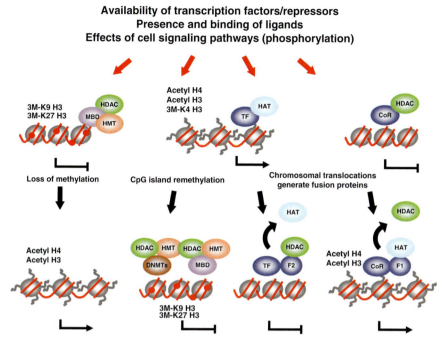

Fig. 1 A comparison of representative mechanisms of epigenetic regulation. In all cases an array of nucleosomes is shown. Histone octamers are represented by grey circles. DNA is represented as a red line in which only methylated CpG dinucleotides are shown (as red circles). Acetylated histone tails are lines protruding from octamers, whereas deacetylated histone tails are not shown. The transcriptional status of a gene is determined by the availability of specific transcription factors or repressors, the downstream effects of cell signalling pathways (which for instance can phosphorylate transcription factors or other chromatin proteins) and presence or absence of specific ligands which bind their corresponding ligand receptors. Methylation by DNMTs determines a particular chromatin status through the direct recruitment of histone modification enzymes, or the binding of methyl binding domain (MBD) proteins which can also recruit HDACs and HMT. In hematological malignancies (central section), generation of fusion proteins through chromosomal translocations can contribute to mistargeting of HDACs or HATs. Changes in DNA methylation patterns occur in both direction, i.e, hypermethylation, which often occurs as a mechanism of aberrant silencing of tumor suppressor genes in cancer, or hypomethylation, which occurs at repetitive sequences in cancer or at specific genes in other diseases

The selective advantage of promoter hypermethylation in this context is provided by multiple examples but three are worth mentioning. First, the cell cycle inhibitor p16INK4a in one allele of the HCT-116 colorectal cancer cell line has a genetic mutation while the other is wild-type: p16INK4a hypermethylation occurs only on the wild-type allele, while the mutated allele is kept unmethylated (Myohanen et al. 1998). The same selectivity of p16INK4a hypermethylation for the wild-type allele, keeping the mutant allele unmethylated, has also been observed in a bladder transitional cell carcinoma cell line (Yeager et al. 1998). A second example is that of APC, the gatekeeper of colorectal cancer which is mutated in the vast majority of colon tumors. When APC methylation occurs in that type of tumors, it is clustered in the APC wild-type cases. And finally, it has been demonstrated that in colorectal and breast tumors from families that harbor a germline mutation in the tumor suppressor genes hMLH1, BRCA1 or LKB1/STK11, only those tumors that still retain one wild-type allele undergo CpG island hypermethylation (Esteller et al. 2001b). These results put CpG island hypermethylation on a par with gene mutation for accomplishing selective gene inactivation.

However, of the most important steps for conferring CpG island hypermethylation a critical role in the origin and progression of a tumor is the demonstration of the existence of relevant biological consequences associated with the epigenetic inactivation of a particular gene. A classical example of this is represented by the hypermethylation of the DNA repair gene O6-methylguanine DNA methyltransferase (MGMT) (Esteller et al. 1999). The MGMT gene product removes the promutagenic O6- methylguanine, generated from the addition of a methyl group to the base guanine, which is then read as an adenine by DNA polymerases and thus may generate G to A mutations. It has been shown that the DNA repair gene MGMT is transcriptionally silenced by promoter hypermethylation in primary human tumors (Esteller et al. 1999b). These tumors might accumulate a considerable number of G to A transitions, some of them affecting key genes, in a similar way that loss of the hMLH1 mismatch repair gene by methylation targets other genes. This information has led to the finding that the hypermethylation- associated inactivation of MGMT gives rise to the appearance of G to A transition mutations in the oncogene K-ras (Esteller et al. 2000b) and the universal tumor suppressor p53 (Esteller et al. 2001c) in human colorectal tumorigenesis. These findings demonstrate that an epigenetic lesion can cause a known genetic lesion in genes that are of key importance in the development of cancer.

Finally, the comprehensive analysis of methylation in many different tumor types and gene promoters has provided evidence for the existence of the tumor-type-specific methylation profile indicated above. In theory, CpG islands should be the most 'attractive' substrate for DNA methylation, since, by definition, they contain a high concentration of CpG-rich sequences. However, under physiological circumstances most CpG island promoters remain unmethylated. It has been speculated on the existence of mechanisms that would normally prevent unscheduled methylation at CpG islands, and for some reasons those mechanisms would lose stringency in cancer cells. Many other questions then arise: Why do CpG islands become methylated in cancer? Why do certain CpG islands become methylated while others do not? Is aberrant hypermethylation a targeted or a random process?

Genome-wide analysis of DNA methylation changes in cancer cells have shed some light on these questions by revealing that tumor-specific methylated genes belong to distinct functional categories, have common sequence motifs in their promoters and are found in clusters on chromosomes (Keshet et al. 2006). These results are consistent with the hypothesis that cancer-related de novo methylation may be specifically targeted through a trans-acting mechanism. Recently, Schlesinger et al. (2007) showed that genes methylated in colon cancer cells are specifically packaged with nucleosomes containing histone H3 trimethylated on K27. The early establishment of this chromatin mark in unmethylated promoter CpG island-containing genes early in development and then maintained in differentiated cell types by the presence of an EZH2-containing Polycomb complex suggests that PcG proteins pre-define genes that are methylated in cancer. In cancer cells, as opposed to normal cells, the presence of this complex brings about the recruitment of DNMTs, leading to de novo methylation. These results suggest that tumor-specific targeting of de novo methylation is pre-programmed by an established epigenetic system that normally has a role in marking embryonic genes for repression (Schlesinger et al. 2007).

As indicated above, DNA methylation and histone modification profiles are mechanistically coupled by multiple mechanisms. In addition to PcG mediated-connections between histone modifications and DNA methylation, other factors have been implicated in DNA methylation-dependent silencing. In this context, MBD proteins have been proposed to play a pivotal role (Ballestar et al. 2003). MBD proteins have the ability to bind selectively to methylated CpGs and recruit different HDAC- and HMT-containing complexes (Ballestar et al. 2005). In addition to the association of MBDs, promoter CpG island hypermethylation has been found to be associated with a decrease in the acetylation levels of histones H3 and H4 and loss of 3mK4 of histone H3 (Ballestar et al. 2003). In contrast, hypomethylation of repetitive sequences in cancer is associated with a loss of monoacecetyl K16 and trimethyl K20 of histone H4 (Fraga et al. 2005a). It has been suggested that this change could be associated with changes in the expression levels of specific histone modification enzymes, like K16 H4-specific HAT MOF (Pfister et al. 2008) or K20 H4-specific HMT Suv4-20h2 (Tryndyak et al. 2006).

The importance of epigenetic mechanisms involved in the pathogenesis of cancer is also revealed by a mechanism frequently found in hematopoietic malignancies. In leukemias and lymphomas, in contrast to most solid tumors, an additional mechanism for epigenetic dysregulation arises from the occurrence of non-random chromosomal translocations that disrupt genes residing in the translocation breakpoint region (Falini and Mason, 2002). In many cases, genes residing at these breakpoint regions are epigenetic enzymes or transcription factors that can themselves recruit epigenetic enzymes and are directly involved in hematopoietic cell differentiation, apoptosis, or proliferation. Therefore, generation of fusion proteins through this mechanism is commonly associated with epigenetic dysregulation at the target sites of the enzymes involved (Fig. 1). These chromosomal translocations indicate how disruptions of the function of the enzymes that control chromatin structure can cause alterations of the histone modification profile in a target-specific fashion, resulting in an altered chromatin structure that affects gene expression at specific loci and ultimately causes cellular transformation. Typical examples of proteins include MLL (mixed-lineage leukemia), a histone H3 K4-specific methyltransferase, RUNX1 (also known as AML1) which is associated with HATs or HDACs, and PML, whose frequent fusion partner (RAR) has been described to interact with various epigenetic modifiers (di Croce, 2005).

Our knowledge on the importance of epigenetic alterations in cancer has greatly increased in the last few years. The contribution of DNA methylation-dependent epigenetic inactivation of tumor suppressor genes is widely recognized. More specifically in hematological malignancies, the epigenetic switch at many genomic sites is also commonly recognized. We need a better understanding on the causes that result in epigenetic deregulation in cancer. Mapping epigenomic changes, at the DNA methylation, histone modification and factor binding level, in cancer cells will surely provide a solid ground to address these issues.

3 Epigenetic Changes in Other Human Diseases

Despite the enormous efforts invested in epigenetics studies, our knowledge on epigenetic alterations in other disease contexts is relatively poor. Epigenetic alterations occur in a wide range of biological scenarios, including the occurrence of genetic defects in the enzymes that regulate the epigenetic balance or epigenetic changes that result from a change in the environment. Although the best studied relationship between epigenetic alterations and disease are in the context of cancer, a number of diseases have proved to exhibit a fundamental epigenetic component. The first group of disorders for which an epigenetic component has been recognized includes diseases for which there is a genetic defect involving proteins implicated in the maintenance of epigenetic regulation. In this group are included a few rare syndromes such as Immunodeficiency-Centromere Instability-Facial anomalies (ICF) syndrome, Rett syndrome or Alpha-thalassemia/mental retardation, X-linked (ATRX).

ICF syndrome, a rare autosomal recessive disorder characterized by the presence of variable immunodeficiency and a unique type of instability of pericentromeric heterochromatin, has been shown to be associated with mutations in DNMT3B. Epigenetic alterations associated with this defect include hypomethylation at various repetitive sequences (Kondo et al. 2000) and chromosomal territory reorganization which may have an impact in alterations of gene expression of many genes (Matarazzo et al. 2007). In Rett syndrome, an X-linked dominant neurodevelopmental disorder affecting almost exclusively girls, mutations in MECP2, the archetypical member of the MBD family, have been found to be present in up to 80% of classical cases (Amir et al. 1999). It has been proposed that loss of function of MECP2 results in the DNA methylation-dependent deregulation of genes (Ballestar et al. 2005), although more recently it has been proposed that binding of MeCP2 outside gene boundaries may organize chromatin into functionally important domains or loops of imprinted regions, thereby modulating gene expression in either a positive or a negative manner (Yasui et al. 2007). In ATRX syndrome, a disorder characterized by alpha-thalassemia, mental retardation and facial dysmorphism, an association with mutations in the SWI/SNF-like protein encoded by the ATRX gene has been found. Mutations in the ATRX gene have been found to yield changes in the pattern of DNA methylation of several highly repeated sequences including the rDNA arrays, a Y-specific satellite and subtelomeric repeats (Gibbons et al. 2000). Mutations in elements of the epigenetic machinery are likely to be involved in the etiology of other diseases. For instance, truncating mutations in one of the primary human HDACs, *HDAC2*, have been identified in sporadic carcinomas with microsatellite instability and in tumors arising in individuals with hereditary non-polyposis colorectal cancer syndrome (Ropero et al. 2006).

In other groups of disorders, genetic defects have been associated with clear distinctive epigenetic defects. This is the case with facioscapulohumeral muscular dystrophy (FSHD) and the imprinting disorders Beckwith-Wiedemann syndrome (BWS) and the Prader-Willi/Angelman syndromes (PWS/AS).

FSHD is a dominantly inherited muscular dystrophy with a distinctive clinical presentation. Despite the identification of a causal deletion on a critical number of repetitive elements (D4Z4) on chromosome 4q35 over a decade ago, the molecular pathophysiology of FSHD remains unclear. Several hypotheses have been developed to connect the contraction of D4Z4 repeats with the inappropriate expression of genes of the 4q35. On one hand, it has been postulated that D4Z4 might impose a heterochromatic structure in its vicinity. Alternatively, it has been suggested that D4Z4 might act as an insulator separating heterochromatic sequences distal to D4Z4 from more open chromatin structures proximal to D4Z4 (Tawil 2004). Interestingly, hypomethylation in shortened D4Z4 repeats has been consistently found in FSHD patients (de Greef et al. 2007) which might be a marker of a less condensed chromatin structure in FSHD-related short arrays.

The best characterized syndromes related to imprinting defects are the BWS and the PWS/AS. BWS is a growth disorder characterized by pre- and postnatal overgrowth, and the occurrence of a variety of minor developmental abnormalities. In contrast, PWS and AS are distinct neurodevelopmental disorders that both map to a common imprinted domain. In these cases, the disease can be associated with a genetic defect that affects specialized regulatory sequence elements involved in the establishment of imprinting at a specific genomic location, the so-called imprinting control regions (ICR). One well-characterized ICR is the regulatory domain of the PWS and AS region which maps on the chromosome region 15q11-13. In PWS, microdeletions occur around the first exon of the paternally expressed SNRPN gene, whereas in AS microdeletions occur 30 kb further upstream of *SNRPN* at a locus of no known function. In the case of BWS, defects also directly involve the ICR within the 11p15.5 chromosomal region. For all of these diseases, ICR deletions abrogate imprinting of the paternally or maternally repressed genes in the neighboring domain resulting in biallelic expression of those genes. During the past few years, analysis of different ICR has shown the accumulation of epigenetic defects (alterations in DNA methylation patterns, histone modifications and associated chromatin factors) in the flanking domains of imprinted genes regulated by the corresponding ICR and associated with defects in imprinted gene control (Arnaud and Feil, 2005).

The existence of an epigenetic component has been suggested for many other diseases for which a direct genetic defect is not obvious or complex genetic patterns have been suggested. This is for instance the case of autoimmune or neurological disorders, and cardiovascular disease. The evidence for an epigenetic component in these diseases has been highlighted by the existence of discordance rates in sets of monozygotic twins (Petronis 2006). Analysis of global and locus-specific differences of DNA methylation and histone modification in a cohort of identical twins has suggested the existence of an age- dependent epigenetic 'drift', which may result from the independent influence of environmental factors (Fraga et al. 2005b). Intuitively, it makes sense that there should be an increasing number of incongruent epigenetic changes in the aging co-twins. It is important to note, however, that the degree of twin discordance for various complex diseases does not necessarily correlate with age of onset.

Our knowledge of the epigenetic contribution to these diseases requires additional research efforts: firstly, a detailed description of the type and extent of epigenetic alterations needs to be done. In addition, identification of the upstream mechanisms that lead to the generation of epigenetic changes should be investigated.

Among this group, various types of disorders are included. An example is represented by autoimmune disorders for which various epigenetic alterations have been described. For instance, in systemic lupus erythematosus (SLE), global loss of methylation has been reported and a number of genes have already been demonstrated to become hypomethylated in SLE (Richardson, 2007) (Fig. 1). The epigenetic component of SLE is also evident through the use of inhibitors of DNMTs and HDACs. Whereas SLE individuals appear to respond positively to the use of HDAC inhibitors, in other individuals the therapeutic use of DNA demethylating agents have been reported to cause the development of autoimmunity (Richardson, 2007).

The availability of novel technologies for the genome-wide analysis of epigenetic alterations and systematic analysis of DNA methylation changes in specific diseases will surely lead to the discovery of specific markers with both basic research and clinical implications. For instance, DNA methylation changes have been described to occur in the estrogen receptor beta gene in cardiovascular atherosclerotic tissues (Kim et al. 2007) or in the membrane-bound catechol-O-methyltransferase associated with a major risk factor for schizophrenia and bipolar disorder (Abdolmaleky et al. 2006).

4 Developing Strategies to Characterize Epigenetic Profiles

Cancer epigenetics research has had an influence on the development of strategies for mapping epigenetic modifications at specific genomic sequences. Despite the multiple interconnections between DNA methylation and histone modification, strategies to investigate these two groups of marks have been developed separately. In the case of DNA methylation changes, the recognition that the promoter CpG islands of specific tumor suppressor genes become hypermethylated in cancer has influenced the development of different approaches to identify genes that have become methylated in cancer. Classical tumor-suppressor genes for which genetic lesions had been described, such as VHL, p73 or p16(INK4a), constituted the major source of candidate genes used for performing analysis on the methylation status of their promoter CpG islands (Esteller et al. 2001a–c). The systematic use of this strategy led to the identification of a number of genes that are epigenetically inactivated in cancer and to the notion that specific DNA hypermethylation patterns occur in cancer in a tumor-specific fashion (Esteller et al. 2001a–c). These candidate gene-based approaches also highlighted the need to develop genomic strategies to obtain comprehensive DNA methylation profiles of cancer cells. Research efforts in this direction have contributed to several methodologies.

The rationale of the first group of approaches was based in the digestion of genomic DNA with restriction enzymes unable to digest the methylated version of their CpG-containing target sites (for a comprehensive review, please read (Esteller, 2007). These strategies allow a direct comparison of differentially methylated sites between two/various cell types. In combination with digestion with methylation-sensitive restriction enzymes, different methods are used to resolve or analyze the resulting fragments. For instance, in restriction landmark genomic scanning (RLGS), fragments resulting from digestion are separated in a two dimensional gel electrophoresis. When comparing two different cell types, differential spots need to be individually analyzed for their methylation status. Other methods use a combination of methylation-sensitive restriction enzymes with ligation-mediated PCR amplification. An excellent example is that of the amplification of intermethylated sites (AIMS). More recent strategies consist in the generation of DNA fragments generated through digestion of genomic DNA with methylation-sensitive restriction enzymes combined with hybridization on genomic microarrays. Again, this method is useful to perform a direct comparison between two different cell types for which differential methylation throughout the genome is expected.

Recently, Weber et al. have developed an immunocapturing approach based on the direct immunoprecipitation of methylated DNA combined with immunoprecipitation on genomic microarrays (Weber et al. 2005). In this assay, named methyl-DNA immunoprecipitation (MeDIP), a monoclonal antibody raised against 5-methylcytidine (5mC) is used to purify methylated DNA. The study of Weber et al. (2005), in which they used MeDIP for the first time, revealed the usefulness of this technique for obtaining high-resolution maps of the human methylome and the possibility of using it to identify genes that suffer DNA methylation changes in response to different biological contexts (Jacinto et al. 2007) (see also Chapters in Part I). For instance, it confirmed that the inactive X-chromosome in females is hypermethylated at CpG islands at a chromosome-wide level. This study also showed for instance that the global distribution of CpG methylation in colon cancer model used is markedly similar to that of primary fibroblasts. It also confirmed that DNA methylation changes in CpG islands of cancer cells primary involves hypermethylation events and that hypomethylation is a rare event.

Regarding histone modifications, chromatin immunoprecipitation (ChIP) assays constitute the basic strategy to investigate both the presence of particular histone modification marks or binding of a particular factor to DNA (Orlando, 2000). For years, ChIP assays were used in individualized studies on the histone modification patterns and transcription factor occupancy of specific loci. The availability of genomic microarrays allowed the possibility of using them for hybridizations with the products of ChIP assays in order to obtain genome-wide maps of histone modifications and factor binding. Parallel studies of MeDIPs and ChIPs combined to hybridization with microarrays allow to investigating correlations between DNA methylation patterns and histone modification marks (Weber et al. 2007).

A novel high-throughput array-based method for analyzing the methylation status of hundreds of pre-selected genes has recently been developed (Bibikova et al. 2006). At the current level of development, this type of array enables the analysis of several thousand genes. The results obtained with this method demonstrate its effectiveness for reliably profiling many CpG sites in parallel, by which informative methylation markers may be identified.

Very recently, massively parallel pyrosequencing technology has been applied for the high-throughput sequencing of bisulfite PCR amplicons from clinical samples (Taylor et al. 2007). This type of approach, known as ultradeep bisulfite sequencing analysis, will continue to contribute to the generation of high resolution maps for the mapping of the DNA methylome in different contexts.

For histone modifications, the possibility of combining ChIP assays with high-throughput sequencing allows the generation of high-resolution maps for the genome-wide distribution of histone modifications (Barski et al. 2007) and transcription factor occupancy.

5 Concluding Remarks

The epigenome of a particular cell type, i.e., the profile of epigenetic modifications and chromatin features through its entire genomic sequence, is the result of the specific events that define which regions need to be expressed in that particular cell type in addition to its temporal and environmental context. Alterations associated with a particular disease are the result of genetic determinants, defects in cell signaling pathways, changes in the environment, and other factors. There are as many epigenomes for an organism as potential biological contexts, including cell and tissue types and all the above factors. The possibility of obtaining high resolution epigenomic maps from a cell is a task of inherent interest in order to profoundly understand regulatory processes and their aberrant behavior in disease.

Acknowledegment ME is funded by the Education and Science (I+D+I MCYT08-03 and Consolider MEC09-05) Department of the Spanish Government and the CANCERDIP FP7 Grant. EB is funded by the BFU2004-02073/BMC (MEC) Grant.

References

Abdolmaleky, H.M., Cheng, K.H., Faraone, S.V., Wilcox, M., Glatt, S.J., Gao, F., Smith, C.L., Shafa, R., Aeali, B., Carnevale, J., Pan, H., Papageorgis, P., Ponte, J.F., Sivaraman, V., Tsuang, M.T., Thiagalingam, S. (2006) Hypomethylation of MB-COMT promoter is a major risk factor for schizophrenia and bipolar disorder. *Hum Mol Genet*. *15*: 3132–3145.

Amir RE, Van den Veyver IB, Wan M, Tran CQ, Francke U, Zoghbi HY. (1999) Rett syndrome is caused by mutations in X-linked MECP2, encoding methyl-CpG-binding protein 2. Nat Genet. *23*:185–188.

Arnaud, P. and Feil, R. (2005) Epigenetic deregulation of genomic imprinting in human disorders and following assisted reproduction. 75: 81–97.

Ballestar E, Paz MF, Valle L, Wei S, Fraga MF, Espada J, Cigudosa JC, Huang TH, Esteller M. (2003) Methyl-CpG binding proteins identify novel sites of epigenetic inactivation in human cancer. EMBO J. 22: 6335–6345.

Ballestar, E., and Esteller, M. (2005) Methyl-CpG-binding proteins in cancer: blaming the DNA methylation messenger. Biochem. Cell Biol. 83:374–384.

Ballestar, E., Ropero, S., Alaminos, M., Armstrong, J., Setien, F., Agrelo, R., Fraga, M.F., Herranz, M., Avila, S., Pineda, M., Monros, E., Esteller, M. (2005) The impact of MECP2 mutations in the expression patterns of Rett syndrome patients. *Hum Genet.* 116: 91–104.

Barreto, G., Schäfer, A., Marhold, J., Stach, D., Swaminathan, S.K., Handa, V., Döderlein, G., Maltry, N., Wu, W., Lyko, F., Niehrs, C. (2007) Gadd45a promotes epigenetic gene activation by repair-mediated DNA demethylation. Nature 445: 671–675.

Barski, A., Cuddapah, S., Cui, K., Roh, T.Y., Schones, D.E., Wang, Z., Wei, G., Chepelev, I., and Zhao, K. (2007) High-resolution profiling of histone methylations in the human genome. Cell 129:823–837.

Bhattacharya, S.K., Ramchandani, S., Cervoni, N., Szyf, M. (1999) A mammalian protein with specific demethylase activity for mCpG DNA. Nature 397: 579–583.

Bauer UM, Daujat S, Nielsen SJ, Nightingale K, Kouzarides T. (2002) Methylation at arginine 17 of histone H3 is linked to gene activation. EMBO Rep. 3: 39–44.

Bestor TH (2000) The DNA methyltransferases of mammals. *Hum Mol Genet.* 9, 2395–2402.

Bibikova, M., Lin, Z., Zhou, L., Chudin, E., Garcia, E.W., Wu, B., Doucet, D., Thomas, N.J., Wang, Y., Vollmer, E., et al. (2006) High-throughput DNA methylation profiling using universal bead arrays. Genome Res. 16: 383–393.

Burgers, W.A., Fuks, F., and Kouzarides, T. (2002) DNA methyltransferases get connected to chromatin. Trends Genet. 18: 275–277.

Chahal, S.S., Matthews, H.R., Bradbury, E.M. (1980) Acetylation of histone H4 and its role in chromatin structure and function. Nature 287: 76–79.

Costello JF, Frühwald MC, Smiraglia DJ, Rush LJ, Robertson GP, Gao X, Wright FA, Feramisco JD, Peltomäki P, Lang JC, Schuller DE, Yu L, Bloomfield CD, Caligiuri MA, Yates A, Nishikawa R, Su Huang H, Petrelli NJ, Zhang X, O'Dorisio MS, Held WA, Cavenee WK, Plass C. (2000) Aberrant CpG-island methylation has non-random and tumour-type-specific patterns. *Nat Genet* 24:132–138.

de Greef, J.C., Wohlgemuth, M., Chan, O.A., Hansson, K.B., Smeets, D., Frants, R.R., Weemaes, C.M., Padberg, G.W., van der Maarel, S.M. (2007) Hypomethylation is restricted to the D4Z4 repeat array in phenotypic FSHD. *Neurology* 69: 1018–1026.

Di Croce L. (2005) Chromatin modifying activity of leukaemia associated fusion proteins. Hum Mol Genet. 14 Spec No 1: R77–R84.

Ehrlich, M. DNA methylation in cancer: too much, but also too little. (2002) *Oncogene 21*: 5400–5413.

Estécio MR, Gharibyan V, Shen L, Ibrahim AE, Doshi K, He R, Jelinek J, Yang AS, Yan PS, Huang TH, Tajara EH, Issa JP.LINE-1 hypomethylation in cancer is highly variable and inversely correlated with microsatellite instability. PLoS ONE. (2007)2(5):e399.

Espada, J., Ballestar, E., Fraga, M.F., Villar-Garea, A., Juarranz, A., Stockert, J.C. Robertson, K.D., Fuks, F. and Esteller, M. (2004) Human DNA methyltransferase 1 is required for maintenance of the histone H3 modification pattern. *J Biol Chem.* 279: 37175–37184.

Esteller M, Lluis Catasus, Matias-Guiu X, Mutter G, Baylin SB, Prat J, Herman JG. (1999a) hMLH1 promoter hypermethylation is an early event in human endometrial tumorigenesis. *Am. J. Pathol.*, 155: 1767–1772.

Esteller, M., Hamilton, S.R., Burger, P.C., Baylin, S.B., Herman, J.G. (1999b) Inactivation of the DNA repair gene O6-methylguanine-DNA methyltransferase by promoter hypermethylation is a common event in primary human neoplasia. Cancer Res. 59, 793–797.

Esteller, M., Tortola, S., Toyota, M., Capella, G., Peinado, M.A., Baylin, S.B., Herman, J.G. (2000a) Hypermethylation-associated inactivation of p14(ARF) is independent of p16(INK4a) methylation and p53 mutational status. *Cancer Res.* 60, 129–133.

Esteller, M., Toyota, M., Sanchez-Cespedes, M., Capella, G., Peinado, M.A., Watkins, D.N., Issa, J.P., Sidransky, D., Baylin, S.B., Herman, J.G. (2000b) Inactivation of the DNA repair gene O6-methylguanine-DNA methyltransferase by promoter hypermethylation is associated with G to A mutations in K-ras in colorectal tumorigenesis. Cancer Res. 60, 2368–2371.

Esteller M, Corn PG, Baylin SB and Herman JG. (2001a) A gene hypermethylation profile of human cancer. Cancer Res *61*:3225–3229.

Esteller M, Fraga MF, Guo M, Garcia-Foncillas J, Hedelfank I, Godwin AK, Trojan J, Vaurs-Barrière C, Bignon Y-J, Ramus S, Benitez J, Akiyama Y, Caldes T, Canal MJ, Rodriguez R, Capella G, Peinado MA, Borg A, Aaltonen LA, Ponder BA, Baylin SB, Herman JG. (2001b) DNA methylation patterns in hereditary human cancers mimic sporadic tumorigenesis.*Human Mol. Genetics*, **10**, 3001–3007.

Esteller, M., Risques, R.A., Toyota, M., Capella, G., Moreno, V., Peinado, M.A., Baylin, S.B., Herman, J.G. (2001c) Promoter hypermethylation of the DNA repair gene O(6)-methylguanine-DNA methyltransferase is associated with the presence of G:C to A:T transition mutations in p53 in human colorectal tumorigenesis. Cancer Res. **61**, 4689–4692.

Esteller, M. (2007) Cancer epigenomics: DNA methylomes and histone-modification maps. *Nat. Rev. Genet.* **8**, 286–298.

Falini B, Mason DY. (2002) Proteins encoded by genes involved in chromosomal alterations in lymphoma and leukemia: clinical value of their detection by immunocytochemistry. Blood. **99**, 409–426.

Feil, R. (2006) Environmental and nutritional effects on the epigenetic regulation of genes. Mutat Res. **600**, 46–57.

Feinberg, A.P. and Vogelstein, B. (1983) Hypomethylation distinguishes genes of some human cancers from their normal counterparts. *Nature* **301**, 89–92.

Fleisher, A.S., Esteller, M., Wang, S., Tamura, G., Suzuki, H., Yin, J., Zou, T.T., Abraham, J.M., Kong, D., Smolinski, K.N., Shi, Y.Q., Rhyu, M.G., Powell, S.M., James, S.P., Wilson, K.T., Herman, J.G., Meltzer, S.J. (1999) Hypermethylation of the hMLH1 gene promoter in human gastric cancers with microsatellite instability. *Cancer Res.*, **59**, 1090–1095.

Fraga, M.F., Ballestar, E., Villar-Garea, A. Boix-Chornet, M., Espada, J., Schotta, G., Bonaldi, T., Haydon, C., Petrie, K., Ropero, S., Perez-Rosado, A., Calvo, E., Lopez, J.A., Cano, A., Piris, M.A., Ahn, N., Imhof, A., Caldas, C., Jenuwein, T. and Esteller, M. (2005a) Loss of acetylation at Lys16 and trimethylation at Lys20 of histone H4 is a common hallmark of human cancer. *Nat Genet.* 37, 391–400.

Fraga, M.F., Ballestar, E., Paz, M.F., Ropero, S., Setien, F., Ballestar, M.L., Heine-Suñer, D., Cigudosa, J.C., Urioste, M. Benitez, J., Boix-Chornet, M., Sanchez-Aguilera, A., Ling, C., Carlsson, E., Poulsen, P., Vaag, A., Stephan, Z., Spector, T.D., Wu, Y.-Z., Plass, C. and Esteller, M. (2005b) Epigenetic Differences Arise During the Lifetime of Monozygotic Twins. *Proc. Natl. Acad. Sci. U.S.A.* 102, 10604–10609.

Futscher, B.W., Oshiro, M.M., Wozniak, R.J., Holtan, N., Hanigan, C.L., Duan, H., and Domann, F.E. 2002. Role for DNA methylation in the control of cell type specific maspin expression. Nature Genet. *31*:175–179.

Gardiner-Garden, M., and Frommer, M. (1987) CpG islands in vertebrate genomes. *J. Mol. Biol. 196*: 261–282.

Gibbons, R.J., McDowell, T.L., Raman, S., O'Rourke, D.M., Garrick, D., Ayyub, H. and Higgs, D.R. (2000) Mutations in ATRX, encoding a SWI/SNF-like protein, cause diverse changes in the pattern of DNA methylation. Nat Genet. *24*: 368–371.

Hendrich, B., and Bird, A. (1998) Identification and characterization of a family of mammalian methyl-CpG binding proteins. Mol. Cell. Biol. *18*:6538–6547.

Jacinto, F.V., Ballestar, E., Ropero, S., and Esteller, M. (2007) Discovery of epigenetically silenced genes by methylated DNA immunoprecipitation in colon cancer cells. *Cancer Res 67*: 11481–11486.

Jaenisch, R., and Bird, A. (2003) Epigenetic regulation of gene expression: how the genome integrates intrinsic and environmental signals. *Nature Genet. 33*: Suppl:245–254.

Jin, S.G., Guo, C., Pfeifer, G.P. (2008) GADD45A does not promote DNA demethylation. PLoS Genet. *4*: e1000013.

Jones, P.A. and Baylin, S.B. (2002) The fundamental role of epigenetic events in cancer. *Nat Rev Genet. 3*: 415–428.

Keshet, I., Schlesinger, Y., Farkash, S., Rand, E., Hecht, M., Segal, E., Pikarski, E., Young, R.A., Niveleau, A., Cedar, H., and Simon, I. (2006) Evidence for an instructive mechanism of de novo methylation in cancer cells. *Nat Genet 38*: 149–153.

Kim, J., Kim, J.Y., Song, K.S., Lee, Y.H., Seo, J.S., Jelinek, J., Goldschmidt-Clermont, P.J., Issa, J.P. (2007) Epigenetic changes in estrogen receptor beta gene in atherosclerotic cardiovascular tissues and in-vitro vascular senescence. *Biochim Biophys Acta. 1772*: 72–80.

Kondo, T., Bobek, M.P., Kuick, R., Lamb, B., Zhu, X., Narayan, A., Bourc'his, D., Viegas-Péquignot, E., Ehrlich M, and Hanash, S.M. 2000. Whole-genome methylation scan in ICF syndrome: hypomethylation of non-satellite DNA repeats D4Z4 and NBL2. Hum. Mol. Genet. *9*:597–604.

Lachner M, O'Carroll D, Rea S, Mechtler K, Jenuwein T. (2001) Methylation of histone H3 lysine 9 creates a binding site for HP1 proteins. Nature *410*:116–120.

Matarazzo, M.R., Boyle, S., D'Esposito, M., Bickmore, W.A.(2007) Chromosome territory reorganization in a human disease with altered DNA methylation. *Proc Natl Acad Sci U S A. 104*: 16546–16551.

Myohanen SK, Baylin SB, Herman JG. (1998). *Cancer Res.*, **58,** 591–593.

Orlando, V. (2000) Mapping chromosomal proteins in vivo by formaldehyde-crosslinked-chromatin immunoprecipitation. *Trends Biochem Sci.* **25**, 99–104.

Petronis, A (2006) Epigenetics and twins: three variations on the theme. *Trends Genet.* **22**, 347–350.

Pfister, S., Rea, S., Taipale, M., Mendrzyk, F., Straub, B., Ittrich, C., Thuerigen, O., Sinn, H.P., Akhtar, A., Lichter, P. (2008) The histone acetyltransferase hMOF is frequently downregulated in primary breast carcinoma and medulloblastoma and constitutes a biomarker for clinical outcome in medulloblastoma. Int J Cancer*122*: 1207–1213.

Rao B, Shibata Y, Strahl BD, Lieb JD. (2005) Demethylation of histone H3 at lysine 36 demarcates regulatory and nonregulatory chromatin genome-wide. Mol Cell Biol. *25*: 9447–9459.

Reik, W., Collick, A., Norris, M.L., Barton, S.C., and Surani, M.A. 1987. Genomic imprinting determines methylation of parental alleles in transgenic mice. *Nature 328*: 248–251.

Reik, W., Dean, W., Walter, J. (2001) Epigenetic reprogramming in mammalian development. *Science 293***:** 1089–1093.

Richardson B. (2007) Primer: epigenetics of autoimmunity. *Nat Clin Pract Rheumatol.* **3**, 521–527.

Robertson, K.D. and Wolffe, A.P. (2000) DNA methylation in health and disease. Nat Rev Genet. *1*: 11–19.

Ropero, S. Fraga, M.F., Ballestar, E., Hamelin, R., Yamamoto, H., Boix-Chornet, M., Caballero, R., Palacios, J., Arango, D., Aaltonen, L., Schwartz Jr. S. and Esteller, M. (2006) A truncating mutation of HDAC2 in human cancers confers resistance to histone deacetylase inhibition. *Nat. Genet.38*: 566–569.

Rundlett SE, Carmen AA, Suka N, Turner BM, Grunstein M. (1998) Transcriptional repression by UME6 involves deacetylation of lysine 5 of histone H4 by RPD3. Nature *392*: 831–835.

Santos-Rosa H, Schneider R, Bannister AJ, Sherriff J, Bernstein BE, Emre NC, Schreiber SL, Mellor J, Kouzarides T. (2002) Active genes are tri-methylated at K4 of histone H3. Nature *419*: 407–411.

Saxonov, S., Berg, P., Brutlag, D.L. (2006) A genome-wide analysis of CpG dinucleotides in the human genome distinguishes two distinct classes of promoters. Proc Natl Acad Sci U S A. *103*: 412–1417.

Schotta G, Lachner M, Sarma K, Ebert A, Sengupta R, Reuter G, Reinberg D, Jenuwein T. (2004) A silencing pathway to induce H3-K9 and H4-K20 trimethylation at constitutive heterochromatin. Genes Dev. *18*: 1251–1262.

Schlesinger, Y., Straussman, R., Keshet, I., Farkash, S., Hecht, M., Zimmerman, J., Eden, E., Yakhini, Z., Ben-Shushan, E., Reubinoff, B.E., Bergman, Y., Simon, I., Cedar, H. (2007) Polycomb-mediated methylation on Lys27 of histone H3 pre-marks genes for de novo methylation in cancer. *Nat Genet*. **39**, 232–236.

Shogren-Knaak, M., Ishii, H., Sun, J.M., Pazin, M.J., Davie, J.R., Peterson, C.L. (2006) Histone H4-K16 acetylation controls chromatin structure and protein interactions. Science **311**, 844–847.

Siegfried, Z., and Cedar, H. (1997) DNA methylation: a molecular lock. Curr. Biol. **7**, R305–307.

Song, F., Smith, J.F., Kimura, M.T., Morrow, A.D., Matsuyama, T., Nagase, H., and Held, W.A. (2005) Association of tissue-specific differentially methylated regions (TDMs) with differential gene expression. Proc. Natl. Acad. Sci. USA *102*: 3336–3341.

Tawil, R. (2004) Facioscapulohumeral muscular dystrophy. *Curr Neurol Neurosci Rep*. *4*: 51–54.

Taylor, K.H., Kramer, R.S., Davis, J.W., Guo, J., Duff, D.J., Xu, D., Caldwell, C.W., Shi, H. (2007) Ultradeep bisulfite sequencing analysis of DNA methylation patterns in multiple gene promoters by 454 sequencing. *Cancer Res*. *67*: 8511–8518.

Tryndyak, V.P., Kovalchuk, O., Pogribny, I.P. (2006) Loss of DNA methylation and histone H4 lysine 20 trimethylation in human breast cancer cells is associated with aberrant expression of DNA methyltransferase 1, Suv4-20h2 histone methyltransferase and methyl-binding proteins. *Cancer Biol Ther 5*: 65–70.

Vire, E., Brenner, C., Deplus, R., Blanchon, L., Fraga, M., Didelot, C., Morey, L., Van Eynde, A., Bernard, D., Vanderwinden, J.M., Bollen, M., Esteller, M., Di Croce, L., de Launoit, Y., Fuks, F. (2004) The Polycomb group protein EZH2 directly controls DNA methylation. *Nature 439*: 871–874.

Wang Y, Fischle W, Cheung W, Jacobs S, Khorasanizadeh S, Allis CD. (2004) Beyond the double helix: writing and reading the histone code. Novartis Found Symp. *259*: 3–17.

Weber, M., Davies, J.J., Wittig, D., Oakeley, E.J., Haase, M., Lam, W.L., and Schübeler, D. (2005) Chromosome-wide and promoter-specific analyses identify sites of differential DNA methylation in normal and transformed human cells. Nat Genet. *37*: 853–862.

Weber, M., Hellmann, I., Stadler, M.B., Ramos, L., Pääbo, S., Rebhan, M., and Schübeler, D. (2007) Distribution, silencing potential and evolutionary impact of promoter DNA methylation in the human genome. Nat Genet. *39*: 457–466.

Wilson, C.B. and Merkenschlager, M. (2006) Chromatin structure and gene regulation in T cell development and function. *Curr Opin Immunol*. *18*: 143–151.

Wolf, S.F. and Migeon, B.R. (1982) Studies of X chromosome DNA methylation in normal human cells. Nature *295*: 667–671.

Wolffe, A.P., Jones, P.L., Wade, P.A. (1999) DNA demethylation. Proc Natl Acad Sci U S A. *96*: 5894–5896.

Yasui, D.H., Peddada, S., Bieda, M.C., Vallero, R.O., Hogart, A., Nagarajan, R.P., Thatcher, K.N., Farnham, P.J., Lasalle, J.M. (2007) Integrated epigenomic analyses of neuronal MeCP2 reveal a role for long-range interaction with active genes. *Proc Natl Acad Sci U S A*. *104*: 19416–19421.

Yeager TR, DeVries S, Jarrard DF, Kao C, Nakada SY, Moon TD, Bruskewitz R, Stadler WM, Meisner LF, Gilchrist KW, Newton MA, Waldman FM, Reznikoff CA. (1998). *Genes Dev. 15*: 163–174.

Cancer Epigenomics

Christine Ladd-Acosta and Andrew P. Feinberg

Abstract Epigenetics is the study of information maintained during mitotic division other than the DNA sequence itself and includes DNA methylation, and modification of chromatin histone tails. Both DNA methylation and chromatin structure are essential to normal growth and development in mammals and regulate diverse functions such as imprinting, genomic stability, and gene transcription. Incorrect establishment, maintenance, or recognition of epigenetic marks can lead to a wide range of human diseases including immunodeficiency, centromeric region instability and facial anomalies syndrome (ICF), Rett syndrome, and cancer. In human cancer, both global hypomethylation of DNA across the genome and locus specific hypermethylation of DNA in promoters are common, thus are hallmarks of malignancy. Changes in transcription of histone tail modifying enzymes have also been well documented in a variety of human tumors. Although a great deal is known about epigenetic changes in cancer at the single gene level, little is known about the cancer epigenome; a genome-wide approach is likely to reveal important new insights that can not been seen from the single gene viewpoint. In this chapter we will describe new technologies used to study the epigenome and review what we have learned about the cancer epigenome using these new approaches.

Keywords Cancer · Chromatin Modification · DNA methylation · Epigenomic

1 Introduction

Cancer is a broad term used to classify a heterogeneous set of diseases that involve uncontrolled cell growth, infinite cell division, and altered cellular function often leading to formation of new blood vessels, known as angiogenesis, invasion of surrounding tissue and metastasis. The classical, most-widely studied model of cancer is the clonal genetic model that hypothesizes cancer results from a single cell

A.P. Feinberg (✉)
Epigenetics Center, Institute for Basic Biomedical Sciences, and the Department of Medicine, Johns Hopkins University School of Medicine, Baltimore, MD 21205, USA
e-mail: afeinberg@jhu.edu

acquiring a series of genetic mutations. Many advances have been made by studying genetic changes in tumors, and numerous mutations in tumor suppressor and oncogenes found however it is not the only important aberration found in cancer. In addition to genetic lesions, numerous types of human malignancies contain epigenetic lesions, changes in DNA methylation density and histone tail modifications, as well. For example, DNA hypermethylation in promoter regions and hypomethylation of promoter associated CpG islands have been associated with many cancers (Feinberg and Tycko 2004). Global DNA hypomethylation has been ubiquitously found in cancer and is present at the earliest stages of carcinogenesis (Feinberg and Tycko 2004). In addition, both an increase and decrease in transcription of histone tail modifying enzymes, such as histone acetyltrasferases (HATs) and histone methyltransferases (HMTs), have been documented in human malignancies (Wang et al. 2007a, 2007b). While great advances have been made analyzing epigenetic aberrations in cancer at the individual gene level, a significant amount of information about the epigenomic landscape of cancer as a whole is lost by looking in isolation at single genes. As a result, many questions still remain such as: How extensive are epigenetic alterations across the genome? Are entire cell signaling pathways epigenetically dysregulated in cancer? Do DNA methylation changes only occur in CpG island or promoter regions? Are gene-specific or epigenomic tests most informative for cancer diagnosis and prognosis? Are gene-specific or epigenome cancer treatments most effective? With recent technological advances, investigators are able to perform genome-wide analysis of epigenetic lesions in cancer and have already begun to answer some of these questions.

2 DNA Methylation Aberrations at the Single Gene Level

DNA methylation (DNAm) is a type of epigenetic mark involving the covalent addition of a methyl group to the C-5 position of the cytosine nucleotide and occurs in mammals at CpG dinucleotides. DNAm is essential for normal development, imprinting, and transcriptional regulation and its disruption is well established in human cancer (Feinberg and Tycko 2004). Since the initial discoveries of aberrant DNA methylation in cancer in 1983 (Feinberg and Vogelstein 1983; Gamasosa et al. 1983), numerous examples of methylation changes, both loss and gain, in gene promoters as well as genome-wide hypomethylation of DNA have been documented. For example, *PAX2* is overexpressed in endometrial cancers and has hypomethylation of the promoter region in tumors compared to normal endometrium (Wu et al. 2005). Similarly, using locus-specific methylation assays the promoter region of *S100A4*, overexpressed in cancer, demonstrated hypomethylation in endometrial, pancreatic, and colon tumors compared to their normal counterparts (Nakamura and Takenaga 1998; Rosty, Ueki et al. 2002; Xie et al. 2007). Tumor suppressor genes, important cell cycle and growth regulators, are often silenced in malignant cells. A common feature of cancer is hypermethylation in tumor suppressor promoters or associated CpG island regions. For example, hypermethylation in CpG islands associated with promoter regions of E-cadherin, p16, p15, and von Hippel-Lindau has been demonstrated in various human cancers (Herman et al. 1996). Some CpG islands are only hypermethylated in a specific type of tumor while others are commonly hypermethylated in multiple types of tumors (Costello et al. 2000); hypermethylation may be secondary to gene silencing (Clark and Melki 2002; Mutskov and Felsenfeld 2004; Stirzaker et al. 2004). In addition to hypermethylation, a number of genes that are overexpressed in cancer have hypomethylated promoter regions in comparison to normal tissue counterparts. For example, *CAGE*, a cancer/testis antigen gene, is hypomethylated in pre-malignant gastric cancers (Cho et al. 2003). Overexpression of cytochrome P450, *CYP1B1*, in prostate cancers is correlated with decreased methylation at the *CYP1B1* promoter compared to normal prostate (Tokizane et al. 2005). Proopiomelanocortin (*POMC*), is overexpressed in thymic carcinoids and associated with hypomethylation of the *POMC* promoter (Ye et al. 2005).

3 Chromatin Alterations at the Single Gene Level

In eukaryotes, chromatin refers to the highly ordered complex of genomic DNA with a small family of histone proteins which form the nucleosome. Five major post-translational modifications of histone tails have been described in humans: (1) acetylation, (2) methylation (3) phosphorylation (4) sumoylation and (5) ubiquitination (Hake et al. 2004). These modifications are important for chromatin remodeling (opening and closing of the higher order structure); they provide a binding platform where nuclear proteins can dock and interact with nucleosomes (Hake et al. 2004). Chromatin remodeling is vital to proper gene transcription, DNA repair, and DNA replication. Aberrations in proteins responsible for "writing", "reading", or "erasing" histone tail modifications, mutations in the protein remodeling machinery, and incorporation of specialized histone variants into the core nucleosome octomer have all been associated with malignancy (Wang et al. 2007a, 2007b).

DNA replication, repair, and accessibility to transcription factors are all regulated by chromatin remodeling. Disruption of chromatin modifications, with the protein remodeling complexes, or changes in the core nucleosome proteins can alter these three vital cellular processes and are associated with carcinogenesis (Wang et al. 2007a, 2007b). At the single gene level, deacetylation of histone H3 and H3K9 trimethylation are associated with hypermethylation of the *MLH1* locus in colorectal cancer cell lines and *GTSP1, RASSF1, RARB2, BRCA1*, and *MGMT* loci in breast cancer cell lines (Fahrner et al. 2002; Ballestar et al. 2003). In addition to finding changes in the histone modifications, alteration of enzymes responsible for "writing" the histone marks have also been found in human cancer. For example, gene expression studies revealed increased transcription of *EZH2*, a histone H3K27 methyltransferase, in mantle cell lymphoma (Visser et al. 2001), bladder cancer (Arisan et al. 2005), and metastatic prostate and breast carcinomas (Varambally et al. 2002; Kleer et al. 2003). Ectopic expression of *EZH2* in multiple myeloma cell lines leads to increased proliferation and terminal differentiation of B-cells (Croonquist and Van Ness 2005). Additionally, a decrease in prostate cell proliferation is observed with decreased EZH2 protein levels using small interfering RNA duplexes (Varambally et al. 2002). Both increased and decreased expression of *HP1*, a methyl-lysine 9 recognition protein important in regulation of heterochromatin, has been linked to genomic instability and aneuploidy (Wang et al. 2007a, 2007b). Similarly, overexpression of proteins that remove histone tail modifications have been associated with various malignancies; overexpression of the H3K9 and H3K36 demethylase, JMJD2C, is common in lung cancer, esophageal tumors, and medulloblastoma (Yang et al. 2000; Ehrbrecht et al. 2006; Italiano et al. 2006). Cellular proliferation, differentiation, and genomic structure are all influenced by specific histone tail modifications; these marks are altered in various cancers.

Not only have expression changes in the "writers", "readers", and "erasers" of histone tails been found in cancer but also in protein remodeling complexes. For example, loss of expression of *SNF5*, a subunit of the SWI/SNF remodeling complex, is commonly found in human rhabdoid tumors (Versteege et al. 1998). A *Snf5* null mouse model causes embryonic lethality however *Snf5* heterozygotes, with one mutated allele and one wild type allele, developed cancer at 15 months of age (Klochendler-Yeivin et al. 2000; Roberts et al. 2000; Guidi et al. 2001). Upon further examination the mice with cancer were found to have acquired a mutation in the wild type allele of *Snf5* (Klochendler-Yeivin et al. 2000). The strong association between SNF5 and aggressive childhood rhabdoid tumors coupled with development of tumors in *Snf5* null mice suggests involvement of chromatin remodelers in carcinogenesis.

Changes in the core nucleosome structure through incorporation of specialized histone variants have also been shown to occur in malignancy. In colorectal cancer, the H3.3 histone variant normally found in regions of transcribed genes, is often replaced by the CENPA histone variant, a specialized H3 protein found only at the centromeres of normal cells (Tomonaga et al. 2003). Overexpression and mistargeting of CENPA to regions other than the centromere could lead to incorrect chromosomal segregation during mitosis thus may play a role in the widespread alterations and instability of chromosomes present in multiple cancers.

While we have learned a great deal about the involvement of histone modifications and aberrant chromatin remodeling in cancer in small scale studies, questions still remain regarding the extent to which these changes occur across the genome and what a global picture may reveal. New approaches to study histone marks and associated proteins on a genome scale have been recently developed and are discussed in detail below.

4 Epigenomic Technology

Commonly used methods to measure DNAm at a single base resolution include sodium bisulfite DNA sequencing, MethyLight, Illumina GoldenGate methylation platform, and methyl-specific DNA karyotyping (MSDK). Sodium bisulfite DNA sequencing involves treating genomic DNA with sodium bisulfite and results in conversion of unmethylated cytosine to uracil (uracil is replaced by thymine during PCR) while methylated cytosines remain unchanged. This post-bisulfite treatment difference between 5-methylcytosine and cytosine is detected at each CpG site as a C/T nucleotide polymorphism during DNA sequencing. While providing single base resolution, the cost of sodium bisulfite DNA sequencing is tens of thousands of dollars to measure ∼40,000 of 28 million CpG dinucleotides in the human genome (Eckhardt et al. 2006), preventing large-scale analysis on this platform with current sequencing costs. MethylLight is a fluorescent-based method which uses real-time PCR to quantify differential annealing of methyl-specific primers to sodium bisulfite treated DNA (Eads et al. 2000). This technique is highly quantitative. Commercial arrays from Illumina and other vendors take advantage of sodium bisulfite conversion, and a modification of genotyping platforms can measure methylation as a C/T SNP using a pair of fluorescent locus-specific probes, one probe (cyanin 5 labeled) corresponds to the methylated and the other probe (cyanin 3 labeled) corresponds to the unmethylated state of a given CpG site (Bibikova, Lin et al. 2006). Methylation specific digital karyotyping (MSDK) discriminates between methylated and unmethylated DNA by using methylcytosine-sensitive restriction enzymes and tagged sequencing to map the fragments back to the genome (Hu et al. 2006). MSDK results in single base resolution but by definition is tailored to the specific restriction enzyme used, e.g. AscI.

Methylation analysis using microarrays consists of initial genomic fractionation followed by array-based sequence identification and quantification. There are three common approaches used to fractionate the genome into methylated, unmethylated, and total DNA fractions: (1) methylation sensitive restriction enzymes such as McrBC, (2) immunoprecipitation using a 5-methylctosine antibody and (3) affinity purification using methyl-binding domain proteins. A model for restriction enzyme-based fractionation methods is McrBC. In comparison to most methyl-sensitive enzymes, McrBC is particularly useful because it recognizes nearly half of all methylated sites in the genome (Sutherland et al. 1992), and includes all CpG islands while most other enzymes are only capable of recognizing a small percent of all possible CpG sites in the human genome. For each sample being analyzed, genomic DNA (gDNA) is split into two fractions, one is digested with McrBC and the other is untreated. High molecular weight gel purification of treated and untreated fractions is performed, DNA is size selected (1.5-3.0kb), and unmethylated (treated) and total genomic DNA (untreated) fractions are obtained. These two fractions are differentially labeled, using cyanin-3 (Cy3) and cyanin-5 (Cy5), and hybridized to high-density microarrays for comparison. Methylcytosine DNA immunoprecipitation (MeDIP) uses an antibody specific for 5-methylcytosine followed by a precipitation procedure to purify methylated DNA from the genome. Immunoprecipitated and total genomic DNA input fractions are comparatively hybridized to microarrays using two dye, Cy3 and Cy5, differential labeling (Weber et al. 2005). A third method for fractionation of genomic DNA into methylated and unmethylated fractions exploits proteins containing methylated DNA binding domains (MBDs). Methyl binding domain protein based recovery (MIRA) uses the MBD2/MBD3L1 complex to isolate methylated DNA across CpG islands in the genome (Rauch and

Pfeifer 2005). Alternatively, CXXC affinity purification (CAP) utilizes the CXXC3 protein domain which has a high affinity for unmethylated CpGs, thus enriching for unmethylated sites across the genome (Illingworth et al. 2008). The coupling of these fractionation methods with hybridization to CpG island and promoter microarrays has resulted in the identification of novel hypermethylated and hypomethylated genes in various types of cancer.

A recent approach termed comprehensive high-throughput arrays for relative methylation (CHARM) has been described and is impartial to fractionation method used. One of the two key components of CHARM is the use of a novel tiling array design which maximizes the number of CpG sites measured on a single array. (Irizarry et al. 2008). Methylation status of neighboring CpGs is often correlated (Eckhardt et al. 2006), therefore CHARM averages small continuous regions represented on the tiling array using genome-weighted smoothing to correct for CpG density and fragment length biases (Irizarry et al. 2008). This approach has proven successful with restriction-enzyme based fractionation methods, HELP and McrBC, as well as 5-methylcytosone immunoprecipitation, MeDIP (Irizarry et al. 2008).

The most widely used genomic technique to measure histone tail modifications and chromatin associated proteins is chromatin immunoprecipitation (ChIP) followed by DNA microarray hybridization, also known as ChIP-chip (Callinan and Feinberg 2006). The first step in this method is crosslinking cellular DNA with associated proteins, *in vivo*, using formaldehyde. This is followed by DNA sonication to randomly fragment the DNA/protein complexes into an appropriate size range, usually 200–1000 bp. Next, immunoprecipitation is performed using an antibody that specifically recognizes the histone modification or nuclear protein of interest. Lastly, the immunoprecipitated fraction undergoes reverse crosslinking and the DNA is purified and hybridized to a microarray containing known probes for location identification. One drawback to this approach is that it requires *a priori* knowledge about what part of the genome should be synthesized on a microarray. A variation on ChIP-chip is ChIP-seq, an unbiased yet costly approach in which immunoprecipitated DNA is sequenced and aligned back to the genome.

5 The Cancer Methylome

With the recent development of whole genome appoaches to examine the epigenome, investigators have begun to examine the landscape of the human cancer methylome. Utilization of promoter and CpG island microarrays following various fractionation techniques resulted in the identification of numerous novel sites of CpG hypermethylation across the genome in various types of tumors. For example, using a CpG island recovery assay and tiling arrays, it was shown that *HOX* gene clusters in primary adenocarcinomas of the lung are preferentially hypermethylated (Rauch et al. 2006; Rauch et al. 2007). HOX genes are important in regulation of gene transcription, differentiation, and development and in controlling cell growth (Cillo et al. 1999); therefore hypermethylation of CpG islands associated with *HOX* genes may be involved in the dysregulation of these cellular functions in cancer.

A second lung cancer study, performed using methyl-sensitive restriction enzyme-based microarray analysis and cell lines, showed 5.7% of gene promoters across the genome are hypermethylated, higher than previously predicted with single gene studies (Hatada et al. 2006). In addition to lung cancer, several CpG islands with hypermethylation in colorectal cancer compared to normal were newly identified using a methylated CpG island fractionation method and CpG island microarrays. A few of the newly identified hypermethylated genes include *DUSP4*, a negative regulator of the MAP kinase family of genes that are associated with cellular differential and proliferation, and *BTG2*, involved in G1/S cell cycle transition (Estecio et al. 2007). It is clear from the functions of these genes they play a key role in differentiation, proliferation, and cell growth thus inappropriate methylation is likely to contribute to dysregulation of these processes in cancer.

Not only has epigenomic technology led to the discovery of numerous new hypermethylated promoters but has also led to the discovery of novel hypomethylated gene promoters and CpG islands. While most promoters and associated CpG islands are unmethylated in normal somatic tissues, 4-8% are normally methylated in at least one type of tissue (Shen et al. 2007; Illingworth et al. 2008). Hypomethylation of normally methylated promoters has been observed in cell lines from 13 different types of common tumors (Shen et al. 2007) and in lung cancer 0.6% of promoters demonstrate loss of methylation in normally methylated promoter regions (Hatada et al. 2006). Both spermatogenesis and oogenesis specific basic helix-loop-helix 2, *SOHLH2*, and ferritin mitochondrial, *FTMT*, gene promoters were hypomethylated in 13 different tumor types including breast, melanoma, leukemia, prostate, and lung compared to their normal counterparts (Shen et al. 2007). The use of promoter and CpG island microarrays has lead to the identification of several novel hyper- and hypomethylated sites across the genome.

In addition to using epigenomic technologies for discovery of genome-wide methylation alterations, DNAm profiles from CpG island and promoter microarrays have been used to classify tumor subtypes. Using microarray-based approach, two subtypes of leukemia, acute myeloid leukemia (AML) and acute lymphoblastic leukemia (ALL), were differentiated from one another using the methylation status of ~250 CpG sites (Scholz et al. 2005). Similarly, methylation signatures obtained using the HELP assay, a methyl-specific restriction enzyme based fractionation method followed by promoter array hybridization, showed distinct DNAm profiles for AML and ALL (Figueroa et al. 2008).

The recent recognition and appreciation of the role tumor microenvironment plays in carcinogenesis combined with high-throughput approaches facilitating measurement of DNAm in multiple samples has led to epigenomic analysis of not only cancerous cells but of the non-malignant cells comprising the tumor microenvironment. Analysis of normal breast epithelium, myoepithelium, fibroblasts and in situ ductal or invasive carcinoma from the same individuals using MSDK demonstrated epigenetic abnormalities in all 3 non-malignant cell types of the breast cancer microenvironment (Hu et al. 2005). Similarly, runt-related transcription factor 3 (*RUNX3*), a tumor suppressor gene frequently silenced in cancer, is aberrantly hypermethylated in the surrounding normal breast epithelia of individuals with breast cancer than that of normal individuals (Cheng et al. 2008), highlighting the existence of epigenetic lesions in the "normal" tumor microenvironment. In addition, different environmental exposure of progenitor cells has shown stable inheritance of DNA methylation alterations in differentiated daughter cells. For example, in-vitro differentiation of normal breast progenitor cells, exposed to estrogen, into breast epithelial cells showed 0.5% of CpG islands in the differentiated cells are hypermethylated in epithelial progeny of exposed progenitors in comparison to unexposed progenitor derived epithelial cells (Cheng et al. 2008). These studies demonstrate important changes in the epigenome occur in the "normal" tumor microenvironment early in carcinogenesis, are stably inherited, and may result in an increased population of epigenetically modified cells in an otherwise normal tissue.

6 Genome-Wide Chromatin Aberrations in Human Malignancy

In addition to aberrant DNA methylation, alteration of chromatin modifying enzymes and histone tail modifications are associated with numerous human malignancies. Until recently, examination of histone tail modifications and histone modifying enzymes was limited to small numbers of genes due to the lack of high-throughput, sensitive, specific, and cost-effective methods available. However, with the development of ChIP-chip and ChIP-seq assays, investigators can now study chromatin and chromatin associated proteins at the genomic level, providing a comprehensive picture of chromatin aberrations in cancer.

The ability to determine patient outcome is often an important clinical tool in oncology. Using ChIP-chip to measure H3K27 trimethylation, a genome-wide signature for men with prostate cancer was defined and proven predictive of patient outcome in terms of survival time (Yu et al. 2007). In addition, an increase in histone H3K27 trimethylation at genes responsible for pluripotency of progenitor cells was observed in men with metastatic disease and poor prognosis (Yu et al. 2007) while men with a good prognosis did not show increased H3K27me3 in these genes.

Epigenomic analysis of histone tail modifications has also shown correlation of specific histone marks and chromatin modifying enzymes with known chromosomal abnormalities such as deletions and translocations, common in leukemia. One particular histone modification, H3K4 trimethylation, is frequently observed near breakpoints in T-cell lymphomas that have undergone translocation events (Barski et al. 2007). Acute promyelocytic leukemia is cytogenetically characterized by a translocation between the promyelocytic (*PML*) and retinoic acid receptor alpha (*RARA*) genes on chromosomes 15 and 17 respectively. The resultant fusion protein, a transcription factor, binds target genes such as CDKN1A, an important cell cycle checkpoint protein, and recruits the histone deacetylase HDAC1. In addition to acetylation changes, target genes of the fusion transcription factor have increased histone H3 lysine 4 and 9 trimethylation. The loss of histone H3 acetylation coupled with gain of H3K4 and H3K9 trimethylation involves chromatin remodeling to a closed transcriptional state (Hoemme et al. 2008).

Using high-performance liquid chromatography (HPLC), high-performance capillary electrophoresis, (HPCE) and liquid chromatography–electrospray mass spectrometry, (LC-ES/MS) techniques, overall cellular levels of histone modifications can be determined. Examination of histone H4 marks in human normal and cancer cells showed an overall loss of lysine 20 trimethylation and lysine 16 monoacetylation in Jurkat cell lines (Fraga et al. 2005). Although individual loci cannot be identified using this approach, it provides a useful global look at histone tail modifications and how they differ in cancer cells. Epigenomic studies of chromatin marks and associated proteins have begun to offer a new understanding of human malignancy.

References

Arisan, S., E. D. Buyuktuncer, et al. (2005). "Increased expression of EZH2, a polycomb group protein, in bladder carcinoma." *Urol Int* **75**(3): 252–7.
Ballestar, E., M. F. Paz, et al. (2003). "Methyl-CpG binding proteins identify novel sites of epigenetic inactivation in human cancer." *EMBO J* **22**(23): 6335–45.
Barski, A., S. Cuddapah, et al. (2007). "High-resolution profiling of histone methylations in the human genome." *Cell* **129**(4): 823–37.
Bibikova, M., Z. Lin, et al. (2006). "High-throughput DNA methylation profiling using universal bead arrays." *Genome Res* **16**(3): 383–93.
Callinan, P. A. and A. P. Feinberg (2006). "The emerging science of epigenomics." *Hum Mol Genet* **15 Spec No 1**: R95–101.
Cheng, A. S., A. C. Culhane, et al. (2008). "Epithelial progeny of estrogen-exposed breast progenitor cells display a cancer-like methylome." *Cancer Res* **68**(6): 1786–96.
Cho, B., H. Lee, et al. (2003). "Promoter hypomethylation of a novel cancer/testis antigen gene CAGE is correlated with its aberrant expression and is seen in premalignant stage of gastric carcinoma." *Biochem Biophys Res Commun* **307**(1): 52–63.
Cillo, C., A. Faiella, et al. (1999). "Homeobox genes and cancer." *Exp Cell Res* **248**(1): 1–9.
Clark, S. J. and J. Melki (2002). "DNA methylation and gene silencing in cancer: which is the guilty party?" *Oncogene* **21**(35): 5380–7.
Costello, J. F., M. C. Fruhwald, et al. (2000). "Aberrant CpG-island methylation has non-random and tumour-type-specific patterns." *Nat Genet* **24**(2): 132–8.
Croonquist, P. A. and B. Van Ness (2005). "The polycomb group protein enhancer of zeste homolog 2 (EZH 2) is an oncogene that influences myeloma cell growth and the mutant ras phenotype." *Oncogene* **24**(41): 6269–80.
Eads, C. A., K. D. Danenberg, et al. (2000). "MethyLight: a high-throughput assay to measure DNA methylation." *Nucleic Acids Res* **28**(8): E32.
Eckhardt, F., J. Lewin, et al. (2006). "DNA methylation profiling of human chromosomes 6, 20 and 22." *Nat Genet* **38**(12): 1378–85.
Ehrbrecht, A., U. Muller, et al. (2006). "Comprehensive genomic analysis of desmoplastic medulloblastomas: identification of novel amplified genes and separate evaluation of the different histological components." *J Pathol* **208**(4): 554–63.
Estecio, M. R., P. S. Yan, et al. (2007). "High-throughput methylation profiling by MCA coupled to CpG island microarray." *Genome Res* **17**(10): 1529–36.
Fahrner, J. A., S. Eguchi, et al. (2002). "Dependence of histone modifications and gene expression on DNA hypermethylation in cancer." *Cancer Res* **62**(24): 7213–8.
Feinberg, A. P. and B. Tycko (2004). "The history of cancer epigenetics." *Nat Rev Cancer* **4**(2): 143–53.

Feinberg, A. P. and B. Vogelstein (1983). "Hypomethylation distinguishes genes of some human cancers from their normal counterparts." *Nature* **301**(5895): 89–92.

Figueroa, M. E., M. Reimers, et al. (2008). "An integrative genomic and epigenomic approach for the study of transcriptional regulation." *PLoS ONE* **3**(3): e1882.

Fraga, M. F., E. Ballestar, et al. (2005). "Loss of acetylation at Lys16 and trimethylation at Lys20 of histone H4 is a common hallmark of human cancer." *Nat Genet* **37**(4): 391–400.

Gama-Sosa, M. A., V. A. Slagel, et al. (1983). "The 5-methylcytosine content of DNA from human tumors." *Nucleic Acids Res* **11**(19): 6883–94.

Guidi, C. J., A. T. Sands, et al. (2001). "Disruption of Ini1 leads to peri-implantation lethality and tumorigenesis in mice." *Mol Cell Biol* **21**(10): 3598–603.

Hake, S. B., A. Xiao, et al. (2004). "Linking the epigenetic 'language' of covalent histone modifications to cancer." *Br J Cancer* **90**(4): 761–9.

Hatada, I., M. Fukasawa, et al. (2006). "Genome-wide profiling of promoter methylation in human." *Oncogene* **25**(21): 3059–64.

Herman, J. G., J. R. Graff, et al. (1996). "Methylation-specific PCR: a novel PCR assay for methylation status of CpG islands." *Proc Natl Acad Sci U S A* **93**(18): 9821–6.

Hoemme, C., A. Peerzada, et al. (2008). "Chromatin modifications induced by PML-RARalpha repress critical targets in leukemogenesis as analyzed by ChIP-Chip." *Blood* **111**(5): 2887–95.

Hu, M., J. Yao, et al. (2005). "Distinct epigenetic changes in the stromal cells of breast cancers." *Nat Genet* **37**(8): 899–905.

Hu, M., J. Yao, et al. (2006). "Methylation-specific digital karyotyping." *Nat Protoc* **1**(3): 1621–36.

Illingworth, R., A. Kerr, et al. (2008). "A novel CpG island set identifies tissue-specific methylation at developmental gene loci." *PLoS Biol* **6**(1): e22.

Irizarry, R. A., C. Ladd-Acosta, et al. (2008). "Comprehensive high-throughput arrays for relative methylation (CHARM)." *Genome Res* **18**(5): 780–90.

Italiano, A., R. Attias, et al. (2006). "Molecular cytogenetic characterization of a metastatic lung sarcomatoid carcinoma: 9p23 neocentromere and 9p23-p24 amplification including JAK2 and JMJD2C." *Cancer Genet Cytogenet* **167**(2): 122–30.

Kleer, C. G., Q. Cao, et al. (2003). "EZH2 is a marker of aggressive breast cancer and promotes neoplastic transformation of breast epithelial cells." *Proc Natl Acad Sci U S A* **100**(20): 11606–11.

Klochendler-Yeivin, A., L. Fiette, et al. (2000). "The murine SNF5/INI1 chromatin remodeling factor is essential for embryonic development and tumor suppression." *EMBO Rep* **1**(6): 500–6.

Mutskov, V. and G. Felsenfeld (2004). "Silencing of transgene transcription precedes methylation of promoter DNA and histone H3 lysine 9." *EMBO J* **23**(1): 138–49.

Nakamura, N. and K. Takenaga (1998). "Hypomethylation of the metastasis-associated S100A4 gene correlates with gene activation in human colon adenocarcinoma cell lines." *Clin Exp Metastasis* **16**(5): 471–9.

Rauch, T., H. Li, et al. (2006). "MIRA-assisted microarray analysis, a new technology for the determination of DNA methylation patterns, identifies frequent methylation of homeodomain-containing genes in lung cancer cells." *Cancer Res* **66**(16): 7939–47.

Rauch, T. and G. P. Pfeifer (2005). "Methylated-CpG island recovery assay: a new technique for the rapid detection of methylated-CpG islands in cancer." *Lab Invest* **85**(9): 1172–80.

Rauch, T., Z. Wang, et al. (2007). "Homeobox gene methylation in lung cancer studied by genome-wide analysis with a microarray-based methylated CpG island recovery assay." *Proc Natl Acad Sci U S A* **104**(13): 5527–32.

Roberts, C. W., S. A. Galusha, et al. (2000). "Haploinsufficiency of Snf5 (integrase interactor 1) predisposes to malignant rhabdoid tumors in mice." *Proc Natl Acad Sci U S A* **97**(25): 13796–800.

Rosty, C., T. Ueki, et al. (2002). "Overexpression of S100A4 in pancreatic ductal adenocarcinomas is associated with poor differentiation and DNA hypomethylation." *Am J Pathol* **160**(1): 45–50.

Scholz, C., I. Nimmrich, et al. (2005). "Distinction of acute lymphoblastic leukemia from acute myeloid leukemia through microarray-based DNA methylation analysis." *Ann Hematol* **84**(4): 236–44.

Shen, L., Y. Kondo, et al. (2007). "Genome-wide profiling of DNA methylation reveals a class of normally methylated CpG island promoters." *PLoS Genet* **3**(10): 2023–36.

Stirzaker, C., J. Z. Song, et al. (2004). "Transcriptional gene silencing promotes DNA hypermethylation through a sequential change in chromatin modifications in cancer cells." *Cancer Res* **64**(11): 3871–7.

Sutherland, E., L. Coe, et al. (1992). "McrBC: a multisubunit GTP-dependent restriction endonuclease." *J Mol Biol* **225**(2): 327–48.

Tokizane, T., H. Shiina, et al. (2005). "Cytochrome P450 1B1 is overexpressed and regulated by hypomethylation in prostate cancer." *Clin Cancer Res* **11**(16): 5793–801.

Tomonaga, T., K. Matsushita, et al. (2003). "Overexpression and mistargeting of centromere protein-A in human primary colorectal cancer." *Cancer Res* **63**(13): 3511–6.

Varambally, S., S. M. Dhanasekaran, et al. (2002). "The polycomb group protein EZH2 is involved in progression of prostate cancer." *Nature* **419**(6907): 624–9.

Versteege, I., N. Sevenet, et al. (1998). "Truncating mutations of hSNF5/INI1 in aggressive paediatric cancer." *Nature* **394**(6689): 203–6.

Visser, H. P., M. J. Gunster, et al. (2001). "The Polycomb group protein EZH2 is upregulated in proliferating, cultured human mantle cell lymphoma." *Br J Haematol* **112**(4): 950–8.

Wang, G. G., C. D. Allis, et al. (2007). "Chromatin remodeling and cancer, Part I: Covalent histone modifications." *Trends Mol Med* **13**(9): 363–72.

Wang, G. G., C. D. Allis, et al. (2007). "Chromatin remodeling and cancer, Part II: ATP-dependent chromatin remodeling." *Trends Mol Med* **13**(9): 373–80.

Weber, M., J. J. Davies, et al. (2005). "Chromosome-wide and promoter-specific analyses identify sites of differential DNA methylation in normal and transformed human cells." *Nat Genet* **37**(8): 853–62.

Wu, H., Y. Chen, et al. (2005). "Hypomethylation-linked activation of PAX2 mediates tamoxifen-stimulated endometrial carcinogenesis." *Nature* **438**(7070): 981–7.

Xie, R., D. S. Loose, et al. (2007). "Hypomethylation-induced expression of S100A4 in endometrial carcinoma." *Mod Pathol* **20**(10): 1045–54.

Yang, Z. Q., I. Imoto, et al. (2000). "Identification of a novel gene, GASC1, within an amplicon at 9p23–24 frequently detected in esophageal cancer cell lines." *Cancer Res* **60**(17): 4735–9.

Ye, L., X. Li, et al. (2005). "Hypomethylation in the promoter region of POMC gene correlates – with ectopic overexpression in thymic carcinoids." *J Endocrinol* **185**(2): 337–43.

Yu, J., D. R. Rhodes, et al. (2007). "A polycomb repression signature in metastatic prostate cancer predicts cancer outcome." *Cancer Res* **67**(22): 10657–63.

Epigenetic Modulation by Environmental Factors

Mark R. Doyle and Richard M. Amasino

1 Introduction

For most organisms the ability to properly sense and respond to environmental cues is critical for survival. Environmental cues come in many different forms. Some cues are cyclical such as those brought about by seasonal change. Because of their regularity and predictability, seasonal cues often play a major role in defining the behavior and life history strategies of organisms. Examples include hibernation and migration in animals and the control of flowering time in many plant species. Other environmental stimuli are erratic in nature. Conditions such as intense heat, cold, flood, or pathogen attack often occur rapidly and unpredictably, so organisms must possess response pathways that are equally as rapid to ensure survival. Given that plants are sessile, they cannot evade harsh environmental conditions. Thus, selection has favored plants which have become quite adept at both sensing and responding to a wide range of predictable and unpredictable changes in the environment.

There are many examples of changes in gene expression that occur in response to changes in the environment. Indeed, the advent of microarray technology has made it possible to catalog the genome-wide changes in steady-state mRNA levels that occur in response to environmental cues (for examples see the datasets available at http://www.arabidopsis.org/portals/expression/index.jsp). Many environmentally induced changes rapidly decay when the signal is no longer present. In contrast, there are situations in which environmental signals induce changes in gene expression that persist for long periods in the absence of the inducing signal. Such cases could be considered examples of epigenetic gene regulation. However there can be no clear line of demarcation to distinguish between transient and persistent. Here we focus on cases where an environmental signal leads to an altered state of gene expression that persists for the remainder of the life cycle of an organism in the absence of the signal.

The word 'epigenetics' was first used to describe the process of differentiation of cellular states during development. Not surprisingly, there are several examples of

---

M.R. Doyle (✉)
Department of Biochemistry, University of Wisconsin-Madison, Madison, WI USA

epigenetic changes in gene expression that are stimulated by developmental cues. One of the best studied examples is the regulation of homeotic gene transcription by polycomb group (PcG) and trithorax group (TrxG) proteins in Drosophila. During embryo development, a series of events occur that define the identity of body segments through the patterned expression of homeotic genes. Perpetuation of homeotic gene expression patterns is essential for development. However, the signals that establish the differential expression of these genes are short lived. It is the role of PcG and TrxG genes to maintain the necessary expression patterns in the absence of developmental cues (Ringrose and Paro 2004). Thus, in Drosophila embryo development, internal cues establish a gene expression pattern that is then maintained epigenetically. There also exist similar examples of epigenetic gene regulation in which the cue is not developmental but environmental in origin. A classic example of this is the vernalization response of many plant species which is discussed below.

2 Epigenetic Programming by Environmental Factors

2.1 *Vernalization*

A number of plant species use prolonged periods of cold temperature as a signal to control the switch from vegetative to reproductive growth through a process known as vernalization. (Henderson et al. 2003, Sung and Amasino 2005). A vernalization requirement in many species is likely to be an adaptation that enables plants to avoid competition with summer-growing species. Vernalization-requiring plants typically become established in the fall season, over-winter and then flower rapidly upon the commencement of spring. Vernalized plants often complete their life cycle before other summer-growing species begin to compete with them (for additional reviews on vernalization see (Dennis and Peacock 2007, Henderson and Dean 2004, Schmitz and Amasino 2007, Sung and Amasino 2005)).

In addition to vernalization, many plants use the relative length of day and night (i.e. photoperiod) as an environmental cue to trigger flowering (Kobayashi and Weigel 2007). In general, plants that respond to photoperiod can be placed into two categories: long-day plants which flower in response to lengthening periods of daylight, and short-day plants which flower in response to lengthening periods of darkness. The response to photoperiod is often quite rapid with flowers being initiated by exposure to just one or two days of the appropriate length. Exposure to the appropriate number of inductive daylengths leads to the production of florigen, a mobile signal that induces flowering. In *Arabidopsis*, florigen appears to be the FLOWERING LOCUS T (FT) protein (reviewed in (Kobayashi and Weigel 2007)). Leaf tissue is the primary source of florigen. Once produced, florigen must move to the shoot apical meristem, the site of flower formation. In *Arabidopsis*, vernalization is responsible for making the meristem competent to respond to FT, and for the ability of young leaves to produce a sufficient amount of FT to trigger rapid flowering (Searle et al. 2006).

Once plants acquire the competence to flower through vernalization, the competent state is most often maintained in the absence of cold. Thus, plants can "remember" prior periods of cold exposure. This was clearly demonstrated in work by Lang and Melchers using a biennial strain of henbane (*Hyoscyamus niger*) which required vernalization followed by long days for flowering to occur. Given this dual requirement, vernalized plants transferred to short days did not flower. However, transfer of these plants to long days, even after extensive periods of growth in short days, resulted in rapid flowering (Lang and Melchers 1947). This key result demonstrated that vernalized plants maintain a "memory" of prior cold exposure.

One fundamental difference between plants and animals is the ease with which plant cells dedifferentiate into cells that can then be used to regenerate entire plants. Using this regenerative ability of plants, another classic experiment showed that mitotically active regions of plants are those that become vernalized. Following a cold-treatment, cells from various tissues of *Lunaria biennis* were used to regenerate plants. Plants regenerated from mitotically active tissue resembled vernalized plants whereas those regenerated from mitotically inactive tissues (such as from an expanded leaf) behaved as if they had never seen cold (Wellensiek 1962, 1964). Recent work has corroborated these results by showing that many of the molecular signatures of vernalization (see below) occur only in mitotically active regions of *Arabidopsis thaliana* (Finnegan and Dennis 2007).

Although the phenomenology is similar, there is considerable variation in both the optimal temperature and the duration of cold needed for the vernalization response in different species (Reeves et al. 2007, Sung and Amasino 2005, Trevaskis et al. 2007). At a molecular level it is also clear that different species have co-opted different genes to regulate flowering time via vernalization (Amasino et al. 2004). The discussion below focuses on work done in the model *Arabidopsis thaliana*. Thus, it is important to note that many of the mechanistic details discussed here may not apply to all plants.

With regards to flowering, different accessions of Arabidopsis range from winter-annuals to summer-annuals. Winter-annual accessions require vernalization for rapid flowering whereas summer-annual accessions do not possess such a requirement. The source of the variation between summer- and winter-annual accessions turned out to be genetically tractable. Crosses between summer- and winter-annual accessions revealed that two dominant loci were responsible for the vernalization requirement, *FRIGIDA* (*FRI*) and *FLOWERING LOCUS C* (*FLC*) (Koornneef et al. 1994, Lee et al. 1993, 1994, Napp-Zinn 1979) (Fig. 1).

In general, rapid-flowering accessions contain one of several mutations in *FRI* (Gazzani et al. 2003, Le Corre et al. 2002, Shindo et al. 2005, Werner et al. 2005). A few accessions which are rapid flowering due to weak alleles of *FLC* have also been described (Michaels et al. 2003). *FRI* encodes a gene of unknown function (Johanson et al. 2000). *FLC* encodes a MADS-box transcription factor that is sufficient to substantially delay flowering (Michaels and Amasino 2001, Sheldon et al. 1999). The cloning of *FLC* provided the first molecular insight into the mechanism of vernalization. Plants containing a functional *FRI* gene are late-flowering due to enhanced expression of *FLC* (Fig. 2). Upon vernalization *FLC* expression

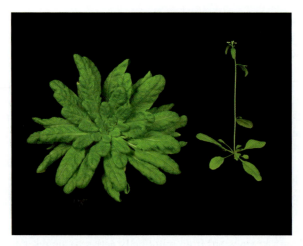

Fig. 1 Variation in flowering time in *Arabidopsis thaliana*. Both of the plants pictured here were grown under identical conditions that did not include cold treatment. The plant on the left behaves as a winter-annual and contains an active allele of *FRIGIDA* (*FRI*) which elevates the expression level of *FLOWERING LOCUS C* (*FLC*). Flowering in *FRI*-containing plants is delayed unless plants experience cold temperature capable of inducing vernalization. The plant on the right carries a mutation in *FRI*. In such plants *FLC* is not induced and plants flowers rapidly without cold

is down-regulated. Following cold treatment, low *FLC* levels are maintained and remain low throughout the rest of the plant's life cycle (Michaels and Amasino 2001, Sheldon et al. 1999).

As noted above, classic studies showed that the vernalized state was maintained following cold exposure suggesting that vernalization occurred via an epigenetic mechanism. The cloning of *FLC* provided a molecular entrée into the mechanism which involves vernalization-induced chromatin modifications.

Much of the progress in understanding vernalization has had a foundation in mutant screens using a parental line that exhibits delayed flowering without cold treatment. One class of mutants flowered rapidly without vernalization and could be placed in one of several classes: alleles of *FLC*, *FRI* or genes involved in *FRI* function, and genes that promote *FLC* transcription in general. In a second class were vernalization-insensitive mutants which flowered late following cold treatment. Not surprisingly, many of the genes identified from both sets of screens were homologous to proteins that modify chromatin.

2.2 FLC Activation

Several histone modifications have been identified that co-localize with regions of active transcription in a range of eukaryotes (Li et al. 2007). Several of these modifications, which include methylation of histone H3 on lysines 4 and 36 (H3K4me and H3K36me), are found at *FLC* when *FLC* is activated. In yeast the Paf1 complex associates with RNA polII and the histone methyltransferases SET1 and SET2

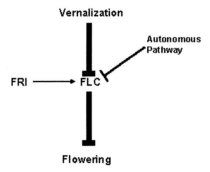

Fig. 2 Hierarchy of *FLC* regulation in *Arabidopsis*. *FLC*, a strong repressor of flowering, is under the control of several pathways. The thickness of the symbol extending from each pathway represents the relative strength of that pathway in the regulation of *FLC*. (1). The autonomous pathway collectively represses *FLC* expression which results in rapid flowering. (2). A functional *FRI*-pathway overrides the repressive ability of the autonomous pathway leading to elevated levels of *FLC* and delayed flowering. This *FRI*-mediated elevation in *FLC* levels is the molecular basis of the vernalization-responsive delay in flowering seen in winter-annual accessions of Arabidopsis. (3). Periods of cold temperatures that result in vernalization are able to repress *FLC* expression in the presence of *FRI*. Prior to cold exposure, *FLC* chromatin contains several histone modifications that are characteristic of active chromatin including methylation of H3K4, and H3K36 and acetylation of H3. After vernalization-mediated repression, the state of *FLC* chromatin changes. Other modifications that are characteristic of silenced chromatin appear including de-acetylation and methylation of H3K9, H3K27, and sH4R3

(Betz et al. 2002, Ng et al. 2003). This results in a record of transcription in the histone code through the deposition of methylation at H3K4 and H3K36. Screens for early-flowering mutants identified several proteins that resemble components of the yeast Paf1 complex. Arabidopsis Paf complex mutants (*elf7*, *elf8*, *vips*) suppress *FLC*-mediated late flowering and display decreased levels of H3K4me at *FLC* (He et al. 2004, Oh et al. 2004).

If the Arabidopsis Paf1 complex functions like yeast Paf1, it must associate with a protein that possesses histone methyltransferase activity. A potential candidate is the SET-domain protein *EFS* (also known as SDG8) (Kim et al. 2005, Zhao et al. 2005). Mutations in *efs* result in early flowering and a decrease in histone methylation at *FLC*; one study reported a decrease in H3K4me (Kim et al. 2005) whereas another study reported a decrease in H3K36me (Zhao et al. 2005).

Another type of chromatin modification involves the incorporation of histone variants into nucleosomes (see Chapter "Epigenetic Profiling of Histone Variants"). A variant form of histone H2A, H2AZ, is often found in regions of active transcription (Santisteban et al. 2000). The presence of H2AZ is thought not to induce transcription *per se*, but instead to poise genes for activation. A chromatin remodeling complex, SWR1, acts to incorporate H2AZ (Kobor et al. 2004, Mizuguchi et al. 2004). As with Paf1, mutants in Arabidopsis SWR1 components are unable to upregulate *FLC* (Choi et al. 2005, 2007, Deal et al. 2005, March-Diaz et al. 2007, Noh and Amasino 2003). Arabidopsis SWR1 components include the genes *PHOTOPERIOD INDEPENDENT EARLY FLOWERING1* (*PIE1*), *ACTIN-RELATED*

PROTEIN6 (*ARP6*), *SERRATED LEAVES AND EARLY FLOWERING* (*SEF*). Several studies have shown that *PIE1*, *ARP6*, and *SEF* interact with one another (Choi et al. 2007, March-Diaz et al. 2007). Arabidopsis contains three homologs of H2AZ all of which interact with SWR1 components (Choi et al. 2007). ChIP studies using an H2AZ-specific antibody revealed enrichment of H2AZ at the 5' and 3' ends of *FLC* in wild type but not in *arp6* or *pie1* mutants (Deal et al. 2007).

It is important to note that components of the Arabidopsis Paf1 and SWR1 complexes do more than activate *FLC*. Mutants in both complexes flower more rapidly than *flc* null mutants. This is due to misregulation of other genes involved in the control of flowering time (He et al. 2004, Kim et al. 2005). Other pleiotropic phenotypes have also been observed in Paf1/SWR mutants including aberrations in leave shape, flower size, and floral organ number (Choi et al. 2005, 2007, Deal et al. 2005, He et al. 2004, March-Diaz et al. 2007, Noh and Amasino 2003, Oh et al. 2004).

The biochemical function of *FRI* is still unknown. However, additional genes have been isolated that may work in conjunction with *FRI* to up-regulate *FLC*. These genes include *FRI-LIKE 1* (*FRL1*), *FRIGIDA-ESSENTIAL-1* (*FES1*) and *SUPPRESSOR-OF-FRIGIDA-4* (*SUF4*) (Kim et al. 2006, Kim and Michaels 2006, Michaels et al. 2004, Schmitz et al. 2005). Mutations in any one of these genes results in complete suppression of the delayed flowering that results from *FRI*-mediated activation of *FLC*. Genetic and biochemical studies suggest that these proteins exist in a complex (Kim et al. 2006, Schmitz et al. 2005). Like *FRI*, *FRL1* does not contain any signatures that point to a particular biochemical function (Michaels et al. 2004). *FES1* contains a CCCH Zn finger domain, but the function of this domain within *FES1* is unknown (Schmitz et al. 2005). *SUF4*, however, contains a C2H2-type zinc finger domain and has been shown to associate with *FLC* chromatin (Kim et al. 2004). Thus, it is possible that *SUF4* confers sequence specificity for the association of a *FRI*-containing complex with *FLC*.

2.3 Endogenous FLC Repression

The autonomous pathway has been defined as a group of genes that act to repress *FLC* (Henderson and Dean 2004) (Fig. 2). Autonomous-pathway mutants are delayed in flowering and are responsive to vernalization. Although the mutants have a very similar phenotype, the genes that comprise the autonomous pathway appear to be quite diverse in function. Several of these genes including *FPA, FCA, FY, LD*, and *FLK* have not to date been shown to be involved in chromatin modification at *FLC* and will thus not be discussed further.

The *FLD* and *FVE* genes repress *FLC* through a chromatin-based mechanism. In *fld* and *fve* mutants, levels of an active chromatin mark, acetylation on histone H3, increases at *FLC* (Ausin et al. 2004, He et al. 2003). Consistent with the mutant phenotype, *FVE* encodes a protein with homology to the yeast MSI protein and the mammalian retinoblastoma-associated proteins RbAp46 and RbAp48 which function in histone deacetylase complexes (HDACs) (Ausin et al. 2004, Kim et al. 2004). *FLD* encodes an Arabidopsis relative of Human Lysine-Specific Demethylase1

(*LSD1*) (Jiang et al. 2007). *FLD* and *FLD*-like genes in Arabidopsis are likely to demethylate H3K4 at *FLC* and other loci and likely work in conjunction with HDAC complexes.

2.4 Repression of FLC by Vernalization

In *Arabidopsis*, downregulation of *FLC* is quantitative in nature with shorter periods of cold repressing *FLC* to a lesser extent than longer periods (Sheldon et al. 2006, Sung and Amasino 2004) (Fig. 2). Forty days of cold treatment nearly saturates vernalization with respect to down-regulation of *FLC* in most accessions of *Arabidopsis*. During cold exposure, *FLC* chromatin undergoes modification. Histone H3 acetylation, a mark often associated with active chromatin, decreases. Conversely, increases in methylation at H3K9 and H3K27 (H3K9me and H3K27me) are observed (Bastow et al. 2004, Sung and Amasino 2004). These marks are typically associated with inactive chromatin. Accumulation of H3K27me3 initiates within the 5' region of the *FLC* gene and then spreads throughout the length of the gene following cold exposure (Finnegan and Dennis 2007).

Screens for mutants that fail to repress *FLC* upon cold treatment led to the discovery of several genes involved in vernalization. *VERNALIZATION 2* (*VRN2*) is required for maintaining low levels of *FLC* expression following cold. In *vrn2* mutants, *FLC* expression decreases in response to cold, but elevated expression levels return in the absence of cold (Gendall et al. 2001). *VRN2* encodes an ortholog of Su(z)12, a component of polycomb repressive complex 2 (PRC2) in Drosophila. In PRC2, Su(z)12 interacts with E(z), a histone methyl transferase with specificity for methylation of H3K27 (Czermin et al. 2002, Muller et al. 2002) (See Chapter "Polycomb Complexes and the Role of Epigenetic Memory in Development"). Likewise, in Arabidopsis, *VRN2* appears to interact with E(z) homologs and is required for H3K27 methylation at *FLC* during vernalization (Bastow et al. 2004, Sung and Amasino 2004, Wood et al. 2006).

Mutants in another gene, *VERNALIZATION 1* (*VRN1*), behave similarly to *vrn2* with regards to *FLC* expression; *FLC* repression is not maintained following cold exposure (Levy et al. 2002). In *vrn2* mutants both H3K9me and H3K27me fail to accumulate during cold treatment; however, in *vrn1* mutants only H3K9me fails to accumulate (Bastow et al. 2004, Sung and Amasino 2004). This suggests that *VRN1* is necessary to maintain levels of H3K9 methylation and likely acts downstream of a plant PRC2-like complex.

In Drosophila and mammals, the H3K27me3 mark is deposited by PRC2 and is then bound by the chromodomain of Polycomb, a component of polycomb repressive complex 1 (PRC1) (Schwartz and Pirrotta 2007). Although plants contain homologs of all components of PRC2, plants do not contain homologs of Polycomb or other members of PRC1. Recent work has shown that the Arabidopsis homolog of HETEROCHROMATIN PROTEIN 1 (HP1), LIKE-HETEROCHROMATIN PROTEIN 1 (LHP1), associates with H3K27me3 and may, therefore, carry out a PRC1-like function (Turck et al. 2007, Zhang et al. 2007). Consistent with this idea, mutants in *lhp1*, like *vrn1* and *vrn2* mutants, are unable to maintain low levels of *FLC* following cold (Mylne et al. 2006, Sung et al. 2006).

Given the epigenetic nature of vernalization and *FLC* repression, it is not surprising that chromatin-modifying proteins such as PRC2 and HP1 homologs play a role in this process. However, many of these proteins are involved in other developmental processes and appear to be expressed without prior cold treatment. Therefore, one or more components should exist that act either directly or indirectly to recruit these factors to *FLC* in a cold-dependent manner. One such component is *VERNALIZATION INSENSITIVE 3* (*VIN3*) (Sung and Amasino 2004). *VIN3* encodes a protein with a plant homeodomain (PHD). This domain is often found in proteins that interact with other chromatin-remodeling proteins. In *vrn1* and *vrn2* mutants *FLC* repression is not maintained following vernalization. In *vin3* mutants *FLC* repression is not initiated and neither H3K9me nor H3K27me accumulation occurs (Sung et al. 2006).

Additional characteristics of *VIN3* further support its role as an initiator of vernalization. First, expression of *VIN3* occurs only during a period of cold that is capable of causing vernalization, and *VIN3* expression rapidly ceases when plants are no longer exposed to cold (Sung and Amasino 2004). In addition *VIN3* has been shown to interact with *VRN2* and other PRC2 components in a high molecular weight complex, and complex formation is partially dependent on temperature (Wood et al. 2006).

VIN3 belongs to a small gene family in Arabidopsis, and a family of *VIN3*-like genes is present in all sequenced flowering plant species. Mutations in a homolog of *VIN3*, *VIN3-LIKE 1* (*VIL1*, also known as *VRN5*) also results in vernalization insensitivity (Greb et al. 2007, Sung et al. 2006). In addition to *VIN3* and *VIL1* being in the same pathway genetically, they also interact in yeast 2-hybrid assays (Greb et al. 2007, Sung et al. 2006). However, *VIL1* expression is not regulated by vernalization, and *VIL1*, unlike *VIN3* is also involved in the photoperiod response (Sung et al. 2006). Collectively, the *VIN3* family appears to be a family of plant-specific chromatin modifiers which may act combinatorially to regulate various processes in plants. In addition the interaction between *VIN3* and the *VRN2*-containing PRC2 complex indicates that the roles of *VIN3*-like genes may involve PRC2-mediated repression of target genes (Wood et al. 2006).

Recently it has been shown that mutations in the Arabidopsis symmetric arginine methyltransferase *AtPRMT5* (also known as *SKB1*) causes late flowering due to elevated levels of *FLC*, and thus *atprmt5* mutants behave like autonomous-pathway mutants (Pei et al. 2007, Wang et al. 2007). However, there are conflicting reports as to whether or not symmetric methylation on lysine 3 of histone H4 (sH4R3me) levels vary between mutant and wild type at *FLC* chromatin. Late-flowering in *AtPRMT5* mutants is fully responsive to vernalization (Pei et al. 2007, Wang et al. 2007) in a Columbia background. However, when the mutant is combined with *FRI*, plants are late flowering even after vernalization (Schmitz et al. 2008). In addition sH4R3 accumulates at *FLC* following cold exposure, and this sH4R3 mark seems to be required for H3K27 methylation at *FLC* in vernalized plants (Schmitz et al. 2008).

Using vernalization in Arabidopsis as a model for the study of epigenetic gene regulation has several advantages. Arabidopsis mutants in many genes involved in chromatin modification are viable which is often not the case in other systems. Second, *FLC*, the primary target of vernalization, appears to be uniquely sensitive to many of these mutations making it an ideal locus for the study of histone modifications. Finally, the fact that the chromatin state at *FLC* is determined by an environmental cue makes it possible to manipulate the state of *FLC* chromatin in the laboratory in a controlled manner.

Many questions remain regarding the molecular mechanisms of vernalization. At our current level of understanding, vernalization begins with the cold-induced expression of *VIN3*. Presumably, *VIN3* is a critical component of a vernalization-specific chromatin-modifying complex that targets *FLC*. Although many components downstream of *VIN3* have been identified, little is known about the actual cold-sensing apparatus that results in *VIN3* induction. Finally, if epigenetic regulation of *FLC* is to occur in subsequent generations, there must exist a resetting mechanism which restores *FLC* chromatin to a pre-vernalized state. The exact developmental phase at which this resetting occurs as well as the underlying molecular mechanism for resetting remains elusive.

3 Maternal Care in Rats

Mechanistically the vernalization response in *Arabidopsis thaliana* is probably the most thoroughly studied case of epigenetic modulation by an environmental signal. However, similar phenomenology has been described in other systems. One such example deals with stress behavior in rats. The environmental signal in this instance is the quality of maternal care given to newborns.

After birth, mother-pup interactions include several quantifiable behaviors such as licking, grooming (LG) and arched-back nursing (ABN). During the first week after birth, natural variation in mother-pup interaction can be classified as either high LG-ABN or low LG-ABN. Following the first week there is no measurable difference in maternal behavior (Meaney 2001).

Stress response and maternal care behaviors in rats can be perpetuated from generation to generation. High and low LG-ABN mothers rear pups that show reduced and enhanced responses to stress respectively. Stress responses can be measured through behavioral assays such as the amount of time rats spend exploring a novel environment or by the relative change in stress-induced hormones while animals are constrained. In addition to stress response behavior, new mothers adopt the type of maternal care that they received as pups. The transmission of these behaviors from mother to pup probably has adaptive value as it may serve to prepare young rats for the type of environmental conditions that may be present outside the relative safety of the nest (Meaney 2001).

Perpetuation of maternal care and stress response behaviors occurs via an epigenetic mechanism. Pup swapping experiments revealed that these behaviors were acquired based on the type of maternal care received. Pups with low LG-ABN biological mothers that were reared by high LG-ABN surrogates acquired high LG-ABN characteristics. The converse was also shown to be true (Francis et al. 1999). Thus, as with vernalization, this system is one in which the effects of an environmental signal persist in the absence of that signal for the remainder of the life cycle of that organism.

The epigenetic nature of the maternal care response is quite clear. In addition there is also data consistent with a putative molecular mechanism to account for this epigenetic phenomenon. Given the effect of maternal care on stress responses, a reasonable candidate for a molecular target of maternal care is the glucocorticoid receptor (GR). Indeed GR expression correlates well with LG-ABN and stress response behaviors (Liu et al. 1997). Individuals reared in a high LG-ABN environment show increased GR expression. High GR expression in the hippocampus leads to increased feedback sensitivity to glucocorticoids and an attenuated stress response (Liu et al. 1997). Thus, as is the case for *FLC* in vernalization, GR expression may be affected by environmental sensing.

The GR gene was analyzed for changes in epigenetic signatures between high- and low-LG-ABN individuals. It was found that DNA methylation at GR varies over developmental time with distinct patterns seen in low and high LG-ABN individuals (Weaver et al. 2004). In rats, DNA methylation in the GR promoter was relatively low prior to birth; however, levels increased in one-day-old pups. Variation in maternal care occurs during the first week following birth. Interestingly at day six low-LG-ABN pups maintained high levels of methylation where DNA methylation in high LG-ABN pups returned to embryonic levels (Weaver et al. 2004). Thus both changes in GR promoter methylation and the exposure to maternal LG-ABN behavior occur coincidently.

If GR is the *FLC* equivalent in maternal care, then what could be the molecular signal that stimulates the epigenetic change; i.e., is there a putative *VIN3* corollary in this example? A high LG-ABN environment correlates with the induction of nerve growth factor-inducible protein A (NGFI-A) in the hippocampus. This likely occurs through a serotonin signaling pathway (reviewed in (Meaney and Szyf 2005)). NGFI-A induction may be significant because one of the differentially methylated cytosines in the GR promoter is within a binding site for NGFI-A, and methylation at this site decreases the binding affinity of NGFI-A at this site (McCormick et al. 2000, Weaver et al. 2004, 2007). In addition, NGFI-A recruits the histone acetyltransferase CBP to GR (Weaver et al. 2007).

The data described above have led the authors to propose a putative molecular mechanism for epigenetic perpetuation of maternal care behavior (Meaney and Szyf 2005, Weaver et al. 2007). At birth all pups exhibit relatively high levels of DNA methylation at the GR promoter in the hippocampus. During the first week after birth, mothers exhibit different degrees of maternal care: high or low LG-ABN. During this period only pups reared by high LG-ABN mothers show an induction of NGFI-A. NGFI-A at first weakly associates with the methylated binding site in the GR promoter; however, recruitment of CBP by NGFI-A activates the chromatin at GR through histone acetylation. This in turn leads to demethylation and stable binding of NGFI-A to the GR promoter and prolonged activation of the GR gene expression (Meaney and Szyf 2005, Weaver et al. 2007).

In the natural world, environmental conditions are in a constant state of flux and selection favors organisms that can best cope with these changes. In addition to coping with rapid environmental change, organisms can also incorporate environmental stimuli into their overall life history strategy. Such stimuli can be seasonal as with vernalization where prolonged periods of cold temperatures are required. Stimuli can also be behavioral like maternal care in rats. In such cases, the response to the stimulus can persist long after the stimulus is gone which invokes the need for a molecular memory of the environmental stimulus. Seasonal responses and behaviors can be found throughout the biological world. As these responses begin to be addressed at a molecular level, it is quite possible that they too will be regulated by mechanisms akin to those described here.

References

Amasino, R., Vernalization, competence, and the epigenetic memory of winter. Plant Cell, 2004. 16(10): 2553–9.

Ausin, I., et al., Regulation of flowering time by FVE, a retinoblastoma-associated protein. Nat Genet, 2004. 36(2): 162–6.

Bastow, R., et al., Vernalization requires epigenetic silencing of FLC by histone methylation. Nature, 2004. 427(6970): 164–7.

Betz, J.L., et al., Phenotypic analysis of Paf1/RNA polymerase II complex mutations reveals connections to cell cycle regulation, protein synthesis, and lipid and nucleic acid metabolism. Mol Genet Genomics, 2002. 268(2): 272–85.

Choi, K., et al., SUPPRESSOR OF FRIGIDA3 encodes a nuclear ACTIN-RELATED PROTEIN6 required for floral repression in Arabidopsis. Plant Cell, 2005. 17(10): 2647–60.

Choi, K., et al., Arabidopsis homologs of components of the SWR1 complex regulate flowering and plant development. Development, 2007. 134(10): 1931–41.

Czermin, B., et al., Drosophila enhancer of Zeste/ESC complexes have a histone H3 methyltransferase activity that marks chromosomal Polycomb sites. Cell, 2002. 111(2): 185–96.

Deal, R.B., et al., The nuclear actin-related protein ARP6 is a pleiotropic developmental regulator required for the maintenance of FLOWERING LOCUS C expression and repression of flowering in Arabidopsis. Plant Cell, 2005. 17(10): 2633–46.

Deal, R.B., et al., Repression of flowering in Arabidopsis requires activation of FLOWERING LOCUS C expression by the histone variant H2A.Z. Plant Cell, 2007. 19(1): 74–83.

Dennis, E.S. and W.J. Peacock, Epigenetic regulation of flowering. Curr Opin Plant Biol, 2007. 10(5): 520–7.

Finnegan, E.J. and E.S. Dennis, Vernalization-induced trimethylation of histone H3 lysine 27 at FLC is not maintained in mitotically quiescent cells. Curr Biol, 2007. 17(22): 1978–83.

Francis, D., et al., Nongenomic transmission across generations of maternal behavior and stress responses in the rat. Science, 1999. 286(5442): 1155–8.

Gazzani, S., et al., Analysis of the molecular basis of flowering time variation in Arabidopsis accessions. Plant Physiol, 2003. 132(2): 1107–14.

Gendall, A.R., et al., The vernalization 2 gene mediates the epigenetic regulation of vernalization in Arabidopsis. Cell, 2001. 107(4): 525–35.

Greb, T., et al., The PHD finger protein VRN5 functions in the epigenetic silencing of Arabidopsis FLC. Curr Biol, 2007. 17(1): 73–8.

He, Y., M.R. Doyle, and R.M. Amasino, PAF1-complex-mediated histone methylation of FLOWERING LOCUS C chromatin is required for the vernalization-responsive, winter-annual habit in Arabidopsis. Genes Dev, 2004. 18(22): 2774–84.

He, Y., S.D. Michaels, and R.M. Amasino, Regulation of flowering time by histone acetylation in arabidopsis. Science, 2003. 302(5651): 1751–1754

Henderson, I.R. and C. Dean, Control of arabidopsis flowering: the chill before the bloom. Development, 2004. 131(16): 3829–38.

Henderson, I.R., C. Shindo, and C. Dean, The need for winter in the switch to flowering. Annu Rev Genet, 2003. 37: 371–92.

Jiang, D., et al., Arabidopsis relatives of the human lysine specific demethylase1 Repress the expression of FWA and FLOWERING LOCUS C and thus promote the floral transition. Plant Cell, 2007. 19: 2975–2987

Johanson, U., et al., Molecular analysis of FRIGIDA, a major determinant of natural variation in arabidopsis flowering time [In Process Citation]. Science, 2000. 290(5490): 344–7.

Kim, H.J., et al., A genetic link between cold responses and flowering time through FVE in Arabidopsis thaliana. Nat Genet, 2004. 36(2): 167–71.

Kim, S., et al., SUPPRESSOR OF FRIGIDA4, encoding a C2H2-Type zinc finger protein, represses flowering by transcriptional activation of Arabidopsis FLOWERING LOCUS C. Plant Cell, 2006. 18(11): 2985–98.

Kim, S.Y., et al., Establishment of the vernalization-responsive, winter-annual habit in Arabidopsis requires a putative histone H3 methyl transferase. Plant Cell, 2005. 17(12): 3301–10.

Kim, S.Y. and S.D. Michaels, SUPPRESSOR OF FRI 4 encodes a nuclear-localized protein that is required for delayed flowering in winter-annual Arabidopsis. Development, 2006. 133(23): 4699–707.

Kobayashi, Y. and D. Weigel, Move on up, it's time for change–mobile signals controlling photoperiod-dependent flowering. Genes Dev, 2007. 21(19): 2371–84.

Kobor, M.S., et al., A protein complex containing the conserved Swi2/Snf2-related ATPase Swr1p deposits histone variant H2A.Z into euchromatin. PLoS Biol, 2004. 2(5): E131.

Koornneef, M., et al., The phenotype of some late-flowering mutants is enhanced by a locus on chromosome 5 that is not effective in the landsberg erecta wild-type. Plant J, 1994. 6(6): 911–919.

Lang, A. and G. Melchers, Vernalisation and devernalisation bei einer zweijahrigen Pflanze. Z. Naturforsch., 1947. 2b: 444–449.

Le Corre, V., F. Roux, and X. Reboud, DNA polymorphism at the FRIGIDA gene in Arabidopsis thaliana: extensive nonsynonymous variation is consistent with local selection for flowering time. Mol Biol Evol, 2002. 19(8): 1261–71.

Lee, I., A. Bleecker, and R. Amasino, Analysis of naturally occurring late flowering in arabidopsis thaliana. Mol Gen Genet, 1993. 237(1–2): 171–176.

Lee, I., et al., The late-flowering phenotype of FRIGIDA and LUMINIDEPENDENS is suppressed in the landsberg erecta strain of arabidopsis. Plant J, 1994. 6(6): 903–909.

Levy, Y.Y., et al., Multiple roles of Arabidopsis VRN1 in vernalization and flowering time control. Science, 2002. 297(5579): 243–6.

Li, B., M. Carey, and J.L. Workman, The role of chromatin during transcription. Cell, 2007. 128(4): 707–19.

Liu, D., et al., Maternal care, hippocampal glucocorticoid receptors, and hypothalamic-pituitary-adrenal responses to stress. Science, 1997. 277(5332): 1659–62.

March-Diaz, R., et al., SEF, a new protein required for flowering repression in Arabidopsis, interacts with PIE1 and ARP6. Plant Physiol, 2007. 143(2): 893–901.

McCormick, J.A., et al., 5'-heterogeneity of glucocorticoid receptor messenger RNA is tissue specific: differential regulation of variant transcripts by early-life events. Mol Endocrinol, 2000. 14(4): 506–17.

Meaney, M.J., Maternal care, gene expression, and the transmission of individual differences in stress reactivity across generations. Annu Rev Neurosci, 2001. 24: 1161–92.

Meaney, M.J. and M. Szyf, Maternal care as a model for experience-dependent chromatin plasticity? Trends Neurosci, 2005. 28(9): 456–63.

Michaels, S. and R. Amasino, Loss of FLOWERING LOCUS C activity eliminates the late-flowering phenotype of FRIGIDA and autonomous-pathway mutations, but not responsiveness to vernalization. Plant Cell, 2001. 13(4): 935–942.

Michaels, S.D., I.C. Bezerra, and R.M. Amasino, FRIGIDA-related genes are required for the winter-annual habit in Arabidopsis. Proc Natl Acad Sci U S A, 2004. 101(9): 3281–5.

Michaels, S.D., et al., Attenuation of FLOWERING LOCUS C activity as a mechanism for the evolution of summer-annual flowering behavior in Arabidopsis. Proc Natl Acad Sci U S A, 2003. 100(17): 10102–7.

Mizuguchi, G., et al., ATP-driven exchange of histone H2AZ variant catalyzed by SWR1 chromatin remodeling complex. Science, 2004. 303(5656): 343–8.

Muller, J., et al., Histone methyltransferase activity of a Drosophila Polycomb group repressor complex. Cell, 2002. 111(2): 197–208.

Mylne, J.S., et al., LHP1, the Arabidopsis homologue of HETEROCHROMATIN PROTEIN1, is required for epigenetic silencing of FLC. Proc Natl Acad Sci U S A, 2006. 103(13): 5012–7.

Napp-Zinn, K., On the genetical basis of vernalization requirement in Arabidopsis thaliana (L.) Heynh, in La Physiologie de la Floraison, P. Champagnat and R. Jaques, Editors. 1979, Coll. Int. CNRS: Paris. 217–220.

Ng, H.H., et al., Targeted recruitment of Set1 histone methylase by elongating Pol II provides a localized mark and memory of recent transcriptional activity. Mol Cell, 2003. 11(3): 709–19.

Noh, Y.S. and R.M. Amasino, PIE1, an ISWI family gene, is required for FLC activation and floral repression in Arabidopsis. Plant Cell, 2003. 15(7): 1671–82.

Oh, S., et al., A mechanism related to the yeast transcriptional regulator Paf1c is required for expression of the Arabidopsis FLC/MAF MADS box gene family. Plant Cell, 2004. 16(11): 2940–53.

Pei, Y., et al., Mutations in the Type II protein arginine methyltransferase AtPRMT5 result in pleiotropic developmental defects in Arabidopsis. Plant Physiol, 2007. 144(4): 1913–23.

Reeves, P.A., et al., Evolutionary conservation of the FLOWERING LOCUS C-mediated vernalization response: evidence from the sugar beet (Beta vulgaris). Genetics, 2007. 176(1): 295–307.

Ringrose, L. and R. Paro, Epigenetic regulation of cellular memory by the Polycomb and Trithorax group proteins. Annu Rev Genet, 2004. 38: 413–43.

Santisteban, M.S., T. Kalashnikova, and M.M. Smith, Histone H2A.Z regulats transcription and is partially redundant with nucleosome remodeling complexes. Cell, 2000. 103(3): 411–22.

Schmitz, R.J. and R.M. Amasino, Vernalization: a model for investigating epigenetics and eukaryotic gene regulation in plants. Biochim Biophys Acta, 2007. 1769(5–6): 269–75.

Schmitz, R.J., et al., FRIGIDA-ESSENTIAL 1 interacts genetically with FRIGIDA and FRIGIDA-LIKE 1 to promote the winter-annual habit of Arabidopsis thaliana. Development, 2005. 132(24): 5471–8.

Schmitz, R.J., S. Sung, and R.M. Amasino, Histone arginine methylation is required for vernalization-induced epigenetic silencing of FLC in winter-annual Arabidopsis thaliana. Proc Natl Acad Sci U S A, 2008. 105(2): 411–6.

Schwartz, Y.B. and V. Pirrotta, Polycomb silencing mechanisms and the management of genomic programmes. Nat Rev Genet, 2007. 8(1): 9–22.

Searle, I., et al., The transcription factor FLC confers a flowering response to vernalization by repressing meristem competence and systemic signaling in Arabidopsis. Genes Dev, 2006. 20(7): 898–912.

Sheldon, C.C., et al., The FLF MADS box gene: a repressor of flowering in Arabidopsis regulated by vernalization and methylation. Plant Cell, 1999. 11(3): 445–58.

Sheldon, C.C., et al., Quantitative effects of vernalization on FLC and SOC1 expression. Plant J, 2006. 45(6): 871–83.

Shindo, C., et al., Role of FRIGIDA and FLOWERING LOCUS C in determining variation in flowering time of Arabidopsis. Plant Physiol, 2005. 138(2): 1163–73.

Sung, S. and R.M. Amasino, Remembering winter: toward a molecular understanding of vernalization. Annu Rev Plant Biol, 2005. 56: 491–508.

Sung, S. and R.M. Amasino, Vernalization in Arabidopsis thaliana is mediated by the PHD finger protein VIN3. Nature, 2004. 427(6970): 159–64.

Sung, S., et al., Epigenetic maintenance of the vernalized state in Arabidopsis thaliana requires LIKE HETEROCHROMATIN PROTEIN 1. Nat Genet, 2006. 38(6): 706–10.

Sung, S., R.J. Schmitz, and R.M. Amasino, A PHD finger protein involved in both the vernalization and photoperiod pathways in Arabidopsis. Genes Dev, 2006. 20(23): 3244–8.

Trevaskis, B., et al., The molecular basis of vernalization-induced flowering in cereals. Trends Plant Sci, 2007. 12(8): 352–7.

Turck, F., et al., Arabidopsis TFL2/LHP1 specifically associates with genes marked by trimethylation of histone H3 lysine 27. PLoS Genet, 2007. 3(6): e86.

Wang, X., et al., SKB1-mediated symmetric dimethylation of histone H4R3 controls flowering time in Arabidopsis. EMBO J, 2007. 26(7): 1934–41.

Weaver, I.C., et al., Epigenetic programming by maternal behavior. Nat Neurosci, 2004. 7(8): 847–54.

Weaver, I.C., et al., The transcription factor nerve growth factor-inducible protein a mediates epigenetic programming: altering epigenetic marks by immediate-early genes. J Neurosci, 2007. 27(7): 1756–68.

Wellensiek, S.J., Dividing cells as the locus for vernalization. Nature, 1962. 195: 307–308.

Wellensiek, S.J., Dividing Cells as the prerequisite for vernalization. Plant Physiology, 1964. 39: 832–835.

Werner, J.D., et al., FRIGIDA-independent variation in flowering time of natural Arabidopsis thaliana accessions. Genetics, 2005. 170(3): 1197–207.

Wood, C.C., et al., The Arabidopsis thaliana vernalization response requires a polycomb-like protein complex that also includes VERNALIZATION INSENSITIVE 3. Proc Natl Acad Sci U S A, 2006. 103(39): 14631–6.

Zhang, X., et al., The Arabidopsis LHP1 protein colocalizes with histone H3 Lys27 trimethylation. Nat Struct Mol Biol, 2007. 14(9): 869–71.

Zhao, Z., et al., Prevention of early flowering by expression of FLOWERING LOCUS C requires methylation of histone H3 K36. Nat Cell Biol, 2005. 7(12): 1256–60.

The Relevance of Epigenetics to Major Psychosis

Jonathan Mill and Arturas Petronis

Abstract Schizophrenia (SZ) and bipolar disorder (BD) are two related psychiatric conditions, together termed major psychosis. As with other complex genetic disease phenotypes, traditional etiological studies of major psychosis have focused primarily on the interplay between genetic (DNA sequence) and environmental risk factors. However, there are many epidemiological, clinical, and molecular peculiarities associated with these disorders that are hard to explain using DNA and environment-based mechanisms. Such observations have led to speculation about the potential importance of epigenetic factors in mediating susceptibility to major psychosis. Epigenetics refers to the heritable, but reversible, regulation of gene expression mediated principally through changes in DNA methylation and chromatin organization. In this chapter we reinterpret a series of epidemiological, clinical, and molecular findings in major psychosis within the framework of epigenetic dysregulation. While epigenetics provides a new perspective on the aetiology of SZ and BD, it would be naïve to expect that applying epigenetic theory to molecular-based studies of psychopathology is a straightforward task that can be achieved without encountering a number of technological and methodological complexities. To date few empirical studies have been performed, but recent large scale epigenomic profiling has begun to highlight associations between specific epigenetic changes and risk for these disorders.

Keywords Epigenetics · DNA methylation · Genetics · Schizophrenia · Bipolar disorder · Complex non-Mendelian disease · Methylome · Microarray

A. Petronis (✉)
Krembil Family Epigenetics Laboratory, Centre for Addiction and Mental Health,
250 College street, Toronto ON M5T 1R8, Canada
e-mail: arturas_petronis@camh.net

1 Traditional Approaches to the Aetiology of Major Psychosis

Schizophrenia (SZ) and bipolar disorder (BD) are two related psychiatric conditions, together termed major psychosis, that affect approximately 2% of the population and contribute greatly to the global burden of disease (Murray and Lopez 1997). SZ is defined primarily by the presence of psychotic symptoms, such as delusions and hallucinations, but is also characterized by disorganisation, dysfunctional affective responses, and altered cognitive functioning. BD presents with episodic swings in mood ranging from extreme mania to severe depression, and is often also accompanied by psychotic symptoms and impaired cognitive function. There is increasing evidence of considerable overlap between SZ and BD, suggesting they are etiologically related (Craddock et al. 2006; Craddock and Owen 2007; Owen et al. 2007), and challenging the validity of the dichotomous classification of the disorders. Despite this, some important phenotypic differences are also apparent, suggesting that certain specific etiological factors are also likely to be important.

The possibility of understanding the origins of human psychopathology is one of the most exciting perspectives of contemporary biomedical research, and the focus of considerable research effort across the world. Traditional etiological studies of major psychosis have focused primarily on the interplay between genetic (DNA sequence) and environmental risk factors. It is well established that SZ and BD aggregate in families, with twin and adoption studies highlighting a strong inherited component to both disorders (Craddock et al. 2005). It is generally assumed that susceptibility is mediated by the action of numerous genes of small effect, interacting additively and/or epistatically with each other and with various environmental factors. Whilst polymorphisms and haplotypes across several loci have been associated with both disorders, association studies are characterized by non-replication, small effect-sizes, and significant heterogeneity (Gershon and Badner 2001; Kato 2007; Riley and Kendler 2006). Recent advances in genotyping technology, and the collection of large sample cohorts, have heralded the advent of whole-genome association studies for disorders like SZ and BD. The results from such studies have, however, been largely underwhelming, with very few polymorphisms reaching genome-wide significance for association, suggesting that few, if any, clinically meaningful sequence changes associated with major psychosis are likely to be discovered in the near future.

As with all complex psychiatric phenotypes, there are many epidemiological, clinical, and molecular peculiarities associated with major psychosis that are hard to explain using traditional DNA- and environment-based mechanisms. For example, despite sharing the same DNA sequence, the concordance rate between monozygotic (MZ) twins for major psychosis is far from 100%: between 41 and 65% for SZ (Cardno and Gottesman 2000) and about 60% for BD (Craddock and Jones 1999). Such phenotypic discordance between MZ twins is often attributed to non-shared environmental factors, although the empirical evidence for such a large environmental contribution to major psychosis is still lacking. It is likely that quantitative genetic studies have overestimated the direct role of the environment in SZ and BD – to date there is little conclusive evidence linking any environmental factor to increased risk for major psychosis (McGuffin et al. 1994; Petronis 2004). Other complexities of major psychosis include a fluctuating disease course with periods of remission and relapse, sexual dimorphism, peaks of susceptibility to disease coinciding with major hormonal rearrangements, and parent-of-origin effects. These observations have led to speculation about the importance of epigenetic factors in mediating susceptibility to both SZ and BD.

2 The Epigenetic Theory of Major Psychosis

Epigenetics refers to the heritable, but reversible, regulation of gene expression mediated principally through changes in DNA methylation and chromatin structure (Henikoff and Matzke 1997). Epigenetic processes are essential for normal cellular development and differentiation, and allow the regulation of gene function through non-mutagenic mechanisms. Of particular interest is the phenomenon of cytosine methylation, occurring at position 5 of the cytosine pyrimidine ring in CpG dinucleotides. This process is intrinsically linked to the regulation of gene expression, with many genes demonstrating an inverse correlation between the degree of methylation at the promoter and the level of expression. The methylation of these CpG sites, over-represented in CpG-islands in the promoter regulatory regions of many genes, disrupts the binding of transcription factors and attracts methyl-binding proteins that initiate chromatin compaction and gene silencing. Histone modification, another epigenetic mechanism mediating gene expression, affects chromatin organization via the processes of histone acetylation, histone methylation, and histone phosphorylation (Jenuwein and Allis 2001). Interestingly, these two broad types of epigenetic mechanism are not mutually exclusive and interact in a number of ways. The methyl-binding protein MeCP2, for example, binds specifically to methylated cytosines, attracting histone deacetylases which hypoacetylate histones (Jones et al. 1998). Transcriptionally competent chromatin is generally enriched with acetylated histones, but transcriptionally silent chromatin is normally deacetylated (Robertson and Wolffe 2000). Recently, a third epigenetic system involving small interfering RNA (siRNA) has been described (Hamilton et al. 2002). It has been shown that siRNA can suppress the activity of specific genes via targeted RNA interference (RNAi), a mechanism likely to be integral to the developmental regulation of gene expression. (Morris 2005) (See also Chapters "Epigenetic Silencing of Pericentromeric Heterochromatin by RNA Interference in Schizosaccharomyces pombe", "Describing Epigenomic Information in Arabidopsis" and "Role of Small RNAs in Establishing Chromosomal Architecture in Drosophila").

We have suggested that the putative epigenetic misregulation of genes may explain numerous epidemiological, clinical, and molecular complexities of SZ, BD, and other complex diseases (Petronis 2000; Petronis 2001; Petronis 2004). The epigenetic theory of complex disease is based on three premises:

(i) Like the DNA sequence, the epigenetic profile of somatic cells is inherited from maternal to daughter chromatids during mitosis, but unlike the DNA

sequence these epigenetic signals are highly dynamic even within an individual (Eckhardt et al. 2006).
(ii) Epigenetic processes are integral in regulating various genomic functions, including gene expression, and such epigenetic regulation can have profound phenotypic effects. Genes, even those containing no mutations or disease predisposing polymorphisms, may be useless or even harmful if not expressed in the appropriate amount, at the right time of the cell cycle or in the right compartment of the nucleus (Jaenisch and Bird 2003).
(iii) It appears that some epigenetic signals are not fully erased and reset during gametogenesis as traditionally believed, and can thus be transmitted transgenerationally (Klar 1998; Rakyan and Whitelaw 2003; Richards 2006). This blurs the demarcation between epigenetic and DNA sequence-based inheritance, and challenges the dominating paradigm of human morbid genetics that is exclusively concentrated on DNA sequence variation.

These three postulates make epigenetic processes particularly relevant to the understanding of various non-Mendelian irregularities of major psychosis and other complex diseases. The following section provides a re-interpretation of a series of epidemiological, clinical, and molecular findings in major psychosis, within a framework of epigenetic dysregulation.

2.1 Non-Mendelian Features of Major Psychosis that are Consistent with Epigenetic Misregulation

2.1.1 Discordance Between MZ Twins

As discussed above, there is considerable discordance between MZ twins for both SZ and BD. Traditionally, most of this discordance is attributed to non-shared environmental influences, but the partial stability of epigenetic signals provides an alternative explanation. A recent study has demonstrated that fairly profound epigenetic differences across the genome do arise during the lifetime of MZ twins, highlighting the dynamic nature of epigenetic processes (Fraga et al. 2005). Interestingly, MZ twin methylation differences have been reported for CpG sites in a number of specific genes that have been associated with major psychosis including the dopamine D2 receptor (DRD2) gene (Petronis et al. 2003) and the catechol-O-methyltransferase (COMT) gene (Mill et al. 2006a). Similarly, genetically identical inbred animals have been shown to demonstrate considerable epigenetic differences that may be linked to gene expression differences resulting in marked phenotypic variation (Rakyan et al. 2002). It is becoming increasingly apparent that many of the observed epigenetic differences between MZ twins and inbred animals may be the result of stochastic events. In tissue culture, the fidelity of the maintenance of methylation in mammalian cells was between 97%–99.9% and *de novo* methylation activity was as high as 3–5% per mitosis (Riggs et al. 1998). Although functionally important promoter regions showed a higher fidelity of methylation pattern with a rate of 99.85–99.92% site/generation (Ushijima et al. 2003), such stochastic epigenetic changes may accumulate over the millions of mitotic divisions occurring during the lifetime of two MZ twins and lead to significant phenotypic differences. It has been proposed that such stochastic epigenetic variation may be more important in complex psychiatric disorders than is currently recognized, perhaps accounting for some of the risk currently attributed to environmental factors (Wong et al. 2005).

Skewed X-chromosome inactivation is another epigenetic process that could partially explain female MZ twin discordance (Craig et al. 2004). Non-random X chromosome inactivation has been observed in a number of disorders, including several X-linked immunodeficiencies, Lesch-Nyhan disease, incontinentia pigmenti, focal dermal hypoplasia, and adrenoleukodystrophy (Willard 2000). It has been demonstrated that approximately half the female carriers of X-linked mental retardation exhibit skewed X inactivation where the activation ratio between the two X chromosomes is 80:20% or higher (Plenge et al. 2002). In the normal population of females without a family history of X-linked disorders, 5–20% of women have constitutional skewing of X inactivation (Belmont 1996). According to other authors, 30–40% of females exhibit ratios 60:40% or more, and 10% of normal females demonstrate even more extreme ratios (Willard 2000). The potential role of skewed X-inactivation in major psychosis was highlighted by a study examining X-chromosome inactivation in a series of 63 female MZ twin pairs concordant or discordant for BD or SZ and healthy MZ controls (Rosa et al. 2007). They found that discordant female BD twins showed greater differences in the methylation of the maternal and paternal chromosome X alleles than concordant twin pairs suggesting a potential contribution from X-linked loci to discordance within twin pairs for BD.

Epigenetic differences existing between MZ twins certainly do not rule out the role of environmental factors in disease susceptibility. Epigenetics does not deny the role of environmental impact; in fact, there is growing evidence that the environment can itself influence the epigenetic status of the genome – either globally or at specific loci (Sutherland and Costa 2003). DNA methylation has been shown to vary as a function of numerous nutritional, chemical, physical, and even psychosocial factors (Feil 2006). For example, it has been shown that DNA methylation is affected by the dietary levels of methyl-donor components contained in substances such as folate (Davis and Uthus 2003). Several studies have demonstrated that maternal dietary methyl supplements during pregnancy can increase global DNA methylation and alter methylation-dependent phenotypes in mammalian offspring (Cooney et al. 2002). In addition, it has been shown that offspring of pregnant rats exposed to the endocrine disruptor vinclozolin, a fungicide used in agricultural crops, have altered DNA methylation profiles across the promoters of several genes and increased rates of prostate disease, kidney disease, immune system abnormalities, and tumor development (Chang et al. 2006). Even the psychosocial environment and stress during key developmental periods early in life can epigenetically mediate gene expression. Meaney and colleagues have shown that postnatal maternal care in rats, as measured by increased pup licking, grooming, and arch-backed nursing, leads to epigenetic modification of a NGF1-A transcription factor binding site in the promoter region of the glucocorticoid receptor gene

(*NR3C1*), directly affecting gene expression and stress-related phenotypes in offspring (Weaver et al. 2004). Because epigenetic changes are inherited mitotically in somatic cells, they provide a possible mechanism by which the effects of external environmental factors can be propagated through development, producing long-term phenotypic changes. The epigenome is known to be particularly susceptible to external disruption during a number of key developmental periods, but is likely to be most vulnerable to the effect of environmental factors during embryogenesis when the rate of DNA synthesis is high and the epigenetic marks needed for normal tissue differentiation and development are being established (Dolinoy et al. 2007). This is interesting, given the role that prenatal environmental insults are postulated to play in mediating risk for major psychosis (Penner and Brown 2007).

In conclusion, epigenetics may provide a direct mechanistic route by which the environment can interact with the genome to bring about long-term changes in gene expression and phenotype. Even more importantly, epigenetic metastability is consistent with the presence of major phenotypic differences in the absence of environmental impact.

2.1.2 Sex Differences

Another non-Mendelian feature of major psychosis is male-female differences in prevalence and disease course; there is considerable evidence – clinical, epidemiological, molecular genetic, and neurochemical – of sex-specific effects in both SZ and BD. For example, while men and women have an approximately equal lifetime risk for SZ, it tends to become manifest in women later than men (Hafner 2003). Most men develop SZ between 15 and 25 years of age. For women, the period of maximum onset is around age 30 with a smaller peak around 50 (i.e. menopausal age). Women also tend to have milder forms of the disease in their younger years than males. Conversely, in later years, symptoms in men tend to decrease in severity while women often have a renewed onset of psychotic symptoms and a worse course of the disease. Similarly, there is evidence that the presentation and course of bipolar disorder differs between women and men (Arnold 2003). The onset of BD tends to occur later in women than men, and women more often have a seasonal pattern of the mood disturbance. Women experience depressive episodes, mixed mania, and rapid cycling more often than men.

In molecular genetic studies, evidence – albeit controversial – for the involvement of sex chromosome genes in major psychosis have been detected (Baron 2001). However, the contribution of sex chromosomes appears to be relatively small compared to that of the autosomes, which in some cases also exhibit sex effects in SZ and BD. One example is *DISC1* (Disrupted in schizophrenia 1 locus), one of the most comprehensively analyzed genes in psychiatric genetics (Harrison and Weinberger 2005). A genetic association study tested 28 single nucleotide polymorphism (SNPs) from 1q42 covering the *DISC1* region in a sample of 458 Finnish families ascertained for SZ and detected a common haplotype (HEP3) to be significantly under-transmitted to affected individuals ($P = 0.0031$) (Hennah et al. 2003). HEP3 represents a two SNP (rs751229 and rs3738401) haplotype spanning from intron

1 to exon 2 of *DISC1*. This haplotype also displayed sex differences in transmission distortion; the under-transmission being significant only to affected females ($P = 0.00024$), suggesting that this haplotype may confer a protective effect against the disease in women (Hennah et al. 2003). Another study investigating Scottish SZ ($N = 394$) and BD ($N = 381$) patients compared to controls ($N = 478$), detected that an extended HEP3 haplotype was significantly over-represented in males affected with BD, but no effect was seen in females (Thomson et al. 2005). Sex effects have been also identified for autosomal genes in other genetic studies of SZ (Shifman et al. 2002), major depression (Abkevich et al. 2003) (Zubenko et al. 2003), and autism (Lamb et al. 2005; Stone et al. 2004).

While sex hormones have been "the usual culprit" in the explanation of gender effects in complex diseases, there are no underlying mechanisms proposed as to how such hormones predispose or protect individuals from a disease relating to the specific molecular mechanisms of hormone action (Kaminsky et al. 2006). One of the potential mechanisms of sex hormone impact is through alteration of the molecular epigenetic signatures of particular chromosomal regions that modulate the access of transcription factors to the transcribed sequences. A number of studies have demonstrated the direct effects of sex hormone administration on epigenetic states. An example is the effect of estradiol administration on the methylation status of various CpG dinucleotides located in an estradiol-mediated regulatory region for the avian vitellogenin II gene (Meijlink et al. 1983; Saluz et al. 1986; Wilks et al. 1984; Wilks et al. 1982). Two of these methylatable cytosines located within the estradiol-receptor binding site are actively demethylated in response to estradiol treatment in hormone responsive tissues in a strand specific manner (Saluz et al. 1986). This DNA demethylation persists after transcription has ended (Wilks et al. 1984; Wilks et al. 1982) resulting in a quicker induction of vitellogenin II mRNA synthesis in response to subsequent estradiol stimulations (Saluz et al. 1986). This finding highlights the fact that hormones can mediate a long lasting epigenetic effect on gene transcription. Numerous more recent studies (Blewitt et al. 2005; Kawakami et al. 2006; Lai et al. 2005; Mani and Thakur 2006; Sarter et al. 2005; Shimabukuro et al. 2006a; Shimabukuro et al. 2006b; Yu et al. 2004) (although not all – e.g. (Eckhardt et al. 2006) detected sex differences in DNA methylation patterns.

Similarly to DNA methylation, chromatin modification can be directly affected by members of the nuclear hormone receptor (NHR) superfamily, and the steroid receptor (SR) subset of NHR is of particular interest, as it contains the androgen and estrogen receptors (Kinyamu and Archer 2004). These sex hormone receptors can have activating or repressing transcriptional activity, dependent on the presence or absence of ligand, respectively (Fu et al. 2004; Xu et al. 1999). Steroid hormone-mediated transcriptional activation or repression results from the SR recruitment of co-activator and co-repressor complexes – protein complexes which associate with various epigenetic modifiers, such as histone deacetylases (HDAC), histone acetyltransferases (HAT), and histone methyltransferases (HMT) (Fu et et al. 2003, 2004). It is these 'co-regulatory complexes' that achieve the epigenetic modification necessary for chromatin remodeling, allowing or restricting access of transcription factors and RNA polymerase II, and thus mediating the epigenetic effects of the sex hormones.

Various studies have demonstrated that tissue specific distribution of the sex hormone receptors varies between the sexes (Azzi et al. 2006), as do the target genes for transcriptional regulation, and thus, the epigenetic modifications mediated through the sex hormone receptors will likely vary by gene and tissue between the sexes. A study investigating the transcriptional regulation of the prolactin gene tested the effects of estradiol administration in GH4 cells (Liu et al. 2005). Estradiol was found to have a stimulating effect on histone H4 acetylation in the promoter region of the prolactin gene (Liu et al. 2005). In agreement with other studies, such histone modifications are implicated as necessary factors in gene transcription via the formation of a euchromatic state of the promoter region (Chakrabarti et al. 2003). Various forms of histone methylation are associated with estradiol binding to the estrogen receptor, affecting the transcription at the target promoter *in vitro* (Kinyamu and Archer 2004; Metivier et al. 2003) and further highlighting that sex hormone regulated gene transcription is associated with the formation of an epigenetic mark.

Based on the above, it can be proposed that for at least some DNA alleles to become risk factors, specific epigenetic changes induced by sex hormones are necessary. In other words, a disease risk factor represents a specific DNA allele, which is epigenetically modified by either estrogens or androgens. If one of the two conditions is not met, i.e. there is a different DNA allele or different sex, no risk factor will be generated. This predicts that the epigenetic status of an identical DNA risk allele in affected individuals is different in comparison to the unaffected individuals of the same sex.

2.1.3 Parent-of-Origin Effects

Another non-Mendelian feature that is commonly observed in studies of major psychosis is a parent-of-origin effect, where disease susceptibility is mediated by parental factors in a sex-specific manner. Parent-of-origin effects are apparent at both a phenotypic level, where the risk to offspring depends on the sex of the affected parent, and also at a molecular level when risk alleles only confer increased susceptibility if they are transmitted from the mother or the father. McMahon et al. (1995), for example, have shown that the risk of developing BD is higher in offspring with affected mothers than in those with affected fathers. Parent of origin-dependent clinical differences were also detected in SZ (Crow et al. 1989; Ohara et al. 1997). Genetic linkage studies, although rarely performed in sex-specific fashion, also reveal parental origin effects in major psychosis (McMahon et al. 1997; Schulze et al. 2003). Several independent chromosome 22 studies in major psychosis have detected that predominantly maternal or paternal alleles contribute to the evidence for linkage. More specifically, the parent of origin-specific extended transmission disequilibrium test revealed that all evidence for transmission disequilibrium of *D22S278* (22q13.1), a marker associated with disease, resulted from the maternal alleles ($p = 0.00005$) but not from the paternal alleles ($p = 0.14$) (Vallada and Collier 1998). Consistent with this finding, parametric linkage analyses in BD revealed that recombination fractions (θ_m; θ_f) of the maximal lod score (Z_{max}) for the distal 22q markers were much higher for male meioses in comparison to female meioses (Kelsoe et al. 2001). Such differences in θ_m and θ_f cannot be explained by differences in the male – female recombination rates of the chromosome 22 region (Dib et al. 1996) but rather argue that maternal alleles predominantly contribute to linkage of chromosome 22q markers to BD, while paternal alleles segregate randomly. Furthermore, a genome scan of over 300 SZ sib-pairs showed that only maternal but not paternal alleles on chromosome 22q demonstrated statistically significant excess sharing (DeLisi et al. 2001). Since parental origin-based linkage studies are less susceptible to false positive errors (Petronis 2000), the findings strongly argue that the parental origin of chromosome 22 is involved in determining the risk of major psychosis. One of the most common mechanisms of parent of origin effect is genomic imprinting (Ferguson-Smith et al. 2003; Paulsen and Ferguson-Smith 2001; Surani et al. 1993). Genomic imprinting refers to parental origin specific regulation of gene activity that is achieved by differential epigenetic modification of maternal and paternal genes. In "classical" cases, imprinted genes exhibit a clear-cut "on/off" type of regulation, i.e. only maternal or paternal genes are expressed but not both. Recent evidence, however, suggests that imprinting may be more widespread and less clear-cut than originally believed (Preis et al. 2003). Imprinting involves both epigenetic mechanisms, namely cytosine methylation within CpG islands and changes in chromatin organization (*ibid.*). Imprinted genes usually accumulate in clusters consisting of maternally and paternally imprinted genes located next to each other (Paulsen et al. 2000). There are two scenarios of how the imprinted gene(s) are involved in SZ and BD. The first possibility is that the pattern of imprinting is disrupted in at least a proportion of SZ or BD patients. Alternatively, the imprinting pattern is intact but the imprinted gene carries a DNA sequence polymorphism or mutation that becomes phenotypically manifest when the allele is not inactivated by genomic imprinting.

2.1.4 The Epigenetic Model of Major Psychiatric Disease

In addition to twin discordance, sex- and parental-origin effects, the epigenetic theory of major psychosis is also consistent with various other features of major psychosis that cannot be explained by more traditional DNA sequence-based mechanisms or hazardous environment. Such include the non-Mendelian mode of inheritance, the presence of familial and sporadic cases, the critical age of susceptibility that follows major hormonal changes in the organism, and the presence of quantitative but not qualitative neurochemical, physiological, and developmental changes in affected individuals (Petronis 2000, 2001, 2004). The heuristic value of the epigenetic model of complex disease lies in the possibility of integrating a variety of unrelated data into a new theoretical framework and providing the basis for new working hypothesis and powerful experimental approaches.

According to the **epigenetic model,** major psychiatric disease is seen to result from a chain of unfavorable epigenetic events that begin with a primary epigenetic defect, or pre-epimutation, occurring in the germline during the error-prone epigenetic-reprogramming process (Flanagan et al. 2006; Jablonka and Lamb 1995). Pre-epimutations increase the risk of developing disease, but unlike the deterministic DNA mutations in Mendelian disorders, a pre-epimutation does not necessarily indicate that the disease is inevitable. Such pre-epimutations may not cause any immediate clinical problems, and thus the age of onset may be delayed for a relatively long time. It may take several decades until the epigenetic misregulation reaches a critical threshold, beyond which the cell (tissue, organ) is no longer able to function normally. The phenotypic outcome depends on the overall effect of a series of pre- and post-natal impacts on such a pre-epimutation. Pre-epimutations are subject to further changes by the multidirectional effects of tissue differentiation, stochastic events, and some environmental factors (Jaenisch and Bird 2003; Petronis 2004; Sutherland and Costa 2003). The epigenetic paradigm in complex diseases allows for, in Kuhn's words, "handling the same bundle of data as before, but placing them in a new system of relations with one another by giving them a different framework" (Kuhn 1962). The epigenetic theory does not reject the role of DNA sequence variation but rather suggests that, in complex diseases, the contribution of epigenetic factors may be substantial, and epigenetic regulation should be investigated in parallel with DNA sequence variation.

3 Approaches to Studying Epigenetics of Complex Psychiatric Disease

While epigenetics provides a new perspective on the aetiology of SZ and BD, it would be naïve to expect that applying epigenetic theory to molecular-based studies of psychopathology is a straightforward task that can be achieved without encountering a number of technological and methodological complexities. The study of epigenetics, especially in complex, non-malignant, diseases, is a relatively new field of research, and optimal laboratory techniques and analysis methods are still being developed. It is vital that laboratory approaches are refined and verified before sweeping conclusions are drawn from experimental data. To date, only a few empirical studies have been performed (see Section 4 of this Chapter), and it is clear that a number of methodological difficulties need to be overcome before large-scale epigenetic studies can be viably executed. Many epigenetic laboratory techniques are labor intensive, expensive, technically difficult, and thus not geared to the high-throughput analyses that will be needed in the hunt for the epigenetic changes associated with disorders like SZ and BD.

3.1 Technological Limitations

Currently the 'gold standard technique' for fine mapping of methylated cytosines is based on the treatment of genomic DNA with sodium bisulfite, which converts unmethylated cytosines to uracils (and subsequently, via PCR, to thymidines), while methylated cytosines are resistant to bisulfite and remain unchanged (Frommer et al. 1992). After sodium bisulfite treatment, one crude method to examine DNA methylation is via methylation-specific PCR (MSP). In this approach two PCR reactions are performed on bisulfite-treated DNA with primer sets specific to (i) methylated DNA and (ii) unmethylated DNA. Such an approach can only investigate methylation at a very small number of CpG sites and gives no quantitative information about the degree of methylation. Furthermore, data from experiments utilizing MSP should be treated with caution given the numerous confounding factors that can affect PCR efficiency on bisulfite-treated DNA. A more rigorous method to investigate DNA methylation is sequencing the bisulfite treated genomic DNA. DNA regions of interest are amplified and sequenced to identify C→T transitions or C positions that have not changed, respectively corresponding to unmethylated and methylated cytosines in the native DNA. Typically, PCR amplicons are either sequenced directly to provide a strand-specific average sequence for the population of DNA molecules, or cloned and sequenced to provide methylation maps of single DNA molecules. An alternative to the laborious and expensive sequencing of cloned bisulfite-PCR products is the use of either pyrosequencing (Tost and Gut 2007) (see also Chapter "Sequencing the Epigenome"), or MALDI-TOF (Coolen et al. 2007) to accurately quantify the degree of CpG methylation. A major problem with the sodium bisulfite approach is that it results in considerable DNA degradation, and relatively large quantities of genomic DNA material are needed if numerous genomic regions are to be profiled – obviously an issue if valuable, relatively inaccessible tissues such as specific populations of neurons or oocytes are investigated. One potential method to overcome problems associated with tissue availability is the use of whole-genome amplification of bisulfite treated DNA (Mill et al. 2006b). In addition, no consensus has yet been reached on how to optimally statistically analyze bisulfite-sequence data. Such analyses are unlikely to be straightforward, especially if the differences observed across individuals are subtle as would be expected for disorders such as SZ and BD. One possibility is to use an approach based on epigenetic distance, which reduces bisulfite sequencing data from cloned PCR products to a binary code for each DNA molecule, and allows patterns of 'epigenetic drift' to be easily ascertained (Flanagan et al. 2006; Yatabe et al. 2001).

These traditional, locus-specific techniques limit the number of the CpG sites that can be feasibly assessed, and thus exclude the possibility of performing a genome-wide 'epigenome-scan' to identify novel regions of importance. In recent years, a number of novel, high-throughput microarray-based methods have been developed, which should enable future epigenetic studies to overcome many of these issues (Huang 1999; Khulan et al. 2006; Lippman et al. 2005; Shi et al. 2003). On the other hand, as we have learnt from the use of gene expression microarrays in psychiatric research, differences in sample preparation, microarray type, sample labeling and data analysis procedures pose a tremendous challenge to the field (Mirnics 2001), and some degree of standardization is needed across epigenetic studies. A major hurdle to the widespread use of methylation microarrays is cost – for example, until recently it has been prohibitively expensive to scan the entire human epigenome of a large sample of major psychosis patients and controls, especially if tissue-specific effects are important and numerous brain regions need to be assessed. Current epigenome methylation studies have been biased by the fact that current microarray designs focus primarily on cDNA, promoters, 5' sequences of known genes only. As array technology advances, however, with the development of commercially produced whole-genome 'tiling' arrays containing dozens of millions of features allowing an unbiased assessment of the entire epigenome, microarray studies have the potential to revolutionize our understanding about the epigenetic mileau of the genome and provide novel insights into the aetiology of major psychosis.

This article has been primarily dedicated to the role of DNA methylation but there is increasing effort to uncover histone modification changes in major psychosis (Akbarian et al. 2005; Stadler et al. 2005). The method used to examine the epigenetic state of histones is chromatin immunoprecipitation (ChIP). One limitation to this approach is the large number of cells needed for each experiment, although recent methodological advances may permit ChIP analysis on as few as 100 cells (O'Neil et al. 2006). Another major problem with histone modification analysis is that, in comparison to DNA modification, histone modifications are far less stable in *post mortem* tissues. In this regard, specific immunoprecipitation protocols applicable to *post mortem* brain tissue need to be developed, and the impact of potential confounds such as autolysis time or tissue pH need to be thoroughly examined (Huang et al. 2006). Once tissue-stability problems have been overcome, however, the use of powerful microarray-based 'ChIP-on-chip' methods, in which DNA isolated from ChIPs is hybridized to a microarray, should allow genome-wide analysis of histone modifications and provide additional epigenetic information to complement data from genomewide DNA methylation studies. The recent development of 'next-generation' sequencing methodologies have taken genomewide analyses of histone modifications to another level, allowing much more detailed investigations of epigenetic variation, via ChIP-seq techniques (Robertson et al. 2007) (See Chapter "Sequencing the Epigenome").

3.2 Sample and Target Tissue

To identify epigenetic changes associated with major psychosis, the ideal experiment would investigate prospectively the dynamics of epigenome–wide changes in the brains of individuals who eventually become affected compared to unaffected control individuals. At the present time, however, limitations with our current range of epigenetic methodologies render such an approach impossible. Since it is not yet possible to perform prospective in vivo epigenetic studies, particularly for tissues like the brain, only retrospective study designs using *post-mortem* brain samples are viable.

Given the role of epigenetics in mediating when and where genes are expressed, an obvious confounding factor in epigenetic studies is tissue heterogeneity. Because different cell types exhibit quite different epigenetic profiles across different genomic regions, specific tissues – i.e. the primary sites of disease manifestation – are deemed preferable for aetiological studies. It is likely that for studies of psychiatric disorders such as SZ and BD, the primary focus of aetiological studies will be the numerous brain regions implicated in the disorder. Even within specific tissue types, however, there is considerable cellular heterogeneity. Tissues like the cortex, for example, consist of numerous different types of neuronal and glial cells, and the detection of cell–type specific epimutations is likely to be difficult unless the epigenetic profile of specific cells can be investigated. This point is highlighted by a recent study identifying epigenetic changes occurring specifically in cortical interneuron cells, suggesting that different cell populations within a single tissue-type can have quite distinct epigenetic profiles (Veldic et al. 2005). Of course, at present it would probably be very difficult, logistically and financially, to perform a microarray-based study focused on various types of cell populations. However, with the rapid technological advances currently taking place, a future line of research could be to search for cell–type specific epimutations using laser capture microdissection technology, which enables the isolation of single cells from whole tissue thus avoiding the confounding effects of cell-type variation (Bahn et al. 2001).

Proving a direct causal link between epigenetic factors and disease is not necessarily straightforward. For example, it is possible that any observed epigenetic differences actually result from psychosis-induced changes in the brain. Alternatively, epigenetic changes could result from the medications used to treat major psychosis. Of relevance to both SZ and BD is the observation that valproic acid, primarily used as a mood stabilizer, is a potent inhibitor of histone deactylating enzymes (Sharma et al. 2006) and induces widespread epigenetic reprogramming (Milutinovic et al. 2007). Tissues that are not the disease site or directly affected by antipsychotic medications could thus actually be very useful in elucidating epigenetic changes associated directly with major psychosis. For example, peripheral blood-based studies may be useful in revealing epigenetic changes resulting from early embryogenesis, or even highlighting inherited epigenetic variation. There is increasing evidence that many epimutations are not limited to the affected tissue or cell type, but can also be detected in other tissues. Good examples are the epimutations at *IGF2* (Cui et al. 2003) in lymphocytes and *MLH1* in sperm cells (Suter 2004), observed in colon cancer patients, and epimutations at *KCNQ1OT1* in the lymphocytes and skin fibroblasts in Beckwith-Wiedemann syndrome (Weksberg et al. 2002). The study of peripheral cells may even have some advantages over the use of brain tissue in that they are likely to accumulate fewer epigenetic changes induced by external factors, such as medications, drugs, and stress, which could all be confounding factors to epigenetic studies. The use of peripheral cells would also allow the longitudinal study of epigenetic changes throughout the life course of individuals diagnosed with major psychosis, providing information about the epigenetic factors associated with the development, remission, and relapse of the disorder.

It has been recently proposed that germline epimutations may be important in disease etiology (Suter 2004), and potentially transmitted between generations. A recent study reported considerable intra- and inter-individual epigenetic variation in male germ cells (Flanagan et al. 2006). However, previous studies of germline epimutations have found that aberrantly methylated cytosines may be present at very low frequencies ($<1\%$) (Suter 2004) and such small changes cannot be accurately detected with current microarray technology. Recent technological advances in DNA methylation analysis, such as the 'deep' sequencing of bisulfite-treated DNA (Taylor et al. 2007), may make the detection of such minute DNA methylation differences more easily detectable.

3.3 Defining a 'Normal' Epigenetic Profile

Despite the current interest in the possible role of epigenetic processes in disorders like SZ and BD, very little empirical research has been performed to characterize what actually comprises a 'normal' epigenome. Before we can systematically investigate the epigenetic changes associated with disease, we must first catalogue the genome-wide DNA methylation patterns in all major tissues. This is one of the targets of the Human Epigenome Project (www.epigenome.org), which aims to map all methylation variable positions (MVPs) in the genome (Eckhardt et al. 2006). Producing a reference map of the entire human epigenome is going to be a gargantuan task, especially given the huge epigenetic differences that are likely to occur both between tissue/cell types, and within a specific tissue/cell type over the course of development. To date, this private/public consortium has released DNA methylation profiles of the major histocompatibility complex (Rakyan et al. 2004) and chromosomes 6, 20, and 22 (Eckhardt et al. 2006).

4 Epigenetic Studies of Major Psychosis

4.1 Candidate Gene Epigenetic Studies in Major Psychosis

Until recently, few studies had investigated the role of epigenetic factors in major psychosis, with the majority focusing on the role of DNA methylation changes in the vicinity of specific candidate psychosis genes. Early studies reported DNA methylation differences associated with SZ in the vicinity of both catechol-O-methyltransferase (*COMT*) (Abdolmaleky et al. 2006) and reelin (*RELN*) (Grayson et al. 2005), although these findings were not confirmed by other groups using fully quantitative methylation profiling methods (Dempster et al. 2006; Mill et al. 2008; Tochigi et al. 2008). Our group recently performed the most thorough study to date of major psychosis candidate gene regions utilizing DNA from the frontal cortex obtained from *post mortem* brain tissues of SZ, BD, and control samples (Mill et al. 2008). Using sodium bisulfite treatment and subsequent pyrosequencing analysis we quantitatively measured the density of methylated cytosines with assays designed to span CpG-rich promoter regions, along with some exonic and intronic regions, across ten candidate genes (*ARVCF, BDNF, COMT, DRD4, DTNBP1, GAD1, GRIN2B, MTHFR, NRG1*, and *RELN*). Little evidence was found to suggest that DNA methylation in these genes is associated with either SZ or BD. Our analyses included the promoter regions of both *COMT* and *RELN* that have been previously shown to be epigenetically altered in psychosis in previous studies (Abdolmaleky et al. 2006, 2005; Grayson et al. 2005). Unlike these studies that report *COMT* hypomethylation and *RELN* hypermethylation in SZ samples, we found no evidence for DNA methylation changes in these genes associated with either SZ or BD. Our data are in agreement with a previous study on *COMT* reporting no association between promoter methylation and major psychosis (Dempster et al. 2006), and a recent study reporting very low levels of methylation across the *RELN* region, and no association with major psychosis (Tochigi et al. 2008). It should be noted that some of the methods used in previous studies of these genes, for example methylation-specific PCR, can lead to biased assessment of methylated cytosines, and are not able to assess epigenetic changes in a truly quantitative manner as is possible with the Pyrosequencing methodology utilized in this study.

One interesting finding from our candidate gene analysis was the observation that a non-synonymous SNP in *BDNF* (rs6265 – val66met), previously implicated in the etiology of major psychosis, was modestly associated with DNA methylation at surrounding CpG sites. 74% of the samples tested were CC (val homozygotes), and 26% were CT or TT (met carriers). Val homozygotes had significantly higher DNA methylation across the exonic region profiled using pyrosequencing (average methylation = 83% *vs* 78% in val homozygotes *vs* met carriers; $p = 0.02$). The observation of an association between genotype at a non-synonymous SNP (rs6265) in *BDNF*, and DNA methylation at surrounding CpG sites in DNA from frontal cortex brain tissue adds to the increasing evidence that DNA sequences can influence epigenetic profiles (e.g. (Flanagan et al. 2006; Murrell et al. 2004). Whilst DNA alleles and haplotypes can be subject to differential epigenetic modification, it appears that epigenetic status cannot be unequivocally deduced from DNA sequence data alone. The notion that epigenetic changes may be associated with DNA sequence variation is relevant to the inconsistent genetic association studies in complex diseases, and suggests that a comprehensive epigenetic analysis of candidate SNPs and haplotypes is warranted.

4.2 Epigenome-Wide Studies Utilizing Microarray Technology

As discussed above, methods to study DNA methylation have been greatly aided by the development of microarray-based techniques that can interrogate the methylation status of thousands of genomic sites in parallel (Huang 1999; Khulan et al. 2006; Lippman et al. 2005; Shi et al. 2003). Despite the obvious benefits of taking an epigenomic approach, to date these methods have not been widely used to identify DNA methylation changes in complex disease phenotypes such as major psychosis (Callinan and Feinberg 2006). The first study to utilize genome-wide methylomic approaches in psychosis investigated DNA methylation differences between MZ twins discordant for BD (Kuratomi et al. 2007). They found evidence for increased methylation in affected twins upstream of the spermine synthase gene (*SMS*) and lower methylation upstream of the peptidylprolyl isomerase E-like gene (*PPIEL*). Whilst DNA methylation upstream of *SMS* was not correlated with expression of the gene, a strong inverse correlation between *PPIEL* gene expression and DNA methylation was observed.

Our group has recently published a comprehensive methylomic study of major psychosis (Mill et al. 2008). This study utilized 105 frontal cortex brain tissue samples obtained from the Stanley Medical Research Foundation. Following enrichment of the unmethylated fraction of genomic DNA, samples were hybridized on 12,192-feature CpG island microarrays to identify DNA methylation changes associated with SZ and BD. We found evidence for psychosis-associated DNA methylation differences in numerous loci, including several genes that have been functionally linked to disease etiology. Consistent with increasing evidence for altered glutamatergic and GABAergic neurotransmission in the pathogenesis of major psychosis (Benes and Berretta 2001; Coyle 2004), we identified epigenetic changes in loci associated with both these neurotransmitter pathways. Glutamate is the most abundant fast excitatory neurotransmitter in the mammalian nervous system, with a critical role in synaptic plasticity. Several lines of evidence link the glutamate system to psychosis, in particular the observation that glutamate receptor agonists can cause psychotic symptoms in unaffected individuals.

In addition, information about lifetime antipsychotic use (in fluphenazine milligram equivalents) was available for 34 SZ samples. Methylation of a promoter CpG island located ~30kb upstream of the gene encoding mitogen-activated protein kinase kinase I (*MEK1*) was found to be significantly correlated with lifetime antipsychotic use in both male ($n = 25$, $r^2 = 0.6$, $p = 6.8E{-}06$) and female ($n = 9$, $r^2 = 0.5$, $p = 0.04$) samples, with higher lifetime antipsychotic use associated with lower DNA methylation. Our observation of a link between epigenetic changes upstream of *MEK1* and antipsychotic exposure in SZ is striking given the involvement of mitogen-activated protein kinase (MAPK) signaling pathways in mediating intraneuronal signaling, and the observation that clozapine, a widely used medication in the treatment of SZ, selectively activates this pathway via an interaction with *MEK1*.

Gene ontology (GO) analysis allows the investigation of functionally-linked biological pathways in microarray datasets (Ashburner et al. 2000). Several interesting GO categories were highlighted by our analysis, including several involved in various epigenetic processes, transcription, and development. In addition we find an association with genes involved in 'brain development' in both female BD and SZ samples and 'response to stress' in male BD samples, consistent with the popular diathesis-stress hypothesis of psychosis susceptibility. In addition, given the postulated link between mitochondrial dysfunction, oxidative stress and psychosis (Prabakaran et al. 2004), it is interesting that a number of mitochondrial GO categories show significantly different distributions in affected individuals. Our methylome results are in close agreement with a parallel microarray-based transcriptomics, proteomics and metabolomics study, also performed on brain tissue obtained from the Stanley Foundation, in which genes/proteins associated with mitochondrial function and oxidative stress responses were the most altered group (Prabakaran et al. 2004).

Traditional etiological studies of complex disease, both genetic and epigenetic, have tended to investigate discrete regions of DNA in isolation. It is plausible, however, that the epigenome, like many other biological systems, comprises a complex network of interacting processes and that DNA methylation in different genomic regions is inter-dependent. Understanding the system-level features of biological organization across the epigenome is an important aspect of elucidating the epigenetic changes associated with disease. In order to investigate if DNA methylation is coordinated across different loci, we utilized a novel network-based approach to test the modularity of our methylome data. In this way, a network comprises of distinct clusters of elements, termed 'modules', which are highly connected within themselves but have fewer connections with the rest of the network (Newman 2006). The study of interaction networks has proven fruitful in many areas of biological research, highlighting distinct modularity in metabolic networks (Ravasz et al. 2002), cellular networks (Rives and Galitski 2003), and protein interaction networks (Spirin and Mirny 2003). Whilst such an approach has not been previously applied to the epigenome, recent evidence suggests the involvement of coordinated epigenetic silencing across large genomic regions in cancer (Frigola et al. 2006).

The goal of our network analysis was twofold: first, to see whether there is modularity in the methylome; second, if such epigenetic modularity exists, to see whether there are any differences between affected and unaffected groups. For both brain and germline DNA, we found evidence for significant epigenetic modularity in both groups analyzed. No modules were observed in a series of simulated 'random' datasets, suggesting that the modular structure of the methylome is a real biological phenomenon and that the epigenome can be split into distinct groups of correlated loci, potentially corresponding to distinct functional pathways and/or physical regions. Whilst DNA methylation in both affected and unaffected groups is clearly modular, the number of interconnections between specific genomic regions is higher in the affected group compared to the control group, resulting in more between-module interference, in both brain and germline DNA. Given that modules within such biological networks are likely to have specific functional tasks, separate to those of other modules (Newman 2006), the lower degree of DNA methylation modularity observed in the major psychosis samples points to some degree of systemic epigenetic dysfunction associated with major psychosis.

5 Conclusions and Future Direction

It is now generally accepted that epigenetic factors may interact with DNA sequence polymorphisms and environmental factors in mediating susceptibility to SZ and BD. In this chapter we have discussed the benefits of including epigenetic theory into models of disease etiology, highlighting how epigenetic mechanisms can account for the many features of major psychosis that are unexplainable using traditional DNA sequence-based and environmental mechanisms. The study of epigenetics, especially in complex diseases, is a relatively new field of research, and optimal laboratory techniques and analysis methods are still being developed. To date few empirical studies have been performed, but there is already mounting evidence that epigenetic changes in several genes are linked to the disorder. Further development of high-resolution epigenome-wide scan for DNA methylation- and histone modification-changes is needed before epigenomic research can be routinely applied to complex disease. Although it would be premature to conclude that epigenetics will lead to revolutionary discoveries in non-Mendelian biology, the study of DNA methylation and histone modifications has the potential to transform our understanding about the molecular etiology of SZ, BD as well as other psychiatric and non-psychiatric complex diseases.

Acknowledgment This project was supported by the National Institute of Mental Health (R01 MH074127-01), Ontario Mental Health Foundation (OHMF), Canadian Institutes for Health and Research (CIHR), NARSAD, and the Stanley Foundation. AP is an OMHF Senior Fellow, JM was supported by a CIHR postdoctoral fellowship.

References

Abdolmaleky HM, Cheng KH, Faraone SV, Wilcox M, Glatt SJ, Gao F, Smith CL, Shafa R, Aeali B, Carnevale J et al., 2006. Hypomethylation of MB-COMT promoter is a major risk factor for schizophrenia and bipolar disorder. Hum Mol Genet 15(21):3132–45.

Abdolmaleky HM, Cheng KH, Russo A, Smith CL, Faraone SV, Wilcox M, Shafa R, Glatt SJ, Nguyen G, Ponte JF et al., 2005. Hypermethylation of the reelin (RELN) promoter in the brain of schizophrenic patients: a preliminary report. Am J Med Genet B Neuropsychiatr Genet 134(1):60–6.

Abkevich V, Camp NJ, Hensel CH, Neff CD, Russell DL, Hughes DC, Plenk AM, Lowry MR, Richards RL, Carter C et al., 2003. Predisposition locus for major depression at chromosome 12q22-12q23.2. Am J Hum Genet 73(6):1271–81.

Akbarian S, Ruehl MG, Bliven E, Luiz LA, Peranelli AC, Baker SP, Roberts RC, Bunney WE, Jr., Conley RC, Jones EG et al., 2005. Chromatin alterations associated with down-regulated metabolic gene expression in the prefrontal cortex of subjects with schizophrenia. Arch Gen Psychiatry 62(8):829–40.

Arnold LM. 2003. Gender differences in bipolar disorder. Psychiatr Clin North Am 26(3):595–620.

Ashburner M, Ball CA, Blake JA, Botstein D, Butler H, Cherry JM, Davis AP, Dolinski K, Dwight SS, Eppig JT et al., 2000. Gene ontology: tool for the unification of biology. The Gene Ontology Consortium. Nat Genet 25(1):25–9.

Azzi L, El-Alfy M, Labrie F. 2006. Gender differences and effects of sex steroids and dehydroepiandrosterone on androgen and oestrogen alpha receptors in mouse sebaceous glands. Br J Dermatol 154(1):21–7.

Bahn S, Augood SJ, Ryan M, Standaert DG, Starkey M, Emson PC. 2001. Gene expression profiling in the post-mortem human brain–no cause for dismay. J Chem Neuroanat 22(1–2):79–94.

Baron M. 2001. Genetic linkage and bipolar disorder: a cautionary note. J Affect Disord 67(1–3): 267–73.

Belmont JW. 1996. Genetic control of X inactivation and processes leading to X-inactivation skewing. Am J Hum Genet 58(6):1101–8.

Benes FM, Berretta S. 2001. GABAergic interneurons: implications for understanding schizophrenia and bipolar disorder. Neuropsychopharmacology 25(1):1–27.

Blewitt ME, Vickaryous NK, Hemley SJ, Ashe A, Bruxner TJ, Preis JI, Arkell R, Whitelaw E. 2005. An N-ethyl-N-nitrosourea screen for genes involved in variegation in the mouse. Proc Natl Acad Sci U S A 102(21):7629–34.

Callinan PA, Feinberg AP. 2006. The emerging science of epigenomics. Hum Mol Genet 15 Spec No 1:R95–R101.

Cardno AG, Gottesman, II. 2000. Twin studies of schizophrenia: from bow-and-arrow concordances to star wars Mx and functional genomics. Am J Med Genet 97(1):12–7.

Chakrabarti SK, Francis J, Ziesmann SM, Garmey JC, Mirmira RG. 2003. Covalent histone modifications underlie the developmental regulation of insulin gene transcription in pancreatic beta cells. J Biol Chem 278(26):23617–23.
Chang HS, Anway MD, Rekow SS, Skinner MK. 2006. Transgenerational epigenetic imprinting of the male germline by endocrine disruptor exposure during gonadal sex determination. Endocrinology 147(12):5524–41.
Coolen MW, Statham AL, Gardiner-Garden M, Clark SJ. 2007. Genomic profiling of CpG methylation and allelic specificity using quantitative high-throughput mass spectrometry: critical evaluation and improvements. Nucleic Acids Res 35(18):e119.
Cooney CA, Dave AA, Wolff GL. 2002. Maternal methyl supplements in mice affect epigenetic variation and DNA methylation of offspring. J Nutr 132(8 Suppl):2393S–2400S.
Coyle JT. 2004. The GABA-glutamate connection in schizophrenia: which is the proximate cause? Biochem Pharmacol 68(8):1507–14.
Craddock N, Jones I. 1999. Genetics of bipolar disorder. J Med Genet 36(8):585–94.
Craddock N, O'Donovan MC, Owen MJ. 2005. The genetics of schizophrenia and bipolar disorder: dissecting psychosis. J Med Genet 42(3):193–204.
Craddock N, O'Donovan MC, Owen MJ. 2006. Genes for schizophrenia and bipolar disorder? Implications for psychiatric nosology. Schizophr Bull 32(1):9–16.
Craddock N, Owen MJ. 2007. Rethinking psychosis: the disadvantages of a dichotomous classification now outweigh the advantages. World Psychiatry 6(2):20–7.
Craig IW, Harper E, Loat CS. 2004. The genetic basis for sex differences in human behaviour: role of the sex chromosomes. Ann Hum Genet 68(Pt 3):269–84.
Crow TJ, DeLisi LE, Johnstone EC. 1989. Concordance by sex in sibling pairs with schizophrenia is paternally inherited. Evidence for a pseudoautosomal locus. Br J Psychiatry 155:92–7.
Cui H, Cruz-Correa M, Giardiello FM, Hutcheon DF, Kafonek DR, Brandenburg S, Wu Y, He X, Powe NR, Feinberg AP. 2003. Loss of IGF2 imprinting: a potential marker of colorectal cancer risk. Science 299(5613):1753–5.
Davis CD, Uthus EO. 2003. Dietary folate and selenium affect dimethylhydrazine-induced aberrant crypt formation, global DNA methylation and one-carbon metabolism in rats. J Nutr 133(9):2907–14.
DeLisi L, Shaw S, Crow T. 2001. A genome-wide scan in 301 families with sibling-pairs diagnosed with schizophrenia of schizoaffective disorder suggests linkage to chromosomes 2pcen and 10p14. American Journal of Medical Genetics (Neuropsychiatric Genetics) 105(7): 561–578.
Dempster EL, Mill J, Craig IW, Collier DA. 2006. The quantification of COMT mRNA in post mortem cerebellum tissue: diagnosis, genotype, methylation and expression. BMC Med Genet 7:10.
Dib C, Faure S, Fizames C, Samson D, Drouot N, Vignal A, Millasseau P, Marc S, Hazan J, Seboun E et al., 1996. A comprehensive genetic map of the human genome based on 5,264 microsatellites. Nature 380(6570):152–4.
Dolinoy DC, Weidman JR, Jirtle RL. 2007. Epigenetic gene regulation: Linking early developmental environment to adult disease. Reprod Toxicol 23(3):297–307.
Eckhardt F, Lewin J, Cortese R, Rakyan VK, Attwood J, Burger M, Burton J, Cox TV, Davies R, Down TA et al., 2006. DNA methylation profiling of human chromosomes 6, 20 and 22. Nat Genet 38(12):1378–85.
Feil R. 2006. Environmental and nutritional effects on the epigenetic regulation of genes. Mutat Res 600(1–2):46–57.
Ferguson-Smith A, Lin SP, Tsai CE, Youngson N, Tevendale M. 2003. Genomic imprinting–insights from studies in mice. Semin Cell Dev Biol 14(1):43–9.
Flanagan JM, Popendikyte V, Pozdniakovaite N, Sobolev M, Assadzadeh A, Schumacher A, Zangeneh M, Lau L, Virtanen C, Wang SC et al., 2006. Intra- and interindividual epigenetic variation in human germ cells. Am J Hum Genet 79(1):67–84.
Flanagan JM, Violeta Popendikyte, Natalija Pozdniakovaite, Martha Sobolev, Abbas Assadzadeh, Axel Schumacher, Masood Zangeneh, Lynette Lau, Carl Virtanen, Sun-Chong Wang, and

Arturas Petronis. 2006. Intra- and Interindividual Epigenetic Variation in Human Germ Cells. The American Journal of Human Genetics 79:67–84.

Fraga MF, Ballestar E, Paz MF, Ropero S, Setien F, Ballestar ML, Heine-Suner D, Cigudosa JC, Urioste M, Benitez J et al., 2005. Epigenetic differences arise during the lifetime of monozygotic twins. Proc Natl Acad Sci U S A 102(30):10604–9.

Frigola J, Song J, Stirzaker C, Hinshelwood RA, Peinado MA, Clark SJ. 2006. Epigenetic remodeling in colorectal cancer results in coordinate gene suppression across an entire chromosome band. Nat Genet 38(5):540–9.

Frommer M, McDonald LE, Millar DS, Collis CM, Watt F, Grigg GW, Molloy PL, Paul CL. 1992. A genomic sequencing protocol that yields a positive display of 5-methylcytosine residues in individual DNA strands. Proc Natl Acad Sci U S A 89(5):1827–31.

Fu M, Rao M, Wang C, Sakamaki T, Wang J, Di Vizio D, Zhang X, Albanese C, Balk S, Chang C et al., 2003. Acetylation of androgen receptor enhances coactivator binding and promotes prostate cancer cell growth. Mol Cell Biol 23(23):8563–75.

Fu M, Wang C, Zhang X, Pestell RG. 2004. Acetylation of nuclear receptors in cellular growth and apoptosis. Biochem Pharmacol 68(6):1199–208.

Gershon ES, Badner JA. 2001. Progress toward discovery of susceptibility genes for bipolar manic-depressive illness and schizophrenia. CNS Spectr 6(12):965–8, 977.

Grayson DR, Jia X, Chen Y, Sharma RP, Mitchell CP, Guidotti A, Costa E. 2005. Reelin promoter hypermethylation in schizophrenia. Proc Natl Acad Sci U S A 102(26):9341–6.

Hafner H. 2003. Gender differences in schizophrenia. Psychoneuroendocrinology 28 Suppl 2:17–54.

Hamilton A, Voinnet O, Chappell L, Baulcombe D. 2002. Two classes of short interfering RNA in RNA silencing. Embo J 21(17):4671–9.

Harrison PJ, Weinberger DR. 2005. Schizophrenia genes, gene expression, and neuropathology: on the matter of their convergence. Mol Psychiatry 10(1):40–68; image 5.

Henikoff S, Matzke MA. 1997. Exploring and explaining epigenetic effects. Trends Genet 13(8):293–5.

Hennah W, Varilo T, Kestila M, Paunio T, Arajarvi R, Haukka J, Parker A, Martin R, Levitzky S, Partonen T et al., 2003. Haplotype transmission analysis provides evidence of association for DISC1 to schizophrenia and suggests sex-dependent effects. Hum Mol Genet 12(23):3151–9.

Huang HS, Matevossian A, Jiang Y, Akbarian S. 2006. Chromatin Immunoprecipitation in Postmortem Brain. J Neurosci Methods 156:284–92.

Huang TH, Perry MR, Laux DE. 1999. Methylation profiling of CpG islands in human breast cancer cells. Hum Mol Genet 8(3):459–70.

Jablonka E, Lamb M. 1995. Epigenetic Inheritance and Evolution: Oxford University Press.

Jaenisch R, Bird A. 2003. Epigenetic regulation of gene expression: how the genome integrates intrinsic and environmental signals. Nat Genet 33 Suppl:245–54.

Jenuwein T, Allis CD. 2001. Translating the histone code. Science 293(5532):1074–80.

Jones PL, Veenstra GJ, Wade PA, Vermaak D, Kass SU, Landsberger N, Strouboulis J, Wolffe AP. 1998. Methylated DNA and MeCP2 recruit histone deacetylase to repress transcription. Nat Genet 19(2):187–91.

Kaminsky Z, Wang SC, Petronis A. 2006. Complex disease, gender and epigenetics. Ann Med 38(8):530–44.

Kato T. 2007. Molecular genetics of bipolar disorder and depression. Psychiatry Clin Neurosci 61(1):3–19.

Kawakami K, Ruszkiewicz A, Bennett G, Moore J, Grieu F, Watanabe G, Iacopetta B. 2006. DNA hypermethylation in the normal colonic mucosa of patients with colorectal cancer. Br J Cancer 94(4):593–8.

Kelsoe JR, Spence MA, Loetscher E, Foguet M, Sadovnick AD, Remick RA, Flodman P, Khristich J, Mroczkowski-Parker Z, Brown JL et al., 2001. A genome survey indicates a possible susceptibility locus for bipolar disorder on chromosome 22. Proc Natl Acad Sci U S A 98(2):585–90.

Khulan B, Thompson RF, Ye K, Fazzari MJ, Suzuki M, Stasiek E, Figueroa ME, Glass JL, Chen Q, Montagna C et al., 2006. Comparative isoschizomer profiling of cytosine methylation: the HELP assay. Genome Res 16(8):1046–55.

Kinyamu HK, Archer TK. 2004. Modifying chromatin to permit steroid hormone receptor-dependent transcription. Biochim Biophys Acta 1677(1–3):30–45.

Klar AJ. 1998. Propagating epigenetic states through meiosis: where Mendel's gene is more than a DNA moiety. Trends Genet 14(8):299–301.

Kuhn TS. 1962. The structure of scienitific revolutions. 172p., editor. Chicago University Press. 172 p.

Kuratomi G, Iwamoto K, Bundo M, Kusumi I, Kato N, Iwata N, Ozaki N, Kato T. 2007. Aberrant DNA methylation associated with bipolar disorder identified from discordant monozygotic twins. Mol Psychiatry.

Lai JC, Cheng YW, Chiou HL, Wu MF, Chen CY, Lee H. 2005. Gender difference in estrogen receptor alpha promoter hypermethylation and its prognostic value in non-small cell lung cancer. Int J Cancer 117(6):974–80.

Lamb JA, Barnby G, Bonora E, Sykes N, Bacchelli E, Blasi F, Maestrini E, Broxholme J, Tzenova J, Weeks D et al., 2005. Analysis of IMGSAC autism susceptibility loci: evidence for sex limited and parent of origin specific effects. J Med Genet 42(2):132–7.

Lippman Z, Gendrel AV, Colot V, Martienssen R. 2005. Profiling DNA methylation patterns using genomic tiling microarrays. Nat Methods 2(3):219–24.

Liu JC, Baker RE, Chow W, Sun CK, Elsholtz HP. 2005. Epigenetic mechanisms in the dopamine D2 receptor-dependent inhibition of the prolactin gene. Mol Endocrinol 19(7): 1904–1917.

Mani ST, Thakur MK. 2006. In the cerebral cortex of female and male mice, amyloid precursor protein (APP) promoter methylation is higher in females and differentially regulated by sex steroids. Brain Res 1067(1):43–7.

McGuffin P, Asherson P, Owen M, Farmer A. 1994. The strength of the genetic effect. Is there room for an environmental influence in the aetiology of schizophrenia? Br J Psychiatry 164(5):593–9.

McMahon FJ, Hopkins PJ, Xu J, McInnis MG, Shaw S, Cardon L, Simpson SG, MacKinnon DF, Stine OC, Sherrington R, Meyers DA, DePaulo JR. 1997. Linkage of bipolar affective disorder to chromosome 18 markers in a new pedigree series. Am J Hum Genet 61(6): 1397–404.

McMahon FJ, Stine OC, Meyers DA, Simpson SG, DePaulo JR. Patterns of maternal transmission in bipolar affective disorder. 1995. Am J Hum Genet 56(6):1277–86.

Meijlink FC, Philipsen JN, Gruber M, Ab G. 1983. Methylation of the chicken vitellogenin gene: influence of estradiol administration. Nucleic Acids Res 11(5):1361–73.

Metivier R, Penot G, Hubner MR, Reid G, Brand H, Kos M, Gannon F. 2003. Estrogen receptor-alpha directs ordered, cyclical, and combinatorial recruitment of cofactors on a natural target promoter. Cell 115(6):751–63.

Mill J, Dempster E, Caspi A, Williams B, Moffitt T, Craig I. 2006a. Evidence for monozygotic twin (MZ) discordance in methylation level at two CpG sites in the promoter region of the catechol-O-methyltransferase (COMT) gene. Am J Med Genet B Neuropsychiatr Genet 141(4):421–5.

Mill J, Tang T, Kaminsky Z, Khare T, Yazdanpanah S, Bouchard L, Jia P, Assadzadeh A, Flanagan J, Schumacher A et al., 2008. Epigenomic Profiling Reveals DNA Methylation Changes Associated with Major Psychosis. Am J Hum Genet 82(3):696–711.

Mill J, Yazdanpanah S, Guckel E, Ziegler S, Kaminsky Z, Petronis A. 2006b. Whole genome amplification of sodium bisulfite-treated DNA allows the accurate estimate of methylated cytosine density in limited DNA resources. Biotechniques 41(5):603–7.

Milutinovic S, D'Alessio AC, Detich N, Szyf M. 2007. Valproate induces widespread epigenetic reprogramming which involves demethylation of specific genes. Carcinogenesis 28(3):560–71.

Mirnics K. 2001. Microarrays in brain research: the good, the bad and the ugly. Nat Rev Neurosci 2(6):444–7.

Morris KV. 2005. siRNA-mediated transcriptional gene silencing: the potential mechanism and a possible role in the histone code. Cell Mol Life Sci 62(24):3057–66.

Murray CJ, Lopez AD. 1997. Mortality by cause for eight regions of the world: Global Burden of Disease Study. Lancet 349(9061):1269–76.

Murrell A, Heeson S, Cooper WN, Douglas E, Apostolidou S, Moore GE, Maher ER, Reik W. 2004. An association between variants in the IGF2 gene and Beckwith-Wiedemann syndrome: interaction between genotype and epigenotype. Hum Mol Genet 13(2):247–55.

Newman ME. 2006. Modularity and community structure in networks. Proc Natl Acad Sci U S A 103(23):8577–82.

Ohara K, Xu HD, Mori N, Suzuki Y, Xu DS, Ohara K, Wang ZC. 1997. Anticipation and imprinting in schizophrenia. Biol Psychiatry 42(9):760–6.

O'Neill LP, VerMilyea MD, Turner B M. 2006. Epigenetic Characterization of the Early Embryo With a Chromatin Immunoprecipitation Protocol Applicable to Small Cell Populations. Nat Genet 38:835–41.

Owen MJ, Craddock N, Jablensky A. 2007. The genetic deconstruction of psychosis. Schizophr Bull 33(4):905–11.

Paulsen M, El-Maarri O, Engemann S, Strodicke M, Franck O, Davies K, Reinhardt R, Reik W, Walter J. 2000. Sequence conservation and variability of imprinting in the Beckwith-Wiedemann syndrome gene cluster in human and mouse. Hum Mol Genet 9(12):1829–41.

Paulsen M, Ferguson-Smith AC. 2001. DNA methylation in genomic imprinting, development, and disease. J Pathol 195(1):97–110.

Penner JD, Brown AS. 2007. Prenatal infectious and nutritional factors and risk of adult schizophrenia. Expert Rev Neurother 7(7):797–805.

Petronis A. 2000. The genes for major psychosis: aberrant sequence or regulation? Neuropsychopharmacology 23(1):1–12.

Petronis A. 2001. Human morbid genetics revisited: relevance of epigenetics. Trends Genet 17(3):142–6.

Petronis A. 2004. The origin of schizophrenia: genetic thesis, epigenetic antithesis, and resolving synthesis. Biol Psychiatry 55(10):965–70.

Petronis A, Gottesman, II, Kan P, Kennedy JL, Basile VS, Paterson AD, Popendikyte V. 2003. Monozygotic twins exhibit numerous epigenetic differences: clues to twin discordance? Schizophr Bull 29(1):169–78.

Plenge RM, Stevenson RA, Lubs HA, Schwartz CE, Willard HF. 2002. Skewed X-chromosome inactivation is a common feature of X-linked mental retardation disorders. Am J Hum Genet 71(1):168–73.

Prabakaran S, Swatton JE, Ryan MM, Huffaker SJ, Huang JT, Griffin JL, Wayland M, Freeman T, Dudbridge F, Lilley KS et al., 2004. Mitochondrial dysfunction in schizophrenia: evidence for compromised brain metabolism and oxidative stress. Mol Psychiatry 9(7):684–97, 643.

Preis JI, Downes M, Oates NA, Rasko JE, Whitelaw E. 2003. Sensitive flow cytometric analysis reveals a novel type of parent-of-origin effect in the mouse genome. Curr Biol 13(11):955–9.

Rakyan V, Whitelaw E. 2003. Transgenerational epigenetic inheritance. Curr Biol 13(1):R6.

Rakyan VK, Blewitt ME, Druker R, Preis JI, Whitelaw E. 2002. Metastable epialleles in mammals. Trends Genet 18(7):348–51.

Rakyan VK, Hildmann T, Novik KL, Lewin J, Tost J, Cox AV, Andrews TD, Howe KL, Otto T, Olek A et al., 2004. DNA methylation profiling of the human major histocompatibility complex: a pilot study for the human epigenome project. PLoS Biol 2(12):e405.

Ravasz E, Somera AL, Mongru DA, Oltvai ZN, Barabasi AL. 2002. Hierarchical organization of modularity in metabolic networks. Science 297(5586):1551–5.

Richards EJ. 2006. Inherited epigenetic variation–revisiting soft inheritance. Nat Rev Genet 7(5):395–401.

Riggs AD, Xiong Z, Wang AG, LeBon JM. 1998. Methylation dynamics, epigenetic fidelity and X chromosome structure. In: Wolffe A, editor. Epigenetics. Chistester: John Wiley & Sons. p 214–227.

Riley B, Kendler KS. 2006. Molecular genetic studies of schizophrenia. Eur J Hum Genet 14(6):669–80.

Rives AW, Galitski T. 2003. Modular organization of cellular networks. Proc Natl Acad Sci U S A 100(3):1128–33.
Robertson G, Hirst M, Bainbridge M, Bilenky M, Zhao Y, Zeng T, Euskirchen G, Bernier B, Varhol R, Delaney A et al., 2007. Genome-wide profiles of STAT1 DNA association using chromatin immunoprecipitation and massively parallel sequencing. Nat Methods 4(8):651–7.
Robertson KD, Wolffe AP. 2000. DNA methylation in health and disease. Nat Rev Genet 1(1):11–9.
Rosa A, Picchioni MM, Kalidindi S, Loat CS, Knight J, Toulopoulou T, Vonk R, van der Schot AC, Nolen W, Kahn RS et al., 2007. Differential methylation of the X-chromosome is a possible source of discordance for bipolar disorder female monozygotic twins. Am J Med Genet B Neuropsychiatr Genet 5;147B(4):459–62.
Saluz HP, Jiricny J, Jost JP. 1986. Genomic sequencing reveals a positive correlation between the kinetics of strand-specific DNA demethylation of the overlapping estradiol/glucocorticoid-receptor binding sites and the rate of avian vitellogenin mRNA synthesis. Proc Natl Acad Sci U S A 83(19):7167–71.
Sarter B, Long TI, Tsong WH, Koh WP, Yu MC, Laird PW. 2005. Sex differential in methylation patterns of selected genes in Singapore Chinese. Hum Genet 117(4):402–3.
Schulze TG, Chen YS, Badner JA, McInnis MG, DePaulo JR Jr, McMahon FJ. 2003. Additional, physically ordered markers increase linkage signal for bipolar disorder on chromosome 18q22. Biol Psychiatry 53(3):239–43.
Sharma RP, Rosen C, Kartan S, Guidotti A, Costa E, Grayson DR, Chase K. 2006. Valproic acid and chromatin remodeling in schizophrenia and bipolar disorder: preliminary results from a clinical population. Schizophr Res 88(1-3):227-31. Epub 2006 Sep 25.
Shi H, Wei SH, Leu YW, Rahmatpanah F, Liu JC, Yan PS, Nephew KP, Huang TH. 2003. Triple analysis of the cancer epigenome: an integrated microarray system for assessing gene expression, DNA methylation, and histone acetylation. Cancer Res 63(9):2164–71.
Shifman S, Bronstein M, Sternfeld M, Pisante-Shalom A, Lev-Lehman E, Weizman A, Reznik I, Spivak B, Grisaru N, Karp L et al., 2002. A highly significant association between a COMT haplotype and schizophrenia. Am J Hum Genet 71(6):1296–302.
Shimabukuro M, Jinno Y, Fuke C, Okazaki Y. 2006a. Haloperidol treatment induces tissue- and sex-specific changes in DNA methylation: a control study using rats. Behav Brain Funct 2:37.
Shimabukuro M, Sasaki T, Imamura A, Tsujita T, Fuke C, Umekage T, Tochigi M, Hiramatsu K, Miyazaki T, Oda T et al., 2006b. Global hypomethylation of peripheral leukocyte DNA in male patients with schizophrenia: A potential link between epigenetics and schizophrenia. J Psychiatr Res 41(12):1042–6.
Spirin V, Mirny LA. 2003. Protein complexes and functional modules in molecular networks. Proc Natl Acad Sci U S A 100(21):12123–8.
Stadler F, Kolb G, Rubusch L, Baker SP, Jones EG, Akbarian S. 2005. Histone methylation at gene promoters is associated with developmental regulation and region-specific expression of ionotropic and metabotropic glutamate receptors in human brain. J Neurochem 94(2): 324–36.
Stone JL, Merriman B, Cantor RM, Yonan AL, Gilliam TC, Geschwind DH, Nelson SF. 2004. Evidence for sex-specific risk alleles in autism spectrum disorder. Am J Hum Genet 75(6):1117–23.
Surani MA, Sasaki H, Ferguson-Smith AC, Allen ND, Barton SC, Jones PA, Reik W. 1993. The inheritance of germline-specific epigenetic modifications during development. Philos Trans R Soc Lond B Biol Sci 339(1288):165–72.
Suter CM, Martin DI, Ward RL. 2004. Germline epimutation of MLH1 in individuals with multiple cancers. Nat Genet 36(5):497–501.
Sutherland JE, Costa M. 2003. Epigenetics and the environment. Ann N Y Acad Sci 983:151–60.
Taylor KH, Kramer RS, Davis JW, Guo J, Duff DJ, Xu D, Caldwell CW, Shi H. 2007. Ultradeep bisulfite sequencing analysis of DNA methylation patterns in multiple gene promoters by 454 sequencing. Cancer Res 67(18):8511–8.

Thomson PA, Wray NR, Millar JK, Evans KL, Hellard SL, Condie A, Muir WJ, Blackwood DH, Porteous DJ. 2005. Association between the TRAX/DISC locus and both bipolar disorder and schizophrenia in the Scottish population. Mol Psychiatry 10(7):657–68, 616.

Tochigi M, Iwamoto K, Bundo M, Komori B, Sasaki T, Kato N, Kato T. (2008). Methylation status of the reelin promoter region in the brain of schizophrenic patients. Biological Psychiatry. 63(5):530–533.

Tost J, Gut IG. 2007. DNA methylation analysis by pyrosequencing. Nat Protoc 2(9):2265–75.

Ushijima T, Watanabe N, Okochi E, Kaneda A, Sugimura T, Miyamoto K. 2003. Fidelity of the methylation pattern and its variation in the genome. Genome Res 13(5):868–74.

Vallada HP, Collier DA. 1998. Genetics of schizophrenia – new findings In: Gattaz WF, Hafner H, editors. Search for the causes of schizophrenia. Berlin, New York: Springer Verlag. p 114–123.

Veldic M, Guidotti A, Maloku E, Davis JM, Costa E. 2005. In psychosis, cortical interneurons overexpress DNA-methyltransferase 1. Proc Natl Acad Sci U S A 102(6):2152–7.

Weaver IC, Cervoni N, Champagne FA, D'Alessio AC, Sharma S, Seckl JR, Dymov S, Szyf M, Meaney MJ. 2004. Epigenetic programming by maternal behavior. Nat Neurosci.

Weksberg R, Shuman C, Caluseriu O, Smith AC, Fei YL, Nishikawa J, Stockley TL, Best L, Chitayat D, Olney A et al., 2002. Discordant KCNQ1OT1 imprinting in sets of monozygotic twins discordant for Beckwith-Wiedemann syndrome. Hum Mol Genet 11(11):1317–25.

Wilks A, Seldran M, Jost JP. 1984. An estrogen-dependent demethylation at the 5' end of the chicken vitellogenin gene is independent of DNA synthesis. Nucleic Acids Res 12(2):1163–77.

Wilks AF, Cozens PJ, Mattaj IW, Jost JP. 1982. Estrogen induces a demethylation at the 5' end region of the chicken vitellogenin gene. Proc Natl Acad Sci U S A 79(14):4252–5.

Willard HF. 2000. The sex chromosomes and X chromosome inactivation. In: Scriver CR, et al., editor. The metabolic and molecular basis of inherited disease. 8 ed. New York: McGraw-Hill. pp. 1191–1211.

Wong AH, Gottesman, II, Petronis A. 2005. Phenotypic differences in genetically identical organisms: the epigenetic perspective. Hum Mol Genet 14 Spec No 1:R11–8.

Xu L, Glass CK, Rosenfeld MG. 1999. Coactivator and corepressor complexes in nuclear receptor function. Curr Opin Genet Dev 9(2):140–7.

Yatabe Y, Tavare S, Shibata D. 2001. Investigating stem cells in human colon by using methylation patterns. Proc Natl Acad Sci U S A 98(19):10839–44.

Yu J, Zhang H, Gu J, Lin S, Li J, Lu W, Wang Y, Zhu J. 2004. Methylation profiles of thirty four promoter-CpG islands and concordant methylation behaviours of sixteen genes that may contribute to carcinogenesis of astrocytoma. BMC Cancer 4:65.

Zubenko GS, Maher B, Hughes HB, 3rd, Zubenko WN, Stiffler JS, Kaplan BB, Marazita ML. 2003. Genome-wide linkage survey for genetic loci that influence the development of depressive disorders in families with recurrent, early-onset, major depression. Am J Med Genet B Neuropsychiatr Genet 123(1):1–18.

Index

A
ANOVA model, 37, 40
Antisense genes, 187, 192
Arabidopsis, 24, 25, 38, 39, 44, 46, 48, 49, 108, 125, 129, 133, 135, 136, 139, 163–171, 178, 275, 329, 332, 333, 398, 399, 401–405, 413
ATP-dependent nucleosome remodelers, 101, 105

B
Bipolar disorder, 378, 411, 412, 416–428
Bisulfite sequencing, 19, 21, 23–25, 27, 28, 380, 421

C
Cancer, 4, 10, 14, 20, 22, 27, 32, 37, 38, 73, 75–78, 93, 344, 345, 347, 349–354, 356, 357, 359–363, 369, 372–379, 385–393, 423, 427
Cancer epigenetics, 75, 369, 378
Centromeres, 91, 102, 105, 106, 109, 132, 149–159, 177, 180, 181, 307, 369, 376, 388
CG dinucleotide, 22, 24, 69, 71, 72, 76, 79, 164, 165, 235
ChIP-on-chip, 3–5, 7–10, 29, 263, 422
ChIP-seq, 3–5, 7, 9, 10, 19, 26, 29–32, 107–109, 111, 112, 167, 238, 247, 272, 343, 390, 392, 422
Chromatin, 3–7, 11, 12, 19, 20, 22, 25, 27–32, 37–42, 44, 45, 50, 51, 55, 57, 62, 70, 71, 75, 76, 85, 86, 95, 101–103, 106–111, 113, 114, 133, 134, 137, 139, 149–153, 155, 157–159, 163, 167–169, 177–183, 187, 198, 200–205, 217–219, 222–226, 229, 238, 239, 243, 255, 260, 261, 271, 272, 283, 286–290, 292, 293, 295, 305–307, 314, 328, 329, 343, 346, 349–353, 371, 373, 375–377, 379, 380, 385, 387, 388, 390, 392, 393, 400–406, 411, 413, 417, 419, 422
Chromatin insulators, 22, 177, 182, 198, 204
Chromatin modification, 30, 31, 37–39, 41, 42, 44, 50, 51, 55, 134, 153, 177, 201, 286, 305, 346, 385, 387, 400–402, 405, 417
Chromatin replication, 217
Chromatin structure, 85, 86, 149, 151, 169, 200–202, 283, 286–290, 377, 385, 413
Complex non-Mendelian diease, 411
CpG island, 10, 14, 26, 57, 69, 74, 75, 78, 79, 192, 291, 371–375, 386, 390, 391, 426
CpG spacing, 85, 92
CpG-methylation, 87, 129, 187, 193, 200, 201, 206, 379, 421
CTCF, 22, 193, 197–200, 202, 204, 288, 289, 292
Cytosine methylation, 21–23, 38, 48, 69–80, 86, 124–126, 129, 133, 134, 139, 164–166, 168, 275, 325, 371, 413, 419

D
Data visualisation, 55, 60, 61
Demethylation, 77, 92, 157, 158, 163, 171, 228, 259–261, 264, 266, 267, 269, 270, 272–274, 370, 406, 417
Differentially methylated regions (DMRs), 10, 14, 57, 60, 61, 92, 93, 235, 236, 244–246, 248, 251–255, 271
DNA methylation, 3
DNA microarrays, 40, 45, 101, 107, 390
DNA sequencing, 59, 101, 275, 388, 389
Dnmt1, 22, 76, 85–89, 165, 198, 201, 253, 260, 270, 347, 370
Dnmt3, 87, 88, 93, 95, 165
Dnmt3a, 22, 76, 77, 85, 86, 88–94, 198, 201, 347, 370

435

Dnmt3b, 22, 77, 85, 88, 89, 91–93, 198, 268, 347, 370, 376
Dnmt3L, 76, 85, 88–95, 198
Drosophila, 4, 105, 106, 108, 110, 111, 150, 168, 177–182, 187, 218–220, 223–225, 227, 229, 262, 268, 307, 329, 332, 351, 398, 403, 413
DXPas34, 187, 189, 190, 193, 194, 196–199

E

EG cells, 261, 263, 265, 266, 272
Embryonic stem cells, 26, 31, 32, 75, 92, 188, 190, 192–202, 204, 218, 228, 229, 239–242, 244–247, 249, 250, 253, 264, 266–269, 271–273, 276
Epigenetic, 3, 4, 9, 10, 15, 19, 20, 22, 24, 28, 29, 32, 33, 37, 38, 46, 49, 50, 55–58, 60, 62, 63, 77, 78, 86, 101–114, 119–140, 149–159, 163–165, 167, 170, 171, 178, 179, 187–207, 217–229, 235, 236, 238, 240, 241, 248, 251–255, 259–270, 272, 283–295, 314, 343, 344, 346, 347, 352, 357, 363, 369–380, 385, 386, 391, 392, 397–407, 411, 413, 414–427
Epigenetic mark, 15, 20, 22, 28, 33, 56, 130, 149, 165, 217, 218, 222, 223, 225, 226, 229, 236, 254, 259, 261, 267, 269, 289, 370, 372, 375, 386, 416, 418
Epigenetic programming, 259, 398
Epigenetics, 19, 37, 62, 87, 120, 163, 217, 236, 283, 343, 344, 347, 369, 376, 378, 385, 397, 411, 427, 428
Epigenome, 3–16, 17–22, 55–63, 69–71, 73, 75, 77–79, 101, 102, 106, 107, 111, 113, 120, 127, 134, 135, 138–140, 149, 157, 238, 263, 270, 271, 275, 343–364, 369–380, 385, 390, 392, 416, 421, 422, 424–427
Epigenomic, 32, 37–51, 55, 62, 70, 73, 74, 78, 79, 101–103, 106, 107, 113, 120, 125, 128, 134, 135, 139, 140, 163–171, 178, 259–276, 376, 380, 385, 386, 388, 391–393, 411, 413, 425, 428
Epigenomics, 16, 37, 38, 75, 113, 135, 138, 267, 347
ES cells, *see* Embryonic stem cells
ESCSs, *see* Embryonic stem cells
Euchromatin, 46, 49, 134, 149, 150, 180, 182

F

Flowering Locus C (FLC), 38, 168, 398–406

G

Genetics, 111, 120, 125, 130, 164, 170, 218, 335, 347, 411, 414, 416
Genome association, 343, 345, 357, 412
Genome browser, 55, 56, 60–62, 245, 264
Genome defense, 166, 321–336
Genome-wide, 9, 10, 19, 22, 29, 49, 57–60, 70, 71, 75, 76, 79, 102, 107, 110, 112, 114, 138, 157, 158, 163, 165–168, 204, 225, 235, 255, 259–263, 265, 268–272, 347, 363, 369, 371, 374, 378–380, 385, 386, 391, 392, 397, 422, 424, 425, 427
Genomic imprinting, 22, 86, 92, 235–255, 311, 369, 419
Genomic imprints, 259
Genomics, 37, 58, 62, 102, 113, 163
Germline reprogramming, 259
Globin, 283–295

H

Heterochromatin, 46
Histone chaperones, 101, 105, 219
Histone code, 70, 240
Histone enzymes, 343, 348–352, 370–373, 375, 385, 386, 423
Histone modifications, 3, 4, 9, 12, 19, 20, 28–30, 37–39, 43, 44, 46, 47, 49–51, 55–58, 60, 62, 70, 74, 76, 85–87, 92, 101, 108, 111, 114, 125, 156, 157, 159, 167, 168, 187, 201, 203, 217, 219, 223, 224, 235, 238–249, 251–255, 259, 261–263, 267, 270, 271, 273, 275, 283, 284, 286, 289, 290, 292, 306, 312, 314, 343, 344, 347–352, 363, 370–373, 375–380, 387, 388, 390, 392, 393, 400, 401, 405, 413, 418, 422, 428
Histone variants, 3, 4, 12, 101–114, 139, 255, 261, 271, 305, 314, 387, 388, 401
Homeotic genes, 180, 217, 220, 221, 226, 227, 229, 398
Human disease, 19, 69, 71, 78, 79, 343–364, 369, 376, 385
Hypermethylation, 10, 27, 49, 164, 193, 265, 271, 272, 363, 369, 372–375, 379, 385–387, 390, 391, 425
Hypomethylation, 23, 74–79, 201, 203, 251, 265, 266, 291, 363, 369, 373, 375–377, 379, 385–387, 391, 425

I

Imprinting, 22, 23, 32, 37, 38, 86, 92, 119–121, 128–130, 197, 235–255, 270, 311, 369, 377, 385, 386, 419

Imprinting control regions (ICRs), 32, 235, 236, 238, 245–250, 253, 254, 260, 377
Infertility, 192, 301–314, 333
Inner Cell Mass, 188, 261, 267, 268, 271
Insulator, 22, 31, 111, 177, 182, 198, 204, 288, 289, 292, 377
iPS cells, 259, 261, 262, 269, 271–273, 276, 344

M

Maize, 119–140
Mammalian DNA methyltransferases, 85, 87
Meiotic sex chromosome inactivation (MSCI), 191, 303–305, 308–313
Meiotic silencing, 192, 301–314, 321, 322, 326, 333, 335
Meiotic silencing by unpaired DNA (MSUD), 303–307, 321, 322, 326, 333–336
Meta-analysis, 37, 39, 42, 44, 47–50
Methyl binding proteins, 69, 263, 329, 343, 413
Methylation, 3, 8–16, 19–28, 31, 32, 37–51, 55, 57–61, 69–79, 85–95, 108, 113, 114, 124–126, 129, 130, 133, 134, 138, 139, 150, 151, 153, 157, 158, 163–171, 180, 182, 187, 193, 198, 200–204, 206, 219, 224–229, 235, 236, 238–240, 242–246, 248, 251–255, 259–275, 284, 286, 289–291, 306, 312, 321–330, 332–336, 343–345, 347, 349, 351, 352, 363, 369–380, 385–392, 400, 401, 403, 404, 406, 411, 413–415, 417–419, 421, 422, 424–427
Methylation arrays, 369
Methylome, 21, 23, 25, 26, 28, 71, 379, 380, 390, 411, 426, 427
Microarray, 4, 7–9, 14, 20, 23, 24, 29, 31, 38–40, 45, 49, 57–60, 70, 71, 75, 106–108, 126, 139, 163, 165, 166, 224, 238, 263, 275, 305, 312, 314, 379, 380, 389–391, 397, 411, 421–423, 425, 426

N

Noncoding RNA, 3, 153, 187, 190, 193, 194, 198, 205, 206
Nucleosomes, 3, 4, 31, 85, 89, 90, 92, 93, 101–105, 108–113, 222–225, 237, 348, 373, 374, 387, 388, 401

P

Pairing sensitive silencing, 177, 179
Paramutation, 119–121, 124, 125, 127, 130–134, 139, 140, 163, 307

piRNA, 177, 189
Pluripotency, 228, 229, 259–261, 264, 266, 267, 269–273, 276, 392
Polycomb mechanisms, 217
Position effect variegation (PEV), 20, 130, 149–151, 180, 287, 288
Profiling, 3–7, 9, 10, 12, 14, 15, 16, 24, 25, 50, 71, 101–114, 134, 139, 140, 259, 269, 274, 380, 411, 424

Q

Quelling, 321, 322, 326, 329, 331–333, 335, 336

R

RIP, 321–330, 332–334, 336
RNA interference (RNAi), 7, 125, 149, 151–159, 165, 169, 177–183, 289, 305–307, 322, 327, 331–333, 335, 413

S

S. pombe, 105, 134, 149–154, 156–159, 178, 329, 413
Schizophrenia, 378, 411, 412, 416
Silencing, 10, 16, 20, 22, 37, 38, 70, 71, 75, 78, 86, 92, 125, 129, 130, 134, 149–159, 164, 166–170, 177–183, 187–192, 194, 197, 201, 202, 204–207, 222, 227, 228, 267, 269, 274, 301–314, 321–324, 326, 329, 331–333, 335, 336, 352, 371, 373, 375, 387, 413, 327
siRNA, 152–156, 166, 168–171, 177, 178, 180, 181, 189, 326, 331–333, 335, 413
Somatic cell nuclear transfer (SCNT), 259, 261, 262, 270–272, 276
Statistical bioinformatics, 37
Subnuclear localization, 283, 293

T

Telomeres, 121, 150, 152, 156, 157, 177, 181
Tiling array, 4, 9, 14, 15, 25, 37, 39, 40, 42, 44–46, 50, 107, 165, 166, 238, 263, 390, 422
Transcription factors (TFs), 4, 8–10, 12, 28, 30, 40, 85, 108, 111, 114, 168, 193, 218, 254, 259, 267, 268, 275, 283, 290, 292–295, 308, 329, 343–346, 348–361, 363, 372, 373, 375, 379, 380, 387, 392, 399, 413, 415, 417
Transgene silencing, 134, 177, 179
Transposons, 74, 120–124, 127, 132, 134, 139, 140, 159, 166, 322, 324, 332, 335

TS cells, 263, 266, 268, 269
Tsix, 187, 189, 190, 192–207

U
Unmethylated histone H3 lysine 4, 85
Unsynapsed chromosomes, 302–308

V
Vernalization, 168, 398–407

X
X chromosome, 22, 86, 113, 179, 181, 187–207, 218, 254, 255, 261, 270, 271, 301–314, 333, 349, 369, 371, 379, 415
X-chromosome inactivation, 22, 86, 187–207, 218, 254, 255, 261, 271, 303, 311, 369, 415
Xist, 187, 189–207, 261, 312, 313
Xit, 187, 189, 190, 192, 194–199, 201, 207